General Surgery for Nurses

Harold Ellis D.M. M.Ch. F.R.C.S.
Professor of Surgery,
Westminster Hospital

Christopher Wastell M.S. F.R.C.S.
Hon. Consultant Surgeon and Reader
in Surgery, Westminster Hospital

General Surgery for Nurses

Including contributions by
Paul Aichroth on Fractures and Orthopaedics
E. H. Miles Foxen on Ear, Nose and Throat
Patrick D. Trevor-Roper on Ophthalmology

Blackwell Scientific Publications
Oxford London Edinburgh Melbourne

© 1976 Blackwell Scientific Publications Osney Mead,
Oxford
8 John Street, London, WC1
9 Forrest Road, Edinburgh
P.O. Box 9, North Balwyn, Victoria, Australia

All rights reserved. No part of this publication
may be reproduced, stored in a retrieval system,
or transmitted, in any form or by any means,
electronic, mechanical, photocopying, recording
or otherwise without the prior permission of
the copyright owner.

ISBN 0 632 095008

First published 1976

Distributed in the United States of America by
J. B. Lippincott Company, Philadelphia,
and in Canada by
J. B. Lippincott Company of Canada Ltd., Toronto.

Photoset and Printed by
Interprint (Malta) Ltd.

Contributors

Paul Aichroth M.S. F.R.C.S.
Consultant Orthopaedic Surgeon,
Westminster Hospital, London S.W.1

Harold Ellis D.M. M.Ch. F.R.C.S.
Professor of Surgery,
Westminster Hospital, London S.W.1

E. H. Miles Foxen F.R.C.S. D.L.O.
Consultant Ear, Nose and Throat Surgeon,
Westminster Hospital, London S.W.1

Patrick D. Trevor-Roper M.A. M.D. B.Chir.(Cantab) F.R.C.S. D.O.M.S. (Eng)
Consultant Ophthalmic Surgeon,
Westminster Hospital, London S.W.1 and
Moorfields Eye Hospital.

Christopher Wastell M.S. F.R.C.S.
Honorary Consultant Surgeon and Reader in Surgery,
Westminster Hospital, London S.W.1

Contents

Contributors *v*

Introduction

1 Infections *1*
  Christopher Wastell

2 Care of the surgical patient *20*
  Christopher Wastell

3 Shock *38*
  Christopher Wastell

4 Burns *43*
  Harold Ellis

5 Tumours; principles of radiotherapy and cytotoxic therapy *51*
  Harold Ellis

6 Chest and lungs *70*
  Christopher Wastell

7 Heart and great vessels *87*
  Harold Ellis

8 Peripheral vascular disease *100*
  Harold Ellis

9 Lymphatics and lymph nodes *124*
  Harold Ellis

10 Central nervous system *132*
  Harold Ellis

11 Stomach and Duodenum *162*
    Christopher Wastell

12 Intestine *198*
    Christopher Wastell

13 Hernia *267*
    Harold Ellis

14 Liver, gall bladder, pancreas and spleen *279*
    Christopher Wastell

15 Urinary tract *312*
    Harold Ellis

16 Endocrine glands *369*
    Harold Ellis

17 Breast *389*
    Harold Ellis

18 Skin *402*
    Harold Ellis

19 Ophthalmology *416*
    Patrick Trevor-Roper

20 Ear, nose and throat *442*
    E. H. Miles Foxen

21 Fractures *482*
    Paul Aichroth

22 Orthopaedics *520*
    Paul Aichroth

23 Transplantation *556*
    Christopher Wastell

Introduction

The surgical nurse today faces the difficult task of coping not only with the heavy responsibilities of the care of seriously ill patients but also with the rapidly expanding corpus of Medical knowledge. New operations, drugs and techniques of treatment constantly appear on the scene, yet as a member of the surgical team, she must be fully aware of these advances and, indeed, play a vital part in their success.

This new text-book attempts to present the essential facts of modern surgical practice in a readable and reasonably compact form. The contributors are actively concerned with lecturing to nurses in training and we have endeavoured to put forward our current teaching into its pages. It has been designed with the S.R.N. and the S.E.N. Diplomas in mind.

We have been greatly assisted in this task by many discussions over many years with the sister tutors at the Wolfson School of Nursing at Westminster Hospital.

Copious illustrations have been used and these have all been specifically selected for the student nurse. Both the figures and the text emphasise the common entities which are seen in hospital today. Much less space has been allowed for the many 'classical' conditions like tuberculosis of bone and joint and poliomyelitis, once so common, but now fortunately almost eliminated from our surgical wards.

We would like to thank our colleagues among the medical and nursing staff at Westminster for their help and to express our appreciation for the encouragement we have received from Mr Per Saugman and his staff at Blackwells.

Westminster Medical School   H.E.
1975   C.W.

Chapter I. Infections

INTRODUCTION

For the whole of our lives we are surrounded by micro-organisms, many of which are capable of gaining entry to the body and causing an 'infection'. Bearing this in mind it is perhaps surprising that significant infection does not occur more commonly. Micro-organisms can be classified as follows:

1. *Viruses*—these are not often concerned with infections of surgical significance but the viruses of measles and mumps can both cause abdominal pain. The latter virus may cause pancreatitis, oophoritis and generalised lymphadenitis. They are too small to be seen by the conventional microscope.

2. *Bacteria*—these are the most common agents in surgical infections and in general may be divided into bacteria that are round, for example streptococci and staphylococci (Figs. 1.1 and 1.2) or rod-like (for example Escherichia coli). Bacteria may be seen, after having been suitably stained, using a microscope. They are further sub-divided depending on their staining properties into, for example, gram positive or gram negative groups and beyond this point other more complex culture procedures are required to differentiate between the different types. The diseases they may be associated with are listed in Table 1.

3. *Fungi*—these are relatively large organisms composed of branching filaments which may be seen using a microscope. An example of this type of organism is candida, which is responsible for the infection known as thrush.

4. *Protozoa*—these are single celled organisms and include plasmodium (responsible for malaria), entamoeba (responsible for amoebic colitis), trichomonas (Fig. 1.3) lamblia and toxoplasma.

Chapter 1

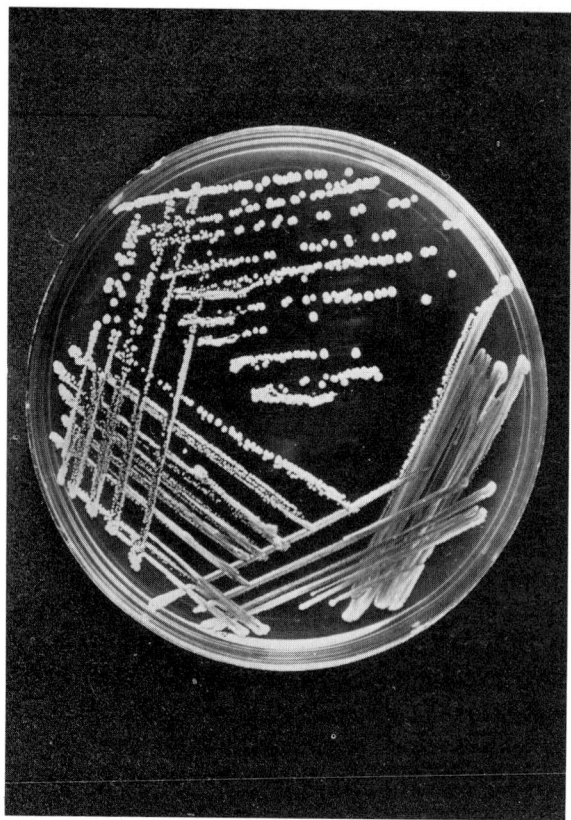

Fig. 1.1. Culture of staphylococcus aureus on blood agar.

For centuries man has searched for specific remedies for specific infections and the whole of art and literature is full of his failure to achieve this goal. In the early 1930's, however, specific chemotherapeutic agents were manufactured which had the effect of interfering with the metabolism of certain bacteria whilst not poisoning the patient. The first of these agents were the sulphonamides, originally produced by May and Baker and for that reason for a long time they were known as 'M & B'. The truly significant departure that these compounds resulted in was the 'systemic' treatment of infection. It was an early observation in 1928 by Dr. Alexander Fleming (later knighted) however, which produced the most profound ecological change the human race has ever seen when he noted inhibition of the growth of staphylococcus aureus on a blood agar plate produced by the mould Penicillium notatum. After some studies on this agent, Fleming concluded that the substance producing this inhibition was so unstable as to defy extraction. It was the work of Professor Florey in Oxford, immediately before the

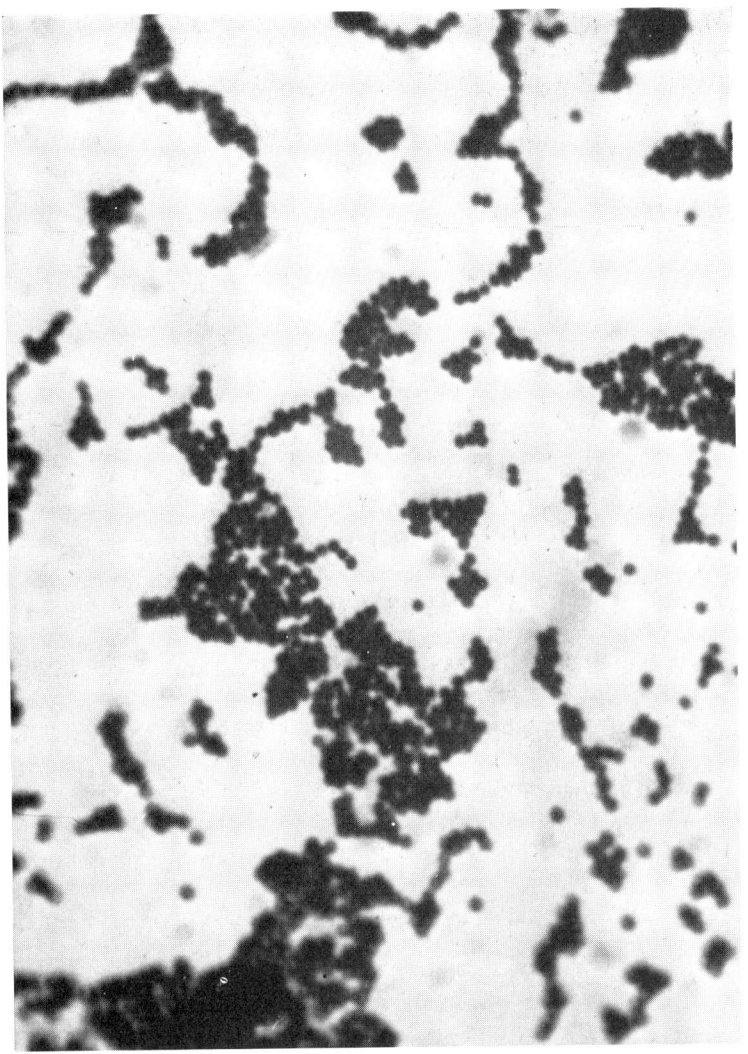

Fig. 1.2. Microphotograph of *Staphylococcus aureus*. These organisms have been stained with gram stain and appear dark blue under the microscope.

second world war in 1939, which resulted in the drug penicillin being extracted in therapeutic quantities. The effect of this work is far reaching when one realises that, for the first time, man had achieved a significant advantage over the micro-organisms of his environment which had all too often swept millions to their death during pandemic infections, such as the great plagues.

The antibiotics, as they become known, are all produced as a result of metabolic processes in micro-organisms, generally fungi but also in bacteria. There is now a large selection of antibiotics, all with specific activities and varying toxic effects. It is perhaps remarkable that penicillin still remains one of the most generally useful antibiotics that we have.

Two definitions

Two terms will repeatedly occur in this chapter and should therefore be defined. The first of these is *pus*, which is defined as 'a collection of dead and alive white cells together usually with dead and alive organisms suspended in serum'. The second is an *abscess*, which is simply 'a collection of pus'.

Mechanisms of infection

Since we are surrounded by micro-organisms, the establishment of an infection depends upon some upset in the balance between our protective mechanism and the infecting organism. If a patient is in a generally reduced state of health by virtue of some other disease, the liability to infection is increased. An example of this is seen in the patient with an advanced malignant disease who dies of bronchopneumonia. The opposite situation also occurs in which a normal patient meets an unusually virulent organism against which he has no protection. The epidemics of Asian 'flu are an example of this phenomenon. Another reason for an infection gaining a foothold is damage to the tissues of the body. If the skin is lacerated, bacteria, such as the staphylococcus, normally resident on the skin, gain entry to the exposed tissues of the body and can multiply. It is also possible for bacteria circulating in the blood to be deposited in tissue damaged by trauma.

One of the general rules of the body is that if a block occurs to a duct, with resulting failure of drainage, infection is likely to occur in the static secretion. Examples of this mechanism are seen in bronchitis when bronchioles are blocked by mucus, upper urinary tract infections which follow obstruction to a ureter or cystitis following obstruction to the urethra.

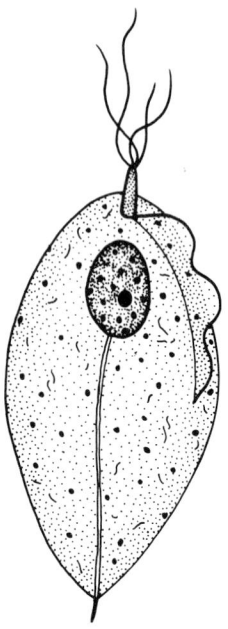

Fig. 1.3. *Trichomonas vaginalis*; a single cell organism with flagellae which allow it to move.

THE SIGNS OF INFECTION

Local. Infected tissue becomes inflamed. This means that the tissue appears to be red and feels hot because of the increased blood supply to it. It is swollen because of oedema fluid resulting from the increased blood supply to the area. There is usually pain due to the increase in tension within the tissues, which is also due to the oedema fluid. Because the tissue is swollen and painful there is also inter-

ference with the normal function of the infected part. These changes are visible when the infection is close to the skin but obviously cannot be seen externally in the case of a deeply placed abscess.
General. The temperature of the patient is raised. The type of pyrexia is often characteristic. When an abscess is present the temperature rises in the evening and falls to normal by the morning; this is known as a 'swinging pyrexia' (Fig. 1.4). Infections of the

Fig. 1.4. Temperature chart exhibiting a swinging pyrexia due to the presence of an abscess. Drainage on the fifth day resulted in rapid resolution of the fever.

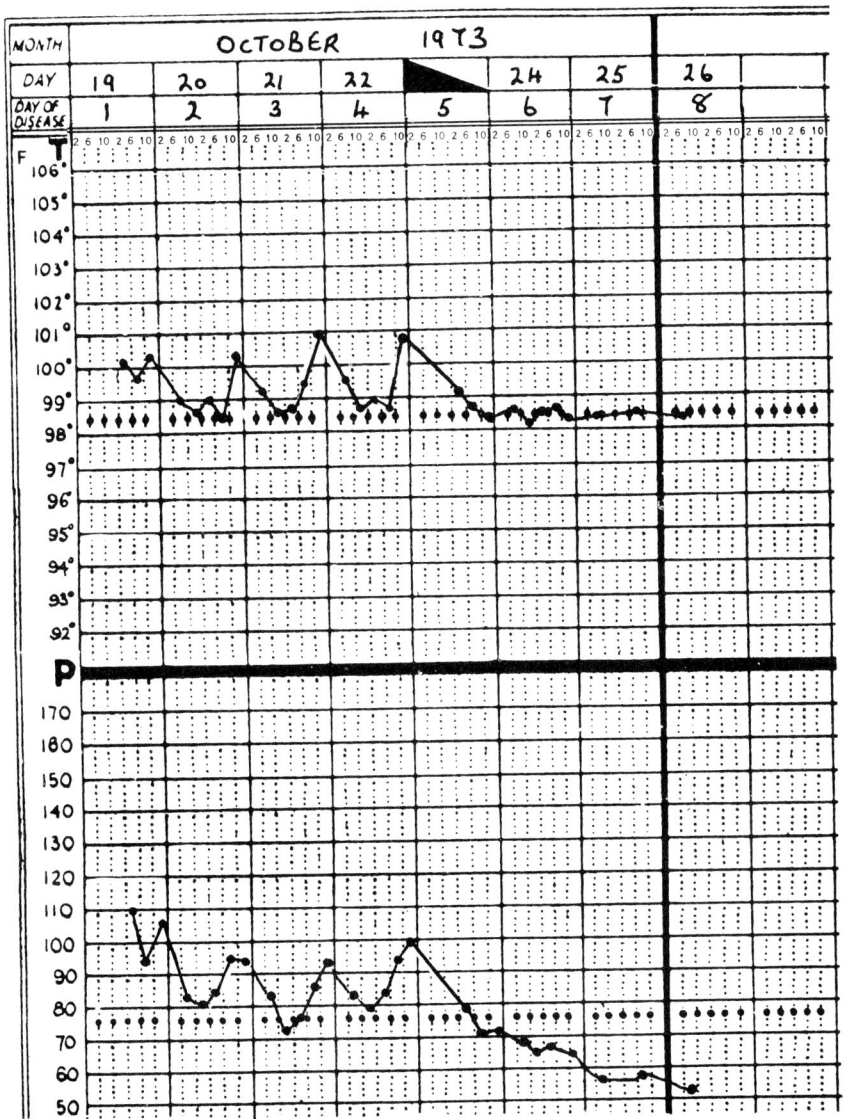

kidney (pyelonephritis) and liver (hepatitis) or of the hepatic ducts (cholangitis) and of the blood (septicaemia), often result in very high pyrexias up to 39° or 40°C associated with a 'rigor'. When a patient has a 'rigor' he shakes uncontrollably. Usually there is an initial subjective impression of coldness. Typhoid fever results in a slowly rising pyrexia over a period of one to two weeks. Pyrexia with a temperature rise of greater than 0.5°C is always significant and unless the cause is known should never be ignored.

Together with the pyrexia the pulse rate also increases. There are no absolute levels above which a pulse rate indicates an infection; it is the day to day change in pulse rate which indicates the course of the infection. A falling pulse rate in a previously infected patient indicates that the infection is getting better.

If a blood count is made during an acute infection a rise in the number of white cells is detected. The first cells to be affected are the polymorpho-nuclear leucocytes, which can be shown to be of the recently formed variety by the small number of lobes on their nuclei. In some chronic infections, for example tuberculosis, the lymphocyte count is raised. It is characteristic of infections by the helminthes (worms) for the eosinophil count to be raised in the peripheral blood.

Measurement of the plasma proteins will indicate a rise in the gamma globulin fraction, which starts approximately ten days after the onset of infection. This is due to the development of antibodies to the infecting organism. One secondary result of this change in the proteins is that the erythrocyte sedimentation rate (E.S.R.) is raised. The E.S.R. may be used as an index for the patient's improvement following infection and is useful in those who have tuberculosis.

Protecting mechanisms

There are two main groups of protecting mechanisms. The first of these are the white cells circulating in the blood; they are capable of ingesting invading bacteria and so destroying them. They have been likened to the policemen of the body, always on duty and ready to deal with trouble. Their response is rapid and they collect in huge numbers around an infected tissue.

The white cells thus mobilised then ingest the bacteria, a process known as phagocytosis. One white cell is able in this way to dispose of many bacteria, which usually are digested and killed, but the white cell itself may be killed. Thus, at the site of an infection there are many white cells, some alive and some dead, bacteria, some of which are also alive and some dead, together with the serum that has exuded into the area: this is *pus*. Pus may assume several characteristics: staphylococcus—yellow; E coli—faecal smelling; pseudomonas—green; streptococcus—watery, and actinomycosis—watery containing yellow flecks known as 'sulphur granules'.

The second is the development of antibodies. These are gamma globulins produced in lymph nodes and other lymphocyte-rich tissues, for example, the spleen. They have the characteristic of combining with the proteins of the invading organism which has itself stimulated their production. Antibodies are highly specific and to give an example, the anti-body to the measles virus will protect against other invasions by that organism but not against other viruses. Whereas the protection afforded by the white cells is immediate, antibodies usually take between 10 and 14 days to be developed. Once a patient has produced antibodies to an organism, subsequent infection with that organism produces an antibody response which is more rapid and of greater magnitude.

Incubation period

The time, in days, from the entry of an infecting organism to the development of the signs of infection is known as the incubation period. This is usually the time taken for the organism to begin multiplying effectively within the body. In general, viruses have an incubation period of between 7 and 21 days. Larger organisms, for example, streptococcus, staphylococcus and other bacteria have a shorter incubation period of 1 to 3 days.

PRINCIPLES OF TREATMENT

The infected part is put to rest. Thus, if a limb has an infection, movement in minimised. The causative organism is identified and, at the same time, the sensitivities to a wide range of antibiotic agents is determined by culture. If it is necessary to treat the infection before the sensitivities have been established (this usually takes 2 days), then the appropriate antibiotic will have to be deduced. An example of this is in the case of peritonitis for which ampicillin, known to be effective against most intestinal organisms, is used. It is quite wrong in most cases, however, to treat an infection with a 'broad spectrum' antibiotic without accurate knowledge as to the type of organism being treated. If pus has formed, then surgical drainage is required. The old dictum: 'Let not the sun go down on unopened pus' still holds good and antibiotics are totally ineffective in the treatment of a pus-filled cavity. If the duct draining a cavity is blocked then drainage either along the duct or by some alternative route has to be secured.

The most efficient form of prophylaxis against infection is by the stimulation of antibody production. This method has been highly

Table 1.1. A list of some bacteria with some of their associated diseases and some of the antibiotics that may be used in their treatment.

Bacteria	Disease	Antibiotic
Staphylococcus aureus	Boils, abscesses wound infections	Penicillin, Ampicillin, Cloxacillin
Streptococcus pyogenes	Cellulitis, lymphangitis	Penicillin, Ampicillin, Cloxacillin, Co-Trimoxazole, Cephalexin
Streptococcus pneumoniae	Lobar pneumonia	Penicillin
Clostridium tetani	Tetanus	Penicillin
Clostridium perfringens (*B. welchii*)	Gas gangrene	Penicillin
Escherichia coli	Some wound infections from intestinal source, urinary infection	Ampicillin, Cephaloridine, Cephalexin, Gentamycin, Co-Trimoxazole
Pseudomonas aeruginosa (*Pyocyanea*)	Infection of burns	Gentamycin
Mycobacterium tuberculosis	Tuberculosis	Streptomycin, Rifampicin

successful in such infections as poliomyelitis, smallpox, tetanus, whooping cough, typhoid, yellow fever and now measles. Some protection can be afforded by the giving of an immune serum, for example in the case of a pregnant woman who has come into contact with German measles and who requires protection for some weeks. Prophylaxis by antibiotics is not so effective, although it is extensively used for patients with chronic bronchitis and in patients undergoing major arterial or cardio-thoracic surgery. One form of prophylaxis which has been shown to be effective is the instillation of antibiotic powder such as ampicillin into operation wounds and there is no doubt that this reduces the incidence of wound infection.

SOME SPECIFIC TYPES OF INFECTION

BOILS

A boil results from the infection of a hair follicle. At first the skin around it is red and painful and then as pus develops the hair follicle appears yellow and the pain increases. As soon as the overlying epidermis ruptures with the release of pus, the pain disappears and the boil is cured. Usually no specific treatment is required. Hot compresses are often soothing and can accelerate the formation of pus. Magnesium sulphate suspension is time honoured when the boil has burst; in reality it probably provides a convenient type of bland dressing more than a specific 'drawing' action. Extraction of the hair with release of tension and pus is the most positive treatment and is always effective.

ABSCESSES

An abscess is a cavity which contains pus. It may occur in almost any site in the body. Depending on the tissue involved, an abscess will cause at least some damage and the longer the process is allowed to continue, the greater this will be. For example, a breast abscess can result in considerable destruction of breast tissue unless treated promptly.

Clinical features

Usually, at least in this country, abscesses form for some identifiable reason: in a fresh surgical wound that has become infected, or around an inflamed organ such as the appendix, Fallopian tube or gall bladder.

There is generally associated pain and a swinging pyrexia develops. The patient usually feels ill. If the abscess is close to the skin a mass may be palpable and if the overlying skin is actually involved, it will be red and oedematous. As an abscess develops and enlarges, the skin becomes stretched over it with the result that the surface of the skin becomes smooth and shiny. If the swelling then regresses the surface of the skin is thrown into small wrinkles. The white cell count is raised.

Treatment

This depends on the site and causation. Superficial abscesses should be drained by having an incision made into the wall, the patient being suitably anaesthetised, usually under general anaesthetic. If the cavity is large, a piece of corrugated latex rubber is inserted so as to ensure free drainage for any pus. Some of the pus is collected on a bacterial swab which is immediately sent to the bacteriology laboratory. Identification of the organism is then undertaken by means of culture for 24–48 hours or more, by staining and other tests. In addition to identification, the bacteriologist is able to measure the effectiveness of a range of antibiotics against that particular organism. All this important work is made impossible if the swab is allowed to dry or if it is left in the refrigerator overnight. Provided that the abscess is draining, no further treatment is required beyond suitably frequent dressing. Generally, antibiotics should never be used once an abscess has become established. If a broad spectrum antibiotic (that is, one effective against a wide range of organisms, a good example being ampicillin) is given, there will be an initial reduction in the surrounding inflammation, which will deceive the attendant into believing that a cure will soon be obtained. Inevitably, however, the process of abscess formation will continue, only having been temporarily slowed down. The reason for identifying the organism is to be able to treat the infection if it spreads generally, beyond the abscess itself.

For abscesses in specific areas, see the appropriate chapters (e.g. breast abscess, page 389, appendix abscess 221).

LYMPHANGITIS

This is an inflammation of the lymphatic channels but the term is reserved for those cases in which the inflammation in the overlying skin can actually be seen. The infecting organism is usually a β-haemolytic streptococcus. The condition is most commonly seen when some part of the hand or forearm is injured and subsequently becomes infected.

Clinical features

There is pain in the infected part, and the pain then extends proximally. When the arm is examined a red line is seen to extend from the wound along the anterior aspect of the forearm to the medial side of the elbow and thence to the axilla. It does occur, although less commonly, in other parts of the body as well.

Treatment

This is with the appropriate antibiotic, which is usually penicillin.

LYMPHADENITIS

This occurs when lymphangitis reaches the lymph nodes. It may be due to the streptococcus, although a very wide range of infecting agents will produce it without first resulting in obvious lymphangitis.

CELLULITIS

If an infection gains access to connective tissue, for example beneath the skin or in the pelvis and then spreads, this is known as cel-

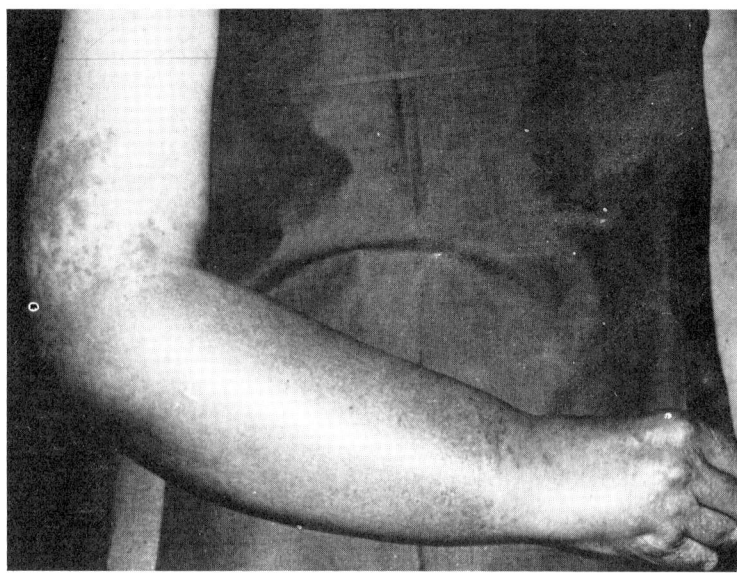

Fig. 1.5. Cellulitis of the arm due to β-haemolytic streptococcus.

lulitis (Fig. 1.5). The most common organism to cause this is again the haemolytic streptococcus, although other organisms, especially staphylococcus, can produce it.

Clinical features

These include pain in the affected part, a raised temperature, pulse rate and white cell count. It is unusual for pus to be formed as a discrete collection, at least in the early stages.

Treatment

The appropriate antibiotic is used. It is unusual to be able to culture the causative organism and the agent used, therefore, should be appropriate for the site. In pelvic cellulitis for example, ampicillin is usually effective.

WOUND INFECTION

One of the complications which may attend any surgical operation is infection of the wound. This is more common when the operation is carried out in an infected area, for example, when the interior of the colon is opened. Usually, wound infections resolve after several days or weeks without causing too much trouble. Occasionally they can be disastrous, particularly in cardiac surgery, orthopaedic surgery, in any surgery that has resulted in the implantation of foreign material within the body or when immuno-suppression is being used in association with organ transplantation. In general abdominal surgery most wound infections resolve without specific treatment, except that if pus is formed deep to the healing skin then free drainage must be encouraged with removal of one, two or three skin sutures. One of the complications of wound infection as it affects the abdominal wall is the later development of an incisional hernia.

TETANUS

Tetanus is an extremely dangerous condition which results from the infection of ischaemic tissue by clostridium tetani. This organism is a gram positive rod and is found in soil and the intestine. Once the organism gains a hold it begins to multiply locally in the tissues and an exotoxin (which is a poison manufactured by the organism) is produced. This rapidly becomes fixed in the nervous system and when this has occurred it cannot be removed by treatment.

Clinical features

The incubation period after injury varies from one day to three weeks. The first symptoms consist of a spastic rigidity in the muscles of the back and neck and also in the muscles of the face and jaw (hence the name 'Lock-jaw'). A curious feature of this disease is that occasionally it is regional; that is, it may affect one group of muscles or one limb, generally the limb that is the site of the infection. If the infection continues unabated, eventually all the muscles become affected and violent spasms with convulsions occur; death then follows because of respiratory failure.

Prophylaxis

Active. It is possible to provide protection against tetanus by injections of tetanus toxoid. This is prepared from cultures of clostridium tetani which are treated so that whilst the exotoxin they produce is rendered non-harmful it retains its capacity to stimulate the production of antibodies. Three injections of toxoid are given at intervals of approximately 4 weeks and confer immunity for a period of 5 to 10 years.

At the time of injury. When an injury is sustained which results in devascularised tissue, the risk of tetanus can be virtually removed by correct care. This includes excision of all dead and devitalised tissue; giving penicillin which is effective against clostridium tetani and for those who have been previously immunised, by giving a booster dose of tetanus toxoid. If previous immunisation has not been given, a full course of toxoid is administered.

Treatment of an established case

Treatment will depend on the severity of the symptoms. In general, the shorter the time from the introduction of the infection to the development of the symptoms, the more severe the attack will be. In all cases an injection of tetanus toxoid is given.

The wound

A swab for culture and identification of the organisms is taken. All dead and devitalised tissue is excised under general anaesthetic and large doses of penicillin are given by intramuscular injection.

The symptoms

If only minor muscle spasms are present, with stiffness of facial and neck muscles, these can be controlled with barbiturates (phenobarbitone 60–200 mgs Im 6 hourly if necessary) and a tranquillizer such as diazepam.

As the condition progresses, more and more muscles become involved in the spastic process until the patient becomes fixed, with back arched (when all muscles go into spasm the position of joints is determined by the strongest muscle groups—in the case of the trunk this is the extensor muscles of the back) in a position known as opisthotonos. When this horrifying stage is reached breathing becomes impossible and respiratory failure ending in death is the result. The treatment now becomes a question of inducing general anaesthesia with intravenous barbiturate (Pentothal) and giving muscle relaxants. So as to maintain respiration, tracheostomy and artificial ventilation is required, a mechanical ventilator being used. Patients have been maintained in this way for 3 weeks, until the effects of the exotoxin on the central nervous system has worn off, after which full recovery has occurred.

GAS GANGRENE

Gas gangrene is due to infection by clostridium. The most common type to cause this disease is clostridium welchii. These organisms are gram positive rods which grow in anaerobic conditions and produce an exotoxin. The organisms are found in soil and in the intestine.

Clinical features

The incubation period varies from 2 to 7 days. The situation that may result in gas gangrene is the implantation of soil or faecal material in a wound that contains tissue whose blood supply has been damaged, for example, a compound fracture.

The main feature of this infection is spreading death of cells with the formation of bubbles of gas. When the infected area is palpated the typical 'crepitations' of small bubbles of gas in tissue are felt. This gas contains hydrogen sulphide and results in the characteristic 'bad eggs' smell associated with this condition. The patient is usually extremely ill, with a rapid pulse rate and high temperature, and if the infection continues unchecked results in death, sometimes within a few hours.

Prophylaxis

The main element here is the recognition and correct care of a wound likely to result in gas gangrene. Thus if tissue has had its blood supply removed then it should be surgically excised under general anaesthetic and all contaminating material removed by washing and swabbing. A bacteriological swab is taken so that any clostridia can be identified.

Treatment

The first treatment that should be carried out is with hyperbaric oxygen at 3 atmospheres for 2 hours. This will stop, dramatically, the further multiplication of the infecting organism. The only other therapeutic agent which there is time to give is a large dose of penicillin (2 mega-units). Following the initial treatment with hyperbaric oxygen, the patient is taken to the operating theatre where all gangrenous tissue is excised. Following this the patient receives a total of seven 2 hour sessions in the hyperbaric chamber at 3 atmospheres and the course of penicillin is continued for a period of 7 days.

TUBERCULOSIS

The organism mycobacterium tuberculosis is responsible for this disease. There are two principal types of organism. The first is the human type and the second is the bovine type. The bovine type is capable of infecting human beings, the usual route of infection being via milk. This type of infection has been virtually eradicated in this country now, due to the rigorous policy of attestation of milk herds. The usual method of infection with the human organism is by droplet from an infected person with pulmonary disease.

In this country, therefore, when a person first comes into contact with tuberculosis it is usually by inhalation of infected droplets. The small infected area in the lung, commonly the right upper lobe, forms a small area of caseation (an abscess that contains tuberculous pus, fancifully likened to Swiss cheese). The regional lymph nodes at the hilum of the lung become enlarged. In the majority of children and young adults so affected, the infection is contained and both the lung lesion and the lymph nodes become calcified. These changes are visible on X-ray and are known as a 'primary' or 'Ghon' focus. In a few patients the infection is not contained and the disease spreads throughout the body to produce miliary tuberculosis.

Primary tuberculous infection results in hypersensitivity to soluble products from cultures of the organism (tuberculin). This is the basis of the tuberculin skin tests for tuberculosis. The two most commonly used are the Mantoux and the Heef tests. A small quantity of dilute tuberculin is injected into the skin with a syringe or special perforating device and if within 48 hours the skin becomes red and swollen, the test is described as positive and the patient is therefore known to have had primary tuberculosis.

The identification of tuberculosis is sometimes difficult. In general the organism is looked for in sputum, urine or tissues (Fig. 1.6) by a stain, carbol fuchsin, which renders the mycobacteria red. This stain has the almost unique characteristic of being acid resistant or 'fast'. Culture of the living organism is difficult; it is carried out on Loewenstein egg/malachite green medium and takes 6 weeks. Another method of culture is to inject infected material into a guinea pig (an animal with no resistance at all to tuberculosis) and then to kill the animal 6 weeks later and examine its organs for signs of infection.

The surgical significance of tuberculosis lies in:

1. Pulmonary disease when one or two lobes become hopelessly damaged. Providing the disease has been localised, the affected lobes are removed.

It is also important to recognise pulmonary tuberculosis when it exists in patients who are undergoing surgical operations. This is one of the reasons that chest X-rays must always be carried out before operations because it is possible for anaesthetic equipment to become infected and so transmit the infection to other patients.

2. Urinary tract infection. The kidney ureter, bladder, seminal vesicles and epididymis may become infected. Once again, if the infection is localised to one kidney or one epididymis then the infected and damaged tissue is removed.

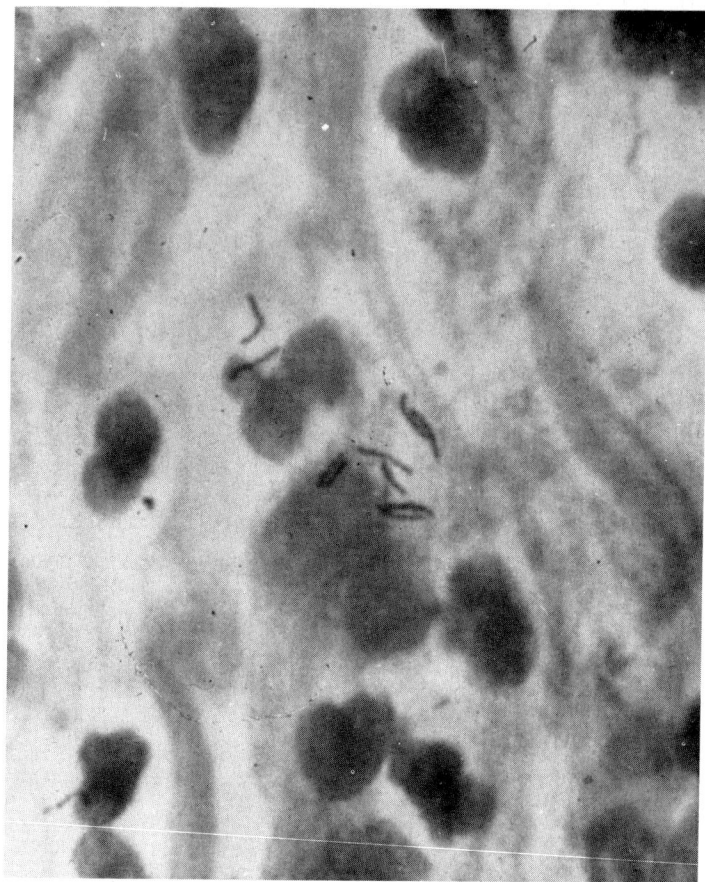

Fig. 1.6. Mycobacterium tuberculosis in the tissues.

3. Tuberculous peritonitis is an acute condition in which the peritoneum becomes covered with miliary tubercles (that is, whitish spots like millet seeds). In this case the condition presents with generalised abdominal pain and can be confused with all the other causes of abdominal pain.

Prophylaxis

It is possible to vaccinate a person who is tuberculin negative with a vaccine prepared from an attenuated bovine strain (Bacille Calmette-Guerin or B.C.G.). This is not considered worthwhile, because of the slight risk attached, in well-developed countries except for subjects in high-risk areas, for example doctors and nurses. In under-developed countries primary tuberculous infection occurs at an early age and B.C.G. vaccination is worthwhile at as early an age as possible to prevent subsequent clinically significant infection.

Treatment

Streptomycin, para-amino salycilic acid (PAS), isonicotinic acid hydrazide (INAH) and rifampicin are the drugs of choice. The organism is killed only by prolonged treatment which, if started, should continue for at *least* 2 years. In order to prevent resistance developing, the drugs are used in rotation.

ACTINOMYCOSIS

Clinical features

This is an infection produced by the fungus actinomyces israeli. It is contracted by contact with infected material, usually of soil origin.

The common places for infection to occur in are the lymph nodes of the head and neck and the tissues of the jaw. The infected area is characteristically very hard and indurated. Eventually it breaks down to discharge a thin pus containing yellowish granules. Several sinuses then tend to form within the indurated area with considerable tissue destruction.

Treatment

This is by incision and drainage of all abscess cavities, with curetting of sinuses. This local treatment is aided by high doses of penicillin to which the organism is partially sensitive.

CANDIDIASIS

This is the commonest fungal infection in man. Candida albicans is a normal inhabitant of the digestive tract and vagina. Occasionally the balance between candida and other micro-organisms becomes upset—for example, by the administration of broad spectrum antibiotics—in favour of the former; clinical 'thrush' is the result. In the mouth and vagina the mucosa becomes inflamed and covered with whitish spots due to the colonies of fungi.

Treatment

This is by the antibiotic nystatin applied topically as a lozenge when the infection involves the mouth and as a pessary when the vagina is affected.

HYDATID DISEASE

This condition is due to infection by the platyhelminth echinococcus granulosus (Fig. 1.7). This is the tapeworm whose host may be dogs, wolves, coyotes and related animals. The adult tapeworm produces eggs which are excreted in the faeces of the dog. If these are deposited on vegetables which are then eaten by the human without being washed, the eggs develop in the intestine into larvae which burrow through the wall to enter the portal bloodstream. In this way the larvae are distributed to the liver, lungs or rarely any of the tissues of the body. They then develop into cysts which may reach a large size. The cyst is lined with a germinal epithelium which produces numerous daughter cysts each capable, if liberated, of independent existence.

Clinical features

The condition should be suspected in any patient living in an area in which the disease is known to exist (for example around the Mediterranean and in some parts of South Wales), who develops a mass in the liver or lungs. Blood count may reveal an eosinophilia. The final confirmation is by the finding of a positive complement fixation test in the patient's serum.

Treatment

If symptoms are being caused by the cyst then a surgical operation is required. The cyst is exposed, some of the fluid is carefully aspirated, making sure that no spillage occurs as it may contain daughter cysts which can become implanted and develop in adjacent tissue. The aspirated fluid is replaced with 2% formalin which will destroy the lining of the cyst together with any contained daughter cysts. After the formalin has been left within the cyst for 10 minutes, the contents of the cyst are removed. There is no need to remove the wall of the cyst which may be deeply imbedded in, for example, the liver.

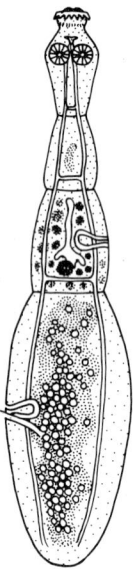

Fig. 1.7. *Echinococcus granulosus.* The two eye-like structures are suckers and the head has two rows of hooks around it. The caudal segment contains eggs. The adult worm is between 5 and 6 mm in length.

AMOEBIASIS

Clinical features

This is due to infection with the protozoa entamoeba histolytica. This is an organism which is very similar in appearance to the amoeba found in ponds. It is contracted by the ingestion of cysts existing in contaminated food and water. Intestinal amoebiasis results in the development of inflammation of the distal part of the colon, the symptoms of which are diarrhoea with the passage of mucus and blood. Extra-intestinal infection is also possible as the organism may spread beyond the confines of the large bowel to infect the tissue around the caecum and the liver (amoebic hepatitis).

Diagnosis is made by the examination of a fresh specimen of stool when the amoebae will be seen moving in their characteristic way.

Treatment

No single drug is completely effective. Intestinal amoebiasis may be treated with tetracyclines combined with emetine. Hepatitis is more difficult to treat and requires the drug chloroquine combined with emetine.

Chapter 2. Care of the surgical patient

PRE-OPERATIVE CARE

INTRODUCTION

The patient who is admitted for surgery, if normal, will be terrified. Calm and sympathetic handling at this stage will often make the difference between a co-operative patient and one who creates difficulties throughout his stay. Anxiety on the part of the patient is often manifest by aggressive behaviour with apparently trivial complaints; for example, patients may object to the form filling that is required, to the food, to members of staff and so on. Sympathetic listening is often the best method of handling such behaviour. Aggression must *never* be matched by aggression and indeed the harsh reply is only justified, and that rarely, in order to achieve a definite objective such as to persuade the patient to accept treatment.

All a patient's symptoms are real. A useful jingle runs as follows:

> 'There was an old lady of Deal,
> Who said that pain wasn't real,
> "But when I sit on a pin,
> And puncture my skin,
> I dislike what I fancy I feel".'

No matter whether the symptoms are physically determined or not, if someone complains of a pain then they have a pain. Scepticism is the province of the Lawyer and has no place in a hospital ward.

The precise nature of the pre-operative 'work-up' depends on what operation will be performed, but certain general rules apply.

The consent form

Informed consent, which consists of a reasonable explanation of the nature and intended purpose of the operation, is required. It is strongly advised that consent be obtained in writing and witnessed by a member of the medical staff, although this is not a legal requirement as situations exist when written consent is impossible to obtain, such as with an unconscious patient.

Over the age of 16 all patients of sound mind can consent for a procedure to be carried out. It is usual to obtain the consent of the legal parent or guardian for all patients between the age of 16 and 18 as the patient is still a minor. Below the age of 16 the consent of the legal parent or guardian must be obtained. An important element in the question of consent is the effectiveness of treatment. If, for some reason or other, consent cannot be obtained for a minor because, for example, the parents cannot be contacted, the administration of life-saving treatment is paramount and delay, simply because the form has not been signed, should not be allowed to occur.

Certain religious sects object to the administration of blood transfusion. A patient who is not a minor is perfectly competent to refuse blood if the refusal is dictated by conscience. In the eyes of the law, therefore, the giving of blood without the patient's consent constitutes an assault. In the case of a minor it is possible, if circumstances justify, for the patient to be taken under the care of the Local Authority (Children's Department) by Magistrate's order and the Authority will then decide whether to consent to blood transfusion and any other necessary procedures.

Labelling the patient

Most hospitals now have a system whereby a label is placed around the wrist of all patients, giving name and hospital number. This prevents the wrong patient being given the wrong blood, for example, particularly when the patient is unconscious.

The surgeons

Some patients will wish to know which surgeon will perform the operation. Discriminating patients will also wish to know which anaesthetist will give the anaesthetic. There is a curious convention that patients often have and this is to assume that the Consultant Surgeon in charge performs all the surgery but when the operation is being discussed with the surgeon, the patient refers to the events in the theatre being carried out by 'them'. Whilst it is true that all patients undergoing an operation are *under the care* of a Consultant (and this is what the term Consultant means) no undertaking is implied or given that he will actually, personally do the operation. In fact the operation may be carried out by the Registrar, S.H.O. or House Surgeon. Within the National Health Service it is only private patients who are able to secure a contractual obligation on the part of the particular surgeon of their choice to carry out their operation.

Nutrition and Diet

Clearly this is of fundamental importance if wounds are to heal. Ideally the patient should be in a normal nutritional state at the time of operation. Four categories of patients exist in which this may not be so. These are:

1. The elderly, who may be short of all food constituents, including particularly vitamin C and iron.
2. Those with wasting diseases such as carcinoma, intestinal fistulae, uraemia and intestinal abnormalities of absorption such as Crohn's disease or ulcerative colitis.
3. Patients with dysphagia.
4. Severe psychiatric problems. Patients with 'food fads'.

If there is doubt about the level of nutrition, help should be sought from the dietician. Often ridiculously simple things may be at fault particularly in the old, such as ill fitting teeth, difficulty in preparing food due to poor eyesight or degenerative diseases of the joints making movement to and from the kitchen difficult.

The haemoglobin should be normal. If it is not and if there is time it should be restored by giving iron or whichever haematinic is appropriate. Vitamin C 100 mg t.d.s. will restore the body's requirements for this within a few hours.

An outline of special diets for particular patients is listed below:
1. *Patients with jaundice* – low fat diet.
2. *Uraemic patients* – diet low in protein.
3. *Diabetic patients* – carbohydrate restricted diet, details of which should always be carried with the patient.

Pre-operative nursing checks

These always include taking and recording the weight, the pulse rate, temperature, respiration rate and an examination of the urine. This latter test is necessary to exclude previously undiagnosed diabetes, renal disease and liver disease and is carried out with Labstix which tests for the following abnormal constituents: glucose, blood, bile and protein. In addition the pH (acidity) and specific gravity of the urine is measured. Cloudiness, particularly of an alkaline urine (pH greater than 7) is common and is due to insoluble phosphates which will clear if the urine is acidified with acetic acid. The findings are recorded on a chart (Fig. 2.1).

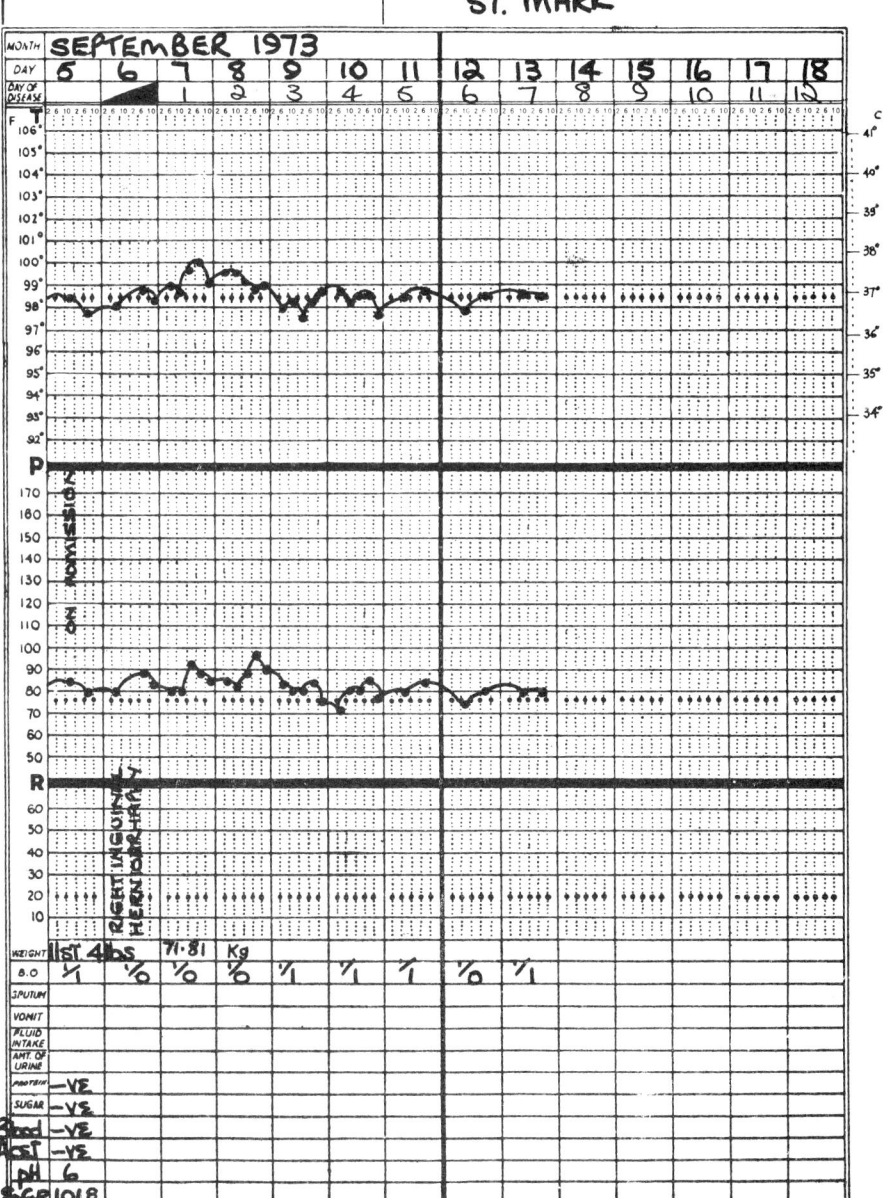

Fig. 2.1. A typical surgical ward chart.

The skin, hair and shaving

An elective operation must be performed through clean skin. If the part to be operated on is hairy, such as the lower abdomen, then shaving of the skin is necessary. But, if the operation cannot reasonably be expected to reach a hair bearing area, shaving is not required. There is no need to perform a pubic shave for operations on the upper abdomen such as cholecystectomy or gastrectomy, providing that an area to at least 3 inches below the umbilicus is clear. Remember that some skin free of hair will be required for dressing and the application of sticking-plaster. If shaving is necessary it must be performed at least on the day prior to operation so that the small ends of hair have time to be cleared from the surface of the skin. Shaving in the theatre is a disastrous failure of pre-operative preparation because small hairs find their way into wounds and are often the cause of infection.

Operating on the head usually requires the scalp to be shaved. A common exception to this is the removal of sebaceous cysts, when the incision is made with an intact head of hair.

Procedures on the face and neck usually do not require any shaving although parotidectomy will mean the loss of the sideboard on that side. Patients for head and neck surgery should have a well fitting plastic cap applied before going to the theatre to keep the hair out of the operative field.

Cystoscopy does not require a perineal shave and, does haemorrhoidectomy.

All patients, for whatever operations, should have a bath on the evening before the operation. It is, of course, quite impossible to sterilise the skin surface and no attempt at this should be made with disinfectants or antiseptics but ingrained dirt from feet and skin should be washed off with ordinary soap and warm water.

For operation on the abdomen the umbilicus should be cleaned and *checked*. This neglected little pit often harbours quite surprising residues of dirt occasionally compacting into an actual lump, called an ompholith or umbolith.

Chest

All patients must stop smoking before operation. It is an extremely interesting observation to ask patients to give just one cough and it is possible on this basis to tell if they are cigarette smokers or not. The larynx, trachea and bronchi are constantly irritated by cigarette smoke and ultimately become irreversibly damaged, giving rise to the husky voice, the productive cough and, in some unfortunate people, cancer of the lung.

In those with a bad chest, physiotherapy will help to clear secretions and will teach patients what is required of them after operation. The sputum should be cultured so that the infecting organism can be isolated and the appropriate antibiotic given if required.

Teeth and other personal effects

False teeth must be removed just prior to the operation and then stored in a cardboard pot marked 'teeth'. If they are wrapped in a paper handkerchief or other unsuitable receptacle they may be thrown away by the ward maid.

With an elective operation attention to dental hygiene is important. Loose, broken teeth should be extracted and the sound remaining teeth cleaned. In an emergency it may be necessary to extract loose teeth before the operation, in the anaesthetic room.

Glasses must be carefully placed in the patient's locker. Contact lenses should be removed and safely stored and false eyes noted. A classic pitfall is to record a fixed, non-moving pupil in a patient recovering from anaesthetic when in reality a very good false eye is the cause!

Artificial legs and arms should be removed and carefully stored.

Rings should either be removed and placed in the safe or should be retained in place with a small strip of elastoplast.

The drugs given as premedication are mainly to allay anxiety. (One of the effective ways of doing this, which should not be neglected, is by sympathetic explanation of the preceding and following procedures). Usually, two types are given, there are opiates or other sedatives such as papaveretum 2 mgm/7Kg body weight with an atropine-like agent, for example, scopolamine 0.4 mgm. Scopolamine is particularly useful because, besides blocking the vagus nerve and causing dryness of the mouth and protecting the heart from vagal overactivity which causes undue bradycardia, it is also an antiemetic and a sedative. The actual dose of these agents depends on the anaesthetist and is tailored to the patient's level of anxiety. Over the age of 65–70 premedicant drugs are often not required at all, and one has to beware of the long-continued sedative effect of a too 'heavy' premedicant continuing long after the operation into the early post-operative phase, causing unwanted respiratory depression.

Children pose a different problem and different drugs are used. Up to the age of approximately 18 months no premedication is required. From 18 months to approximately 8 years trimeprazine tartrate (Vallergan) 3 mgm/Kg body weight is a useful drug as it can be given orally and is a very effective sedative. Over the age of 8 an adult type of premedication is given with due reference to dose in relation to the child's weight.

No elective operation must be performed with either food or fluid in the stomach. For this reason 6 full hours must be allowed to elapse between the last meal or drink and the onset of anaesthesia. If this is not adhered to there is a danger of the inhalation of gastric contents on induction of the anaesthetic. If any doubt exists it is safer to pass a nasogastric tube and to empty the stomach by this means prior to anaesthetic. This is also the safest way to ensure an empty stomach in emergency operations.

Bowels

A universal finding is that the normal daily bowel rhythm is interrupted on admission to hospital. Most patients, except those for very minor procedures, benefit from the administration of a small disposable enema to clear the rectum and lower colon on the night before operation.

Bowel preparation for colonic surgery is a procedure that takes 5 days to carry out. The most important part of the preparation is the removing of all faecal matter from the interior of the colon. The steps are as follows:

			Phthalyl sulphathiaziole 2 gms 6 hourly	Mist-magnesium sulphate 10 ml t.d.s.	
Day 1	Low residue diet	enema			
Day 2	,,	—	,,	,,	
Day 3	,,	—	,,	,,	
Day 4	,,	—	,,	—	Neomycin 1 gm 6 hrly
Day 5	Fluid diet	wash out	,,	,,	,,

AFTER OPERATION

Recovery from the anaesthetic and pain relief

Nowadays, nearly all hospitals have recovery wards. It is therefore possible to ensure that the anaesthetised patient recovers coughing and eyelid reflexes whilst in the theatre area under continuous care. If the patient is deeply anaesthetised in the recovery room, then he should be nursed in the semi-prone position until the coughing reflex returns. Oxygen, 28% via a Ventimask, should be given for 1–4 hours and the pulse, respiration and blood pressure measured and recorded every 15 minutes. Only when the patient has fully recovered consciousness should he be allowed to make the journey back to the ward. Once in the ward the degree of surveillance can be slackened a little but pulse, respiration and blood pressure should be recorded every 30 minutes until they have become stable. There is frequently a post-operative fall in blood pressure which is physiological and providing that the extremities are warm and well perfused with blood this should cause no anxiety. It is difficult to provide an absolute lower permitted level of systolic blood pressure but in general this should remain above 100 mm Hg.

At first, for 1–2 hours, the patient should be nursed flat but, as recovery proceeds, a sitting up position should be arranged as soon as this can be managed without difficulty. This allows easier breathing and coughing with better aeration of the bases of the lungs.

It is at this stage that the patient usually first becomes aware of pain. The pain which results from an operation can be extremely intense and adequate relief is essential. The typical drugs used to secure this are papaveretum 20 mgs or pethidine 100 mgs (for an average sized adult). Both these drugs result in some respiratory depression and to some extent adequate analgesia is a compromise with not too profound depression of breathing. Generally 4 hourly intramuscular injections of either of these drugs for up to 3 or 4 doses will be sufficient to make the patient comfortable.

Some anaesthetists will ensure a controllable area of local anaesthesia by the use of an epidural catheter. This nylon catheter is introduced to the outside of the spinal dura mater and lignocaine can be injected down it to spread for a limited distance up and down the outside of the emerging spinal roots. By siting the tip of the catheter at just the desired level and by varying the volume of lignocaine injected so can the area of anaesthesia be controlled. This technique is particularly applicable to thoracic operations or operations on the abdomen when it is essential that there is no inhibition of breathing and coughing, because of pain, for example in patients with very bad chests.

Usually by 24–48 hours after operation little in the way of pain relief is required.

The post-operative care of the chest

Pre-operative physiotherapy should have ensured a clear chest by the time the operation is performed. Smoking before and after operation is banned. After operation the physiotherapist will carry out deep breathing exercises and coughing. Coughing is essential to clear the bronchi of any plugs of mucus. It is a useful manoeuvre to teach the patient to hold the incision with his hand during coughing in order to minimise jerking of the wound with consequent pain. If these mucus plugs are allowed to remain, the lung distal to them is no longer aerated and will become infected. This is the origin of the post-operative pulmonary collapse and pneumonia which is so commonly seen in cigarette smokers.

Inhalation of steam with tinct. benz. co. is helpful or if the mucus is very tenacious the detergent properties of Alevaire used as an inhalation are useful.

Fluids and the care of 'drips'

For a procedure that does not involve an intestinal anastomosis or an abdominal operation, oral fluids can be allowed directly on recovery from the anaesthetic. All patients are thirsty and will tend to drink too much if allowed. This often results in abdominal distension, nausea and vomiting. Therefore, at first, drinking should be of plain water in small quantities in the range of 30 ml hourly. As the effects of the anaesthetic wear off the volume of fluid allowed can be increased rapidly.

If the operation has been on the abdomen with opening of the peritoneal cavity, there will be a post-operative paralytic ileus. In this case fluid will not pass from the stomach to the duodenum and small bowel and will not be absorbed. Even so, sips of water are allowed to keep the mouth moist and comfortable.

In the absence of peritonitis, paralytic ileus recovers within 48 to 72 hours. On listening to the abdomen with a stethoscope bowel sounds will be heard. Patients often complain of cramping 'wind pains' at this stage. The most satisfactory indication that all is well with the bowel is the passage of flatus per anum. When this happens the intravenous infusion may be taken down and oral feeding progressively increased towards normal.

Generally the fluid intake in the absence of renal failure should be such that at least 1,000 ml of urine are produced in a 24 hour period. For the first 24 hours therefore, in an average man, as much as 4000 ml of intravenous fluid may be required. Some of this will go to make up the deficit that will have resulted from the pre-operative deprivation of fluids; some will be secreted into the small bowel where it will be sequestered away and where it will not be available until the paralytic ileus recovers, and some will be used for the normal daily fluid requirement. For a patient with normal kidneys, lungs and heart (which includes the majority of surgical patients), an excess of water and sodium is an advantage as the kidney excretes the excess and the metabolic processes of the body are thus well supplied with the raw materials for maintaining normal acid-base relationships and serum electrolytes. A typical fluid balance after major abdominal surgery is shown in Table 2.1.

Table 2.1. Typical fluid balance for the 1st 24 hours after a major abdominal operation, a nasogastric tube having been left in place.

IN		OUT	
Oral sips only	100 ml	Urine	1,000 ml
Intravenous—N. Saline	2,000 ml	Faeces	nil
Dextrose Saline	2,000 ml	Gastric aspirate	100 ml
		Insensible loss	1,000 ml
Totals	4,100 ml		2,100 ml
Positive balance 2,000 ml			

Notes A. The apparently large positive balance will be distributed between (1) The deficit that resulted from the pre-operative fluid deprivation, and (2), the fluid pooling in the small bowel due to paralytic ileus.
B. Oral sips of water are allowed in spite of the paralytic ileus to keep the mouth moist and comfortable.
C. Insensible loss is made up of water vapour in the breath and sweat from the skin. It increases in fever and in hot weather.

On a more practical level, intravenous infusions or drips must be constantly maintained. If they are allowed to stop then the blood in the needle or the catheter in the vein will thrombose. In this case it is often possible to restart them by flushing out the needle with normal saline (which must be suitable for intravenous injection). Some intravenous fluids are more prone to produce damage to the vein endothelium than others with consequent venous inflammation and thrombosis. For example, concentrated solutions such as 30% or 40% laevulose and solutions of amino-acids and carbohydrates tend to produce venous thrombosis in the superficial vein into which they are placed and the patient will actually experience pain while the fluid is being infused.

Skin and pressure areas

Patients may not be able to move after an operation because of pain. Because of this, many hours may be spent in one position. The whole of the body's weight is then transmitted through four areas; the two heels and the two buttocks. If the patient is simply allowed to lie without movement, pressure sores will develop. The heels and buttocks will become sore and eventually the skin will break down

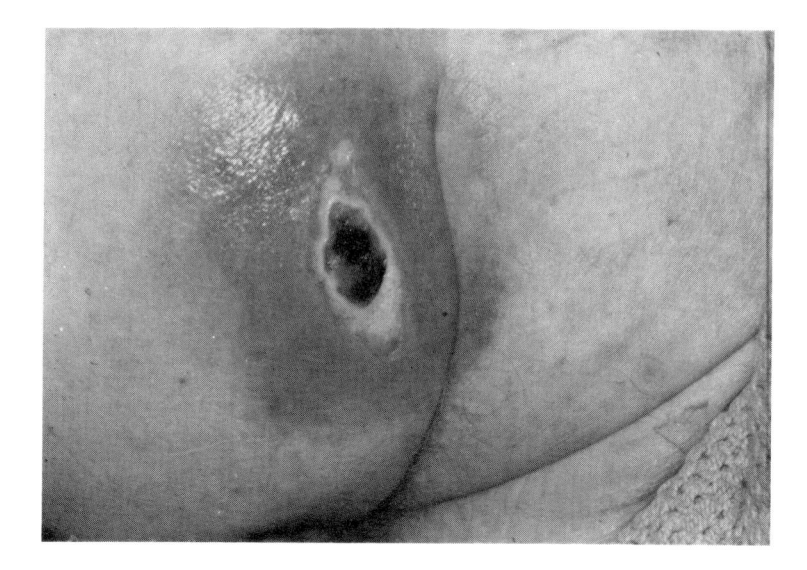

Fig. 2.2. A buttock bedsore.

to form a pressure sore (Fig. 2.2). Therefore the patient must be moved every 2 hours from one position to another.

Even in patients who have undergone quite major abdominal procedures it is an advantage for them to stand out of bed during bed-making. In old patients this encourages the maintenance of balance and righting reflexes that can so easily be lost for ever.

Drains

Drains are left in wounds for one of four reasons:
1. To drain a potential space; for example following splenectomy or resection of any other intraperitoneal organ.
2. To provide a track to an anastomosis that may subsequently leak; for example, colonic anastomoses.
3. To drain away fluid which it is known will otherwise collect, for example the lymph which appears beneath a mastectomy incision.
4. To drain a pus-filled cavity, e.g. after incision of an abscess.

Drains used in the abdomen are commonly of the corrugated plastic type and should have a radio-opaque stripe so that their position can readily be identified on X-ray (Fig. 2.3). They require suitable dressing externally so that any serum or blood can be absorbed as it is discharged onto the surface of the skin. It is unwise to leave most drains in place for more than 5 to 7 days and they should be gradually withdrawn over a period of several days. They do not cause pain even when they are being removed.

Drains used to provide a track should remain in place for 5 days

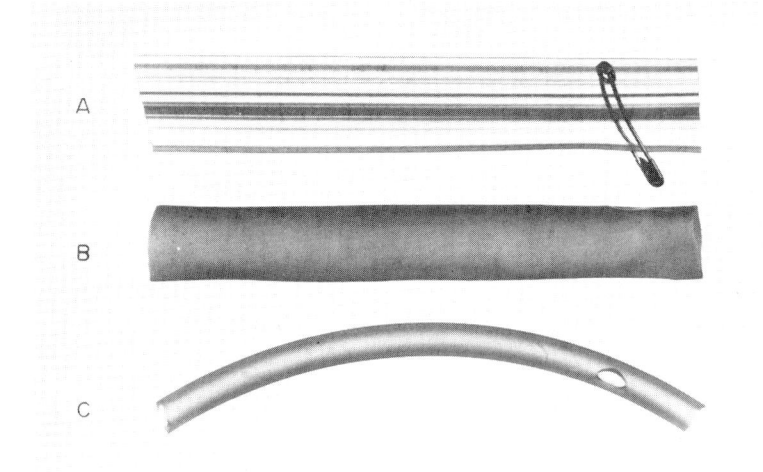

Fig. 2.3. Wound drains. A corrugated, B Penrose and C plastic tube.

and then be withdrawn. To prevent the tip of the drain causing pressure necrosis of underlying bowel it should be withdrawn by one inch on the second day.

Chest drains are dealt with later, as are 'T' tube drains of the common bile duct and suction drainage following mastectomy.

Urethral catheters

Urethral catheters are of two main types. The first of these is a plain tube, usually plastic, which is inserted into the bladder and after all the urine has drained, is removed. The second type is the self-retaining catheter and the most common of these is the Foley balloon catheter (see Fig. 15.38). When a self-retaining catheter has been placed in the bladder it should be connected to a plastic drainage bag, using full sterile precautions. Once the system has been set up it must be left undisturbed and the tube must *never be disconnected* as this is the point at which infection so commonly enters the bladder and urinary tract. Most plastic urine bags now have a tap whereby they can be emptied, thus obviating the need for disconnection of the tubes (see Fig. 15.34).

A plastic Foley catheter can be left in the bladder for 2–3 weeks at a time. When this situation obtains it is essential to ensure that no infection is allowed to enter the urine and all patients should therefore receive a suitable antibacterial agent such as sulphadimidine or ampicillin.

If the catheter is left in place for several weeks or if it is permanent then it should be changed regularly (every 2–3 weeks) because deposits tend to form on it.

Wound care

A clean wound, properly dressed in the operating theatre, is probably best left alone. If, however, the dressing becomes soaked with blood or serum it will need to be changed. A wide variety of dressings are available as well as those made up by nurses consisting of gauze and adhesive tape. The main function of a dressing is to prevent the wound from suffering physical trauma—although it should in addition be bacteriologically sterile when applied, it is impossible to provide a complete bacteriological barrier since bacteria live in the depths of the skin at the edge of the wound.

Wound healing is a complex process that proceeds for many months. Sutures are removed when they are no longer required to hold the edges of the skin together. The length of time for this varies with the particular skin incision. In the case of the abdomen and limbs, sutures should be left for 10 days. If there is any tension, such as in mastectomy scars, they may be left for considerably longer; up to 21 days. On the face and neck sutures should be removed much earlier to prevent ugly cross scarring. In this case the wound is sewn up with deep sutures which result in the skin edges staying together almost without skin sutures at all. Alternate sutures are removed on day 2 and the rest on day 3. Naturally sutures are only removed if the wound edges appear to be safely united.

Different methods are used to secure wounds. The most usual is with a simple through-and-through suture using black silk or monofilament nylon. Very long wounds, such as those resulting from operations to peripheral arteries, are often sewn up with a single continuous black silk suture. Wounds in babies can be sewn up with subcuticular sutures in which the edges of the skin are held together with a suture placed just beneath the surface. This suture may be of monofilament nylon, which will have to be removed on day 10, or it may be of catgut, in which case removal is not required. Some wounds can be sewn up with catgut, for example incisions in the scrotum, the stitches being allowed to fall out spontaneously after about 2 weeks.

Even though sutures are removed on the 10th day, the wound as a whole has very little strength at this stage, being united mainly by epithelial cells; immature collagen and fibrin. Patients with laparotomy wounds should be advised not to strain for 3 months and thereafter to increase gradually the stress applied over another period of 3 months. Then at 6 months from the operation the strength of the scar approximates fairly closely to the pre-operative state.

A common question after operation is 'When is it safe to drive a car?' Experiments conducted with a simulator indicated that 2 weeks should be allowed to elapse from the time of the operation in the majority of cases; providing the car is no more than a small family saloon the average patient should be able to handle it satisfactorily at this stage.

Swimming beyond the depth of the patient should not be permitted until 3 months from operation.

Wound infection

Operations can be divided into 'dirty' and 'clean'. In dirty operations known contamination of the wound occurs and cannot be prevented. An example of this is when a laparotomy for peritonitis is carried out. Wound infection in this circumstance is extremely common, in the region of 30%. A clean operation is one in which no known contamination occurs. In this case wound infection is very rare, being less than 2%. When clean operations are performed the whole ritual of the theatre is designed to ensure that no bacteria are implanted in the wound. If a wound infection occurs in this case the possible sources of the bacteria are as follows:

1. The patient's skin.
2. Infection introduced in theatre by:
    (a) bacteria in the theatre atmosphere;
    (b) droplet infection from the nose, mouth, hair, skin or clothes of doctors or nurses;
    (c) poor theatre technique that allows non-sterile materials to come into contact with the open wound, for example, inadequate drapes.
3. Bacteria circulating in the patient's blood stream.
4. Poor technique in wound care in the ward.

Whatever the cause, the patient will complain of pain and develop a temperature and all the signs of inflammation in the wound itself, which will become red, hot, tender and swollen. Later pus may be formed.

When a wound infection develops a swab should be taken so that the organism can be identified. If pus has formed this should be allowed to escape by removing one or more sutures to permit the skin edges to gape slightly. When the pus is discharged there is usually a great feeling of relief. Indeed, the principle of infected wound care is the same as for an abscess. The infection will clear providing free drainage is allowed.

Deep vein thrombosis

A much feared post-operative complication is thrombosis within the deep veins of the leg and in the pelvic veins. The danger is not so much from the thrombus itself as from the risk of detachment of the thrombus into the blood stream with its passage to the heart and thence into the pulmonary artery, where it lodges as an embolus (see below).

In the post-operative period the patient has a peculiarly increased predisposition to venous thrombosis in the veins of the calf muscles, the main deep venous channels of the leg and the pelvic veins due to a number of factors. These include:

1. An increased thrombotic and clotting tendency produced by an increase in the blood platelets and in the serum fibrinogen.
2. Increased stagnation within the veins resulting from immobilization in bed and depression of respiration. There is particularly slow venous circulation when the patient lies on the operating table paralysed with curare and having artificial ventilation.
3. Damage to the vein walls in the leg may be produced by pressure of the mattress or the hard operating table against the calves. Or there may be direct damage at operation and this is particularly so in the case of the pelvic veins during gynaecological procedures.

Clinical features. The peak incidence of deep vein thrombosis clinically is during the second post-operative week but it may be earlier or later. Earlier thrombosis is particularly likely to occur when the patient has already been immobilized in hospital for some time before the operation. Recent studies using radio-iodine labelled fibrinogen, which is deposited as fibrin in the developing thrombus and where it can be detected by scanning the leg, suggests that the thrombotic process usually commences at, or soon after, the operation.

The patient complains of pain in the calf, and on examination there is tenderness of the calf and swelling of the foot, often with oedema and with dilatation of the superficial veins of the leg. This is accompanied by a mild pyrexia. If the pelvic veins or the femoral vein are affected, then there is massive swelling of the whole lower limb.

Treatment. Prophylaxis comprises active mobilization of the patient and breathing exercises in the immediate post-operative period. In the established case, anticoagulant therapy with intravenous heparin is commenced in order to prevent the formation of further clot. Once anticoagulated, the patient can be mobilized with the lower limb supported by an elastic stocking. If the thrombosis occurs in the immediate post-operative period, there is a very difficult decision to be made whether or not to anticoagulate the patient, since the former carries with it the serious risk of haemorrhage. If this occurs, then the heparin must be immediately discontinued and the antidote, protamine sulphate, given intravenously in the dose of 1 ml of a 1% solution for each 1,000 units of heparin.

Ligation of the major veins is a procedure which very rarely has to be performed when recurrent episodes of pulmonary embolization occur in spite of adequate anticoagulant therapy. The heparin must be continued after ligation, otherwise further clot forms above the site of venous interruption.

Pulmonary embolus

This occurs when a clot from a vein in the lower limb or the pelvis detaches and becomes lodged in the pulmonary arterial tree.

Clinical features. A massive embolus obstructs the right heart output and causes rapid death from heart failure. Less severe cases present with shock, breathlessness and cyanosis, often accompanied by pain behind the sternum. Still milder episodes present with pleural pain, (which is felt in the chest wall and is aggravated by taking a deep breath), dyspnoea and frequently haemoptysis.

If the patient survives the embolus, then dissolution of the clot will occur and the patient can make a complete recovery even after a most serious episode.

It may be difficult to differentiate between a pulmonary embolus and a chest infection or a post-operative coronary thrombosis. A chest x-ray in the early stages is often quite normal although within a few hours patchy shadowing of the affected segment of the lung takes place. An E.C.G. may help in differentiating between an embolus and a coronary thrombosis. In the former, there will be the changes of right heart strain.

It is important to know that a pulmonary embolus may occur without any preceding warning signs of thrombosis in the leg. This applies to the great majority of fatal emboli. Indeed, once there are obvious clinical features of deep vein thrombosis, detachment of an organized and adherent clot from the limb is unlikely, provided that anticoagulant therapy has been commenced so that fresh clot formation is inhibited.

Treatment. Morphia is given for the pain, oxygen administered and heparin treatment commenced if the patient is not already on anti-coagulants. It will be obvious that this regime will do no harm even if a coronary thrombosis has been misdiagnosed as a pulmonary embolism.

In some selected cases in special cardiac units, embolectomy may be performed to remove the obstruction in the pulmonary trunk with the assistance of a heart-lung by-pass machine.

Wound dehiscence

Very occasionally a wound bursts. If the wound is a laparotomy wound this is disastrous because the abdominal contents are forced out. Often the first indication that such an event is about to occur is the escape of a small quantity of blood stained fluid from the wound (the 'pink fluid sign'). A minor strain, such as moving in bed or coughing, is then the final act which results in rupture of all the layers of the wound.

Certain conditions are associated with poor healing and these are:
1. Disseminated neoplastic disease, especially in the presence of jaundice and anaemia.
2. Uraemia.
3. Scurvy (Vitamin C deficiency).
4. Poor general nutrition.
5. High doses of steroids.

In patients with any of these conditions special precautions must be taken. Pre-operative care should be designed to return the patient to as normal a state as possible. At the operation, deep-tension sutures, which are those that are placed through all layers of the abdominal wall, may be required. If there is any doubt as to the healing of the wound it is wise to leave sutures in place and only to remove them cautiously, perhaps on 3 separate occasions.

If an abdominal wound bursts, the intestines literally pour into the bed. The first aid in this situation is to wrap the intestine gently in a sterile towel against the abdomen. Arrangements are then made for the immediate resuture of the abdominal wall in the operating theatre. Amazing as it may seem patients rarely come to harm and the abdomen then heals well.

Visiting

There was a time when visitors were considered to be a nuisance. In these more enlightened days it is realised that a patient's family is of paramount importance to his return to full health. There is absolutely no need to exclude children rigidly from an adult ward. The main consideration is the mental trauma that children may suffer when confronted with sick people. However, children are more resilient than we tend to think and are well able to assimilate what is, in fact, a part of life. It seems foolish to protect children against all such sights and sounds and smells and there is no doubt that a mother, father or grandparent can have the vital strength to recover revivified by the visit of a beloved small child.

After operation there is no reason why a close relative should not visit briefly only an hour or two after the completion of the procedure. What relatives sometimes do not appreciate in this circumstance is that a patient at such a time does not remember anything of the visit. From day one onwards visiting is best organised to fit in with the routine of the ward. Relatives should be encouraged to visit often for short periods of time, say only 10 minutes at first. Undoubtedly long visits can be exhausting and very difficult for a patient to terminate whilst still preserving the social graces.

Telling the patient

This subject always engenders much discussion. In general terms patients should be told precisely, in a way that they can understand, what is wrong with them, what operations they should have or have had and what the likely outcome will be. The exception to this simple rule is in the case of a cancer. If a patient is told bluntly that he has cancer, English usage being what it is, this is equated with a sentence of death and removal of hope is an unkind and usually unnecessary act. Other synonyms such as a 'growth' or 'tumour' do not carry the same connotation and can therefore be used with caution. Complete frankness is necessary with relatives, whose co-operation must be sought in this aspect of the management of the patient.

Certain patients must be told of impending death for their peace of mind. These include devout Roman Catholics, priests and nuns. In these people this information usually produces a state of great calm.

Rehabilitation

This is the single most important part of being in hospital. It is the point of the whole exercise of becoming better. With minor procedures such as hernias or varicose veins, little difficulty will be experienced. With more major operations, however, patients are often extremely anxious and fearful of their capacity to perform their job. If a man is off work for a year there is a considerable risk that he will never be fit for employment again.

For physical defects, such as follow amputation, departments of rehabilitation are available to advise as to suitable occupations and to help with appliances that aid the patient. A good example of a device in use for many years in patients who have undergone amputation of the hand, is the simple forked hook with which many patients become extremely dextrous.

Often the thing that counts most is the counsel of the bedside conversation with a wise and experienced nursing sister. Many patients owe their re-establishment into their lives to such an informal talk.

Chapter 3. Shock

Shock is of extreme importance to the surgeon. One of the reasons for the reduction in operative mortality in major surgical procedures in recent years is our greater knowledge of the aetiology and management of this condition. Most major hospitals now have Intensive Therapy Units which are primarily concerned with the treatment of shocked patients.

Clinical features

Shock is the term used to describe a very typical clinical state which comprises:
1. Pale, cold, and sweating skin with peripheral cyanosis.
2. Rapid, low volume pulse. As the shock state progresses the pulse may become impalpable at the wrist.
3. Low blood pressure. This is a relatively late feature and indicates serious failure of the body's compensating mechanism.

In severe cases there may also be dyspnoea, thirst, nausea or vomiting. The patient may be confused and restless.

Aetiology

Shock is produced by a wide variety of circumstances, all of which result in a state in which there is a failure of perfusion of the tissues with blood.

In the pump mechanism that makes up the cardiovascular system, it is obvious that three basic circumstances can produce this state of affairs:

1. Loss of fluid to prime the pump; this is termed *hypovolaemic shock*
2. Dilatation of the peripheral vessels. This increases the capacity of the vascular tree, and so reduces the effective blood volume available for tissue perfusion; this is termed *normovolaemic shock*.
3. Heart failure, which reduces the effectiveness of the cardiac pump; this is *cardiogenic shock*.

Hypovolaemic shock

Hypovolaemia is the condition which occurs when fluid is lost from the circulation and is not replaced; it simply means that there is insufficient blood to fill the vascular system. It occurs in severe haemorrhage, or when large quantities of plasma leak from the skin as the result of severe burns, or when water and electrolytes are lost in profuse vomiting or diarrhoea.

When the blood volume is reduced, the following chain of events will take place. There will be a reduction in the amount of blood returning via the veins to the right side of the heart; the pressure in these veins (that is the *central venous pressure*), falls. Since it is obvious that the heart can only pump the blood that arrives to it from the veins, there will be a reduction in the amount of blood pumped into the peripheral arterial circulation and there will therefore be a fall in the cardiac output. At first this is compensated for by constriction of the peripheral arteries of the body, which is partly a sympathetic reflex mechanism, and partly due to the secretion of adrenalin and noradrenalin from the adrenal medulla. These hormones produce peripheral arterial constriction and acceleration of the heart rate. This combination of sympathetic over-action and adrenal secretion is the explanation of the cold, pale, sweating extremities and rapid pulse seen in patients with hypovolaemic shock. This mechanism at first maintains the blood pressure and therefore the blood flow to the vital organs, but progressive fluid loss eventually reaches the stage at which compensation can no longer be maintained, and the blood pressure then falls.

A continued low blood pressure may produce a series of irreversible changes, so that the patient may die in spite of later fluid replacement. The oxygen lack affects all the vital organs; there may be damage to the brain, the heart may fail due to inadequate coronary perfusion, there may be tubular necrosis of the kidney resulting in renal failure, and there may be damage to the liver and the adrenals. In the tissues themselves inadequate blood flow may produce capillary paralysis and dilatation, so that copious fluid loss occurs into the interstitial spaces.

Normovolaemic shock

In this condition the blood volume is normal, but the capacity of the blood vessels is increased. This may be seen in the *vasovagal syndrome*, which is the simple faint which may follow severe pain or emotional disturbance. The mechanism of this is a reflex dilatation of the blood vessels in muscle together with vagal cardiac slowing. This syndrome may be recognised because the shock picture is accompanied by slowing of the heart and responds to the simple measure of lying the patient flat with the legs elevated.

In surgical practice normovolaemic shock may be seen in septicaemia (particularly when caused by gram-negative organisms). Here the picture may be complicated because, in addition to dilatation of peripheral vessels, there may also be fluid loss from vomiting, etc., and the effect of chemical or bacterial toxins on the heart.

Cardiogenic shock

If the heart is unable to pump blood around the body obviously adequate tissue perfusion with blood becomes impossible. Such a situation may arise following a large myocardial infarct due to coronary artery occlusion, or may occur in an extensive pulmonary emobolism.

STAGES OF SHOCK

These are divided into the following:
1. Early.
2. Reversible.
3. Refractory.
4. Irreversible.

In early shock, although some of the signs described above are present, they are rapidly corrected by prompt treatment.

Reversible shock means that the patient can be returned to normal, provided that rapid adequate restoration of the circulation is secured.

In refractory shock careful and skilled handling is required if the patient is to recover, and there are often complications, such as renal tubular necrosis, which require management over several weeks before full recovery is achieved.

Irreversible shock, as its name implies, means that prolonged and severe impairment of tissue perfusion has produced irreversible changes in vital organs so that, even though adequate tissue perfusion is eventually restored, the patient succumbs.

Treatment

The treatment for the shocked patient obviously depends on diagnosis.

Where haemorrhage is the cause of the shock, further bleeding must be arrested; this may require direct pressure to a wound, the application of an artery forceps to a spurting vessel in a laceration, or surgical exploration where continued bleeding is the result of a peptic ulcer haemorrhage, a ruptured spleen, or an ectopic pregnancy.

Hypovolaemic shock requires rapid restoration of the blood volume. The appropriate fluid should be replaced; blood in the case of haemorrhage, plasma in severe burns, and saline in profuse vomiting and diarrhoea. In severely shocked patients it is useful to set up a caval drip; a long (60 cm) nylon catheter is introduced into the superior vena cava via one of the veins in the arm. This catheter serves a double function. The first of these is to introduce the appropriate fluid as quickly as possible into the circulation, and the second is to allow measurement of the central venous pressure (Fig. 3.1). In hypovolaemic shock, the central venous pressure is low, but as the transfusion of fluid becomes adequate it will rise and should be maintained at a level of between +2 and +8 cm of water, measured from the upper border of the heart. This is marked by the junction between the sternum and the manubrium (the angle of Louis), when the patient is in the lying position. The measurement of the central venous pressure protects the patient against over-transfusion and therefore cardiac failure.

In order to measure the effects of treatment, it is essential to make frequent recordings of pulse, blood pressure, the central

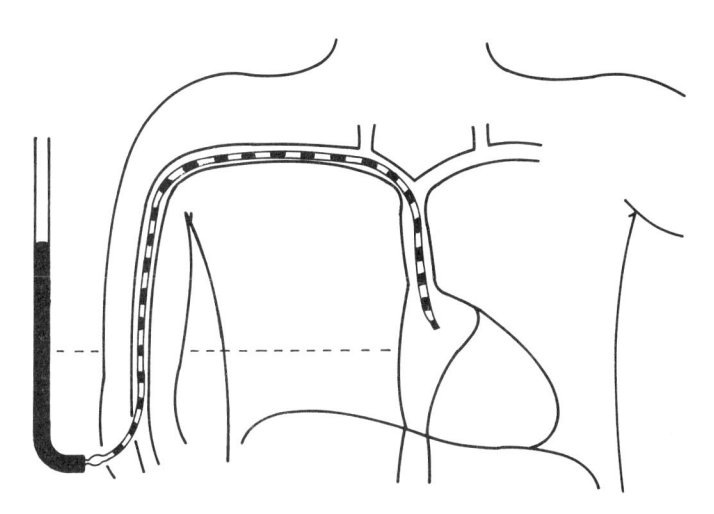

Fig. 3.1. Diagram of a central venous pressure catheter. This is passed into the superior vena cava via an arm vein. The manometer is filled with saline; the C.V.P. is the height in centimetres of the water level in the manometer above the base line, which is taken as the junction of the sternum and the manubrium.

venous pressure, urinary output, and the general appearance of the patient. Often the most sensitive index of recovery will be the return of colour to the periphery together with a rise in skin temperature. If the skin is pink, dry and warm, then it is likely that adequate tissue perfusion is taking place.

In order to measure urinary output a self-retaining catheter is introduced into the bladder, and the volume of urine secreted each hour is measured. As a rough guide this should be equal to, or more than, 1 ml per minute

Relief of pain by means of an injection of morphia is necessary where pain is a marked feature. Obviously, any fracture should be splinted to reduce pain from this source, as well as to prevent further injury.

Excessive warmth should be avoided; this produces vasodilatation of the skin vessels, thereby diverting available blood from vital organs. Oxygen is not usually required since the arterial blood is fully oxygenated, unless there is an associated chest injury or respiratory depression due to a head injury.

When a patient is extremely ill, and multiple procedures are being carried out rapidly, it is important to chart precisely when therapy is started, what is given, and to note the patient's general condition, as well as recording pulse, blood pressure, central venous pressure, and urinary output. Quite apart from absolute values, the trend of the patient is often of importance in judging response to treatment.

Treatment of septicaemic shock

The measures outlined for the patient with hypovolaemic shock should all be carried out in this condition, with the difference that the infecting organism must be eliminated with the appropriate antibiotic. The condition can be extremely confusing in its early phase because peripheral vasodilatation takes place, so that often the periphery is warm, in contrast to the usual picture of cold, pale, extremities seen in the more common hypovalaemic shock. Diagnosis is confirmed by blood culture, and while waiting for the result to come back, a broad spectrum antibiotic, such as ampicillin, is commenced, although the drug regime may have to be altered when the sensitivity of the organism has been checked by the bacteriologist.

Plasma or dextran is given by drip in order to fill the increased capacity of the dilated vascular system.

In long continued stress due to shock it may be necessary to give hydrocortisone 100 mg 6 hourly intravenously to combat failure of the adrenal cortex.

Chapter 4. Burns

Major burns still present serious problems for the surgical and nursing team. The mortality of extensive deep burns remains high, with infection still the commonest ultimate cause of death. The patient presents a unique problem in nursing care, quite different from other emergency situations. He is often the causative factor in his own catastrophe—the few exceptions in peace-time being the innocent victims of air disasters and road crashes. From being a normal healthy person he is suddenly converted into someone faced by an illness which may last for many months and which he knows may produce extensive disfigurement. He is often unable to help or feed himself. He is smelly, unclothed, isolated, subjected to frequent painful (or at least uncomfortable) surgical and nursing procedures and he makes slow progress, often beset by setbacks. A great part of his burden must be shouldered by a sympathetic, knowledgeable and skilled nursing staff.

PATHOLOGY

Burns are classified into partial or full thickness, depending on whether or not the deep germinal layer of the skin is intact or destroyed (Fig. 4.1).

A partial thickness burn may be quite superficial, the skin being erythematous (reddened) due to capillary dilatation. If rather more severe, areas of blistering are produced by exudation of plasma beneath coagulated epidermis. The underlying germinal layer of the epithelium is intact and complete healing takes place within a few

44
Chapter 4

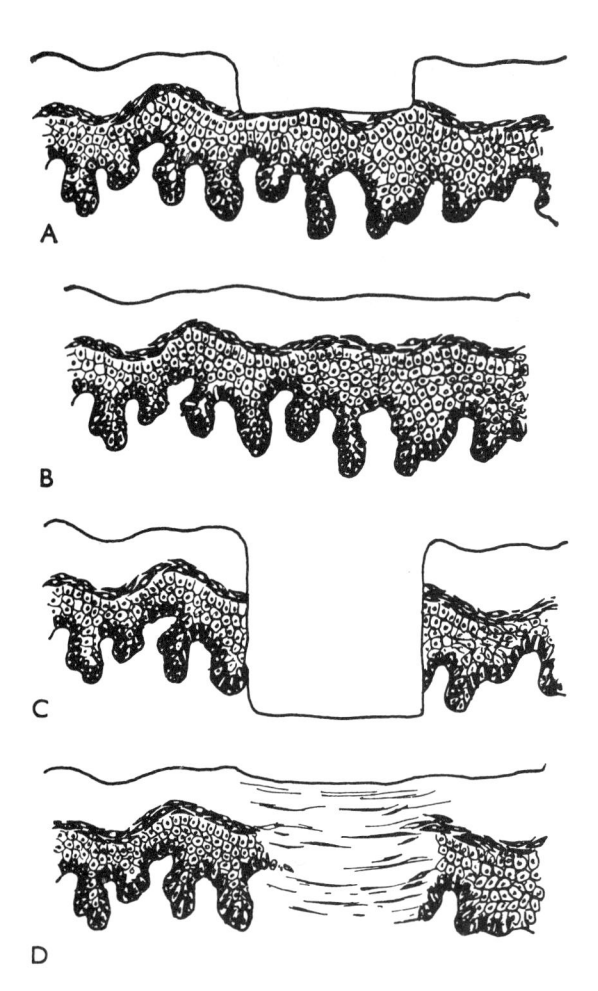

Fig. 4.1. A partial thickness burn (A) leaves part or whole of the germinal epithelium intact and therefore complete healing takes place (B). However, a full thickness burn (C) destroys the germinal layer and therefore heals by scar tissue (D).

days. Deeper partial thickness burns extend down to the germinal layer and may partially destroy it. There is intense blistering, which is followed by the formation of a slough. This scab separates after about 10–17 days, leaving healthy newly formed epithelium.

Full thickness burns completely destroy the epithelium. There may be initial blistering, but this is soon replaced by a coagulum or slough; more often, this is present from the onset in an intense deep burn. Unlike more superficial burns this slough separates only slowly over 3 or 4 weeks, or longer, to leave an underlying surface of granulation tissue (Fig. 4.2). Unless grafted, this will heal only by dense scar tissue, with consequent contractures and deformity (Fig. 4.3).

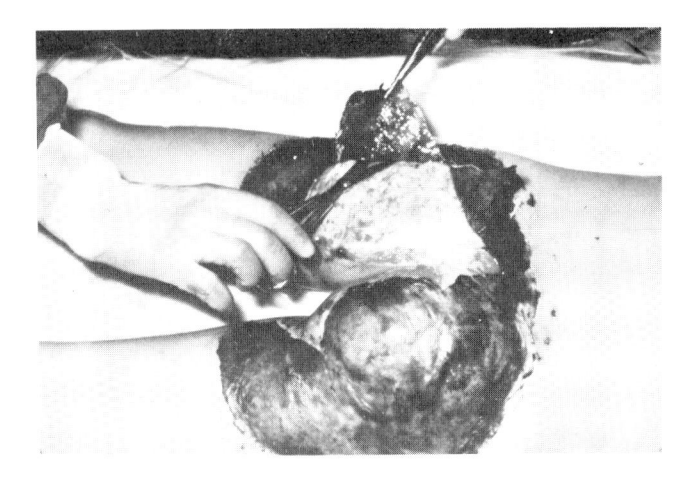

Fig. 4.2. A full thickness burn of the buttock undergoing excision three weeks after the accident. As the slough is cut away with scissors the underlying granulation tissue is revealed.

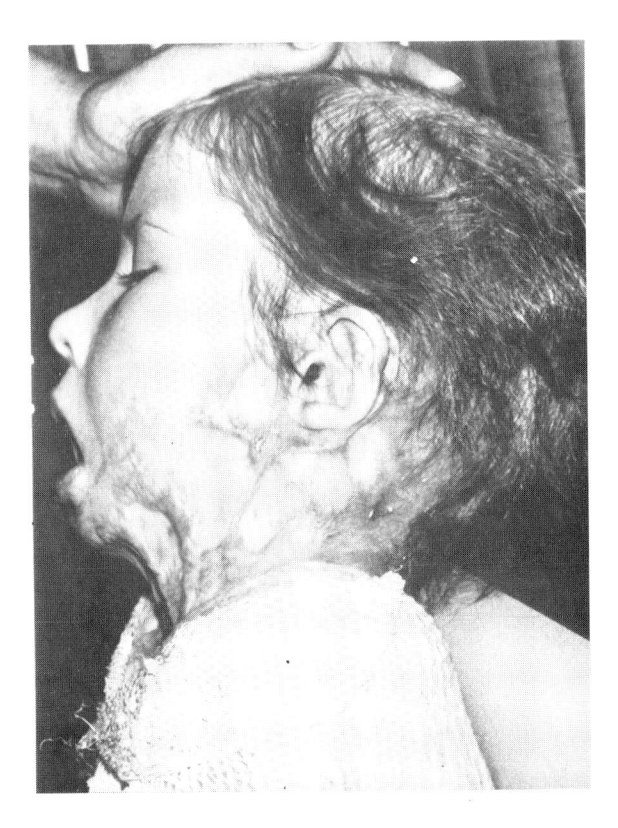

Fig. 4.3. The gross deformity produced by the contracting fibrous scars of a full thickness burn.

THE GENERAL EFFECTS OF BURNS

As well as local tissue destruction, the following general phenomena may be present in the extensively burnt patient:

1. *Pain*

This is due to the stimulation of numerous nerve endings in the damaged skin. It is more severe in superficial burns and, indeed, deep burns may be relatively painless because the nerve endings are to a great extent destroyed as they lie beneath the germinal epithelium.

2. *Plasma loss*

The damaged capillaries in the burnt skin allow plasma to exude through their walls, especially during the first 24 hours of an injury. This loss ceases by the time a coagulum has formed over the burn, a process which takes about 48 hours. As a direct result of this plasma loss from the blood stream, the circulatory volume falls and, in an extensive burn, the patient passes into oligaemic shock with rapid pulse and low blood pressure (see chapter 3). Since shock is a direct result of plasma loss, it is therefore proportional to the surface area of the body which is burnt. The loss of the plasma fraction of the blood is demonstrated by a rapid rise in the haematocrit reading of the blood, which is estimated by spinning down a blood sample in the centrifuge. The blood from a severely shocked burnt patient will have a much higher haematocrit level than normal, due to the increased proportions of red blood corpuscles compared with the plasma.

3 *Anaemia*

This results partly from destruction of the red cells within involved skin capillaries and partly from toxic inhibition of the bone marrow if infection of the burnt area takes place. It is therefore particularly marked in deep, infected burns.

4 *Stress reaction*

The body shows the typical stress reaction which follows any severe injury and which is due to an excess secretion of hormones from the adrenal cortex. There is comparative retention of water and sodium chloride, together with an excess breakdown of tissue protein and loss of potassium in the urine. Occasionally stress ulcer of the stomach and duodenum may develop (*Curling's ulcer*), with perforation or haemorrhage.

5. *Toxaemia*

This is a combination of factors which include biochemical disturbances, plasma loss and infection (the latter sometimes complicated by septicaemia). It is rather less common now that burns are treated adequately.

TREATMENT

The principles underlying the treatment of burns are:
1 *General*, to mitigate the more widespread effects of burns listed above.
2 *Local*, to prevent infection and to promote healing of the epithelium, either spontaneously or by skin grafting.

General treatment

1. *Pain* is relieved with morphia, and this is best given initially by slow intravenous injection.
2. *Oligaemic shock due to plasma loss*. This is treated by replacement with either plasma or plasma substitutes such as dextran. The amount of plasma to be given and its rate of administration depend on careful and repeated assessments of the patient. If the patient is being overtransfused there may be congestion of the neck veins, cyanosis and a fall in the haematocrit reading below normal, showing that too much haemodilution is taking place. Too little replacement is suggested by a rapid thready pulse, a low blood pressure, low urinary output and a high haematocrit level. During transfusion the patient must therefore be kept under strict observation, on a quarter or half hourly shock chart, the urinary output must be carefully charted (if necessary a catheter is inserted in the bladder) and the haematocrit level is estimated four hourly or at even more frequent intervals. As a guide to the amount of fluid replacement 'the rule of nine' is helpful. The body is divided into zones of percentage of surface area as follows (Fig. 4.4):

Head and neck	— 9%
Each arm	— 9%
Each leg	— 9% × 2 = 18%
Front of trunk	— 9% × 2 = 18%
Back of trunk	— 9% × 2 = 18%
Perineum	— 1%

As a rough rule, the patient's hand is approximately 1% of his surface area. In adults, as a guide, 1 litre of fluid is required for each 9% of the body affected per 24 hours.

In children special charts are available which equate size of the patient with area of burn and amount of fluid replacement required. If the burns are full thickness, approximately one third of the fluid replacement may be given as blood in order to restore the extensive red cell destruction within the affected area. Subsequent anaemia, if present, may also require blood transfusion.

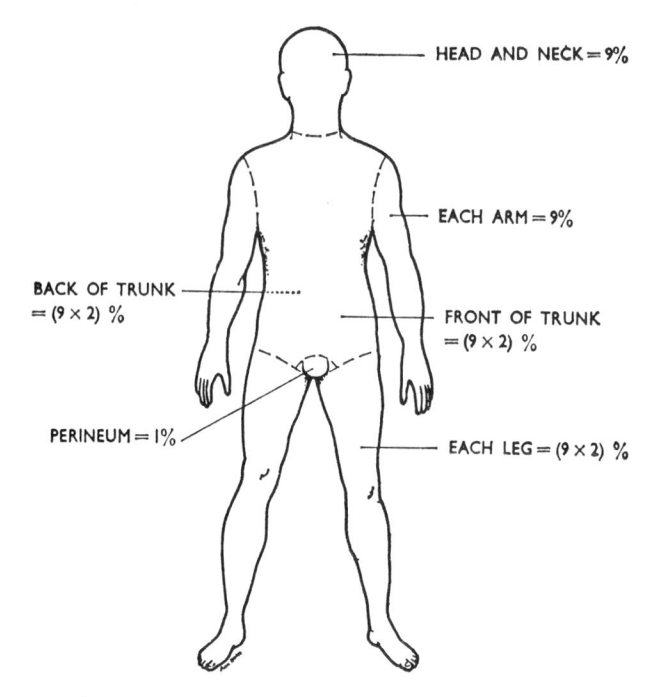

Fig. 4.4. 'The rule of nine', a useful guide to the estimation of the area of a burnt surface.

HEAD AND NECK = 9%
EACH ARM = 9%
BACK OF TRUNK = (9 × 2) %
FRONT OF TRUNK = (9 × 2) %
PERINEUM = 1%
EACH LEG = (9 × 2) %

These rules are useful guides but must be interpreted in the light of the patient's response to transfusion.

Local treatment

A burn at the moment at which it is sustained is sterile—our duty is to try and keep it so. The immediate first aid treatment of a burn is to wrap the area in sterile dressings during transfer to hospital. The treatment of major burns may be either by the *open* or the *closed* method. Sometimes a combination of the two is required.

The open or exposure method

This is based on the principle that bacteria cannot grow on the dry coagulum which rapidly forms over the exposed burn surface. The patient is therefore completely exposed in a warm isolated room. Elevation is used wherever possible to reduce oedema. It is excellent for the face, the limbs (apart from the fingers), or where only the front or the back of the trunk is involved. It is obviously a difficult technique to apply to circumferential burns of the trunk outside special burns units, and is best avoided for burns of the fingers. It has the advantage of simplicity and comparative freedom from discomfort for the patient (Fig. 4.5).

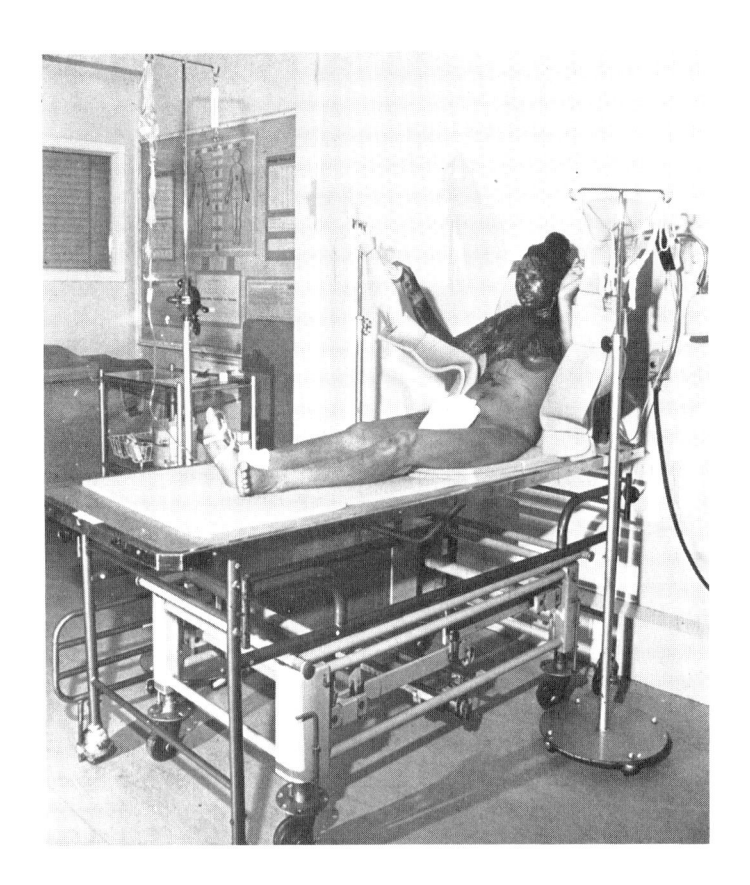

Fig. 4.5. Exposure treatment for severe burns of the face, chest and arms.

The closed treatment

This aims at excluding bacteria from the burnt areas by means of sterile dressings which are supplemented by antibiotics or chemical antiseptic agents. The burn is cleaned with a mild detergent, covered with an antibiotic cream, Vaseline gauze and thick layers of sterile dressings, which must be changed if they become soaked with plasma (Fig. 4.6). Recently a sulphonamide preparation termed maphenide acetate in a water soluble cream (sulphamylon) has been introduced with good results. It requires twice daily application, but unfortunately it is painful and drug sensitivity may occur. Gentamycin sulphate as a 1% cream may also be used but, again, toxic reactions may occur and some strains of pseudomonas are resistant to this antibiotic. Silver nitrate as a half per cent aqueous solution is relatively painless to use with no local sensitivity, but it has to be repeatedly applied as wet dressings which require re-soaking every 2–4 hours and it is not effective in the treatment of infected burns. The silver stains normal skin and the sheets, as well as pretty well

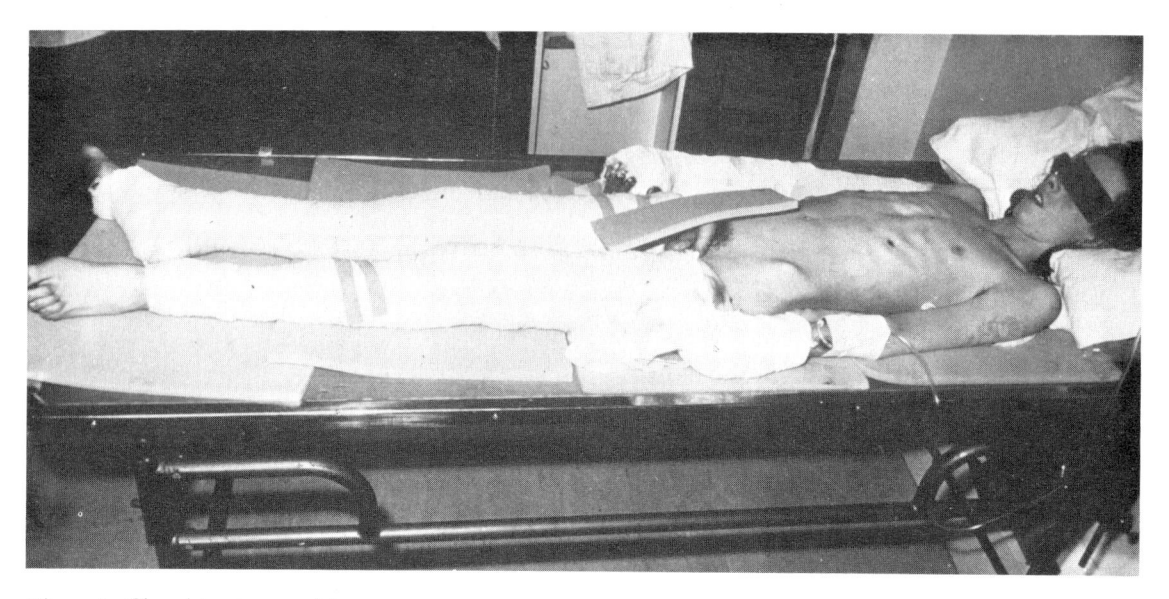

Fig. 4.6. Closed treatment of burns using topical antibiotic and bulky sterile dressings.

everything else with which it comes into contact. Recently silver sulphadiazine cream has been introduced, which eliminates some of these disadvantages.

At the end of about 10 days in both methods of treatment the slough will separate from superficial burns to leave an underlying healthy healed pink epithelium and no further local treatment is then required. In contrast, the slough over a full thickness is still adherent and attempts to remove it will produce bleeding (see Fig. 4.2). Full thickness burns are therefore excised at about 14 to 17 days and covered with split skin grafts (Fig. 4.7).

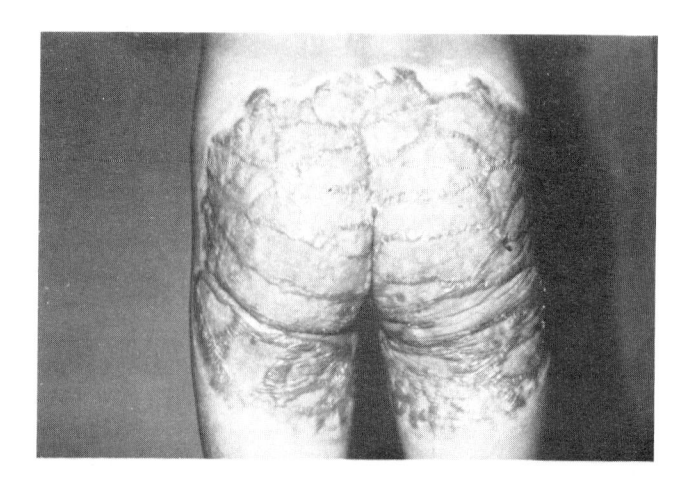

Fig. 4.7. Extensive full thickness burns of the buttocks which have been excised and grafted with split skin. (A later stage in the treatment of the patient shown in Fig. 4.2)

Chapter 5. Tumours; Principles of radiotherapy and cytotoxic therapy

INTRODUCTION

The word 'tumour' literally means a swelling, but for practical purposes the term is now used to describe a new growth or neoplasm. All the cells in the body, apart from the nerve cells within the central nervous system, are undergoing reproduction throughout life and in some organs, especially the bone marrow, the epithelia of the skin, alimentary canal and the reproductive organs, this is occurring very rapidly indeed. In a normal person this cell division merely keeps pace with the wear and tear of the tissues; under some circumstances there may be sudden very rapid bursts of cell division, for example in a healing wound or in the rapid growth of a fetus within the uterus, yet such growth is controlled and is in response to some need of the organism. In complete contrast to this, a tumour may be defined as 'an uncontrolled new growth of tissue' and it is a characteristic feature of such growths that they develop without any relationship to the requirements of the body. Indeed often their development may be harmful or even lethal.

CLASSIFICATION OF TUMOURS

Tumours are divided into *benign* and *malignant* and it is to this second group that the term 'cancer' is applied. It should be noted that some tumours are intermediate in their behaviour between benign and malignant neoplasm (a neoplasm means literally 'new growth') and that sometimes malignant change can take place in a benign tumour.

The pathological terms used to describe tumours at first sound complicated but, in fact, in the majority of cases, the technical name of the tumour tells us its tissue of origin and whether or not it is benign or malignant. Throughout, the termination '-oma' means 'some sort of tumour'. Next, tumours are divided according to their tissue of origin, depending on whether they arise from epithelium (skin, the lining of the alimentary canal and its associated glands, the kidney and the genito-urinary tract), or from the connective and supporting tissues of the body (bone, cartilage, muscle etc.).

Epithelial tumours

Benign epithelial tumours are termed *papillomas* when they derive from a simple epithelium, for example a papilloma of the bladder, but the term *adenoma* is used for benign epithelial tumours which arise from glands or a gland-bearing epithelium; for example a benign tumour of the pancreatic ducts would be termed a pancreatic adenoma. All malignant tumours arising from epithelia are termed *carcinomas*, to which is added the organ in which they originate; thus we talk about a carcinoma of the stomach or a carcinoma of the rectum where we mean a malignant tumour arising from the epithelial lining of these organs.

Supporting tissue tumours

Benign tumours of connective and supporting tissues are designated by the suffix 'oma' preceeded by the name of the cell of origin. Thus 'lipoma' means a benign tumour of fat, 'chondroma' a benign tumour of cartilage. Malignant tumours have the suffix 'sarcoma' preceded by the name of the cell of origin—'liposarcoma' and 'chondrosarcoma' are thus malignant tumours of fat and cartilage respectively. Sometimes, two or more types of cell are found in the same sarcoma thus a fibro-liposarcoma contains elements of both fibrous tissue and fat.

Not all tumours fall into this neat classification and a number of special groups exist. Among the more common of these are the tumours of lymphoid tissue termed the *lymphomas*, which include Hodgkin's disease and lymphosarcoma, the *leukaemias*, which can be thought of as malignant disease of the white cells, the *melanomas* (both benign and malignant) which originate in the melanin-producing cells (melanocytes) of the skin and elsewhere, and the *teratomas* which are derived from a number of different cell types, which occur particularly in the testis and ovary and which may contain bone, glandular tissue, muscle and other structures in conglomeration.

Differentiation between benign and malignant tumours

As a general rule malignant tumours grow faster than benign neoplasms and this is mirrored in their microscopic appearance. A benign tumour shows only an occasional cell undergoing division and its appearance is very similar to that of its parent tissue (Fig. 5.1A). In contrast, a highly malignant tumour viewed under the microscope will show numerous cell divisions and the malignant cells themselves are often grossly abnormal, with large nuclei and relatively little cytoplasm. Instead of having the microscopic appearance of their tissue of origin, malignant tumours may simply show sheets or columns of rapidly dividing cells spreading through the parent organ (Fig. 5.1B).

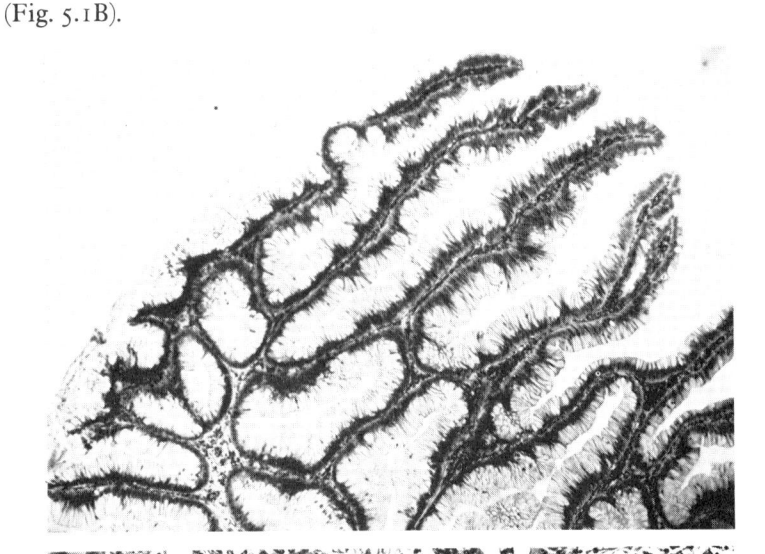

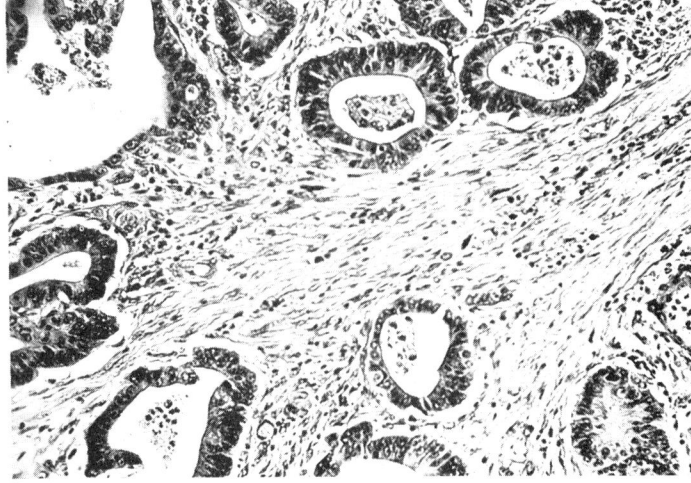

Tumours: Radiotherapy and cytotoxic therapy

Fig. 5.1. (A) A well differentiated and (B) a poorly differentiated (anaplastic) carcinoma of the large intestine viewed under the microscope.

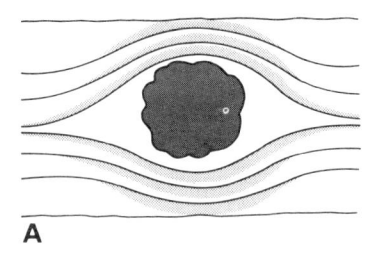

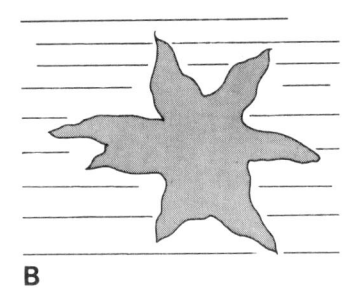

Fig. 5.2. (A) A benign tumour compresses and pushes aside surrounding tissues. (B) A malignant tumour invades surrounding structures.

Fig. 5.3. Benign epithelial tumours tend to become pedunculated (A) whereas the malignant surface tumours tend to be sessile (B).

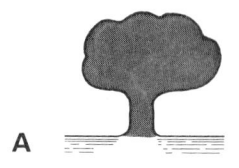

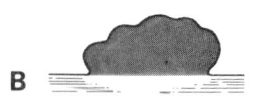

Although both benign and malignant tumours grow without regard to the needs of the body, they have very different behaviour in their relationship to surrounding tissues. A benign tumour simply compresses and pushes aside surrounding structures as it enlarges and these tissues may become compressed to form a fibrous capsule around the tumour. In contrast, a malignant growth invades its surrounds as a result of which no capsule is formed (Fig. 5.2). The tumour will grow along the paths of least resistance, easily tearing through soft connective tissues but halting for a time when it encounters bone or large blood vessels, although these in turn may eventually be invaded and destroyed. Cartilage is relatively resistant to tumour invasion so that, for example, when cancer deposits occur in the vertebral column the bones themselves may be almost destroyed but the cartilaginous intervertebral discs remain intact. This invasion is very typical of malignancy and indeed the word 'cancer' literally means 'crab', and describes the crab-like processes which the malignant growth sends into adjacent tissues (Fig. 5.2B).

Benign epithelial tumours tend to project outwards and often to develop a pedicle. Only when they reach a very large size will such pedunculated tumours ulcerate. Epithelial carcinomas, in contrast, usually form a flat mass, to which the term 'sessile' is applied (Fig. 5.3). Such a tumour rapidly outgrows its blood supply and often undergoes ulceration (Fig. 5.4). All malignant tumours possess the properties of local invasion. Many, in addition, have another feature which differentiates them from benign tumour, this is the ability to spread elsewhere in the body with the formation of *secondary deposits* or *metastases*. This spread may occur along the lymphatics to regional lymph nodes, a property which is possessed by carcinomas but not by sarcomas. However, both carcinomas and sarcomas may invade through the blood stream to produce deposits, which are especially likely to be found in the liver, lungs, the skeleton and the brain (Fig. 5.5). For some mysterious reason they are rare in the spleen and the heart.

Carcinomas within the chest and abdominal cavities may seed and spread over these pleural and peritoneal surfaces, a process termed *transcoelomic spread*. Pleural effusion and ascites are the usual clinical manifestations of this phenomenon (Fig. 5.6).

Very few things in nature fall into neat classifications and it is a general rule that most natural phenomena show a gradation from one end of a continuous spectrum to the other. Tumours are no exception. At each end of the scale are undoubtedly benign and undoubtedly malignant growths, but in the middle are those which have a rather untidy intermediate behaviour. Adenomas of the parotid gland, for example, do not have a well defined capsule and if

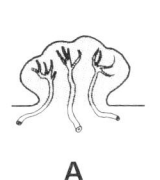

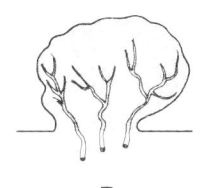

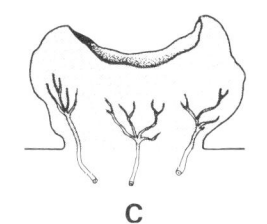

Fig. 5.4. As tumours enlarge they tend to outgrow their blood supply and therefore ulcerate. Note that this explains the usual raised and everted edge of a malignant ulcer.

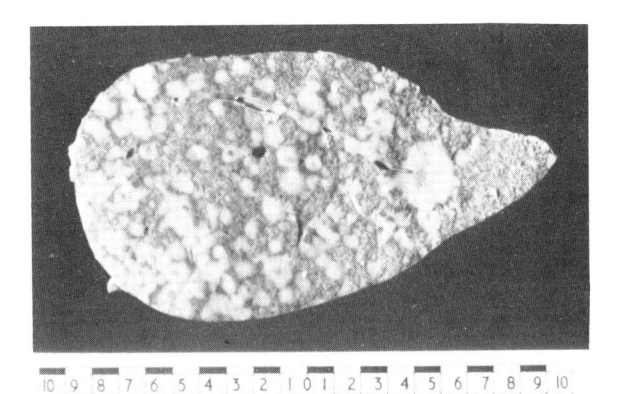

Fig. 5.5. Metastases in the liver from a patient dying of carcinoma of the breast. These secondaries result from blood stream spread.

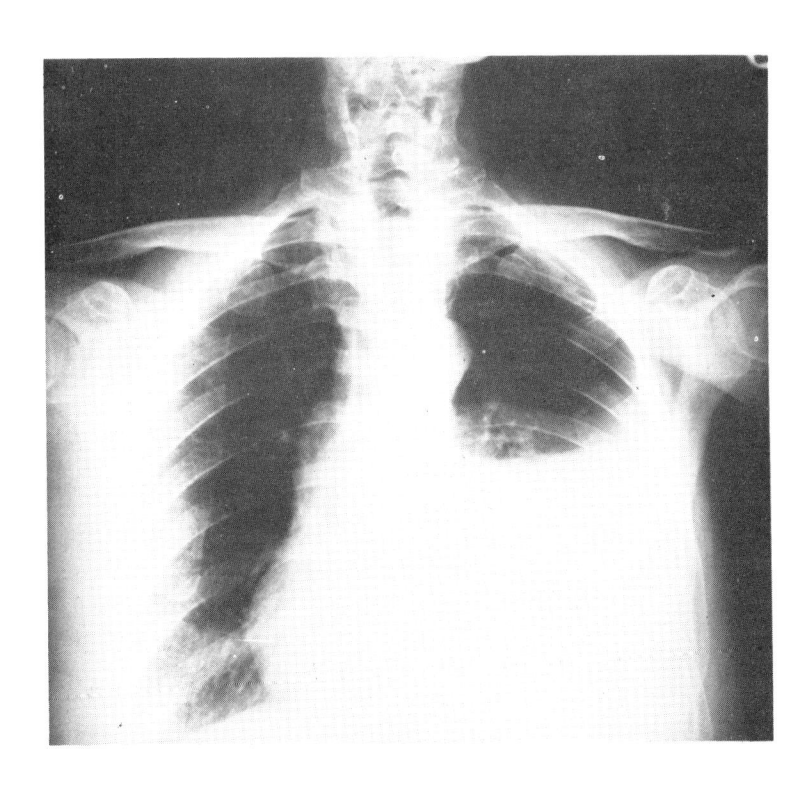

Fig. 5.6. Chest X-ray showing a large left pleural effusion in a patient with breast cancer. This results from transcoelomic spread in the pleural cavity.

simply enucleated by the surgeon they tend to recur locally in the operation wound; moreover, long-standing tumours may undergo frank malignant change. Papillomas of the urinary tract may deposit on other parts of the lining epithelium, may seed into the surgical scar when removed at operation and may also eventually turn into a typical carcinoma.

Obviously a malignant tumour which spreads throughout the body may harm and eventually kill the patient. The majority of benign tumours are little more than a nuisance but it should not be thought that this is always so and there are situations where benign tumours may be just as dangerous as a malignant growth. For example, a small benign growth within the rigid framework of the skull may produce fatal brain compression, or a benign tumour within the bowel or urinary tract may cause serious haemorrhage or obstruction. Adenomas of the endocrine glands may produce excessive and harmful hormone secretion; examples are Cushing's syndrome which results from an adenoma of the cortex of the adrenal gland, or hypoglycaemia produced by excessive secretion of insulin from an adenoma of the islet cells of the pancreas.

There is little doubt, also, that benign tumours occasionally undergo malignant change. This may occur in melanomas of the skin, adenomas of the bowel and urinary tract and even occasionally in the commonest benign tumour of all, the subcutaneous lipoma which very rarely becomes a liposarcoma.

THE CLINICAL FEATURES AND DIAGNOSIS OF MALIGNANT DISEASE

There are three ways in which a malignant tumour may draw attention to itself:

1. *By the effects of the primary tumour*; for example, a woman may feel a lump in her breast and this proves to be a carcinoma, or a man coughs up blood from his lung cancer.

2. *By the effects produced by secondary deposits*; for example, the woman with the carcinoma of the breast may have overlooked the lump itself, but comes to the doctor because of back pain due to the presence of secondary deposits in her vertebrae, or the patient with the lung cancer may report because he has noticed a mass above the clavicle which is a clump of secondarily involved supraclavicular lymph nodes.

3. *By the general effects of malignant disease*; these patients report with loss of weight, loss of appetite, anaemia and general debility (Fig. 5.7). In its most advanced stages, this is termed *malignant cachexia*.

It should be noted that a patient may present with features which fall into one, two or all three categories—for example, a patient with a carcinoma of the stomach may complain of having noticed a lump in his abdomen (the primary tumour), and of having become jaundiced (from the secondaries in his liver), and may also have noticed that he has become pale and has lost a considerable amount of weight (the general effects of the tumour).

Now it is a general rule that the diagnosis of any condition in the whole of medicine and surgery follows three logical steps. First, a history is taken, then the patient is examined and then, if necessary, certain special investigations are carried out in the laboratory and X-ray department.

Let us now apply these three steps to the diagnosis of a cancer, bearing in mind the three ways in which a tumour may present that we have already mentioned. As an example, let us take the commonest killing cancer in this country, carcinoma of the lung:

The history

(a) *The primary tumour* may present with cough, haemoptysis, breathlessness or chest pain.
(b) *Secondary deposits* may bring the patient to the doctor with the complaints of enlarged glands in the neck, back pain or pathological fractures due to bone deposits, headaches or drowsiness from cerebral metastases, or jaundice from liver deposits.
(c) *General effects of malignant disease*—the patient may present with lassitude, anorexia, loss of weight or anaemia.

Examination

(a) *The primary tumour* may produce physical signs in the chest which can be detected by percussion or by auscultation through the stethoscope.
(b) *Secondary deposits* may cause enlarged lymph nodes, enlargement of the liver or obvious bony deposits.
(c) *The general effects of malignant disease* may be suggested by clinical anaemia or cachexia.

Special investigations

(a) *For the primary tumour*—a chest X-ray may reveal a suspicious shadow in the lung, microscopic examination of the sputum may show the presence of malignant cells and the tumour itself may be

Tumours: Radiotherapy and cytotoxic therapy

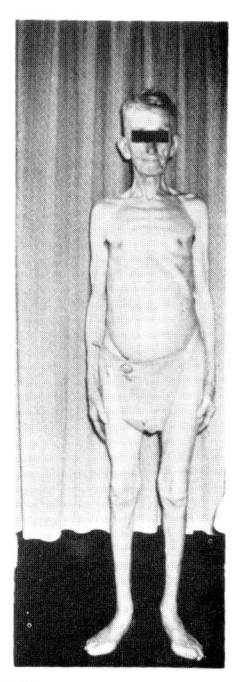

Fig. 5.7. Malignant cachexia in a patient with an advanced carcinoma of the stomach. Note that the abdomen is distended with ascites.

visualised directly at bronchoscopy, at which time a biopsy of the growth may be obtained for microscopic examination.

(b) *For secondary deposits*—X-rays of the skeletal system may demonstrate secondary deposits in the bones and special radioactive scanning techniques may reveal deposits in liver or brain.

(c) *For general manifestations of malignant disease*—a blood count may reveal anaemia.

This simple scheme can be applied to any of the principal malignant tumours and will be employed throughout this book.

GENERAL PRINCIPLES OF TREATMENT

The majority of benign tumours require simple surgical removal. The patient may not like the cosmetic appearance of the lump and in any case is worried by it. Furthermore, the surgeon cannot be entirely certain of the nature of the lump, even though he suspects that it is benign, and it is safer to have it removed and put it under the microscope. Some tumours may undergo malignant change, so that their removal before this can happen is obviously a wise prophylactic measure. In other situations, the benign tumour may produce unpleasant effects due to obstruction, bleeding, pressure on adjacent organs, or, in the case of the endocrine glands, symptoms due to hormone over-secretion. In all these cases, surgical removal is indicated.

Turning now to the treatment of malignant tumours, these must always be considered under two headings: First, *curative* in which an attempt is made to remove the disease entirely and second, *palliative* where, although the disease is incurable or has recurred after an attempt at curative treatment, steps can still be taken to ease the patient's symptoms.

In this chapter the possible lines of treatment will be dealt with in general and, in subsequent chapters, the management of the main tumours of specific organs will be considered in more detail.

Curative treatment

There are two methods by which at present an attempt can be made to cure a patient of cancer. The first is *surgical excision*, in which the tumour, often together with adjacent draining lymph nodes, is widely excised. The surgeon hopes to diagnose the cancer before metastases have developed, and, by complete excision, prevent the possibility of later dissemination. Typical examples of such a treatment are mastectomy, in which a carcinoma of the breast is removed together with surrounding breast tissue, the overlying skin and the adjacent axillary lymph nodes, or resection of a carcinoma of the colon when the growth is removed together with adjacent bowel wall clear of the cancer and a generous wedge of the mesocolon containing the draining lymph nodes. The second method is *radiotherapy* which is usually employed to destroy tumours which are not readily accessible to surgical removal, for example, cancers of the mouth and pharynx. Later in this chapter the principles underlying radiotherapy will be considered in more detail.

In some circumstances a combination of surgery and radiotherapy is employed.

Palliative treatment

In many cases the patient presents too late for any attempt at cure; by now the tumour has widely disseminated and there are obvious metastases elsewhere in the body which preclude curative treatment. In other instances, the patient returns to hospital after an attempted cure by surgery or radiotherapy carried out months or even years before but has now developed recurrence of the original disease or metastases elsewhere. Although the patient is now beyond cure, a number of measures are available which may prolong life and provide freedom or relief from pain. The types of therapy can be listed as follows:

1. *Surgery.* Even though secondary deposits may be present it may still be worthwhile carrying out a palliative excision of the primary tumour. For example, a patient with an obstructing carcinoma of the colon may be treated by partial colectomy to remove the primary growth even though secondary deposits are already present in the liver. He will be relieved of his obstructive symptoms and may live for many months or even years in comfort before eventually dying of his liver metastases. An inoperable obstructing tumour of the oesophagus or the upper end of the stomach may be intubated by means of a plastic tube so that dysphagia can be relieved. Although the patient is doomed to die of his cancer, at least he will be able to swallow comfortably for the rest of his days (Fig. 5.8).

2. *Radiotherapy.* This is extremely valuable in the treatment of localised irremovable disease, for example, painful secondary deposits in bone, advanced irremovable breast tumours, inoperable lymph node metastases etc. The principles of radiotherapy are considered in the section below.

3. *Cytotoxic therapy.* A large number of cytotoxic agents are available which may temporarily produce regression of tumours. The principles of this treatment are considered in a section later in this chapter.

Fig. 5.8. Some of the tubes which are available for pallatiave intubation of inoperable carcinomas of the oesophagus and cardia. From above down, these are: A Mousseau-Barbin tube, a short and a long Souttar's tube, and a Celestin tube.

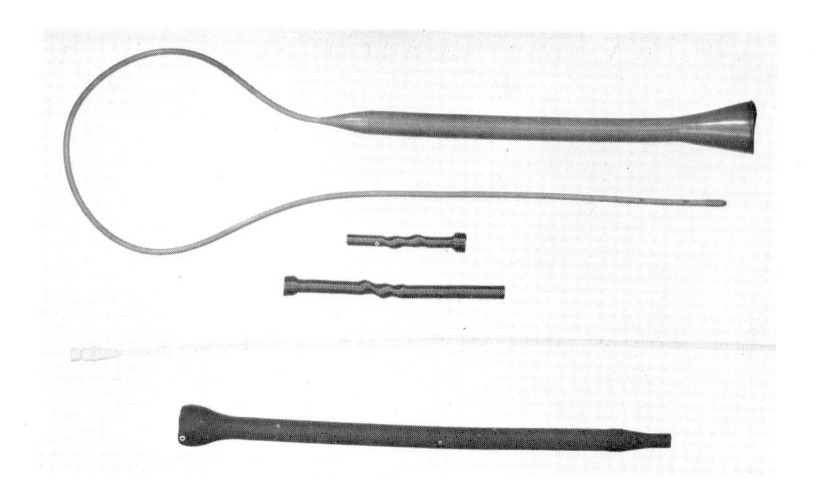

4. *Sex hormone and endocrine surgery.* Two carcinomas, those of the breast and the prostate, are often sensitive to changes in the sex-hormone environment and may respond either to the administration of sex hormones (e.g. stilboestrol) or to removal of the sex hormone secreting glands (the gonads and/or the adrenals) or the pituitary gland which controls their secretion. Further details will be found in the chapters on breast and prostrate.

5. *Pain relief.* This is extremely important in patients with advanced cancer. The judicious use of pain relieving drugs may be supplemented by employing tranquilising agents and anti-emetics, among which chlorpromazine is particularly valuable. Nerve blocks by means of phenol or alcohol may anaesthetise the conduction pathways from a painful inoperable tumour.

6. *Maintenance of morale.* An essential part of the nursing treatment of patients with advanced cancer is a kindly understanding and yet cheerful attitude of the medical and nursing staff, coupled with the difficult nursing care of a patient who is often bed-ridden and in pain.

PROGNOSIS IN MALIGNANT DISEASE

One of the most difficult tasks facing doctors and nurses is when the patient who knows he has malignant disease, or his relatives, ask for the prognosis. It must be realised that we can only give the chances, or possibilities, in each particular case. If we say, for example, that the patient has a 90% chance of cure, we must remember that he may be unfortunate enough to fall into the 10% who are to suffer a

fatal recurrence of the disease. In any particular patient we have four main features upon which prognosis depends:
1. The extent of spread of the tumour
2. Its microscopic appearance
3. Its anatomical situation
4. The general condition of the patient.

The extent of spread

The prognosis of any tumour deteriorates in proportion to the extent of invasion and dissemination which has taken place. For example, a cancer of the bowel which is confined to the mucosa has a better prognosis than the same tumour which has invaded through the wall of the bowel and this, in turn, has a better outlook than a tumour which has spread to the draining lymph nodes. Prognosis is worst of all if metastases have spread to the liver or other organs (Fig. 5.9). A woman with a small tumour confined to the breast has, on average, a much better prognosis than a woman of the same age and same type of tumour which has disseminated to the lymph nodes in her axilla, or, worse still, widely to the liver, bones and lungs. Clues about the extent of the spread may be found in the pre-operative examination of the patient, where, for example, enlarged lymph nodes or a nodular swollen liver may be found, or this may be determined at the time of surgical exploration. Finally the microscopic examination of the specimen may reveal involvement of

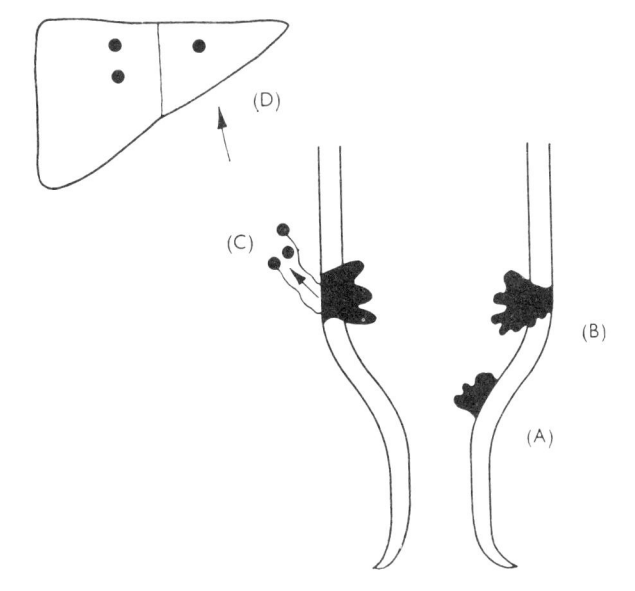

Fig. 5.9. Diagram to show the progressive stages of a tumour of the large bowel. A, confined to the bowel wall; B, penetrating the wall; C, involvement of regional lymph nodes; D, distant spread to the liver. Each stage is associated with progressive worsening of the prognosis.

lymph nodes which had not been detected clinically, or of microscopic extension of the growth to the very edges of the resected specimen with consequent worsening of the outlook for the patient.

Microscopic appearance

The pathologist's examination of a biopsy of the tumour or of the resected surgical specimen is valuable in telling us the degree of differentiation of the tumour. As a general rule, the more actively growing the tumour, and the more primitive its cells (to which the term 'de-differentiation' or 'anaplastic' is applied) the worse the prognosis.

These two factors, the spread of the tumour and its degree of differentiation, should always be taken in conjunction with each other. A small tumour, with no apparent spread, may still have a relatively poor prognosis if it is highly anaplastic, whereas an extensive tumour is not incompatible with long survival if microscopic examination reveals that it is very well differentiated and therefore tends to be slowly growing.

Anatomical situation

The situation of the tumour is of some prognostic significance, because on this may depend whether or not the lesion is easily accessible to surgical removal. A brain tumour located in the frontal lobe may be resected, whereas a similar tumour buried deeply in the brain stem would be a hopeless surgical proposition. An anteriorly placed cancer of the rectum in a male, which is invading into the prostate and bladder base, is usually considered irremoveable, whereas a similar state of affairs in the female in which the tumour is invading the posterior vagina is still amenable to abdomino-perineal excision of the rectum in which the posterior wall of the vagina can also be sacrificed.

The general condition of the patient

This is something that must be taken into consideration in giving the prognosis of any surgical condition. Although the tumour itself in a particular patient may be curable, it may, in practical terms, be inoperable because of the poor general condition of the patient. For example, gross congestive cardiac failure may render what is technically an operable carcinoma of the rectum a hopeless surgical risk. In dealing with an elderly unfit patient the surgeon, in consultation with the anaesthetist, has to weigh up in each case the risks of the operation against the suffering the patient is likely to undergo if left untreated.

PRINCIPLES OF RADIOTHERAPY

Each year the number of patients attending the radiotherapy departments of our hospitals increases. The nursing care of these often very sick and very anxious people is a considerable responsibility and it behoves the nurse to have a clear understanding of the basic principles underlying radiotherapeutic treatment.

Radiotherapy may be used in the primary treatment of cancer, especially where the tumour is deeply placed and relatively inaccessible (e.g. the mouth, pharynx, larynx, and for extensive tumours of the bladder) or it may be used as a pre-operative treatment to shrink down a tumour and render it more amenable for operation. In its most widespread use, radiotherapy is employed in the management of inoperable or recurrent cancers in order to give palliative relief of symptoms.

Three main techniques are currently available:
1. Supervoltage or cobalt beam therapy.
2. Implants into tissues or cavities such as the uterine canal of radioactive materials—for example, radium, caesium or radioactive gold.
3. Radioactive isotopes administered orally or by injection.

X-rays were discovered by Wilhelm Roentgen in 1895 as mysterious rays of a very short wave-length found to be emitted from the anode (positive electrode) when this is struck by cathode rays (a stream of negatively charged electrons) passed through a vacuum tube (Fig. 5.10). These X-rays were found to penetrate human tissues and then

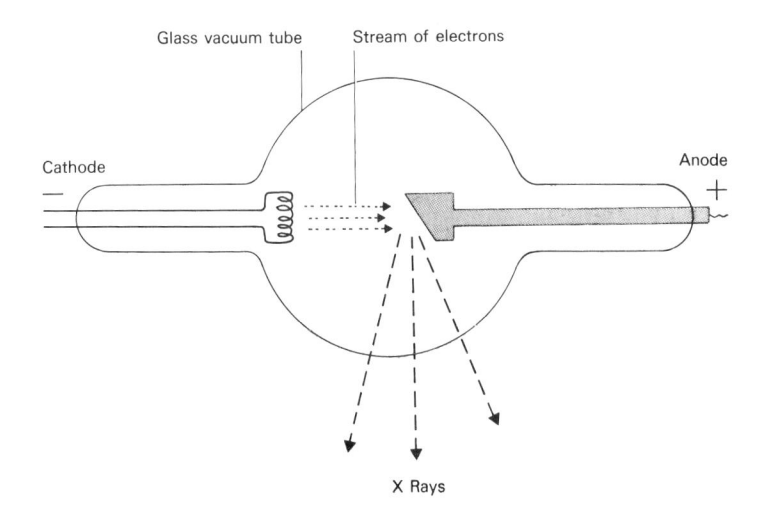

Fig. 5.10. Diagram of an X-ray tube.

to be picked up on photographic paper—the basis of modern radiology. But powerful X-rays, produced by increasing the voltage applied between the electrodes, also cause tissue damage, which is now harnessed in our therapeutic use of X-rays. Rays of intense penetration are produced by using a linear accelerator at 4 to 6 million volts as the source of the electron beam (Fig. 5.11).

In 1896 Bequerel discovered by chance that photographic plates placed near a mineral called pitchblende, (from which uranium is obtained) become fogged; obviously this contained some 'radio-active' substance. Madame Marie Curie, a Polish scientist working in Paris, succeeded, 2 years later, in the difficult task of extracting a newly discovered element from pitchblende—she named this 'Radium'.

Radium and radioactive isotopes of other elements are unstable and break down with the liberation of radiant energy.

Fig. 5.11. The 4 million volt linear accelerator at Westminster hospital.

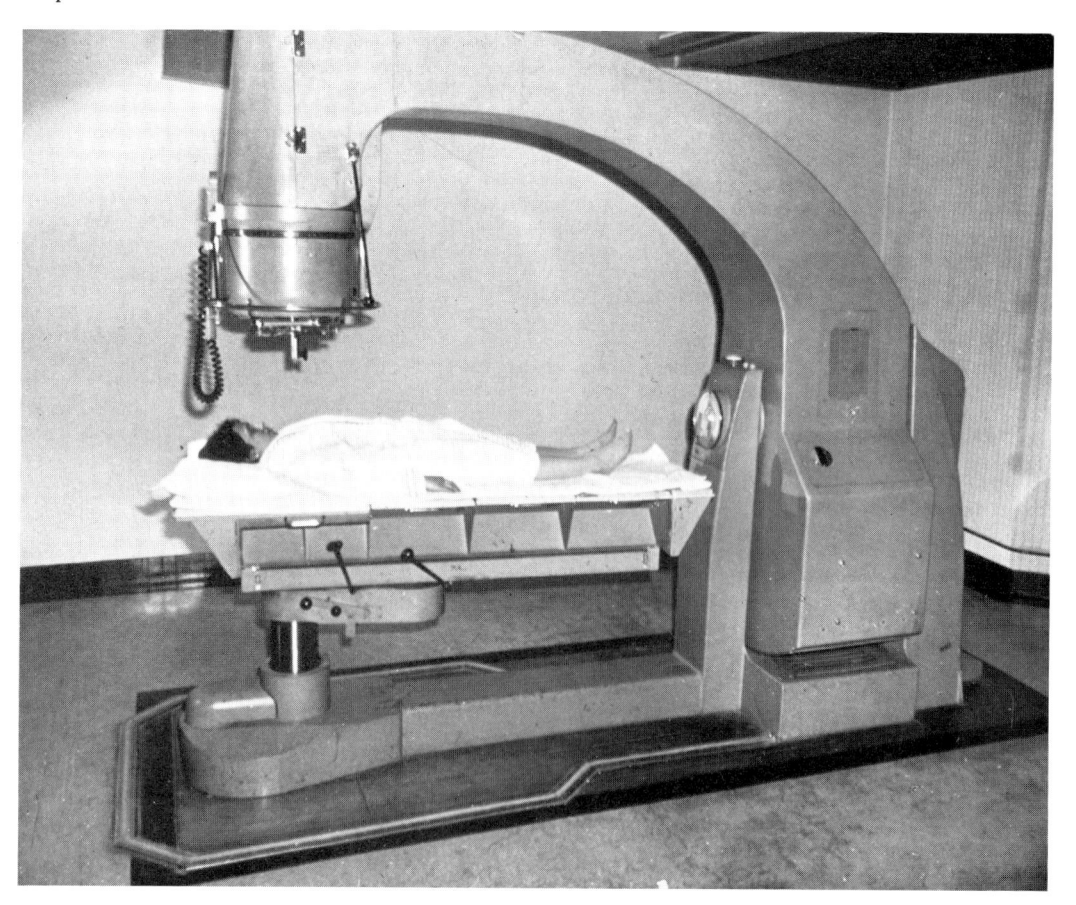

This radiation is made up of three components:
1. *Alpha particles*, which are positively charged helium nuclei. These move at high speed, but are large particles and are readily stopped, for example, by a sheet of paper.
2. *Beta Particles*, which are electrons travelling at nearly the speed of light. These can be absorbed by a thickness of lead of about 1 mm, by spectacles, or a 1 cm thick piece of perspex, and can penetrate the body tissues to a depth of about 1 cm.
3. *Gamma rays*, which are short wave length electro-magnetic waves and which can penetrate several centimetres of lead.

There is no practical difference between X-rays produced in high voltage X-ray machines and the gamma rays emitted by some radioactive elements such as Cobalt 60.

X-ray therapy is now usually employed at very high voltage and short wave lengths (mega voltage X-rays in a range of 2 or more million volts).

Radium is employed in the form of gold or platinum coated needles. The coating filters off the alpha and beta particles, allowing the gamma radiation to be used by implantation of the needles into the tissues (for example, tongue cancer) or else as an intra-cavitory application, for example in the treatment of carcinoma of the cervix or body of the uterus (Fig. 5.12).

Radioactive isotopes may occur naturally, for example isotopes of uranium, or they may be produced artificially by bombarding an element in a nuclear reactor. Radioactive isotopes may be employed in the form of a solution to be injected into the pleural or abdominal cavity to control malignant effusions (radioactive gold, which utilises beta ray emission, is used for this purpose) or as a radioactive implant directly into tissues (e.g. radioactive tantalum wire) or, perhaps most important of all, certain radio isotopes such as Cobalt 60 and Caesium 137 produce extremely powerful gamma radiation which can be used instead of megavoltage X-rays in external radiotherapy.

The effects of irradiation

Electro-magnetic radiation (X-rays and gamma rays) or particulate beams of alpha or beta rays produce their effect by causing ionisation in the living tissues through which they pass. Ionisation is the process in which atoms throw off negatively charged electrons which in turn bombard other atoms to produce more ionisation. Alpha rays, with their small penetration, can only be used in therapy if in direct contact with cancer cells as a surface application. Beta particles produce dense ionisation but only for up to 1 cm penetration into

Fig. 5.12. X-ray of patient who has radium needles implanted into a carcinoma of the tongue.

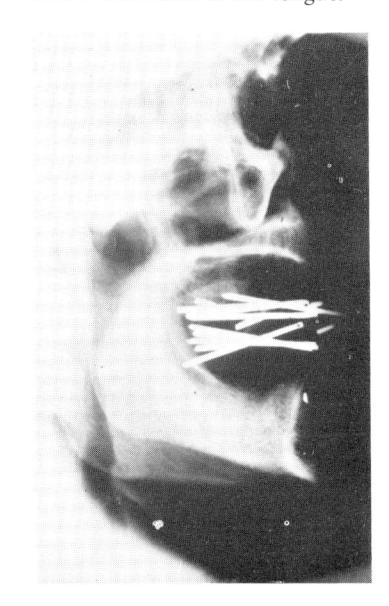

the tissues, whereas x-rays (particularly supervoltage) and gamma rays can penetrate deeply into the body.

When cells are irradiated, both the nucleus and cytoplasm are damaged so that the cells are killed. This rarely takes place immediately but the cells appear to die after one or more further divisions. Irradiation of sufficient dosage will destroy any tissue but its use in the treatment of cancer depends on the fact that cells are damaged differentially by the irradiation. Those cells which are rapidly growing tend to be far more sensitive than slowly growing cells. When we irradiate a rapidly growing malignant tumour we try to adjust the dosage so that the cancer cells are destroyed without too much damage to surrounding normal structures.

Complications of irradiation

Patients undergoing radiotherapy may develop a number of general and local side effects. The general complications include *radiation sickness*, in which the patient becomes nauseated or vomits, and complains of lassitude and anorexia. This syndrome is particularly liable to occur when large fields of radiation are used, for example, in the treatment of intra-abdominal or intra-thoracic disease. This phenomenon is seen at its worst in people who have been injured in nuclear explosions or accidents and who have therefore received whole-body irradiation. The most important general effect is damage to the bone marrow; there is a drop in the white cell count, affecting first the lymphocytes and then the polymorphs. The platelet count falls and the patient becomes anaemic. The depressed white cell count (which may fall below 2,000) is accompanied by a low resistance to infection and the fall in platelets produces a bleeding tendency, which may be associated with haemorrhages into the skin and other tissues. The white cell count is quite a sensitive guide to the tolerance of a patient undergoing large field irradiation and regular blood counts are therefore carried out in the radiotherapy department in patients undergoing extensive treatment.

The skin in the area irradiated usually becomes red (erythema) and, following high dose irradiation, often undergoes moist desquamation. This is followed by local pigmentation of the skin, atrophy, or the development of telangiectases. During treatment any irritation of the skin in the irradiated area must be carefully avoided and this includes exposure to sunlight, constricting clothing, soap and water and cosmetics.

Radiotherapy to the brain is followed by loss of scalp hair (depilation); it usually recovers in about 6 months.

The affected skin remains more sensitive than normal for many years; it may break down if subjected to subsequent trauma, producing an area of *irradiation necrosis* and it may not heal well after subsequent surgery. It is dangerous to give further irradiation to a previously treated area because of the risk of skin necrosis. Occasionally malignant change may occur in the skin long after exposure to heavy irradiation.

It should be noted that the problems of skin reaction, which were very serious in the days of conventional X-ray therapy, are less severe now that megavoltage therapy is used. This is because modern high voltage therapy and gamma treatment spare the skin and produce maximal effect in deeper tissues, so that the very badly affected skin that we used to see following irradiation is now seldom encountered.

Irradiation of deep structures may be followed by damage to adjacent tissues, so that, for example, pulmonary fibrosis can result from treatment of the lung and too high a dose of radiotherapy to the pelvis may cause stricture formation or fistula involving the intestine, bladder or ureter.

Modern, accurate supervoltage irradiation has the advantage of sparing skin and of not being differentially absorbed by bone. The cosmetic results of treatment are thus much improved and the morbidity of irradiation greatly reduced. It has become a particularly useful weapon in our armoury in the treatment of cancer.

CYTOTOXIC THERAPY

The word 'cytotoxic' means 'injurious to cells'. The dream of this type of therapy would be the discovery of some drug, completely innocuous to normal cells, which would, however, seek out the cancer cells in the body, enter into their metabolic process and destroy them. This would resemble, let us say, the injection of a dose of penicillin into a patient invaded by streptococci—the bacterial cells are destroyed but the patient's own tissues are unaffected. Unfortunately, at present, an ideal anti-cancer drug is still to be discovered. None of the vast number of substances at present available in the treatment of malignant disease is specifically toxic to tumour tissues, but every one of them attacks all rapidly dividing cells, whether malignant or normal. The latter include specially the bone marrow, the mucosa of the gastro-intestinal tract, the skin and fetal tissues. The inevitable damage to normal cells explains why the use of cytotoxic drugs is so dangerous and so replete with side effects and complications.

The cytotoxic drugs fall into four main groups:

1. Anti-metabolites.
2. Alkylating agents.
3. Antibiotics.
4. Miscellaneous.

1. *The anti-metabolites* resemble in chemical structure substances which are normally present in cells, or else they compete for metabolites required by the cells for their normal function. In this way essential chemical processes within the cell are disturbed, with lethal consequences. A good example of an anti-metabolite is *Methotrexate* which resembles folic acid, which itself is essential for the enzyme system used in the synthesis of DNA and therefore of cell reproduction. *5-Fluorouracil* is a pyrimidine antagonist and *6-Mercaptopurine* is a purine antagonist; both these substances block the synthesis of nucleic acid by substituting themselves for essential chemicals in its manufacture.

2. *Alkylating agents* are compounds which are capable of replacing a hydrogen atom in another molecule with an alkyl radical. They alter the essential components of cells (nucleic acids, proteins, cellular enzymes), leading to cell death. These drugs include *Nitrogen Mustard*, *Chlorambucil*, *Cyclophosphamide*, *Melphalan* and *Thiotepa*.

3. *Antibiotics.* As part of the search for antibacterial substances produced by bacteria and fungi, a group of substances have been discovered which have anti-tumour activity. These include *Actinomycin D* and *Mithramycin*.

4. *The miscellaneous group* include alkaloids extracted from the periwinkle (*Vinca rosea*) which are termed *Vinblastine* and *Vincristine*. These block mitoses in dividing cells. Other drugs in this ever-enlarging group include *Urethane*, and derivatives of *Colchicine*.

Modes of administration

At present the clinician chooses a cytotoxic drug for a particular case out of this bewildering variety of available substances in a rather arbitrary manner based on previous clinical experience. For example, 5-Fluorouracil seems to be the most useful drug in the treatment of advanced cancer of the large bowel. It may be that in future we shall be able to grow a portion of the particular tumour under treatment in tissue culture and test it against a variety of cytotoxic drugs to see which ones are especially effective against it, just as now the bacteriologist tests organisms in culture for their sensitivity of resistance to a variety of antibiotic agents. In some cases several cytotoxic drugs are used in combination in order to attack the cancer cells from different metabolic aspects. For example, in quadruple therapy, cyclophosphamide, methotrexate, vincristine and 5-Fluorouracil are used sequentially.

Most drugs can be given orally, although some, such as 5-Fluorouracil, must be given by intravenous injection. Cytotoxic drugs may also be instilled into the pleural or peritoneal cavities in treatment of malignant effusions at these sites. Tumours confined to a limb or to the head and neck may be treated on occasion by perfusion via the feeding artery in order to provide a high local dosage in the tumour area and less effect on normal structures elsewhere.

Indications for use

Cytotoxic drugs are of particular value in the reticuloses—Hodgkin's disease, leukaemia, and disseminated lymphosarcoma. Two solid tumours, chorioncarcinoma of the uterine cavity and Burkitt's lymphoma, a tumour seen particularly in African children, are particularly sensitive to cytotoxic therapy and long term cures have now been reported. For solid, disseminated tumours results are far less good so that cytotoxics are usually only employed when other methods have failed, but remissions of many months, or occasionally, even years, may sometimes be obtained.

Side effects

These are very similar to those mentioned under the general effects of radiotherapy, and, indeed they result in the main from the same underlying cause—damage to cells in those normal tissues which are undergoing rapid cellular division. The most important in this respect is the bone marrow; an early sign of toxicity from any of the cytotoxic drugs is a fall in the white cell count and in the blood platelets. If the total white count drops below 3000, drug treatment must be stopped at once. Other toxic effects are nausea and vomiting, oral and intestinal ulceration due to damage to the mucosa of the alimentary canal, secondary monilial (thrush) infection of the mouth and gut, loss of hair, skin rashes, and haemorrhages into the skin and other tissues, the last resulting from depletion of the blood platelets.

Chapter 6. Chest and Lungs

ANATOMY

The chest wall is composed of 12 ribs on either side that articulate posteriorly with the transverse processes and the bodies of the vertebrae. The upper 7 are joined anteriorly to the sternum by cartilaginous joints; 8, 9 and 10 articulate with the cartilage of the rib above and 11 and 12 are free anteriorly, ending in the layers of the abdominal muscles. The ribs are joined together by the intercostal muscles (Fig. 6.1).

Nerves and vessels run beneath each rib from the spinal cord, aorta, azygos and hemi-azygos veins respectively to supply the muscles and the overlying skin. The chest is separated from the abdominal cavity by a muscular and tendinous sheet, the diaphragm. This arrangement permits the cavity of the chest to expand and contract, altering its volume by as much as 2 litres in an adult male.

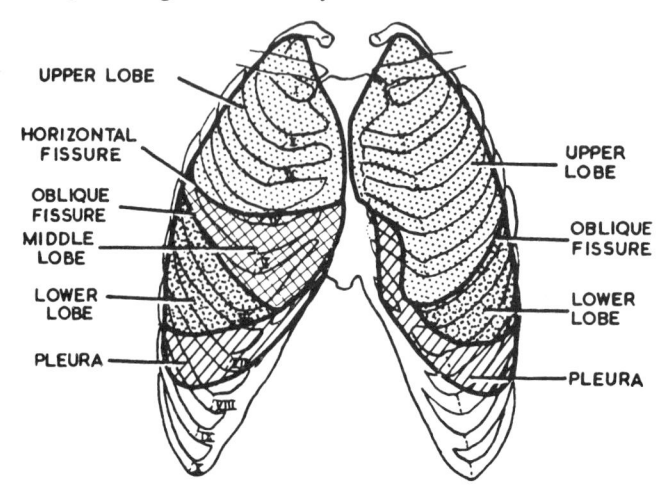

Fig. 6.1. The chest wall, lungs and pleura.

The right ventricle of the heart pumps blood into the lungs. The lungs are elastic structures which allow intimate contact between the oxygen in the inspired air and blood, separated by only one cell. If a lung is removed from the body it will contract down to a small ball of tissue, but it is kept in an expanded state in the thorax by the integrity of the chest wall. The chest is lined by a thin, smooth and shining membrane, which is termed the *parietal pleura*. The *visceral pleura* covers the lungs and the mediastinum in an exactly anagalous way to the peritoneum in the abdomen. Thus, during respiration, expansion and contraction of the lungs within the chest is possible without friction.

Air is drawn into the lungs via the pharynx, trachea and left and right main bronchus which then divide into bronchi (Fig. 6.2) which supply the lobes of the lungs (3 on the right and 2 plus the lingula on the left). Each lobe of the lung is further subdivided into segments.

The heart, great vessels (that is aorta and venae cavae) and the root of the lungs occupy a central position in the chest termed the *mediastinum*.

PHYSIOLOGY

Respiration, that is the process whereby blood is oxygenated, requires:
1. Normal inspired air.
2. A clear airway.

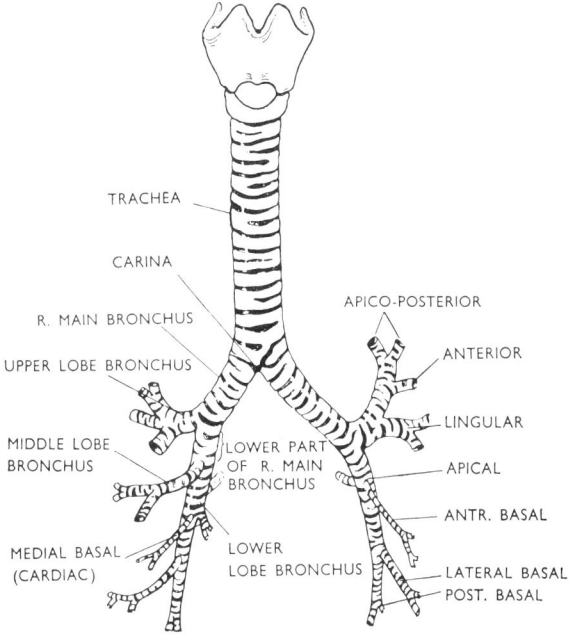

Fig. 6.2. The trachea and main bronchi.

3. Efficient neuromuscular co-ordination to move the chest.
4. An intact chest cavity.

In addition to oxygenation, the lungs are one of the routes for the clearance of carbon dioxide as gas, water as vapour (a mechanism whereby the body is cooled and the most important in the dog) and certain volatile compounds and drugs, for example alcohol and Fluothane.

The nervous control of respiration is a complex function which can be interfered with by certain drugs and by alteration in consciousness. For example, deep surgical anaesthesia depresses respiration to the point at which it will completely cease and an overdose of barbiturate kills the suicide by depressing respiration to the level at which insufficient oxygen and carbon dioxide exchange occurs. On these occasions it is possible to pass a tube through the larynx into the trachea (an endotracheal tube) and inflate the lungs rhythmically with oxygen. This process is called intermittent positive pressure respiration (IPPR). This can be carried on indefinitely mechanically using a ventilator until such time as normal respiratory control is established; the endotracheal tube can then be removed.

FRACTURED RIBS

Normal ribs may be fractured by direct external violence, for example, when the chest strikes the steering wheel in a road accident. They may also be fractured by excessively severe coughing. Ribs that are diseased by, for example, osteomalacia or by malignant deposits may be fractured by slight coughing or moderate external trauma.

The symptoms associated with a rib fracture are pain, which is aggravated by breathing, and coughing and which is localised to the area of the fracture. Compression of the chest wall by the hand will cause intense pain. If a number of ribs are fractured on one side the pain may be so intense as to prevent the patient being able to draw in breath and he may thereby become cyanosed.

STABLE FRACTURES

Treatment

If only one or two ribs are fractured and respiration is satisfactory this is known as a stable fracture and the only treatment required is a suitable analgesic. Strapping of the chest with adhesive plaster is usually not effective and if too efficiently applied will so reduce respiratory movement as to compromise bronchial clearing and may precipitate pneumonia. The ribs are splinted one by the other and will heal quite rapidly if left alone.

Some patients may suffer fracture of the ribs and have some underlying lung disease, such as occurs in chronic smokers. In this case, it is important to establish normal respiratory and coughing movements rapidly. It is possible to achieve complete analgesia by the use of an epidural local anaesthetic; a small catheter is introduced to the side of the spinal dura mater and local anaesthetic can be injected around the posterior nerve roots as they emerge to pass around the chest. This extremely effective and elegant technique is often successful in allowing the patient to be managed without IPPR in a borderline case.

UNSTABLE FRACTURES

If ribs are fractured on both sides of the chest or at both their extremities it is possible for there to be a loose segment of chest wall. This results in a condition known as *'flail chest'*. In this case when the chest expands the flail segment instead of moving out is drawn in. Air is not sucked into the trachea and respiration is thereby interfered with (Fig. 6.3).

Treatment

In this case the patient will require endotracheal intubation with IPPR together with full doses of analgesic, for example morphia 15 mg or pethidine 100 mg and basal narcosis to reduce awareness using such drugs as diazepam to permit tolerance of the tube in the conscious state. After 48 to 72 hours the chest usually stabilizes by clot and fibrin sufficient for the patient to be 'weaned off' the ventilator.

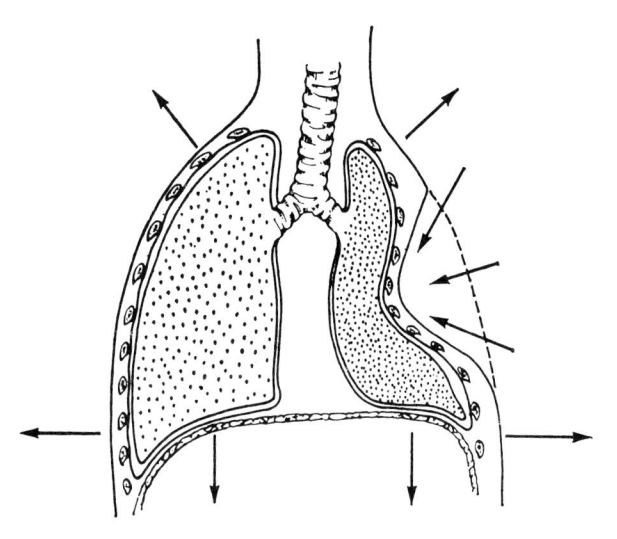

Fig. 6.3. Flail chest. On inspiration the detached segment of the chest wall is sucked inwards, producing paradoxical movement

PNEUMOTHORAX

Pneumothorax is the condition that occurs when air is introduced between the layers of visceral and parietal pleura—the lung on that side then collapses and is not aerated by the respiratory movements. There are a number of causes:

1. By a leak from the lung tissue via the bronchus (bronchopleural fistula). This is a common cause and results when a lung cyst or bulla ruptures. It occurs in young people for no known reason (Fig. 6.4).

Occasionally the leak is associated with a flap of pleura which forms a valve which permits air to enter the pleural space without being able to return to the bronchus. This results in a *tension pneumothorax*. The particular danger of this condition is that the mediastinum is pushed across to the other side of the chest with compression of the other lung. Unless the air is allowed to escape from the pleural cavity, the patient will asphyxiate (Fig. 6.5).

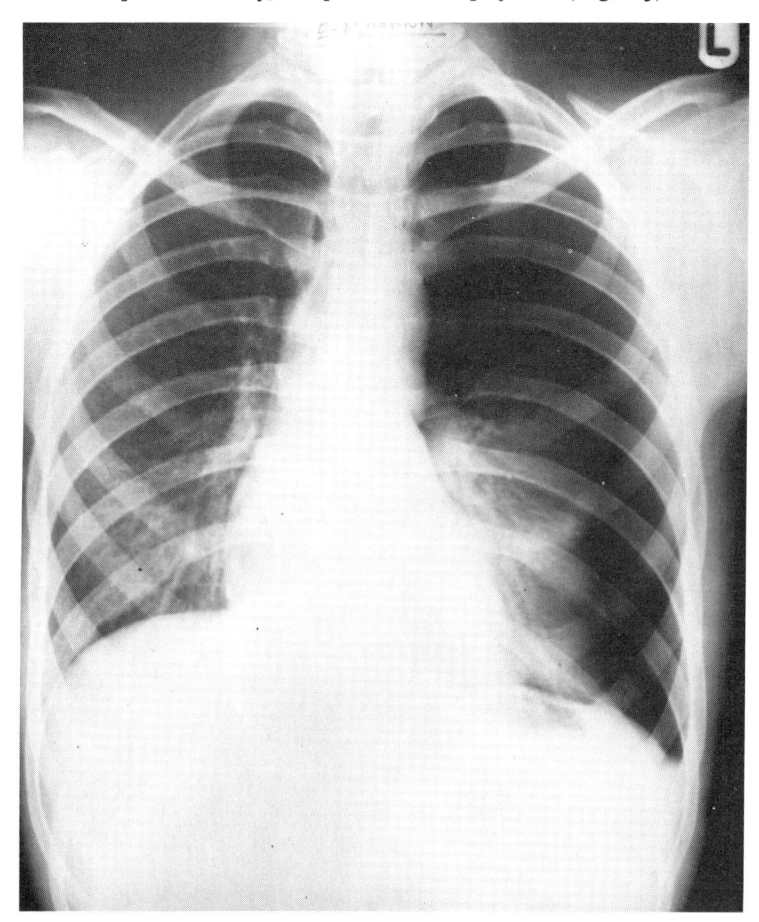

Fig. 6.4. Chest X-ray showing a left-sided pneumothorax.

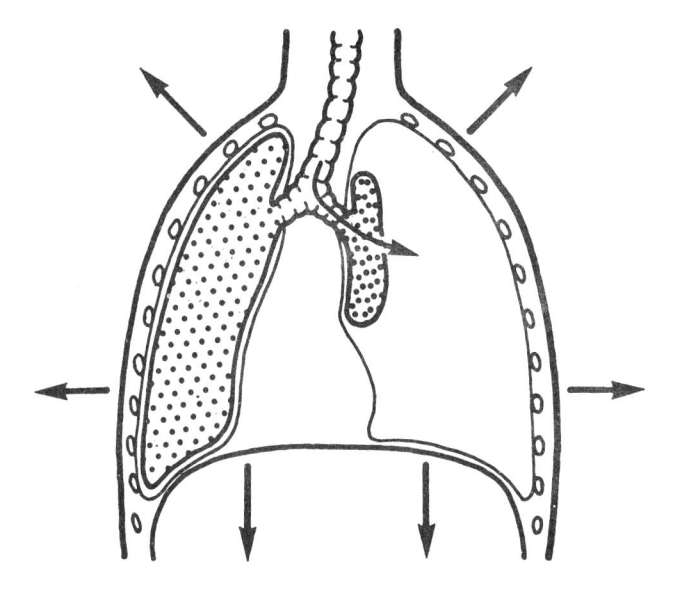

Fig. 6.5. Tension pneumothorax produced by a valvular tear in the lung. Air is sucked into the pleural cavity on inspiration and cannot excape on expiration.

2. By rupture of the bronchus in an accident. This is rare.
3. By an external puncture of the chest wall such as might occur in a stab wound. If the hole in the chest wall is large, air is sucked in and out of the pleural cavity with the movements of respiration. This is known as a *'sucking pneumothorax'*. The puncture may also rupture the lung with a further leak of air.
4. In error when a pleural effusion is tapped. In this case a quantity of air may be allowed to enter the chest.
5. Post-operatively. When operations on the chest wall or the underlying lung are carried out inevitably air enters the pleural cavity and has to be expelled at the completion of the operation.

The diagnosis of pneumothorax is confirmed by chest X-ray.

Treatment

If the pneumothorax is small and the chest wall is intact, the lung can usually be relied on to seal itself and the air will absorb spontaneously from the pleural cavity. No active treatment is required therefore, other than regular surveillance by chest X-ray to confirm that re-expansion of the lung is occurring. If on the other hand there is a persistent bronchopleural fistula or if the chest wall is punctured, then drainage of the pleural cavity via an underwater drain is required. If in spite of this the lung does not re-expand, a pump will have to be applied to the system to draw the air out. Occasionally when the hole joining the pleural cavity to the bronchus is large, **operative** closure is required.

It is a matter of life and death to treat a tension pneumothorax rapidly. All that is required is for a large bore needle to be plunged into the chest wall through an intercostal space. Following this emergency measure drainage of the pleural cavity via an underwater drain will usually result in cure of the condition (Fig. 6.6).

Haemothorax

This is a collection of blood in the pleural cavity. It is usually the result of trauma or it may occur post-operatively. If the bleeding is only of moderate severity, the treatment is aspiration of the effusion, blood replacement and observation; if the bleeding is severe operative treatment is required to control the source of the haemorrhage.

Hydropneumothorax

This is the condition that obtains when there is both liquid and air within the pleural cavity. Diagnosis is confirmed by chest x-ray and treatment follows the same general lines as for haemothorax.

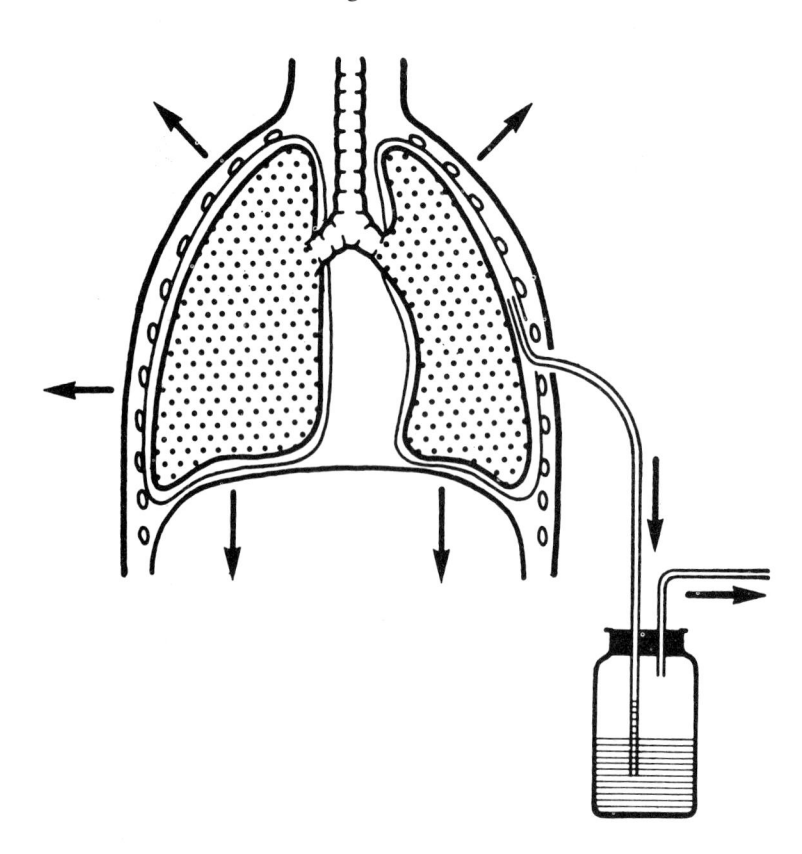

Fig. 6.6. Underwater seal chest drain in the treatment of a pneumothorax. Air escapes from the pleural cavity on expiration but cannot be sucked back through the water seal on inspiration.

LUNG INFECTIONS

Post-operative pneumonia—see p. 28.

LUNG ABSCESS

This is usually due to one of a variety of causes:
1. Inhaled foreign body, for example a peanut.
2. Infected pulmonary embolus.
3. Failure of pneumonia to resolve.
4. Distal to an obstructing carcinoma of the bronchus.
5. As part of a staphylococcal or other septicaemia.

Clinical features

The symptomatology is that of an abscess anywhere, that is a raised white cell count, swinging pyrexia, plus local pain in the chest if the parietal pleura is involved and cough if the abscess communicates with the bronchus. Diagnosis is confirmed by chest X-ray, with tomography if required (Fig. 6.7).

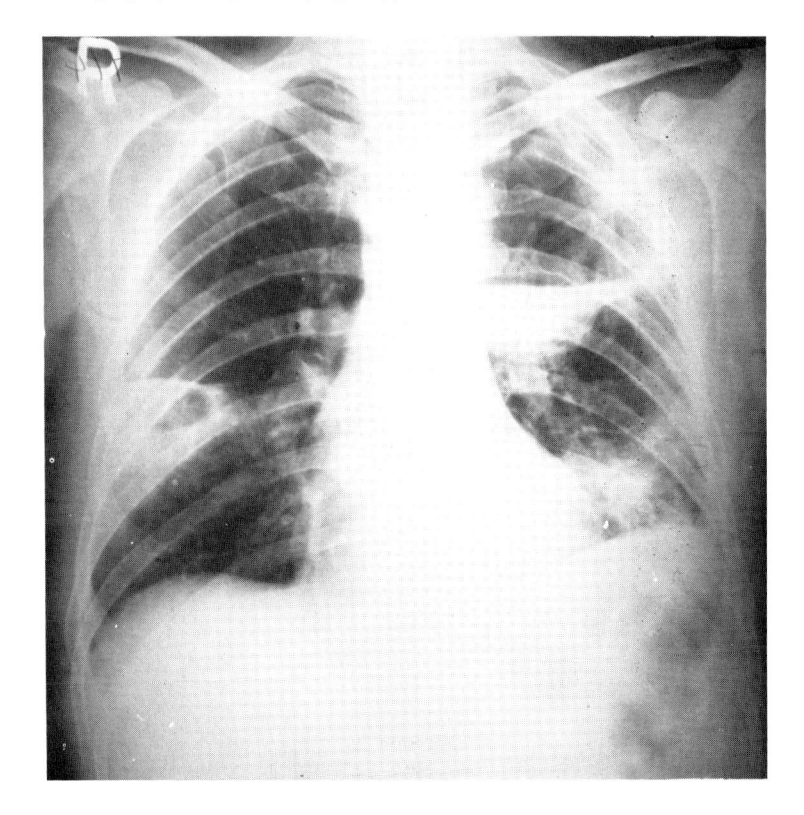

Fig. 6.7. Chest X-ray of a patient with bilateral lung abscesses. Note that each has a fluid level at the interface between air and pus in the abscess cavity.

Treatment

The majority of abscesses point into the bronchus and drain that way. The patient experiences a rush of offensive material which is expelled by expectoration and soon feels better. In this case all that is required is for the pus to be cultured for micro-organisms and their sensitivities determined. The patient is then tipped by the physiotherapist so as to encourage drainage via the bronchus. Antibiotics are usually unnecessary. The underlying condition that caused the abscess in the first place must be treated; e.g. if a foreign body is present it must be removed.

An important complication of a lung abscess is rupture into the pleural cavity and production of an empyema which is a collection of pus in this space. It will then require external drainage.

PULMONARY TUBERCULOSIS

A few years ago most people in this country contracted a primary tuberculous pulmonary infection. This was usually overcome by the defences of the body and left no more than a slight trace at the apex of one or other lung visible on X-ray. Nowadays with control of the infection in the population and in the milk supplies, this primary infection is not so common.

If a virulent mycobacterium infects a person who has no previous experience of the disease, a generalised pulmonary infection may result. The chest X-ray in this case shows the lung fields to be covered by a multitude of small white spots (Fig. 6.8). This condition of miliary tuberculosis, if left untreated, is rapidly fatal after a short period of a wasting disease which lasts for a few days or a few weeks at the most. If treatment is adequate with antituberculous therapy there is a high chance that cure will result.

Usually, however, the infection will become localised to one lobe or segment of a lobe. In this case the lung tissue breaks down and a cavity is formed (Fig. 6.9). The cavity usually drains via the bronchus and results in copious expectoration of sputum. It is very common for such patients to cough up blood, which is bright red and frothy.

Treatment

This is similar in principle to that of any infection but is complicated by the fact that the mycobacterium of tuberculosis takes approximately 6 weeks to culture.

After sputum has been sent for culture the patient is given 'rotating' therapy with streptomycin 1.0 gm daily INAH 100 mgm three times per day and PAS. Nowadays there is a tendency in this

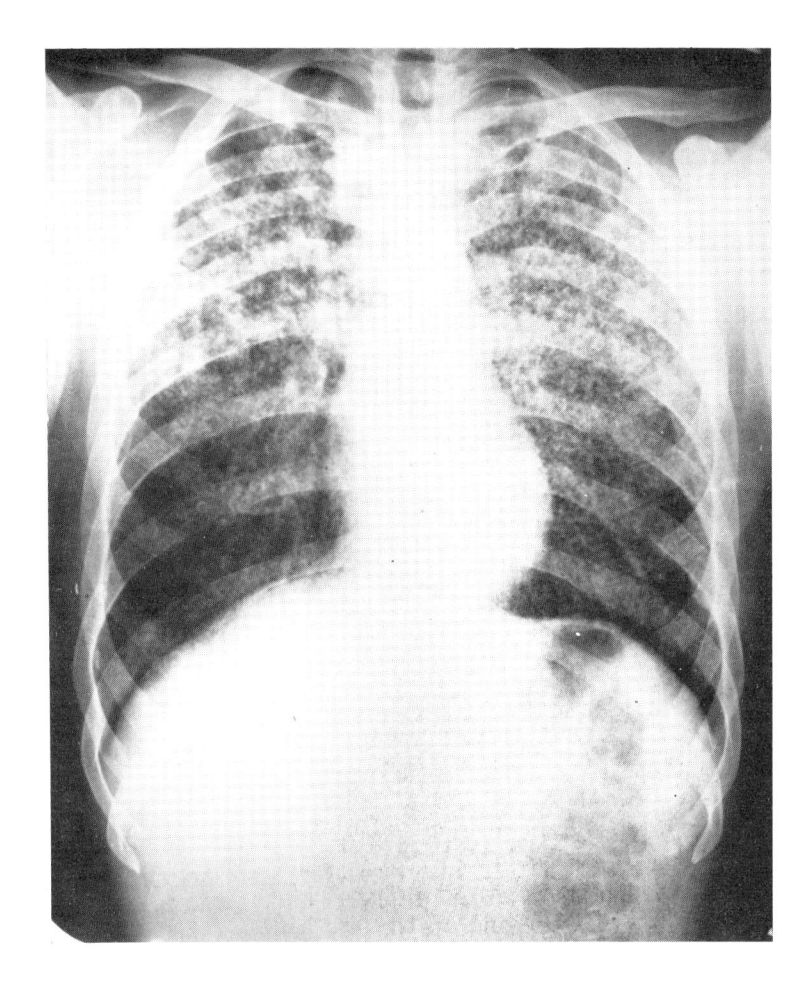

Fig. 6.8. Chest X-ray of a patient with miliary tuberculosis. Note the myriad of small white deposits throughout the lung fields.

country for PAS to be replaced by rifampicin but this has the disadvantage of being more expensive. Six weeks from the onset of treatment the sensitivities of the infecting mycobacterium are known in some cases and therapy can be gauged accordingly. It is unusual to continue with streptomycin for more than six to twelve weeks, rifampicin and INAH being continued for a total period of 2 years. The exact length of treatment is a subject of several trials at the present moment but it is hoped that with the greater use of rifampicin the total length required will be reduced.

If pulmonary tuberculosis is treated prior to the development of cavitation complete resolution of the disease can be expected. If cavitation has occurred then there will be residual damage to the lung tissue. If this is slight no harm will result but if it is gross then there will be some danger of a lingering infection which could be re-

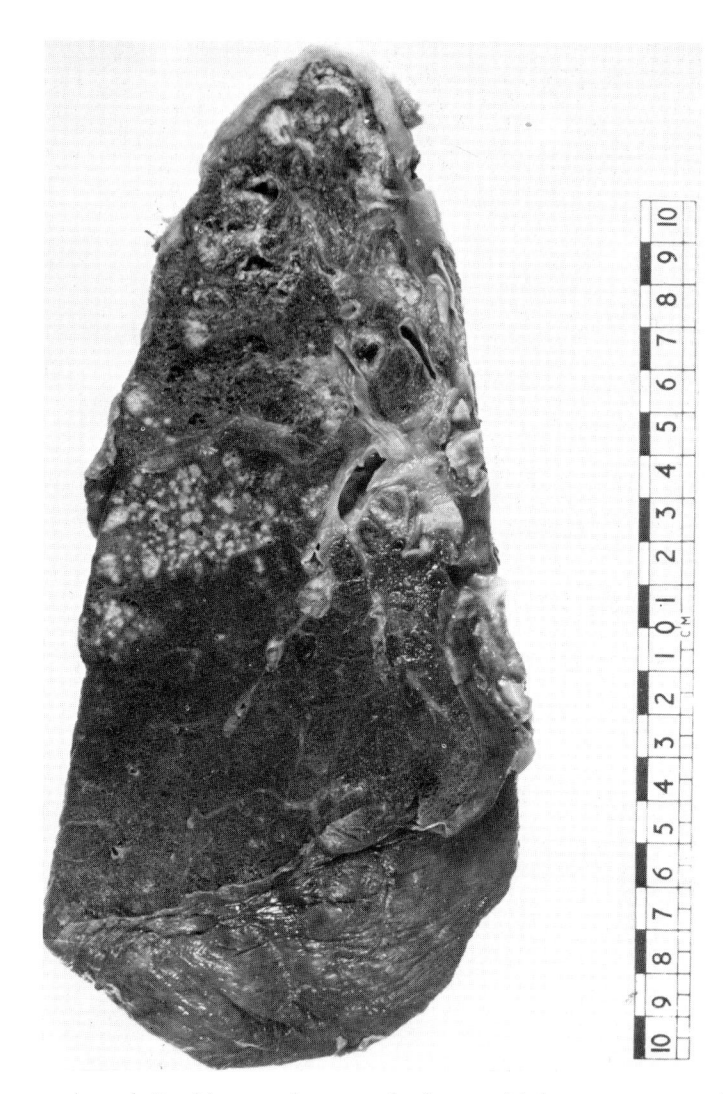

Fig. 6.9. Severe tuberculosis of the upper lobe of the lung (post-mortem specimen).

activated. In this case the severely damaged lobe or segments of the lung are removed, (lobectomy or segmental lobectomy).

BRONCHIECTASIS

This is a condition associated with areas of dilatation of the bronchi and may follow such disease as whooping cough. It gives rise to the production of large quantities of infected sputum and results in a progressive destruction of lung tissue due to the effects of infection which is never completely eradicated. It is also a common cause of haemoptysis.

The most satisfactory method to confirm the diagnosis is by performing a bronchogram (Fig. 6.10).

Treatment

If the disease is localised to one lobe only of the lung and if it is severe then surgical excision by lobectomy is indicated. The majority of cases however are managed perfectly satisfactorily by postural drainage together with the use of an appropriate antibiotic to cover a phase of significant infection.

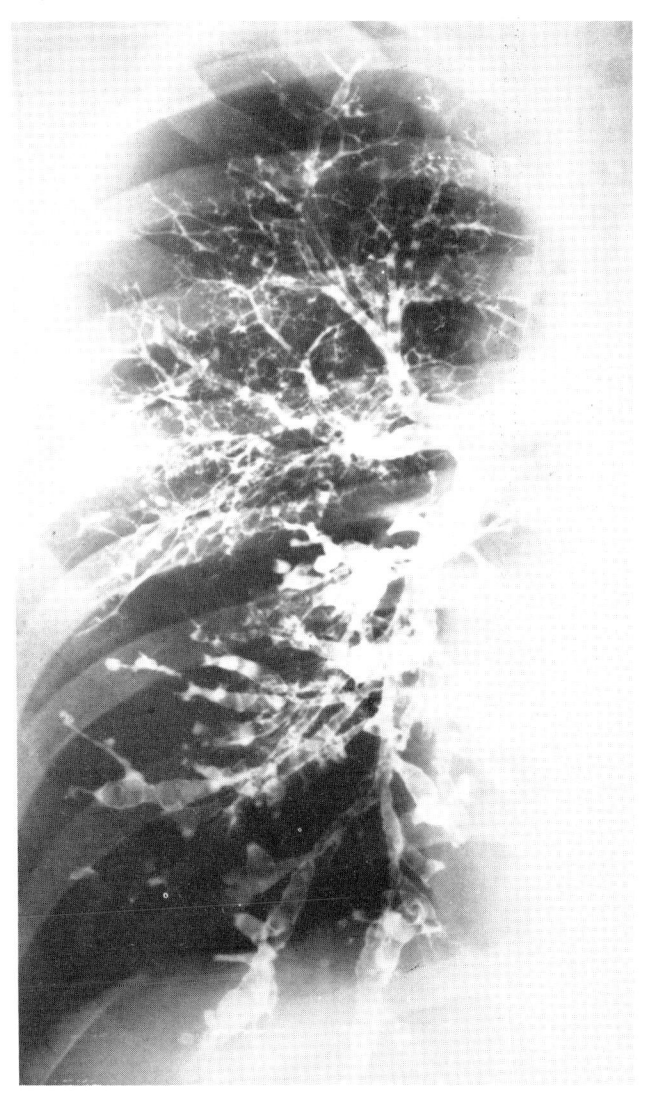

Fig. 6.10. A bronchogram of the right lung. This patient has a moderate degree of bronchiectasis of the right lower lobe.

EMPYEMA

This term means that there is a collection of pus within the pleural cavity. It may be caused in a number of ways:
1. Extension of infection from the lung.
2. By extension of infection from beneath the diaphragm, for example from a subphrenic abscess.
3. By penetrating injuries of the chest wall.
4. Following operations which involve the chest wall.
5. Spread of infection from the mediastinum, for example following rupture of the oesophagus.
6. By blood stream spread.

Clinical features

The patient with an empyema is usually ill with a raised temperature and gives a history consistent with the cause of the empyema. There is usually pain on the affected side of the chest which is aggravated by breathing. The white cell count is raised. Diagnosis is confirmed by chest X-ray which will indicate an effusion within the pleural cavity (Fig. 6.11).

Treatment

The treatment is similar to that for a collection of pus anywhere in the body, that is, the pus has to be drained. A needle is inserted into the chest under local anaesthetic and the fluid in the pleural cavity is removed. Some of this fluid is sent to the laboratory for culture so that the causative organism can be identified and its sensitivity to antibiotics established. One million units of soluble penicillin are inserted in the pleural cavity through the needle before it is withdrawn. Aspiration is continued on a daily basis so long as it is possible to evacuate completely the pleural cavity. If the pus becomes too thick to aspirate it will then become necessary to insert a drain and this is done by resecting a small portion of rib. The tube that is inserted need not be connected to an underwater drain because the visceral pleura is stuck to the parietal pleura in the region of the empyema, making pulmonary collapse impossible. Thereafter the tube is dressed each day in the usual way. So as to check that the cavity is becoming obliterated, a sinogram is performed at approximately 2 weekly intervals.

Sometimes, particularly in the case of tuberculosis, the visceral pleura becomes covered with a thick layer of fibrin. Normal function will never be established in this case and it is necessary to peel this layer off at operation, a procedure known as *decortication*.

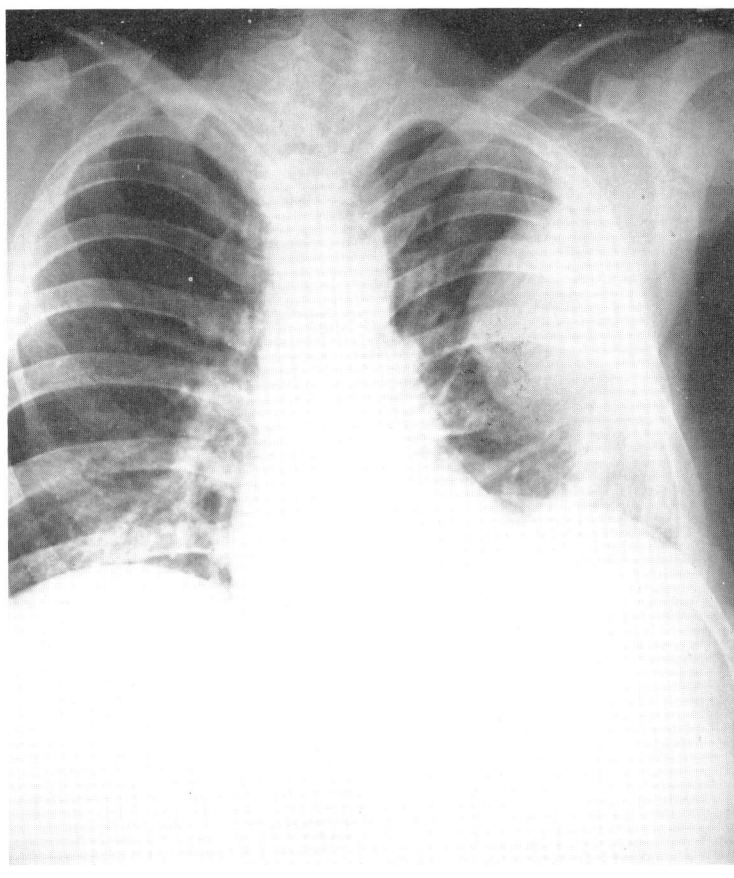

Fig. 6.11. Chest X-ray of a patient with an empyema. Note the opaque effusion in the left pleural cavity.

NEOPLASMS OF THE LUNG AND BRONCHI

These may be either benign or malignant, and the malignant neoplasms may be either primary or secondary. By far the most important group of neoplasms are the primary malignant carcinomas of the bronchus.

Benign lung neoplasms

These are rare and include adenomas of the bronchus, carcinoid tumours, which may produce the hormone 5 hydroxytryptamine, which results in attacks of flushing and diarrhoea.

CARCINOMA OF THE BRONCHUS

Pathology

This is the commonest primary malignant tumour in males in this country and results in 27,000 deaths in England and Wales per year. There is now no doubt that one of the factors involved in its causation is the smoking of cigarettes. The fact that the incidence continues to rise may also be a reflection on atmospheric pollution by industry. It is a condition that is more common in men than women, although the incidence in women is rising and it is suggested that this is due to the increasing number of women who smoke.

In approximately half of those affected the tumour arises in one or other of the main bronchi and in the other cases it arises peripherally. The tumour spreads by infiltration and to the regional lymph nodes at the hilum of the lung as well as disseminating widely in the bloodstream. If the tumour is situated in a main bronchus it can enlarge and eventually block the bronchus with subsequent collapse of the lung distal to the obstruction (Fig. 6.12).

Clinical features

If the tumour ulcerates it very commonly bleeds and this gives rise to one of the most common presenting symptoms, namely, haemoptysis. Other presenting features include cough, shortness of breath,

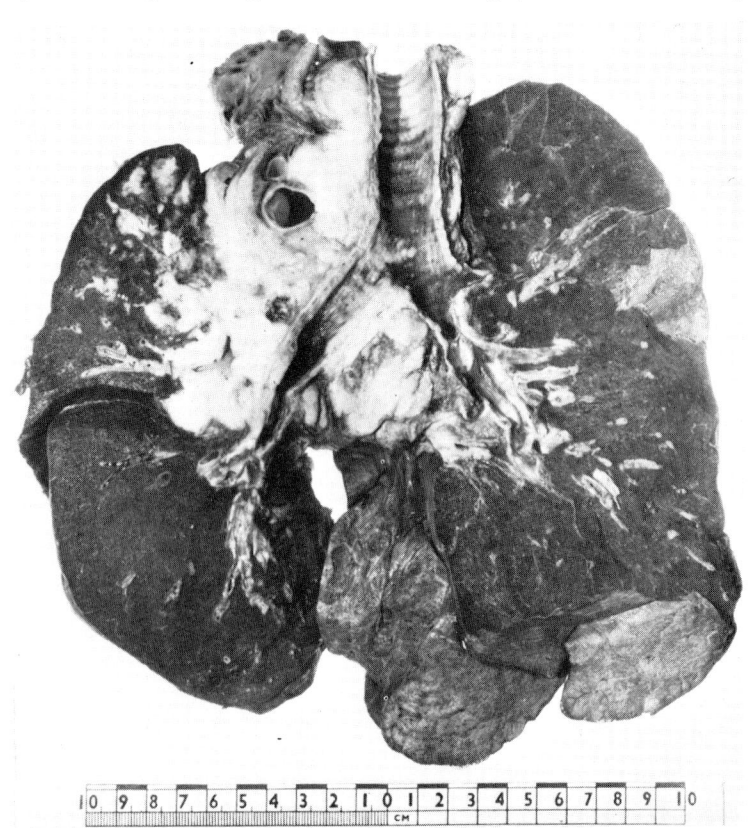

Fig. 6.12. Specimen of lung showing an extensive carcinoma. The patient was a heavy cigarette smoker.

lung abscess or secondary deposits in distant tissues, for example, the liver which may become enlarged, bones producing pathological fractures, enlarged lymph nodes in the neck, and cerebral metastases with psychiatric presentation. Patients with bronchial carcinoma which has metastasised lose weight and appear to be ill. Some patients may have a silent carcinoma which is only discovered on chest X-ray either of the mass miniature type or being carried out for some other purpose. (See also page 57).

Special investigations

Diagnosis is confirmed by chest X-ray, which often shows a shadow in the lung (Fig. 6.13) but absolute confirmation of diagnosis is only obtained by bronchoscopy and biopsy of the tumour.

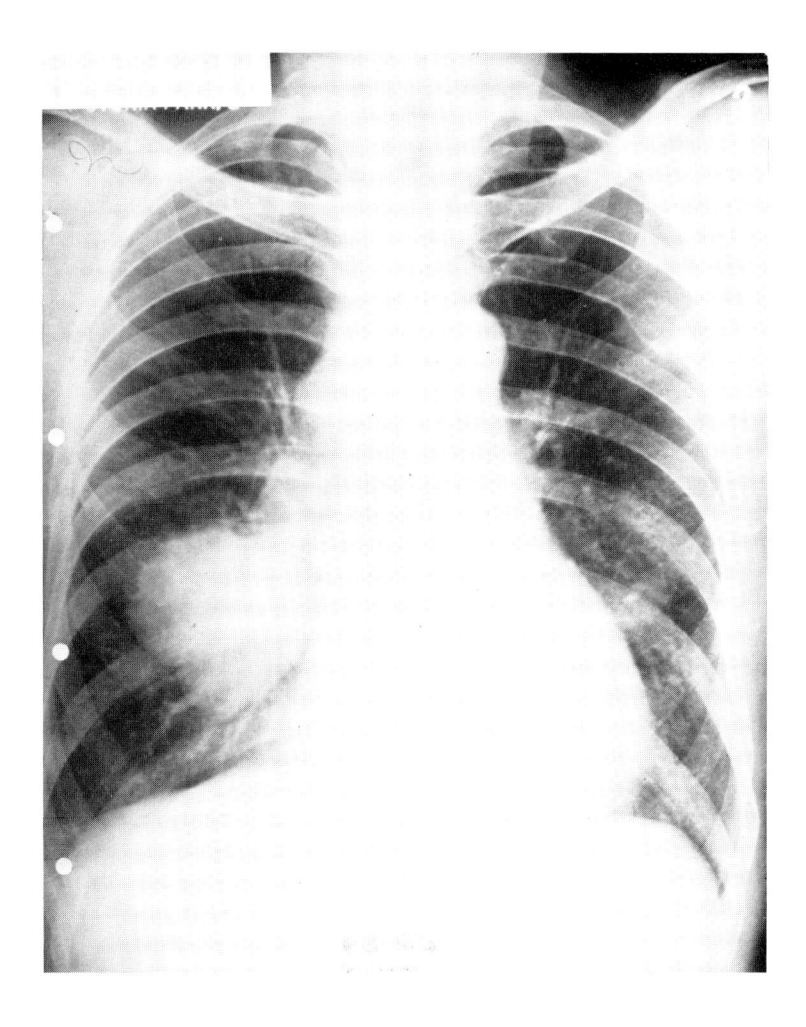

Fig. 6.13. Chest X-ray showing an extensive carcinoma of the right lung.

Treatment

Unfortunately carcinoma of the lung is often one of the most malignant tumours and by the time diagnosis is made in the majority of patients the disease has spread beyond the local confines of the primary tumour. As soon as distant spread occurs surgical excision is no longer possible. Nevertheless the ideal method of treatment in a suitable case is surgical excision of the primary tumour together with the lobe or lobes of the lung which are involved; this is only possible in 1 in 20 of the patients who present with the disease. Of these patients operated on, only 1 in 5 can expect to be alive and free of disease 5 years later.

In the inoperable case radiotherapy is of some help in controlling the local spread of the tumour and in providing palliation for painful secondary deposits, for example, those which occur in bones. Chemotherapy is now being used more often and in some cases produces a good response.

Secondary neoplasms of the lung

These are particularly common from non-epithelial tumours, for example, osteogenic sarcoma of bone and melanoma. Deposits also occur however from other carcinomas of, for example, breast or kidney.

Chapter 7. Heart and great vessels

ANATOMY

The heart is a remarkably effective pump which functions day and night and without attention for 70 or more years, altering its rate and output to the body's requirements. It is made up of striated but involuntary muscle fibres. Essentially it is in two halves, one to deliver oxygenated blood at high pressure to the systemic circulation, and the other to perfuse the deoxygenated blood at low pressure through the lungs.

The heart is irregularly conical in shape (Fig. 7.1) and is placed obliquely in the mediastinum. It is invested in the tough fibrous pericardium and possesses four chambers and four valves. *The right atrium* (Fig. 7.2) receives deoxygenated venous blood from the superior and inferior venae cavae as well as the coronary sinus, which drains the heat muscle itself. It communicates with the *right ventricle* through the tricuspid valve, while the right ventricle empties into the pulmonary trunk guarded by the pulmonary valve. *The left atrium* has the four pulmonary veins opening into it, and communicates with the *left ventricle* via the mitral valve. The left ventricle opens into the aorta, the orifice being guarded by the three semi-lunar cusps of the aortic valve. The openings of the right and left coronary arteries, which supply arterial blood to the heart wall, open immediately above the aortic valve.

The atria are thin walled in contrast to the thick ventricles. The inner aspect of both the ventricles is marked by the presence of a number of irregular muscular elevations (trabeculae carneae) from some of which the papillary muscles project into the lumen of the ventricle and find attachment to the free borders of the cusps of both

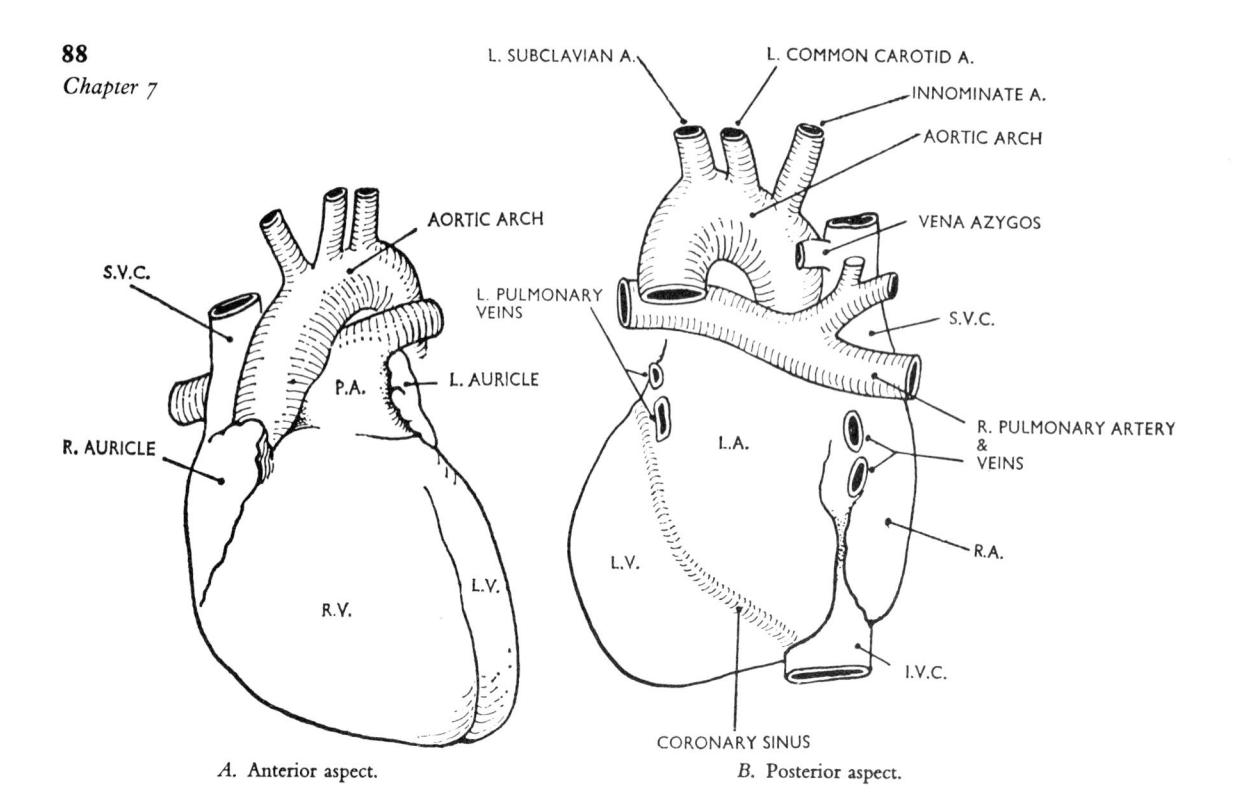

Fig. 7.1. The heart and great vessels.

A. Anterior aspect.

B. Posterior aspect.

the tricuspid valve (on the right) and mitral valve (on the left) by means of the chordae tendineae (Fig. 7.3).

The atria are separated from each other by the interatrial septum which contains an oval depression termed the *fossa ovalis*. This represents the foramen ovale of fetal life since, in the embryo, much of the blood returning from the umbilical veins along the inferior vena cava is shunted through this directly into the left side of the heart and hence into the systemic blood vessels, rather than perfusing through the non-functional lungs.

The interventricular septum, which divides the two ventricles, is muscular in its lower part and its upper portion is fibrous. Septal defects are a relatively common congenital abnormality and are specially likely to occur in the region of the fossa ovalis and in the membranous upper portion of the interventricular septum.

PRINCIPLES OF CARDIAC SURGERY

Much of surgery comprises the closing of defects and the relieving of obstructions. It is now possible to carry out these procedures on the heart and great vessels. Operations on the pericardium, the main

89
Heart and great vessels

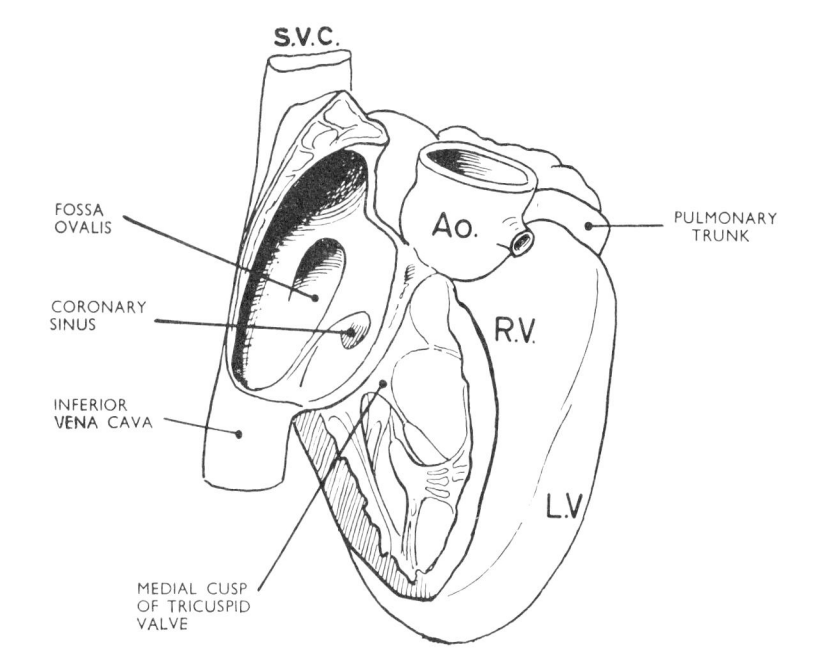

Fig. 7.2. The interior of the right atrium and ventricle

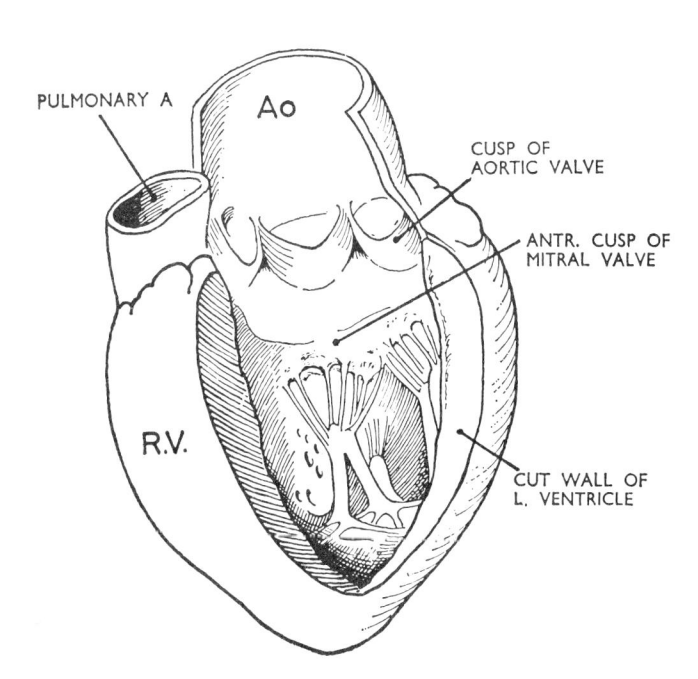

Fig. 7.3. The interior of the left ventricle.

vessels emerging from the heart, and some relatively simple cardiac procedures, such as splitting of the mitral valve for stenosis, can be performed without interruption of the circulation. However, major cardiac surgery can only be carried out in a relatively bloodless field produced by temporary cardiac arrest.

There are two main techniques at present employed, hypothermia and cardio-pulmonary bypass.

Hypothermia

If the circulation is stopped at normal body temperature the brain undergoes irreversible changes after 3 minutes. The liver, heart muscle and kidneys are also extremely susceptible to ischaemia, but may tolerate between 30–60 minutes of cardiac arrest. Hypothermia reduces the metabolic requirements of the tissue and thus allows prolongation of the period of permissible circulatory arrest. At 28°C up to 10 minutes of arrest can be tolerated, whereas in deep hypothermia (10°C or lower) arrest can be carried out for periods of up to one hour. Conventional hypothermia is produced by surface cooling of the body whereas profound hypothermia requires the circulation of blood through a heat exchanger.

Cardio-pulmonary bypass

In this technique the heart-lung machine takes over the functions of pumping and oxygenation of the blood. Catheters are inserted into the venae cavae or the right atrium so that blood returning to the heart from the systemic venous circulation is siphoned off and pumped into an oxygenator (Fig. 7.4). There are 3 main types; the blood may be spread over rotating discs as a thin film in an oxygen chamber, or may be passed over the surface of a permeable membrane, or may have oxygen bubbled directly through it.

Once oxygenated, the blood is pumped back into the aorta, either through the femoral artery or directly through the ascending aorta. This technique will perfuse the whole body with oxygenated blood at an adequate pressure while shunting it away from the heart and lungs. If the aorta is cross-clamped it may be necessary, in addition, to perfuse the coronary arteries separately, and to drain the returning blood from the heart by means of a catheter in the coronary sinus.

At present the heart-lung machine is the more commonly used method.

Fig. 7.4. Cardio-pulmonary by-pass ('The heart-lung machine') in diagram form.

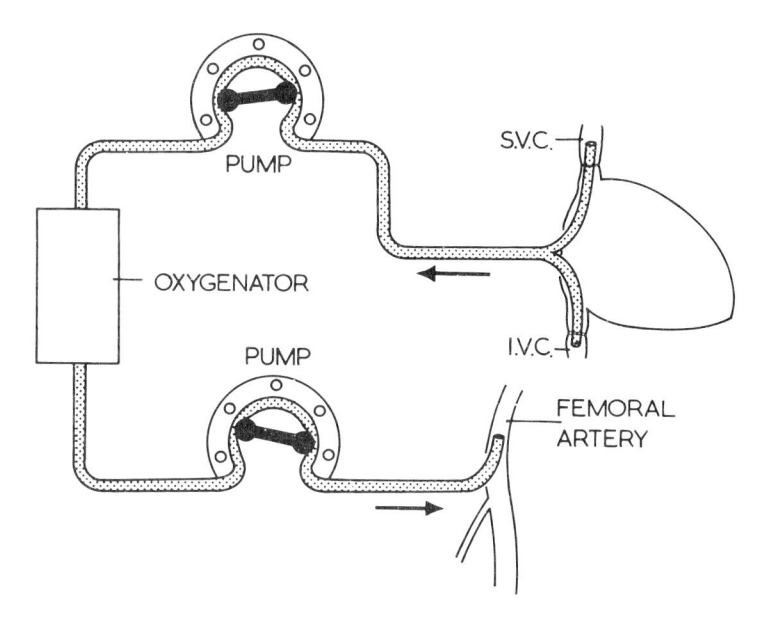

SURGICAL DISEASES OF THE HEART AND GREAT VESSELS

For convenience of further discussion, these can be subdivided into 3 main groups:
1. Diseases of the Great Vessels.
2. Congenital Defects of the Heart.
3. Acquired Cardiac Diseases.

DISEASES OF THE GREAT VESSELS

Diseases of the great vessels include persistent ductus arteriosus, coarctation of the aorta, aortic stenosis and aortic aneurysm.

PATENT DUCTUS ARTERIOSUS

Normally this channel between the aorta and the pulmonary artery closes at the time of birth. If it persists, (Fig. 7.5) blood will be shunted from the high pressure systemic circulation into the pulmonary low pressure circulation, with resultant pulmonary hypertension.

Fig. 7.5. Patent ductus arteriosus.

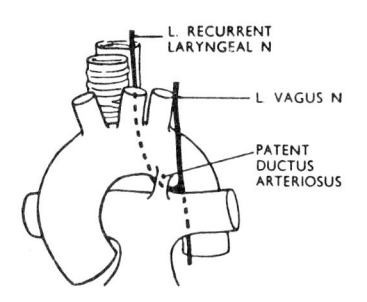

Clinical features

The patient is often asymptomatic and diagnosis is made because the doctor finds the characteristic machinery-like continuous murmur in the upper chest on routine examination with the stethoscope. If the condition is allowed to persist, the abnormal strain on the heart may lead to cardiac failure.

Any congenital abnormality of the heart or its great vessels may become infected with the *Streptococcus viridans* with resulting *subacute bacterial endocarditis*.

Special investigations

Chest X-ray usually shows enlargement of the left ventricle and increased pulmonary arterial markings.
Angiocardiography will outline the patent ductus.

Treatment

Surgical treatment should be carried out as soon as possible after the age of one year to prevent heart failure and the possibility of infection of the duct. Ligation and division is preferable where possible to mere ligation, because of the possible risk of recanalisation in the latter case.

COARCTATION OF THE AORTA

Pathology

This is a congenital narrowing of the aorta (Fig. 7.6) and is usually in the region of the ductus arteriosus; indeed, on occasions, a patent ductus may also be present. The stenosis is usually extreme, and only a pinpoint lumen remains. Blood reaches the lower aorta through anastomotic channels, but only at grossly diminished pressure. The patient develops hypertension which results not from the blockage of the aorta itself, but in a large part is due to the relatively poor blood supply to the kidneys. Renal ischaemia causes a release of renin, which is a potent hypertensive agent. The danger of coarctation is due to the effects of this raised blood pressure, which may result in cerebral haemorrhage or heart failure. Another risk is the development of subacute bacterial endocarditis.

Clinical features

The diagnosis is usually made because hypertension is discovered in a child or young adult. A characteristic physical sign is absent or diminished femoral pulsations in contrast to the bounding pulses in the upper limbs.

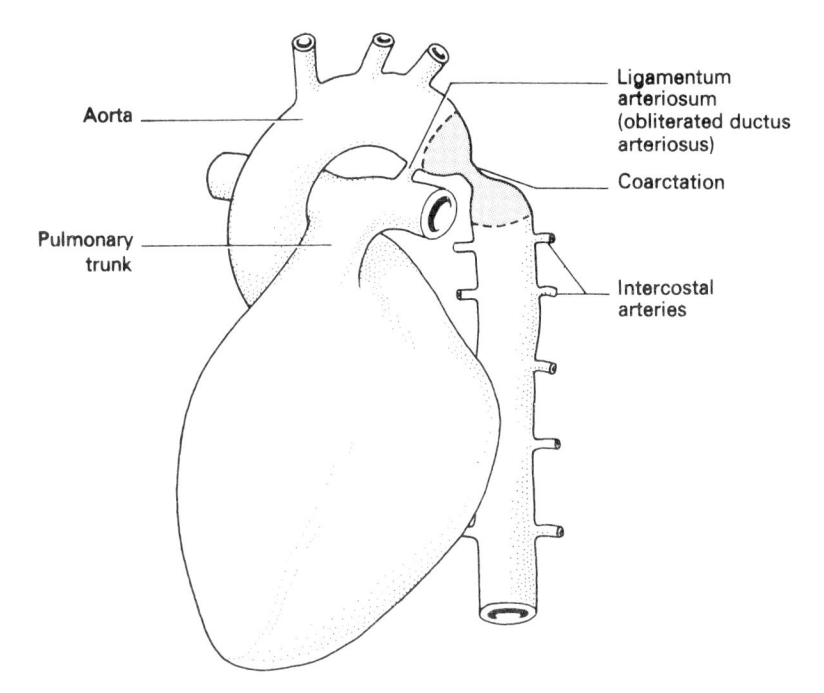

Fig. 7.6. Coarctation of the aorta. The dotted lines represent the segment which is resected in surgical correction of this condition.

Special investigations

Chest X-ray will demonstrate hypertrophy of the left ventricle and often the ribs are seen to be notched by the large intercostal collateral arteries shunting blood around the stenotic area.

Treatment

The stenotic segment is excised and an end to end anastomosis performed. If the gap is too great, an arterial graft is used to join the two ends.

AORTIC STENOSIS

This may be congenital or may follow rheumatic heart disease. The damaged valve becomes grossly distorted and is liable to calcification.

Clinical features

Because the flow of blood into the aorta is diminished, the coronary blood flow is consequently reduced and the patient experiences angina pectoris. The left ventricle hypertrophies proximal to the stenosis and the patient may develop left ventricular failure with pulmonary oedema.

Attacks of syncope (unconsciousness) are common.

Treatment

Initially dilatation of the stenosed valve was used by a blind technique through the wall of the left ventricle or through the ascending aorta. Nowadays valve replacement is carried out under cardio-pulmonary by-pass.

AORTIC ANEURYSM

The subject of aneurysm is considered in Chapter 8, but here we must note that aneurysms may involve the thoracic part of the aorta. These are commonly syphilitic, but may occur in Marfan's syndrome. Arteriosclerotic aneurysms may occur in the descending part of the thoracic aorta, but these are more likely to involve the abdominal aorta.

Dissecting aneurysm is especially likely to occur in the region of the aortic arch.

Direct repair of aneurysms in this region require heart by-pass.

CONGENITAL CARDIAC DEFECTS
SEPTAL DEFECTS

Pathology

Congenital defects in the atrial or ventricular septal walls allow blood to shunt from the systemic into the pulmonary circulation. The effect may be negligible with a small defect, but a large one may be associated with considerable flow. As the pressure rises in the pulmonary system (pulmonary hypertension) there may eventually be reversal of flow with deoxygenated blood passing into the left atrium, so that the patient becomes cyanosed. The situation is complicated by the fact that other congenital abnormalities of the heart may coexist, particularly stenoses of valvular outflow tracts.

Clinical features

These vary from the asymptomatic patient, who is found to have a cardiac murmur on examination, to the cardiac cripple with cyanosis and heart failure. The situation may be complicated by infection of the defect (*subacute bacterial endocarditis*).

Special investigations

A chest X-ray may show dilatation of the heart.
Cardiac catheterisation and angiography may be used to demonstrate the size of the shunt, the degree of pulmonary hypertension and whether there are other associated congenital abnormalities.

Treatment

Although small symptomless atrial septal defects may be kept under observation, other defects with considerable shunting of blood require repair by open operation, using either hypothermia or cardiopulmonary by-pass (Fig. 7.7).

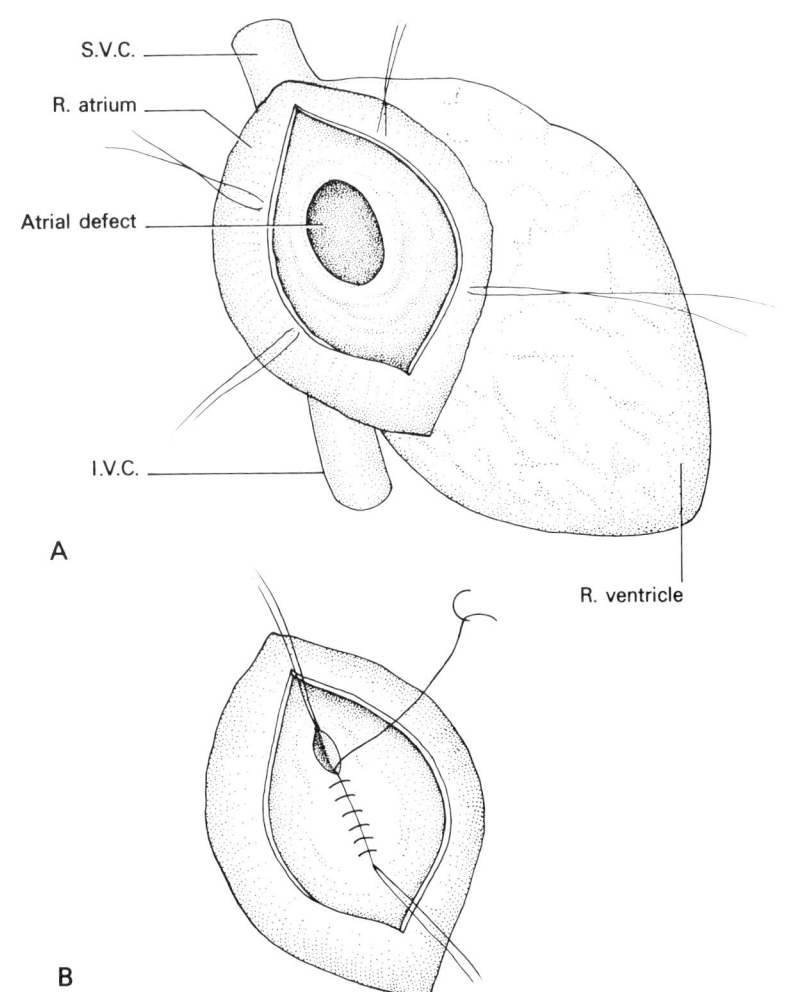

Fig. 7.7. Surgical closure of an atrial septal defect.

FALLOT'S TETRALOGY

This is a relatively common congenital cardiac lesion (Fig. 7.8) which is associated with cyanosis. It comprises:
1. pulmonary stenosis.
2. a ventricular septal defect.
3. an aorta whose orifice overlies the right as well as the left ventricle.
4. right ventricular hypertrophy, which results from attempts to force blood through the stenosed pulmonary trunk.

The cyanosis results from the aortic blood becoming mixed with venous blood returning to the right heart, and which fails to enter the pulmonary circulation for oxygenation.

Clinical features

Cyanosis is usually present from birth. The child is breathless, is stunted in development, adopts a characteristic squatting position at rest and has clubbing of the fingers and toes. The heart is usually grossly enlarged on its clinical examination and a murmur can be heard at its root.

Special investigations

The chest X-ray confirms the enlargement of the heart, which has a characteristic boot shape.
Cardiac catheterisation and angiocardiography are necessary to delineate the abnormality.

Treatment

A major break-through in the treatment of congenital abnormalities of the heart was the development by Blalock of Boston of his operation in which an anastomosis was made between the left subclavian

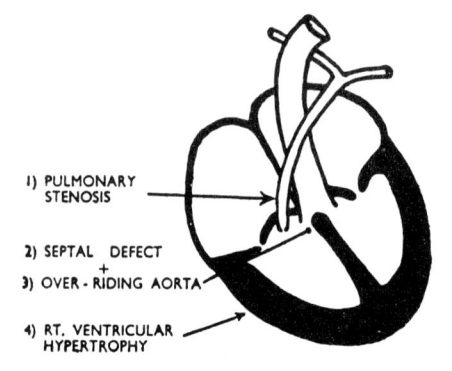

Fig. 7.8. The tetralogy of Fallot.

artery and the pulmonary artery. This resulted in blood being shunted into the pulmonary circulation beyond the region of the stenosis. Today the condition is dealt with by open heart surgery in which the interventricular defect is closed by suture or graft and the pulmonary stenosis relieved.

ACQUIRED DISEASES OF THE HEART
CONSTRICTIVE PERICARDITIS

Gross fibrosis and even calcification of the pericardium may result from a number of conditions—tuberculosis, rheumatic pericarditis, virus pericarditis, or fibrosis in a previous haemopericardium. The inelastic jacket which results impedes both the cardiac action and venous return to the heart. The patient develops ascites and hepatomegaly.

The chest X-ray may reveal calcification in the pericardium and on screening the pulsations of the heart are seen to be grossly impaired.

Treatment

The thickened pericardium is excised.

MITRAL STENOSIS

Pathology

Mitral stenosis commonly follows rheumatic carditis. The cusps of the mitral valve become thickened, fibrosed, and eventually calcified, so that the orifice of the valve becomes grossly narrowed. There may be associated involvement of the aortic valves.

Clinical features

The condition usually affects patients between the 20th and 40th year, females more commonly than males.

The damming up of blood proximal to the stenosed mitral valve produces pulmonary oedema with breathlessness and haemoptysis. Eventually the right ventricle goes into failure, with resultant hepatomegaly, ascites and oedema.

The complications of this condition include right heart failure, auricular fibrillation, peripheral arterial embolism from thrombus which forms in the dilated fibrillating left atrium, and subacute bacterial endocarditis from infection of the diseased valve.

Treatment

In the absence of mitral regurgitation, calcification of the valves or emboli, the closed operation is used. The original procedure was to insert the finger through the left atrium to split the valve, but it is now more satisfactorily achieved by means of a dilator inserted through the wall of the left ventricle while a finger palpates the valve through the left atrium.

If the valves are calcified, or if there is regurgitation, or if the left atrium is full of clot giving rise to emboli, then open operation is preferable with replacement of the diseased valve by means of a prosthetic (Fig. 7.9) or homograft valve.

ANGINA PECTORIS

Severe angina due to myocardial ischaemia may be treated surgically in selected cases. It may be possible to improve the cardiac blood supply by implantation of the internal mammary artery directly into the heart muscle (*Vineberg's Operation*). In some cases a localised segment of arteriosclerosis in the coronary artery may be removed by endarterectomy or bypassed with a saphenous vein graft from the aorta.

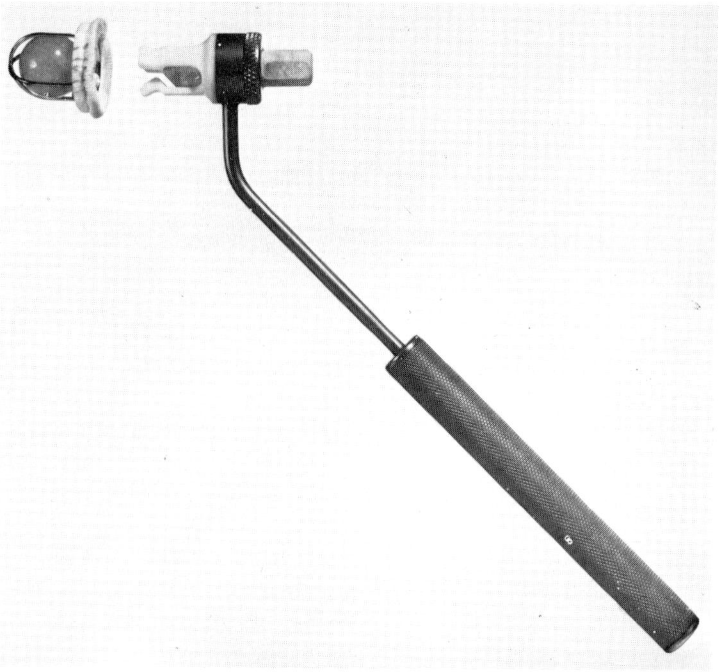

Fig. 7.9. A Starr-Edwards prosthesis for heart valve replacement, with introducer.

CARDIAC TRANSPLANTATION

The place of cardiac transplantation in the treatment of severe myocardial disease is still the subject of world-wide controversy. At present there seems no doubt that such operations should only be carried out in one or two highly specialised centres where full assessment of the advantages and disadvantages of such a procedure can be assessed.

Chapter 8. Peripheral vascular disease

PERIPHERAL ARTERIAL DISEASE

Introduction

The function of the arteries is to convey nourishment and oxygen to the tissues. If the flow of blood in major arteries supplying a limb is diminished the first tissue to be affected is muscle, since this is the structure within the limb which has greatest demands on oxygen and metabolites, far more than skin or subcutaneous tissue which, in turn, require a better blood supply than relatively inert bone and tendon.

When a muscle is exercised its demand for oxygen and glucose is increased and its production of waste products of metabolism are proportionally higher. If insufficient blood is reaching the muscle, these products accumulate in the tissue and produce pain. This can easily be reproduced on oneself if the arm muscles are vigorously exercised while a sphygmomanometer cuff is applied to the upper arm and pumped up above the arterial pressure. Very soon a severe cramp-like pain is felt in the forearm muscles, which disappears as soon as the cuff is let down. This is because fresh arterial blood sweeps through the forearm muscles and washes away the pain-producing chemicals produced in the course of muscle action. This same pain is experienced by a patient whose major arteries in the lower limb are obstructed. He will complain of severe cramp, particularly in the back of the calf (where the muscles are especially bulky), which comes on after a few yards of walking and which disappears again when he has rested for a time. Such episodes of pain on exercise receive the term *intermittent claudication* from the Latin word Claudicare, which means 'to limp'. Nurses who remember their history will recall that the Emperor Claudius, who ruled in Rome in the first Century A.D., was so called because he had a severe limp, probably due to poliomyelitis acquired in infancy.

As the degree of arterial obstruction increases, so the claudication distance correspondingly diminishes and the period of time the patient must rest before the pain disappears becomes longer. Eventually the blood supply to the muscles is insufficient to wash away the metabolic breakdown products produced even when the muscles are inactive; the patient now complains of 'rest pain', often sufficiently bad to prevent sleep at night.

The normal pink appearance and warm feel of the fingers and toes is due to their perfusion by oxygenated blood through dilated arterioles and capillaries. If the amount of blood entering the limb is grossly limited by severe obstruction of the major arteries or if the peripheral small vessels are clamped down in severe spasm as in Raynaud's disease, the digits become cold and pale. If the limb is held dependent, it will demonstrate peripheral cyanosis, since the circulation is so slow through it that blood in the small vessels stagnates, becomes deoxygenated and therefore dark blue in colour. Eventually the blood supply to the skin is so impaired that death of tissue takes place and gangrene supervenes. Often this is precipitated by some very minor trauma. For example, the toe may become gangrenous following a nick produced in cutting the toe nails, or the pressure of the mattress against the heel may produce gangrene of the skin over this region (Fig. 8.1).

Note that the complete loss of blood supply to any tissue must inevitably result in its death, but *gangrene* implies the macroscopic (visible) death of tissue accompanied by infection. If a patient has a severe obstruction of one of the coronary arteries, for example,

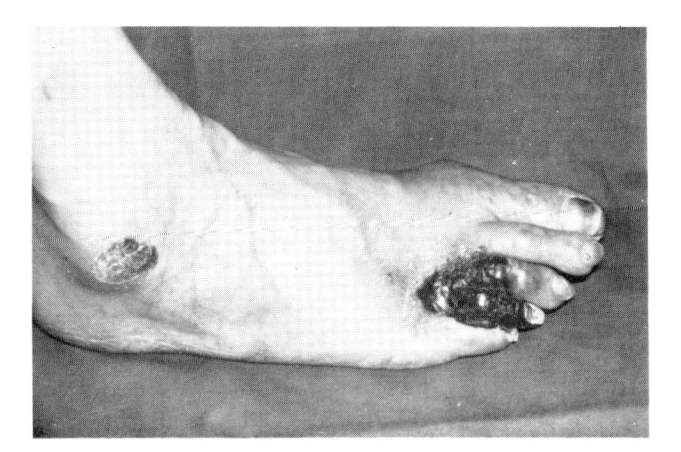

Fig. 8.1. Gangrene of the toes in arterial obstruction. Note that there is also an area of gangrene over the lateral malleolus.

the cardiac muscle supplied by that vessel will undergo necrosis and die. This takes place in the absence of bacteria and gangrene of the heart muscle does not supervene. However, whenever the blood supply is cut off in the presence of organisms, these will invade the necrotic tissue. Typical examples are the gangrene which take place in acute appendicitis or in strangulated intestinal obstruction. Similarly, when a finger or toe has its blood supply cut off, inevitably the tissues will be invaded by bacteria entering through minute cracks or cuts in the skin, so that gangrene then ensues.

The causes of impaired limb circulation

There are a large number of conditions which can cause impaired arterial blood flow to the limbs and these include:
1. Injury to vessels by trauma, heat, cold or chemicals.
2. Atherosclerosis with superadded thrombosis.
3. Embolism.
4. Small vessel spasm (Raynaud's phenomenon).
5. Diabetes, either by itself or complicating atherosclerosis.
6. Buerger's disease.
7. Ergot poisoning.

The common conditions seen in this country are, first and foremost atherosclerosis, far outstripping the other conditions, although peripheral embolism and Raynaud's phenomenon are also common. Diabetes frequently complicates atherosclerotic disease.

ARTERIAL INJURY

Peripheral arteries may be injured by closed or open trauma.

Closed injuries may complicate fractures and dislocations, the ones most likely to be associated with arterial injury being supracondylar fracture of the humerus with damage to the brachial artery and dislocation of the knee or fracture of the lower end of the femur implicating the popliteal artery. Arterial injury may also occur from too tight application of a plaster of Paris splint to an injured limb or from a tourniquet which has been left on for more than an hour. Vessel damage from such closed injuries may take the form of spasm, thrombosis, rupture, or, in some cases of comminuted fracture, a direct tear of the artery by a spicule of bone.

Open injuries are not common in civilian practice in this country, although from time to time a butcher will be admitted whose knife will have slipped during the cutting up of a joint and who has stabbed himself in the femoral artery at the groin. In Spain the bull-fighter may be damaged in the same place by the bull's horn. In less civilised parts of the world, stab wounds and gunshot wounds are more common. The damaged artery may go into spasm, or undergo thrombosis. It may be divided, and such division may either be partial or complete. Interestingly enough a partial division tends to bleed more furiously than a complete tear because, in the latter case, spasm may completely close the vessel.

Occasionally the damaged wall of the artery gives way to form an aneurysm (see below).

Clinical features

Arterial damage in an open wound is suggested by severe bright red bleeding. In a closed injury there may be the production of a massive haematoma. Major arterial interruption is accompanied by the signs of distal ischaemia which can easily be remembered since they all begin with the letter P:

Pain (due to extreme ischaemia of the muscles of the limb)
Pallor (due to lack of blood flow through the skin capillaries)
Pulselessness (the pulses below the point of injury disappear)
Paraesthesia (pins and needles due to peripheral nerve ischaemia)
Paralysis (due to loss of blood supply to the affected muscles)

Recently a colleague of ours in Dublin added a sixth P to the list—*'Perishing with cold'*, and certainly the ischaemic limb rapidly cools.

Treatment

Any obvious compression, such as a tight plaster or obstructing tourniquet, is removed. If vascular damage accompanies a closed fracture or dislocation, this must be reduced under a general anaesthetic and the stretched or spastic artery may then return to normal. If this does not occur rapidly, say within the next half hour, the artery must be explored. If found to be in spasm it may respond to the local application of a 2.5% solution of Papaverine, which is the only effective local antispasmodic. If the artery is found to be torn it will require repair, usually by means of a vein graft.

In an open injury associated with arterial bleeding the haemorrhage can usually be controlled by direct pressure and it is rarely necessary to use a tourniquet or pressure on a pressure point. A blood transfusion is arranged and the wound explored in the operating theatre under a general anaesthetic. Small peripheral arteries (below the elbow or the knee) can be treated by ligation but major vessels should be repaired, or, if the ends cannot be brought together, grafted. A suitable vessel to use is the patient's own saphenous vein so that most of us carry our own artery bank with us.

ANEURYSM

Definitions

An aneurysm is a sac communicating with the lumen of an artery. The following types may occur (Fig. 8.2):

1. *True aneurysm.* This is an actual dilatation of the wall of the artery itself. It may be *fusiform*, when the whole circumference of the artery is expanded, or *saccular*, when one side of the artery is dilated and communicates with the arterial wall through a comparatively narrow neck.

2. *False aneurysm.* This occurs when an artery is perforated by a puncture wound so that a cavity is produced which communicates with the lumen of the artery and which is lined by clot and fibrous tissue.

3. *An arterio-venous aneurysm* is formed by a communication between an artery and a vein. It may be congenital or traumatic in origin.

4. *A dissecting aneurysm* is formed when there is a tear in the inner coat of an artery (almost invariably the aorta) and blood dissects the wall of the vessel to form a second channel. This may either rupture back into the main arterial lumen or else burst through the outer coat of the vessel, with disastrous results.

Aetiology

A wide variety of pathological processes may produce an aneurysm. These include:

1. *Congenital.* The commonest example of this is the berry aneurysm which occurs on the branches of the internal carotid or vertebral arteries within the skull at the base of the brain on the circle of Willis (Fig. 8.3). This may rupture and is a common cause of subarachnoid haemorrhage. Much less common are congenital arterio-venous aneurysms, often multiple, which may occur between major vessels in the upper or lower limb.

2. *Traumatic.* Aneurysms are common in times of war and in areas where stabbings and shootings are everyday occurrences. The wall of the artery may be damaged by a penetrating wound and the weakened area may subsequently distend into an aneurysm. Puncture wounds may produce false aneurysms or, if the injury goes through both the artery and vein, an arterio-venous aneurysm may result.

3. *Inflammatory.* Patients with subacute bacterial endocarditis may develop an infective arteritis in peripheral arteries which leads to aneurysm formation. Syphilis may involve the thoracic part of the aorta but fortunately this once common occurrence is now rare in this country, thanks to early treatment of the disease.

ANEURYSMS

TRUE
(a) SACCULAR
(b) FUSIFORM

FALSE

ARTERIO-VENOUS

DISSECTING

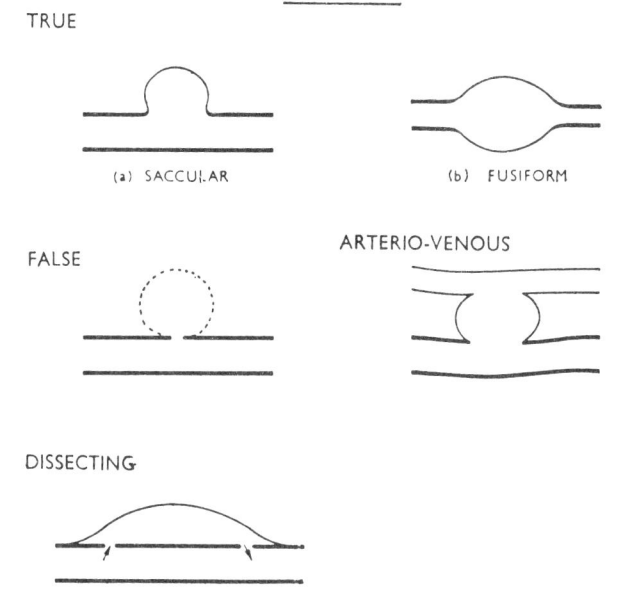

Fig. 8.2. The types of aneurysm.

4. *Degenerative disease.* In modern practice atherosclerosis is the commonest cause of aneurysm. Degeneration of the arterial wall may result in a true aneurysm of the fusiform type and this is especially seen in the abdominal aorta, the iliac vessels, the femoral artery at the groin and the popliteal artery immediately behind the knee. It is also responsible for dissecting aneurysm of the aorta.

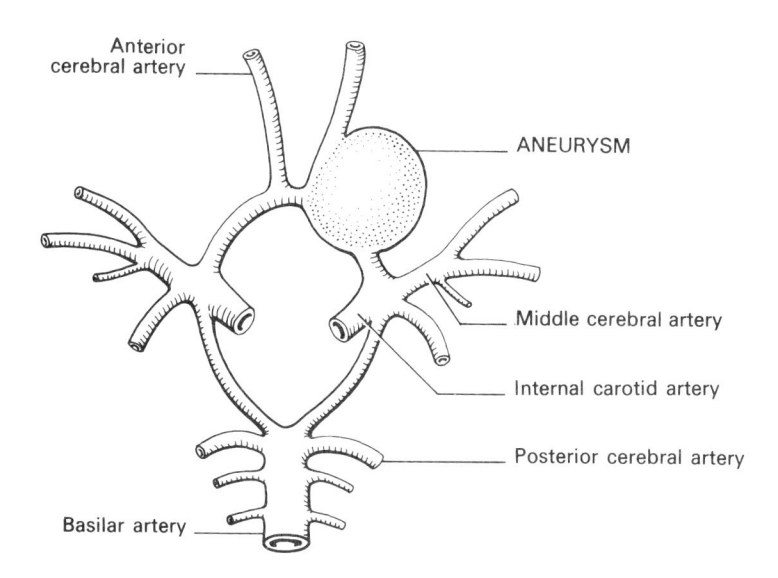

Fig. 8.3. A berry aneurysm on the circle of Willis at the base of the brain.

Clinical features

It is usually easy to diagnose an aneurysm. There is a dilatation along the course of an artery, which can be felt to pulsate. Pressure on the artery proximal to the aneurysm may reduce both its size and pulsation and it may also be possible to diminish its size by direct compression. If the entering artery has a narrow orifice, a thrill may be felt if the fingers are gently rested on the aneurysm because of the turbulent flow of blood within it. By the same token, a bruit (a rushing sound) may be heard over it by means of a stethoscope.

The commonest differential diagnosis is from a dilated, tortuous atherosclerotic artery, which is not uncommon in elderly subjects. It may also be mistaken for a highly vascular tumour, which because of its enormous blood supply may be felt to pulsate. In doubtful cases it may be necessary to perform an arteriogram to clinch the diagnosis.

Left untreated, an aneurysm may rupture into surrounding tissues, may thrombose, with impairment of the peripheral arterial circulation, may produce pain from pressure from an adjacent structure or, rarely, may become infected.

Treatment

Small peripheral aneurysms can be excised without endangering the peripheral circulation. More major aneurysms are removed and continuity of the artery restored by means of a graft (Fig. 8.4). In

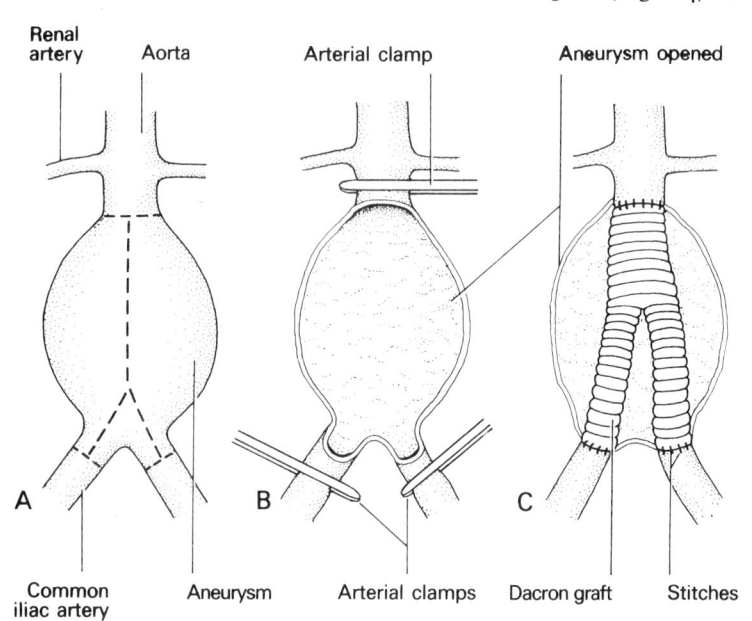

Fig. 8.4. Steps in the excision and grafting of an aortic aneurysm.

some situations the artery is ligatured proximal to the aneurysm sac in order to induce thrombosis and obliteration of the aneurysm; ligation of the carotid artery, for example, may be used to thrombose an intracerebral aneurysm.

ATHEROSCLEROTIC DISEASE

Pathology

Atherosclerosis (arteriosclerosis) is the commonest non-malignant killing disease of modern civilisation. Not only does it affect the peripheral arteries but it also involves the coronary and cerebral vessels which give rise to the potentially lethal complications of coronary and cerebral thrombosis. In spite of considerable research the aetiology of this condition is unknown. Its incidence and severity increase with advancing age and it is especially likely to be found in obese, diabetic subjects who are heavy smokers and who have a high blood cholesterol level.

In the initial stages, there are deposits of fatty material in the artery wall which may then become thickened, calcified and even ulcerate. Actual obliteration of the lumen of the artery is brought about by deposition of platelets on the damaged intima of the artery wall to produce a thrombus (Fig. 8.5).

Clinical features

Many patients with quite severe atherosclerosis of peripheral vessels have no symptoms because sufficient blood is able to reach the periphery through the narrowed arteries themselves, or along the collateral arteries. However, as the disease progresses, and particularly as arteries become completely occluded with thrombus, the deficient blood supply to the leg may first produce symptoms of claudication and, in the most severe cases, gangrene (see above).

Treatment

The treatment of patients with atherosclerotic disease of the legs must be sub-divided into the management of claudication, which is for the most part conservative, and the treatment of gangrene, which often requires surgical intervention.

Claudication

Since the principle disability is limitation of walking because of pain, it is often possible to keep a claudicating patient at work simply by altering his job. For example, a postman may have to change from delivering letters to office employment. If the patient is overweight,

Peripheral vascular disease

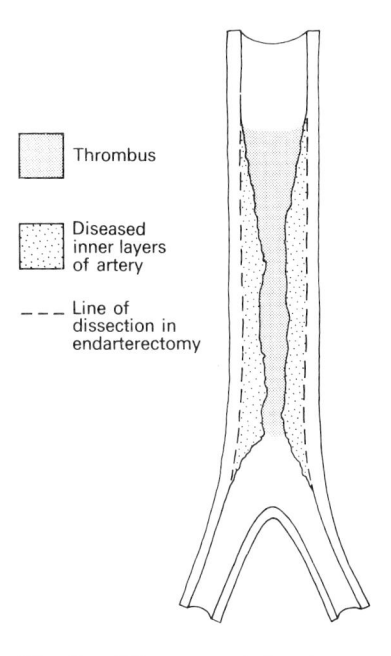

Fig. 8.5. Diagrammatic longitudinal section through an atherosclerotic artery. The lumen is obliterated with thrombus. The dotted line demonstrates the plane along which the diseased inner part of the artery together with the thrombus is removed in the operation of endarterectomy.

this must be corrected, since obesity gives added work to the muscles of the leg. It is quite unusual for patients with claudication not to be heavy smokers and it is essential for this habit to stop at once. Cigarette smoking produces spasm of the small blood vessels, increases the tendency for thrombosis to occur and, furthermore, replaces the oxy-haemoglobin in the arterial blood with carboxy-haemoglobin due to the inhalation of carbon monoxide in the cigarette smoke. We tell our patients that while they are smoking, coal gas rather than oxygen reaches the tissues of their limbs!

Careful chiropody is essential since gangrene can commence from the trauma produced by inexpert cutting of the nails or of a corn.

If a patient with atherosclerosis has diabetes it is extremely important that this is satisfactorily controlled since in addition to the impaired circulation due to atheroma, the diabetic is especially likely to develop gangrene, partly as a result of his increased tendency to infection and partly due to the associated diabetic neuritis, which may lead to trophic ulceration in the anaesthetic foot.

Naturally the patient is apprehensive that he is going to lose his leg. He should be told that, provided he carries out the above instructions, particularly with regard to complete cessation of cigarette smoking, he has a 90% chance that the claudication will remain at its present level or even improve; only approximately 10% of patients eventually develop gangrene.

Unfortunately, atherosclerosis is a generalised disease and many of these patients are going to succumb from the other major complications of this condition—coronary or cerebral thrombosis.

Arterial reconstructive surgery should only be considered when claudication is so severe that the patient can hardly walk and can no longer carry on his work. The details of such operations are given under the treatment of gangrene below.

We may summarise the treatment of claudication as follows:
1. Learn to live within the claudication distance and change job if necessary.
2. Lose weight—less effort for the leg muscles.
3. Stop smoking completely.
4. Take care of the feet to prevent minor trauma which may lead to gangrene.
5. Treat diabetes if present.
6. Consider reconstructive surgery if symptoms are severe and do not respond to conservative treatment.

GANGRENE

Once the patient has severe pain in the leg even at rest or has developed an area of gangrene on the foot, the intensity of the symptoms usually forces the surgeon to consider more active treatment. Provided that the patient's general condition is reasonable, an arteriogram is carried out in order to determine whether some sort of reconstructive operation is possible. If the popliteal artery and its branches are blocked then reconstruction is virtually impossible, but if the x-rays show that there is a good 'run-off' beyond the block in the iliac or femoral artery then an attempt can be made to shunt blood from above to below the obstruction (Fig. 8.6).

Two main types of operation may be carried out:
1. *Thromboendarterectomy.* In this the surgeon cores out the inner part of the diseased artery together with its contained thrombus, either through one long incision or through several small openings in the artery using a special ring stripper (Fig. 8.7). The incisions

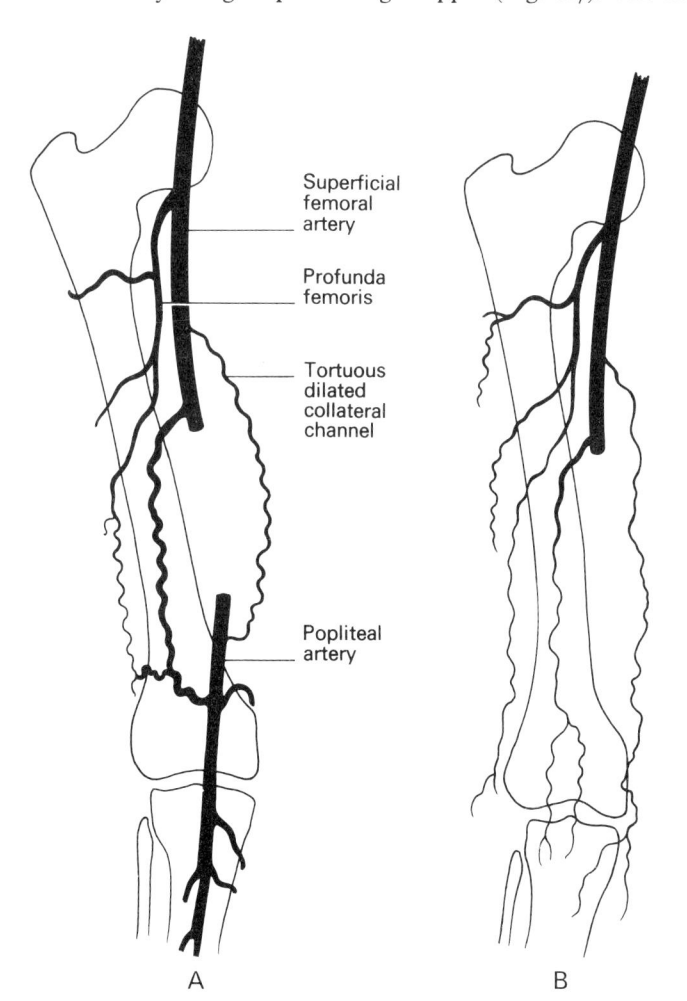

Fig. 8.6. Tracings of arteriograms which demonstrate A. an example of a good 'run off' with a patent popliteal artery; this is suitable for reconstructive surgery. In B, however, the main arterial tree is obliterated and reconstruction cannot be carried out.

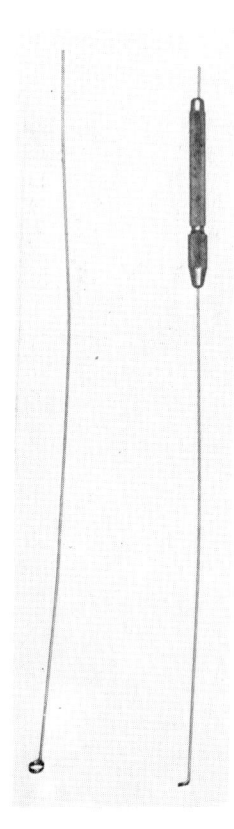

Fig. 8.7. A Cannon ring stripper, used in endarterectomy.

in the artery wall are then sutured with fine arterial stitches or else repaired by means of a patch graft taken from one of the superficial veins. This has the advantage of widening the diseased artery wall (Fig. 8.8).

2. *By-pass*. In this the diseased part of the artery is left intact and a shunt inserted from above to below the block. The graft most commonly employed is the patient's own saphenous vein which must be reversed so that its valves do not impede the flow of blood. Less commonly, a plastic dacron tube or a preserved cadaver artery may be employed (Fig. 8.9).

If it is impossible for anatomical reasons to perform any kind of reconstructive surgery, it may be possible to abolish rest pain in the leg and occasionally to improve the circulation by means of a *lumbar sympathectomy* or by blocking the lumbar sympathetic chain by means of an injection of phenol, but these procedures are usually only successful in relatively mild cases.

Major amputation

If pain cannot be controlled by sympathectomy, or sympathetic block, or if reconstructive surgery is impossible or has failed, then the only remaining treatment is amputation of the limb. Obviously this is a serious undertaking in an old feeble patient and the nursing care of such cases is of paramount importance. A constant anxiety is the healing of the amputation flaps in tissues which are obviously depleted of blood supply. There is therefore a compromise which has to be made—the higher the amputation, for example, mid-thigh, the better the chances of wound healing, but against this must be placed the fact that amputation above the knee joint means that rehabilitation of the patient is going to be much more difficult and many of these elderly people are never able to learn to walk using an above knee prosthesis. Another serious risk in patients with atherosclerosis is gas gangrene infection of the amputation stump due to Clostridium welchii. This results from inoculation of the

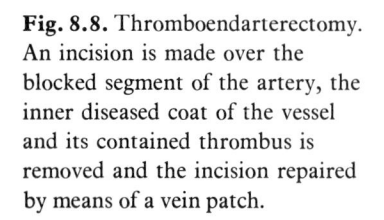

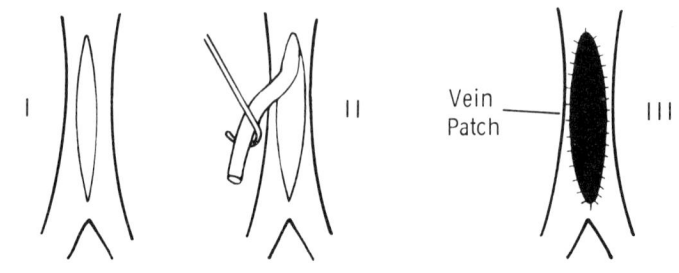

Fig. 8.8. Thromboendarterectomy. An incision is made over the blocked segment of the artery, the inner diseased coat of the vessel and its contained thrombus is removed and the incision repaired by means of a vein patch.

relatively ischaemic muscles of the amputation stump with these organisms which may be present on the faecally contaminated skin of the lower limb. An essential prophylaxis in such cases is a course of intramuscular penicillin, which should be commenced a day before amputation and continued for seven days after operation.

Following amputation, an active programme of rehabilitation is carried out with early fitting of a prosthesis as soon as the wound has healed. With this technique a proportion of patients can be taught to walk satisfactorily using their artificial limb.

ARTERIAL EMBOLISM

Definition

An *embolus* is a foreign body which circulates in the blood and which may become lodged in a vessel to form an *embolism*. If a segment of tissue is deprived of its blood supply as a result of this an *infarct* results.

An embolus is usually made up of a detached thrombus, but less common emboli include, air, fat, tumour tissue, and parasites. These will not be considered further in this section.

In attempting to establish the source of an embolus, it is useful to consider the possible sites of origin from the heart and the major vessels:

1. *The left atrium*—stasis and consequent thrombosis within this chamber of the heart may occur in atrial fibrillation with mitral stenosis.
2. *Valves*—thrombi may detach from the aortic or mitral valves affected by subacute bacterial endocarditis.
3. *Left ventricular wall*—after a coronary thrombosis infarction may extend up to the lining of the ventricle, on which a mural thrombus may deposit and then become detached as an embolus.
4. *Aorta*—thrombi may detach from an aneurysm of the aorta or from areas of atheroma on its wall.
5. Very rarely a *paradoxical embolus* may occur; This arises in the veins of the leg and then passes via a septal defect in the heart into the arterial system rather than lodging, as usually happens, in the lung as a pulmonary embolus. (see page 35).

Emboli tend to lodge at branches in the arteries and their danger will depend on the anatomical situation. An embolus in the central artery of the retina, for example, produces sudden blindness, in the cerebrum it results in a stroke, in the superior mesenteric artery it results in extensive infarction of the small intestine. In this section we are particularly concerned with emboli which lodge in the limb arteries.

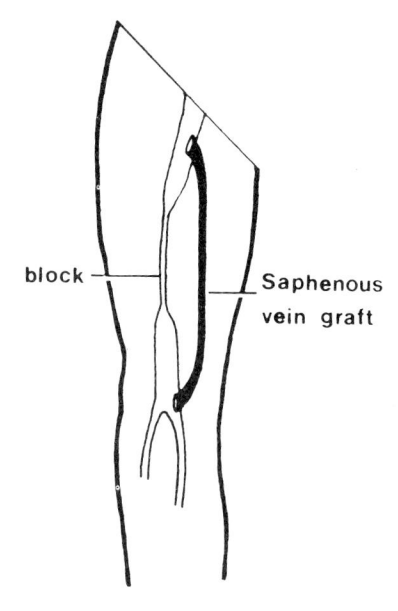

Fig. 8.9. A saphenous vein by-pass graft.

Clinical features

There is often a preceding cause for the embolus. Acute obstruction of a major artery in the limb produces sudden pain and the limb becomes white and cold. Sensation may disappear and the muscles may become rapidly paralysed ('Pain, Pallor, Pulselessness, Paraesthesiae, Paralysis, Perishing with cold').

Treatment

A small peripheral embolus in a limb may be treated conservatively, since there is sufficient collateral circulation to maintain viability. Heparin is given in order to prevent propogation of clot from the site of blockage and the limb kept cool to reduce its oxygen requirements.

An embolus which blocks a major artery and produces acute ischaemia in the limb is a surgical emergency since the success of embolectomy is directly proportional to the time interval from the onset of the block to the operation.

The operative treatment is relatively simple; the vessel is exposed above the site of embolism and the clot removed by means of a special inflatable Fogarty balloon catheter (Fig. 8.10). This is passed beyond the embolus, the balloon distended and pulled back. The procedure is repeated on several occasions until all the block is removed and back-bleeding occurs. If the embolus has lodged at the aortic bifurcation, the catheter is passed in a retrograde manner upwards from the femoral arteries exposed at each groin. This saves the necessity of carrying out a laparotomy in a gravely ill patient

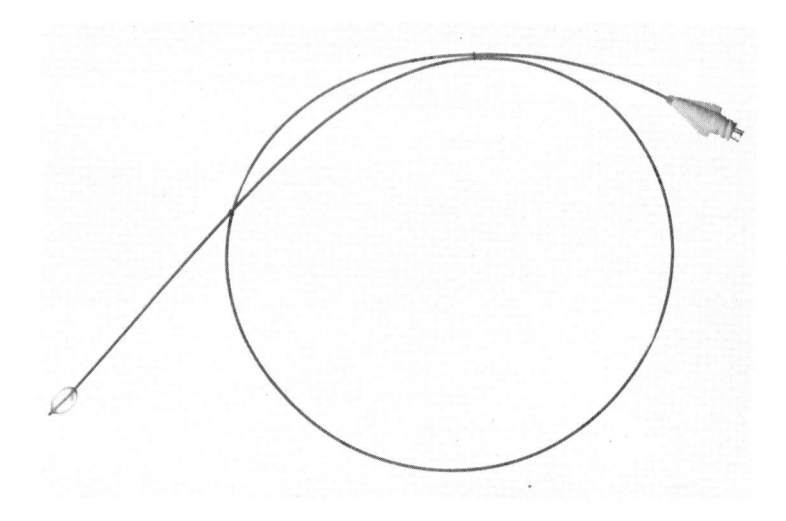

Fig. 8.10. The Fogarty balloon catheter for removal of an embolus. (The balloon has been distended).

and can, if necessary, be performed under local anaesthesia. It is therefore possible to remove an embolus even in elderly patients with serious co-existent medical conditions such as heart failure.

RAYNAUD'S DISEASE

This is a condition usually found in young women in which the small arteries of the fingers and, to a lesser extent, the feet, nose and ears, go into spasm. The limbs become cold and blue, especially in cold weather, and in severe cases, patches of gangrene may appear on the tips of the digits.

Treatment

The management is initially conservative. The limbs are kept warm with gloves and fur-lined boots. Vasodilator drugs may improve the symptoms. In more severe cases sympathectomy is employed but unfortunately its effects may not be longlasting.

VARICOSE VEINS

A varicose vein is one that has become dilated, elongated and tortuous. Although veins in various situations in the body become dilated, by common usage, when we talk of varicose veins without qualifying the site everyone knows that we mean varicose veins of the leg.

Anatomy of the leg veins

The veins of the lower limb can, for convenience of description, be divided into two systems, the first is the superficial system and lies just beneath the skin, and the second is the deep system which lies deep to the deep fascia of the leg and thigh. These two systems of veins communicate with each other at a number of points.

(a) *Superficial veins* (Fig. 8.11)

The dorsal venous arch can be seen on the dorsal aspect of the foot. Radiating from its convex lower surface, veins pass to the toes. The medial end is continuous with the *long saphenous vein* and the lateral end is continuous with the *short saphenous vein*.

The long saphenous vein passes upwards, immediately in front of the medial malleolus, runs up alongside the medial aspect of the knee to the medial part of the front of the thigh and thence the groin. Here it pierces the deep fascia to enter the femoral vein.

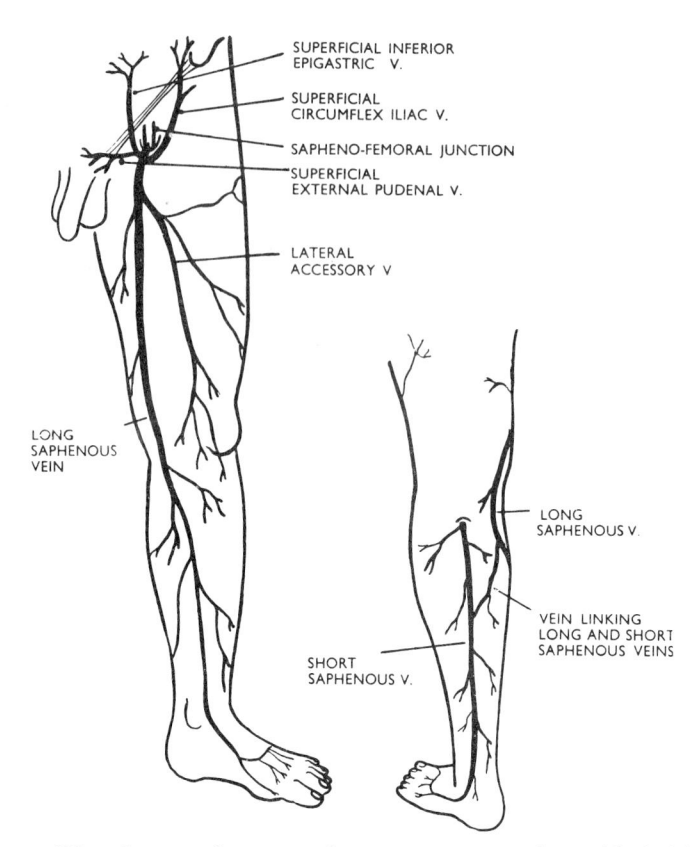

Fig. 8.11. The superficial veins of the lower limb.

The short saphenous vein commences at the ankle behind the medial malleolus, runs up over the back of the calf and then pierces the deep fascia just below the popliteal fossa to terminate in the popliteal vein. One or more branches run upwards and medially from it to join the long saphenous vein.

(b) *Deep veins*

The deep veins commence as wide channels or 'lakes' in the muscles of the calf. They then accompany the corresponding major arteries and behind the knee coalesce to form the popliteal vein. This drains proximally and in the thigh becomes the femoral vein, in turn becoming the external iliac vein as it passes beneath the inguinal ligament.

(c) *Communications between deep and superficial systems* (Fig. 8.12)

The long saphenous communicates with the femoral and the short saphenous with the popliteal vein. In addition, approximately halfway down the thigh the long saphenous vein has a tributary which

Fig. 8.12. Communications between the deep and superficial veins of the legs.

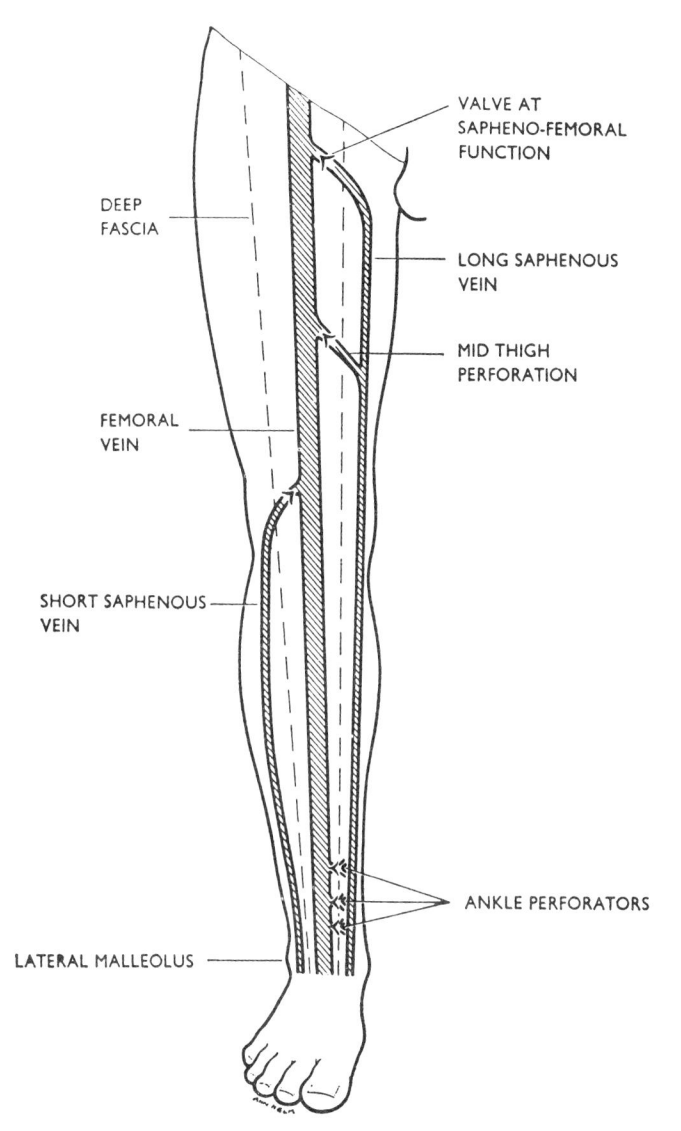

again joins the femoral vein, the so-called 'mid-thigh perforator'. There may be a further communication between the long saphenous vein and the deep venous system just below the knee joint. There are usually three communicating veins which pass from the superficial venous plexus on the medial aspect of the leg approximately one finger's breadth behind the posterior border of the tibia through the deep fascia to the deep venous system. There is, in addition, a further communicating vein also from the superficial venous plexus of the skin below the lateral aspect of the leg just below the knee joint. These communicating veins, with the exception of the upper ends of the saphenous veins, are variable in site and number.

Physiology of the leg veins

The deep and superficial system of veins are divided from each other by the investing deep fascia of the leg, a tough sheet of fibrous tissue that functions rather like a strong elastic stocking placed beneath the skin of the leg. Both the superficial and the deep veins are provided with valves which are made up of two cusps. Valves are also present in the communicating veins which pass from the superficial to the deep system. The valves allow free flow of blood,
(1) from the periphery towards the heart, and
(2) from the superficial system to the deep system.

Any attempt to force blood in a retrograde direction closes the valves. The presence of efficient, competent valves in the veins is necessary for effective return of blood from the lower limb. As the muscles of the leg contract within their rigid sheet of deep fascia, the pressure in the deep veins rises above that in the superficial veins. Blood cannot pass into the latter because of the valves guarding the communicating veins. During this high pressure phase, blood is therefore pumped by the muscular action towards the heart from the deep veins, thus emptying the blood from the muscles of the leg. When the muscles relax, the pressure in the deep veins falls below that of the superficial veins, thus allowing blood to pass from the superficial system via the communicating veins along this pressure gradient. Venous return from the lower limb may also be assisted, of course, by gravity when the subject elevates the legs.

Provided that the venous valves are competent, return of blood to the heart is assured. However, the pressure to which these valves may be subjected can be very high. When standing, the pressure in the lower leg is equivalent to a column of blood extending from ground level to the level of the heart, roughly equivalent to about 100 cm of water in an average adult man. When the leg is exercised and the deep muscles of the leg contract hard, the pressure in the deep venous system rises to very much higher levels.

Aetiology of varicose veins

The cause of varicose veins is always incompetence of one or more of the valves that connect the deep system with the superficial system. Once blood is allowed to leak from the deep veins back into the superficial veins through these incompetent valves, the veins of the superficial system are subjected to a constant high pressure and thus become distended. This distension renders further valves incompetent so that the process tends to become progressively worse. Once the superficial veins become dilated, they elongate and become tortuous.

There are two main types of varicose veins and the first of these is due to incompetence of the valve at the junction between the long saphenous and femoral veins. In this case, the long saphenous vein itself and its immediate tributaries become dilated and these are the very obvious varicosities which are seen over the medial aspect of the thigh and calf. In the great majority of these cases there is no obvious reason for this incompetence. It may be something to do with the upright posture of man, since varicose veins do not occur in four-legged animals. Another possibility is that patients with varicose vein have some sort of congenital weakness of the valves, and it is interesting that in many cases the condition is familial.

The second type follows a previous thrombosis of the deep veins of the leg. In this case the thrombotic process extends into the communicating veins, which become temporarily obstructed. The clot then organises and eventually is removed as the process of recanalisation proceeds. Unfortunately, although the communicating vein redevelops a lumen, the valves are not perfectly reconstructed and become incompetent. The communicating veins particularly prone to this are those on the medial aspect of the leg. In these cases there may be no visible varicose veins at all, but the venous circulation of the leg is disturbed with consequent disruption of the supply of blood to the superficial tissues, and skin. The leg becomes swollen and there are subcutaneous changes so that the tissues feel hard. Because there is stasis in the superficial veins, blood pigments become deposited in the tissues which are consequently stained brown. As the condition progresses the nutrition of the skin begins to suffer, with the consequent development of a scaly dermatitis, the so-called 'varicose eczema'. If this is allowed to continue, a varicose ulcer will eventually occur.

Clinical features (Fig. 8.13)

Varicose veins, particularly when due to sapheno-femoral incompetence, may first become obvious in teenagers, particularly if there is a history of several other members of the family having the same condition, thus suggesting a congenital valve weakness. More often, however, varices are seen in middle-aged or elderly people and are three or four times as common in women as in men. There

Fig. 8.13. A gross example of varicose veins.

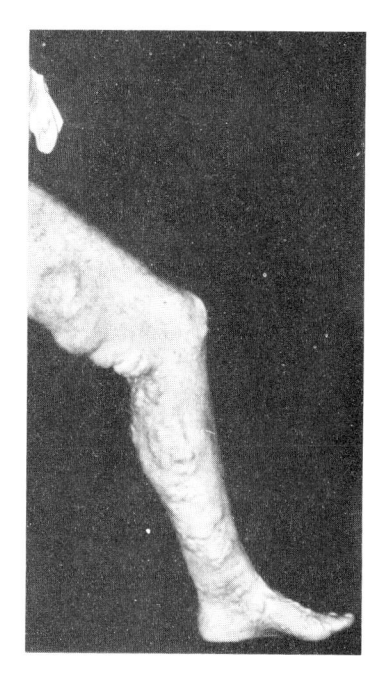

may be some association with sex hormones as a considerable proportion of female patients complain of discomfort in their veins just before menstruation and many women develop varicose veins during pregnancy which then regress after delivery. Although this may represent a hormonal effect, another contributory factor could be that the venous pressure in the lower limbs is raised due to the presence of the pregnant uterus pressing against the iliac veins.

The most common complaint of patients with varicose veins is their unpleasant appearance. As the veins become more dilated the patient may then complain of aching and heaviness of the limb during prolonged periods of standing; doctors and nurses often complain of their veins, possibly for this reason. As the veins become progressively worse, the venous circulation of the legs becomes more abnormal, and swelling of the ankles occurs.

Treatment

There are three possibilities, some or all of which may be appropriate to the particular patient. These are:
1. Surgical treatment.
2. Injection treatment
3. External support, for example by the use of elastic stockings.

1. *Surgery*. When a patient has incompetence of the valves in the long saphenous vein just as it joins the femoral vein, surgery is required. The saphenous vein is exposed at the groin through a small incision and is tied and disconnected together with all its tributaries at its junction with femoral vein (Trendelenburg operation). The operation of stripping of the long saphenous vein is no longer performed except in the rare instance of an incompetent mid-thigh perforator, when the long saphenous vein is stripped down to, but not below, the knee.

There are other methods of surgical treatment, such as multiple ligations, but the same effect is achieved much more simply by the use of injection sclerotherapy.

It must be explained to a patient undergoing a Trendelenburg operation that the visible varicosities in the leg will persist, but the origin of the increased pressure in the veins has been removed and if she wears an elastic stocking for approximately six weeks, the varicosities will tend to regress, particularly if there are no other incompetent communicating veins in the leg. Six weeks after operation, if there are any remaining varicosities these are treated by injection.

2. *Injection treatment*. (Fig. 8.14). This involves the injection of a sclerosant solution (the most commonly used is a 3% solution of

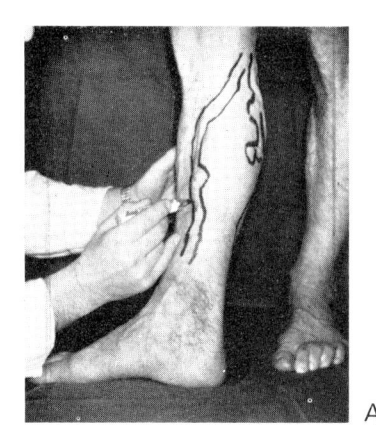

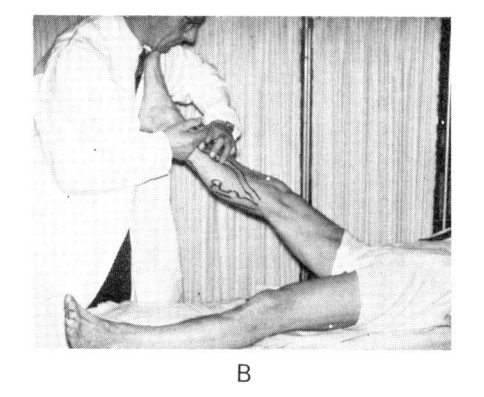

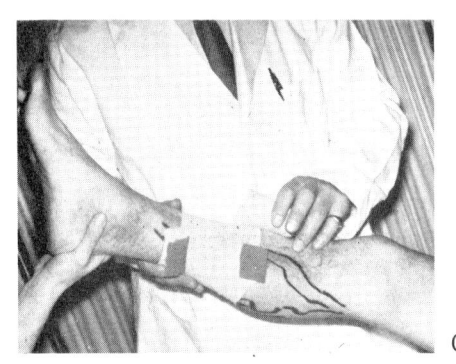

Fig. 8.14. Injection treatment. The veins are marked out (A), injected at the sites of perforation into the deep veins (B) and firm compression is then applied (C).

sodium tetra-decyl-sulphate, S.T.D.) at the points where the varicosities drain into the deep veins as they come through the deep fascia, a technique introduced by Professor George Fegan of Dublin. The principle is to inject the visible vein at the point at which the communicating vein emerges from the deep fascia. A fine needle is inserted into the vein, the leg is then elevated so that the vein is emptied, the segment of vein to be injected is isolated between fingers and 0.5 ml of S.T.D. is injected. This injection site is then kept in a compressed state so that the vein is kept empty by means of a bandage and a rubber pad. The S.T.D. is an intense irritant which damages the lining of the vein so that thrombosis occurs and scar tissue forms within it, thus producing obliteration of the varicosity and of the communicating vein. In order to be effective, the vein must be kept empty during the period of fibrous tissue formation, and this is achieved by firm compression bandaging maintained for a period of six weeks. A firm elastic stocking is worn over the bandage which holds the pad in place, and the patient is instructed to walk for at least three miles each day of the treatment period.

It is quite common for there to be pigmentation of the skin over a varicose vein. A successful injection of a varicose vein usually results in brown pigmentation in the line of the vein. This is usually stated by the patient to be bruising, this however is not the case. It is due to the deposition of blood pigments in the skin after a successful, therapeutically induced, thrombosis.

3. *External support.* In elderly or unfit patients a firm, full-length elastic stocking will compress the veins, give relief from the aching experienced by the patient on prolonged standing and reduce the oedema of the leg. As previously mentioned, when the pressure in the varicosities has been reduced by Trendelenberg operation, the wearing of an elastic stocking will assist the regression of the veins. If a patient has a tendency to varicose veins it is a good idea to wear elastic tights during the later stages of pregnancy.

Apart from the above, the main place of external support is in the treatment of a varicose ulcer which is described below.

The complications of varicose veins

There are three important and common complications:
1. Haemorrhage.
2. Thrombophlebitis.
3. Ulceration.

1. *Haemorrhage.* This usually follows some quite trivial injury. The dilated vein is close to the skin surface, thin-walled and contains blood under high pressure, when the patient is in the upright position or if the leg is hanging down.

Treatment: emergency treatment is extremely simple; the patient lies flat on the back with the leg elevated and a pressure bandage is applied, although the bleeding will stop if the tip of the thumb or finger is applied to the correct place. There is a recorded case of a woman patient who bled to death after one of her chickens pecked her varicose vein. This sad outcome would bave been prevented had she not panicked and had simply applied a little pressure over the bleeding point.

Once the emergency is over, the varicose veins should be treated either by injection or by operation.

2. *Thrombophlebitis.* Thrombosis may occur spontaneously in the stagnant column of blood within a varicose vein or may be secondary to trauma of the leg. Thrombosis is intentionally induced, of course, by the sclerosing fluid used in the injection treatment of varicose veins. The affected segment of vein becomes tender and hard and the overlying skin may be red and hot. There is often a mild pyrexia

and malaise. This is not an infective condition but is due simply to the tissue reaction to the segment of blood clot within the vein. Bacterial infection is only seen when an infected injection or intravenous infusion has been given into the vein.

Treatment: since this is a chemical and not a bacterial reaction, there is no indication at all for antibiotic therapy. The patient requires bed rest if the condition is very severe, with the foot of the bed elevated and a mild pressure bandage applied to the leg. Generally, however, the condition is not sufficiently serious to require bed rest and will respond to the use of an elastic stocking and a suitable analgesic, for example Paracetamol. Anti-coagulant therapy is never indicated because the thrombus is adherent to the wall of the vein and there is no risk of its detachment with the formation of a pulmonary embolus.

3. *Ulceration.* An ulcer may be defined as an area where epithelium has been lost, and the commonest ulcer by far is the so-called varicose ulcer. A better name is a 'gravitational ulcer' since this includes the concept of the cause of the condition as the high venous pressure within the leg veins. The immediate precipitating factor which may result in an ulcer is a trivial injury to the affected skin (Fig. 8.15).

A rare complication of a longstanding ulcer is malignant change in its edge with the result that this becomes raised above the surface (Marjolin's ulcer).

Treatment: the high venous pressure within the incompetent veins and the superficial venous system can be abolished by putting the patient to bed with the foot elevated. Under these circumstances the venous abnormality is corrected and tissue health is improved. However, this simple treatment is not always a practical one as quite often the patients are elderly and prolonged recumbency will carry with it the dangers of venous thrombosis, pressure sores and chest infection. The other way to abolish the high venous pressure is to use elastic bandaging of the leg from the toes to the knee. This acts by emptying the superficial dilated veins, thus enabling the muscles of the leg to pump the venous blood back towards the heart. There is absolutely no need to place exotic ointments on the ulcer and antibiotics should at all costs be avoided; indeed, all that is required is some bland dressing to apply to the ulcer itself in order to prevent the Elastoplast from sticking to it. The most commonly used dressing is Viscopaste, although other preparations are available if this does not suit the patient. If the skin of the patient is badly affected by varicose eczema, Icthopaste may be used or if there is an extensive scaly eruption of the skin, coal tar paste is the dressing of choice. The technique involved in dressing the leg is

Peripheral vascular disease

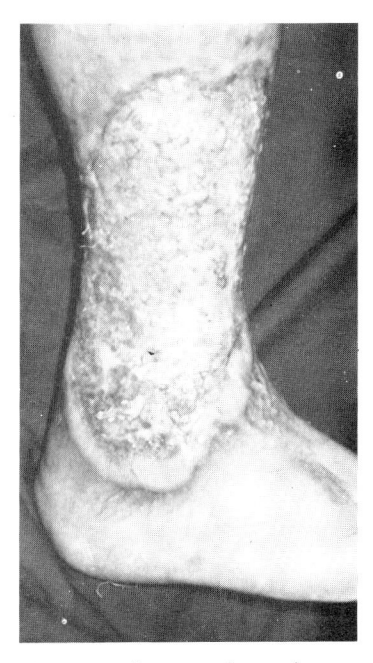

Fig. 8.15. An extensive varicose ulcer.

important. The bland bandage dressing is applied without wrinkles and then over the top of this Elastoplast is applied in smooth circular sweeps so that an even and firm pressure is applied to the whole of the leg and foot to the level of the knee (Fig. 8.16).

Once the elastic bandage has been applied to the leg, the patient should be advised to sleep with the foot of the bed elevated to encourage venous return, and should also walk about as much as possible to encourage muscle pumping. The first bandage is removed after a week, because there will often have been considerable oozing through the dressing. Once this has ceased, the next bandage can be left on for two or sometimes three weeks and progressive healing will be seen to take place. Small ulcers will heal in a few weeks, although larger ulcers will take several months of patient dressings before epithelialisation is complete.

Occasionally, very extensive ulcers may require skin graft and

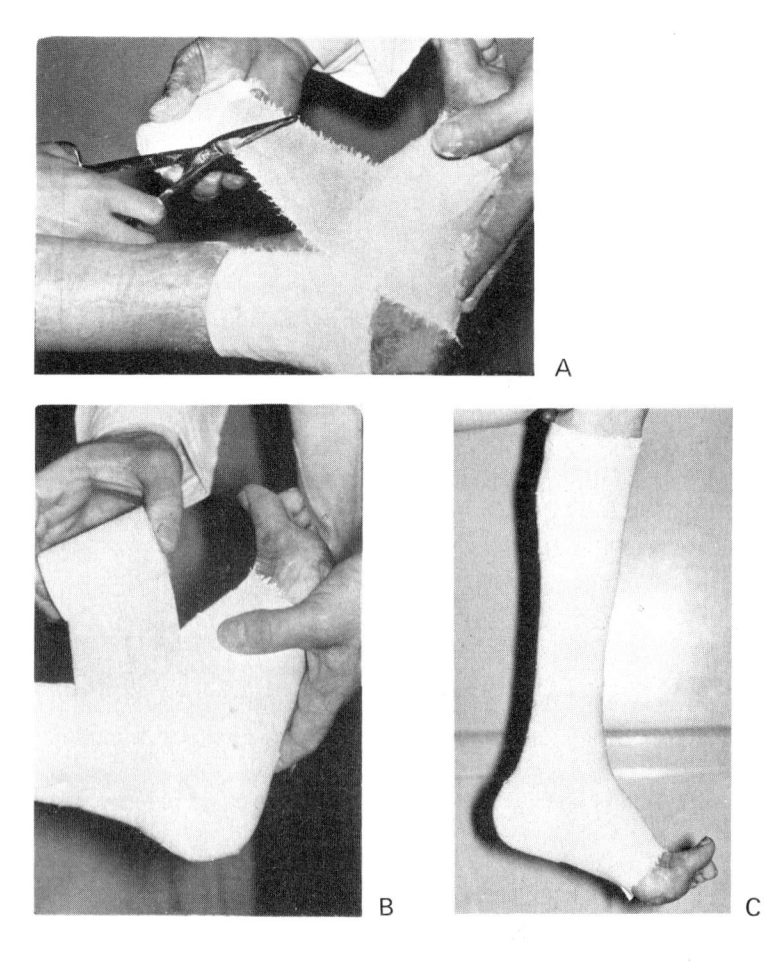

Fig. 8.16. Steps in the bandaging of a varicose ulcer. A sterile gauze dressing is placed over the ulcer and the eczematous skin is protected with a Viscopaste bandage (A). Elastoplast bandaging is commenced distally (B) and continued to below the knee (C).

now and again ulceration is so extensive with destruction of the underlying tissues and fixing of the ankle joint that patients are advised to submit to below-knee amputation.

Other causes of ulcers of the leg

Gravitational ulcers account for 9 out of every 10 ulcers seen in this country. The most important of the others is the ischaemic ulcer due to impaired arterial blood supply. This should be diagnosed if the foot is felt to be cold and pale, the patient complains of intermittent claudication on walking and the peripheral pulses are absent. An ulcerated tumour may be a breaking-down melanoma or a squamous carcinoma of the skin, but this often arises in a pre-existing chronic ulcer. A gumma in advanced syphilis used to be common, but it is now only rarely seen. Ulcers may complicate some medical diseases including ulcerative colitis, rheumatoid arthritis and acholuric jaundice. From time to time we see self-inflicted ulcers on the leg, and this should be suspected if the ulcer has a peculiar shape such as an exact square and also if the patient has an unusual psychological make-up.

Chapter 9. The lymphatics and lymph nodes

INTRODUCTION

The lymphatics are fine, thin walled tubes which ramify through all the tissues of the body with the exceptions of the central nervous system and cartilage. They are concerned with the circulation of tissue fluid, which passes into the lymphatics and is then shunted into the venous system. In addition, lymphatics can take up fine particulate matter and this is of particular importance in the intestine, where the bulk of fat is absorbed in this manner into the lymphatics of the gut wall. The lymphatics filter through the lymph nodes, which number approximately 800, and which are found particularly in the neck, axillae, groin, the mesenteries of the alimentary canal and in the mediastinum. The lymph drains back into the blood stream principally via the thoracic duct, which opens into the commencement of the left innominate vein at the root of the neck, and the smaller lymph ducts, which open in the major veins (subclavian and jugular) on the right side of the neck.

The lymph nodes serve the following functions:

1. As filters for bacteria and other foreign particles, including cancer cells.
2. As the sites of production of lymphocytes.
3. As centres which respond to foreign proteins (*antigens*) to produce *antibodies* from the plasma cells and to develop sensitised lymphocytes. These two processes are the fundamentals of the immune response to any foreign proteins, which include bacteria, viruses, transplanted tissues, such as kidneys, and probably also cancers.

ACUTE LYMPHADENITIS

The particulate material which may be taken up by the lymphatics includes bacteria, and these organisms may produce an acute inflammation of the lymphatics draining an infected area (*acute lymphangitis*). This is especially likely to occur with streptococcal infection and is characterised by the appearance of red streaks along the skin which correspond to the lymphatic channels. At the same time, the draining lymph nodes become swollen and tender (*acute lymphadenitis*) and these may indeed suppurate, with abscess formation.

Treatment

This condition, once extremely serious, can now be treated very satisfactorily with antibiotic therapy. Rapid resolution takes place, provided that the organism is sensitive to the antibiotic employed. The wound itself or the regional nodes, if either or both are the site of abscess formation, will require surgical drainage.

Fig. 9.1. Congenital lymphoedema of the right leg and the scrotum.

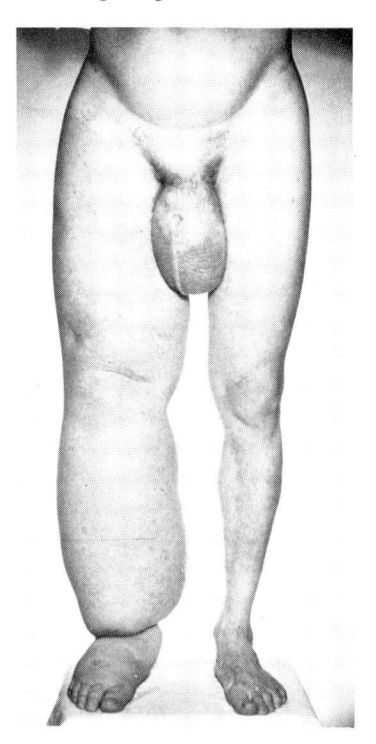

LYMPHOEDEMA

Obstruction of the lymphatic flow from any cause results in the accumulation of fluid in the affected region, for which the term *lymphoedema* is applied. The common causes of lymphoedema are:

1. *Congenital abnormality of the lymphatics of the lower limbs*
Lymphoedema in these patients may be present at birth but usually develops early in adult life. Females are more affected than males, and the conditions may run in families (Fig. 9.1).

2. *Post-inflammatory*
Repeated attacks of acute lymphangitis may result in obliteration of the lymphatics by fibrous tissue.

3. *Filariasis*
A tropical disease due to the nematode worm Filaria bancrofti which is transmitted by the mosquito. The filaria infects the lymphatics with consequent fibrotic lymphatic obstruction. This results in gross lymphoedema, especially of the lower limbs and the genitalia.
Chylous ascites may also complicate this condition—the peritoneal cavity becoming filled with milky lymphatic exudate.

4. *Following radical surgery*
Extensive removal of the lymphatics, for example block dissection of the groin or the neck in the treatment of malignant disease, may be followed by lymphoedema.

5. *Post-irradiation fibrosis*

Heavy irradiation in the treatment of malignant disease may obliterate the lymphatics in the treated area, and this state of affairs may be aggravated by previous radical surgery. Lymphoedema of the arm, for example, may be seen after an extensive radical mastectomy, in which the axillary lymph nodes have been removed, and which has then been followed by a full course of irradiation.

6. *Malignant disease*

Extensive secondary deposits in the lymph nodes frequently produce sufficient lymphatic obstruction to result in lymphoedema. Late oedema of the upper limb after mastectomy is often indicative of massive recurrence of tumour in the axilla, occluding any residual lymphatic pathways (Fig. 9.2).

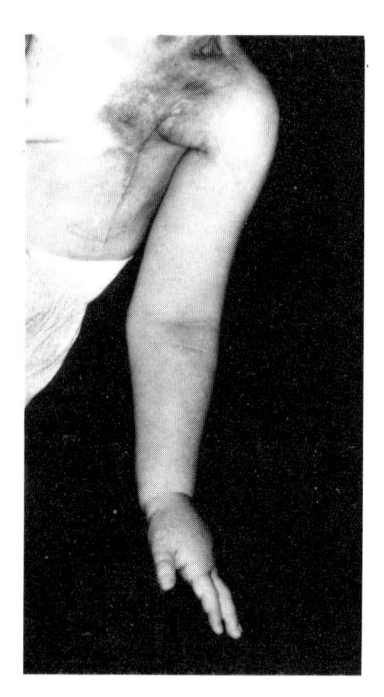

Fig. 9.2. Lymphoedema of the arm. The patient has had a previous mastectomy and radiotherapy and has now developed recurrent tumour in the axilla and supraclavicular fossa.

Differential diagnosis

There are, of course, many other causes of oedema apart from disturbance of lymphatic drainage. Increased venous pressure, either from venous obstruction or from congestive cardiac failure, causes transudation of fluid into the tissues as a result of high pressure in the capillary vessels. Conditions which lower the plasma protein (starvation, the nephrotic syndrome, cirrhosis, etc.) produce a lowered osmotic pressure of the plasma which results in decreased fluid take up of tissue fluid through the capillaries.

Treatment

The treatment of lymphoedema naturally depends to a great extent on its aetiology. Conservative treatment comprises elevation of the affected limb and the use of elastic compression by means of either an elastic bandage or stocking. Gross cases of congenital lymphoedema may be treated surgically by excision of the oedematous subcutaneous tissue. This will restore the contour of the leg, but leave it with considerable scarring.

The massive brawny arm or leg that is seen in late cases of malignant obstruction of the lymphatics is a serious and intractable condition which can only be helped slightly by limb elevation, elastic bandages and analgesic drugs.

THE LYMPHADENOPATHIES

This is a convenient term for the group of conditions characterised by enlargement of the lymph nodes, the causes of which can be classified as follows:

1. Acute infection.
2. Chronic infection.
3. Neoplastic—due to secondary spread of tumour.
4. The reticuloses.
   (a) Hodgkin's Disease
   (b) Lymphosarcoma and reticulum cell sarcoma
   (c) Lymphatic leukaemia.

Enlarged lymph nodes may also be seen in sarcoidosis and rheumatoid arthritis.

The acute infective causes may be due to some local infection. The commonest example of all is the cervical lymphadenopathy secondary to tonsillitis, which nearly everybody has experienced at some time. But lymph nodes draining any area where there is an acute infection may become inflamed.

A generalised infection associated with enlarged lymph nodes is *glandular fever* (infective mononucleosis) which is a viral infection associated with enlarged lymph nodes, fever, a sore throat, a rash, and sometimes enlargement of the spleen. The blood film shows a raised total count, in the region of 15,000 white cells, the majority of which are monocytes.

Of the chronic infections, *tuberculosis* is the commonest and is considered below. Enlarged lymph nodes are found in the area draining a primary syphilitic chancre and a generalised enlargement of lymph nodes may occur in the secondary stage of syphilis.

Neoplastic nodes are hard and, as they enlarge, may become matted together and eventually ulcerate through the skin. Common examples are the enlarged axillary nodes found in carcinoma of the breast or the cervical nodes associated with cancer within the oral cavity.

The reticuloses usually produce rubbery enlarged nodes, frequently affecting more than one anatomical site. The liver, spleen and other organs may be involved and enlarged.

TUBERCULOUS LYMPHADENITIS

With a general decline in tuberculosis, this once common lesion (mainly of children) is now quite unusual in this country. However, the incidence has shown some rise recently, particularly among immigrants. The cervical nodes are most commonly involved, the bacilli having entered via the tonsil. The organisms may be human or bovine, the latter due to the ingestion of milk contaminated with tubercle bacilli. Occasionally enlarged cervical nodes are found in elderly patients who usually have active tuberculosis of the lung apex.

It is quite common on routine X-rays of the chest and abdomen to see calcified nodes in the mediastinum or mesentery. These represent burnt out tuberculous disease resulting from a previous pulmonary inoculation in the case of the mediastinal nodes, or the ingestion of bovine organisms in contaminated milk with subsequent take-up by the intestinal lymphatics in the case of the mesenteric nodes. Tuberculous lymphadenitis in the neck commences as a group of small discrete painless nodes, usually found in the upper part of the neck in the carotid triangle. As they enlarge they become matted together, break down into a tuberculous abscess, which then bursts through into the subcutaneous tissues. This is a chronic abscess and, unlike the usual acute affair, there is very little pain and although the skin may be reddened it does not feel hot to the touch. For this reason the term *'cold abscess'* is applied to this lesion (Fig. 9.3). Left untreated, the abscess will discharge spontaneously onto the skin with the formation of a chronic tuberculous sinus. Fig. 9.4 shows diagrammatically the stages of the progression of this condition.

Solid nodes must be differentiated from acute lymphadenitis, from secondary deposits or from one of the reticuloses. At the stage of a breaking down abscess the differential diagnosis is from a branchial cyst. Diagnosis is assisted by an X-ray of the neck, because usually the chronic tuberculous nodes show flecks of calcification, which are not seen in other causes of lymph node enlargement.

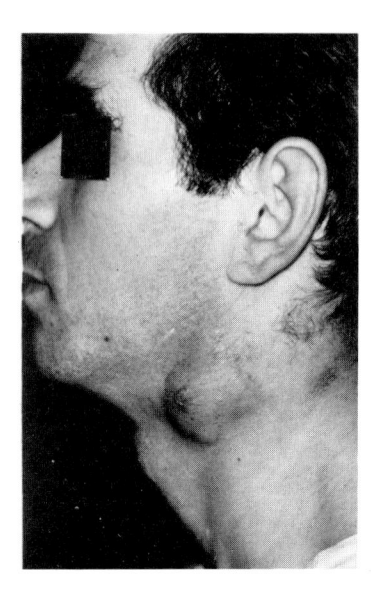

Fig. 9.3. A tuberculous 'cold abscess' of the neck.

Treatment

If the patient is seen at an early stage, before abscess formation has occurred, it is possible to excise the enlarged node. If the patient presents with an abscess already present, the pus is evacuated and the underlying breaking down tuberculous nodes evacuated by curettage. Once the diagnosis has been confirmed by pathological examination of the node and bacteriological study of the pus, a full course of anti-tuberculous chemotherapy is commenced. This normally comprises an initial three months of triple therapy with streptomycin, PAS and INAH followed by a further nine months in which the latter two drugs only are administered. In addition, the patient's general condition is improved by a full diet and fresh air.

SECONDARY CARCINOMA

One of the commonest causes of enlarged lymph nodes is the presence of secondary deposits from a primary carcinoma which lies in the area of lymphatic drainage of that particular group of nodes. Thus nodes in the groin may derive from a tumour situated anywhere

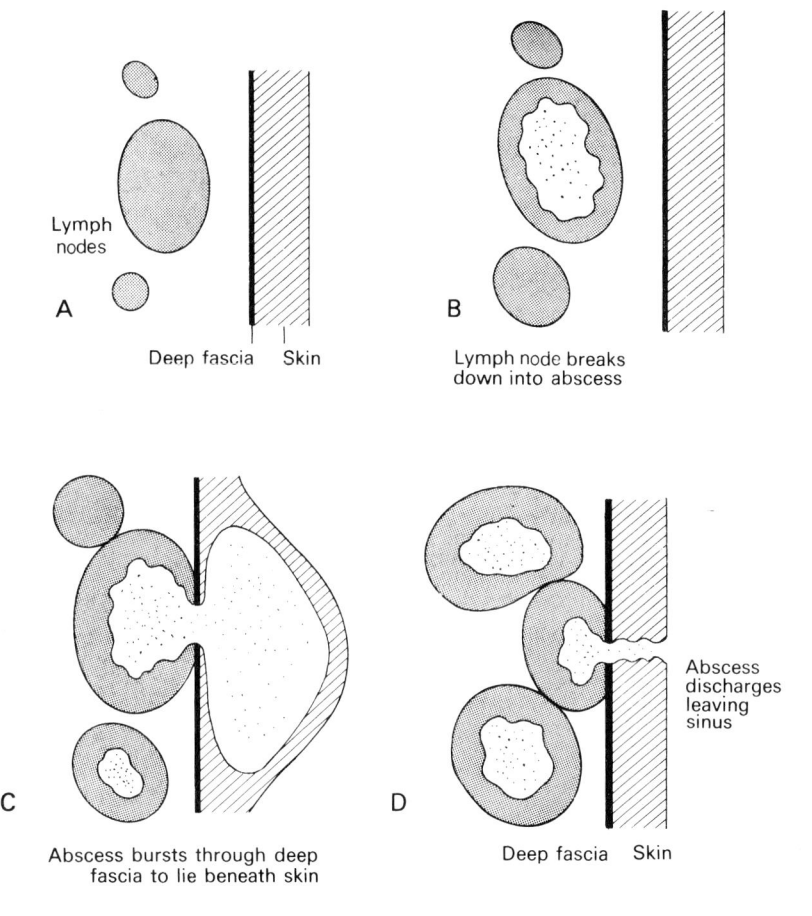

Fig. 9.4. Tuberculous infection of cervical lymph nodes leading to a 'cold abscess' and eventually a chronic sinus.

along the leg, buttock, lower abdominal wall, external genitalia, or lower part of the anal canal; axillary nodes may be involved from a primary of the upper limb or breast, and enlarged cervical lymph nodes may be secondary to a primary growth of the face, the mouth, larynx, pharynx, oesophagus, bronchus, breast, or thyroid. The cervical nodes may also be involved via the thoracic duct from the primary tumour situated in the breast, stomach, large intestine, or the testis (Fig. 9.5).

Treatment

The treatment of secondarily involved lymph nodes in the common tumours is dealt with in the appropriate sections, but here we may sum up by saying that, as a rule, enlarged superficial nodes which are mobile may be removed by block dissection provided that the

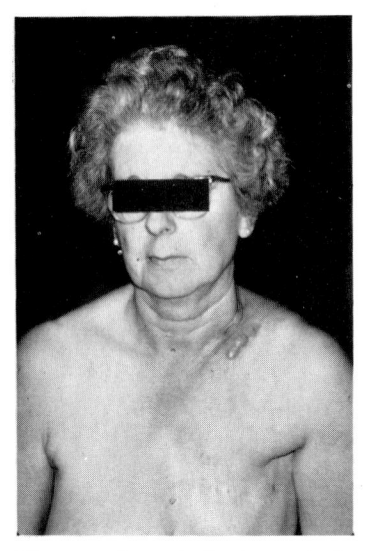

Fig. 9.5. Secondaries in cervical lymph nodes following a mastectomy for carcinoma of the left breast.

Fig. 9.6. Hodgkins' disease affecting the right cervical lymph nodes.

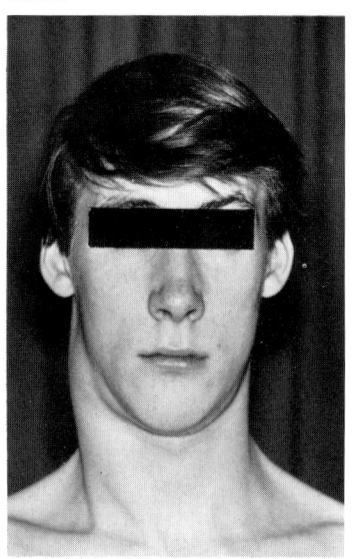

primary tumour is either operable or can be treated effectively by radiotherapy. For example, a patient with a carcinoma of the tongue may have this treated by a radium implantation, following which block dissection of a group of enlarged but mobile nodes in the neck may be carried out. If the primary tumour is inoperable because of fixation and invasion, or if the nodes themselves have now reached the stage where they are matted and fixed to surrounding structures, then obviously radical surgery is out of the question, and usually palliative radiotherapy is employed. A frequent cause of death in such circumstances is ulceration of the lymph nodes, leading to lethal haemorrhage from invaded adjacent blood vessels.

THE RETICULOSES

Primary tumours of lymphoid tissues are termed the reticuloses or malignant lymphomas. The most important of these are:
1. Hodgkin's Disease.
2. Reticulum cell sarcoma.
3. Lymphosarcoma.
4. Chronic lymphatic leukaemia.

These conditions usually present with lymph node enlargement, particularly the cervical nodes, but any group or groups of lymph nodes may be affected, including the mediastinal, abdominal or retroperitoneal groups. Spread from one lymph node group to another frequently occurs, and there may be involvement of spleen, liver, bone marrow and other tissues. Males are more often affected than females. Hodgkin's disease particularly affects young adults, whereas the other reticuloses are more often seen in more elderly patients (Fig. 9.6).

The differential diagnosis between the various types depends on the microscopic examination of a lymph node taken at biopsy.

Hodgkin's disease is characterised by replacement of the normal lymph node architecture by pleomorphic tissue made up of mononuclear cells, giant cells (containing several nuclei), lymphocytes, eosinophils and fibrous tissue, although there is wide variation in the microscopic appearance of this condition.

Reticulum cell sarcoma is made up of undifferentiated cells which, on special staining, show interspersed reticulin fibres.

Lymphosarcoma is made up of darkly staining lymphoid cells. Chronic lymphatic leukaemia gives the same histological picture as lymphosarcoma, but is characterised by the presence of large numbers of abnormal lymphocytes in the blood, the count rising to between 30,000 and 300,000.

Treatment

Some examples of localised lymphoma, for example, Hodgkin's disease confined to one group of superficial nodes, or a lymphosarcoma localised to a segment of intestine, may be treated by surgical excision. In the main, treatment depends on radiotherapy and/or cytotoxic therapy.

Chapter 10. The central nervous system

HYDROCEPHALUS

The circulation of the cerebro-spinal fluid (C.S.F.)

Hydrocephalus is gross distension of all or part of the ventricular system of the brain by cerebro-spinal fluid. It is therefore essential to understand the production, circulation and absorption of C.S.F. if the mechanism and treatment of this condition is to be understood.

C.S.F. is produced by the choroid plexuses of the lateral, third and fourth ventricles (Fig. 10.1). These plexuses are made up of vascular folds derived from the lining epithelium of the ventricles. The fluid escapes from the 4th ventricle through a mid-line and two lateral foramina into the subarachnoid space surrounding the brain. About four fifths of the fluid is reabsorbed via the arachnoid villi; these are minute projections of the arachnoid mater which pierce the dura covering the venous sinuses to lie immediately

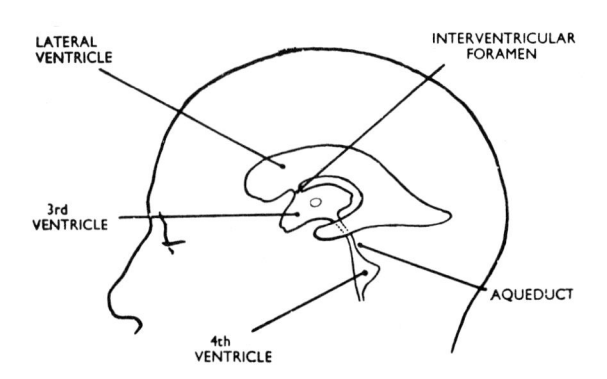

Fig. 10.1. The ventricular system.

beneath their endothelium and pump C.S.F. back into the venous blood stream. The remaining one fifth of the C.S.F. is absorbed by the arachnoid villi in the spinal segment of the dural sheath or else escapes along the spinal nerve sheaths to be absorbed in the lymphatics.

The C.S.F. itself is a water-clear fluid containing electrolytes similar to those in the blood plasma together with glucose.

The total quantity of C.S.F. in the adult is about 150 ml and approximately 500 ml of this fluid is produced daily.

Obstruction anywhere along the C.S.F. pathway produces a rise in pressure and then dilatation within the system proximal to the block. This resulting hydrocephalus can be divided into:

1. *Obstructive.* Here the fluid cannot escape due to blockage within the duct system. This may be produced by a congenital abnormality, a chronic abscess, scarring from previous trauma, or by pressure from a tumour. One form of congenital stenosis is the *Arnold-Chiari malformation* which is a congenital downward protrusion of the cerebellum through the foramen magnum of the skull. There is consequent occlusion of the foramina of the 4th ventricle, and hydrocephalus ensues. Frequently this condition is associated with spina bifida.

2. *Communicating.* C.S.F. can escape from within the brain but absorption via the villi is prevented by obliteration of the subarachnoid channels. This may be the result of meningitis, birth trauma, or perhaps congenital failure of development of the arachnoid villi.

Clinical features

From the clinical point of view hydrocephalus may be sub-divided into two important groups: the first comprises the congenital type, and the second the acquired variety who present with features of raised intracranial pressure as described later in the chapter.

Congenital hydrocephalus is usually of the communicating type but may be produced by congenital stenosis within the ventricular system of the brain or the Arnold-Chiari malformation (See above).

The enlargement of the head may occur before birth and may be a cause of obstructed labour. After birth rapid enlargement of the head takes place and produces a typical clinical picture (Fig. 10.2). The head is large, the fontanelles are wide, tense and fail to close at the normal times, the skin is stretched over the skull and dilated cutaneous veins are present over the scalp. Typical of the condition is the downward displacement of the eyes, and the brow overhangs

Central nervous system

Fig. 10.2. Congenital hydrocephalus. Note the dilated cutaneous veins over the enormous skull.

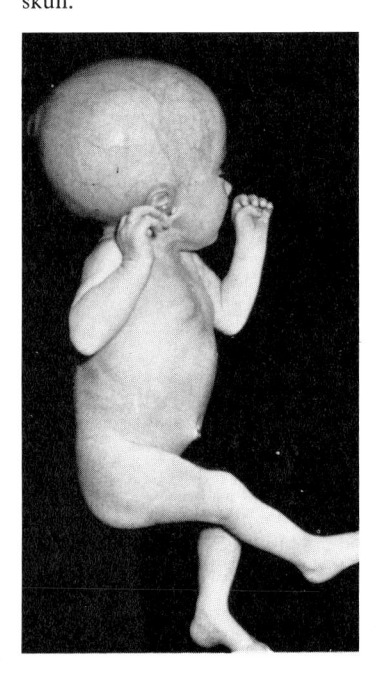

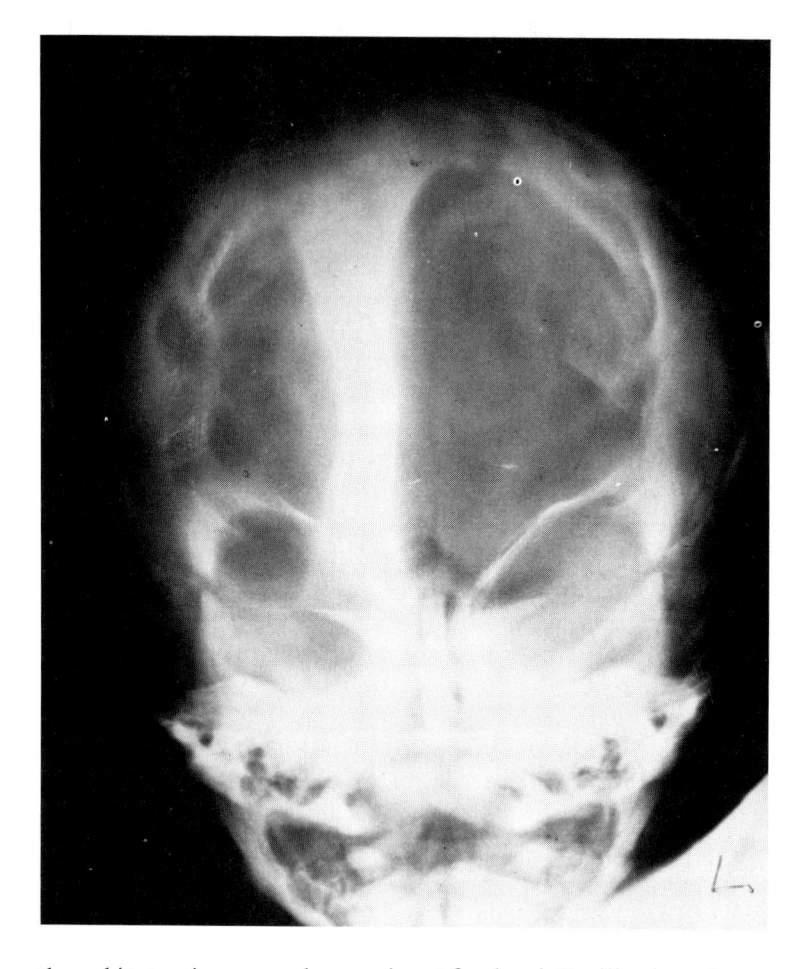

Fig. 10.3. X-ray of the skull of a child with hydrocephalus. The cortex of the brain is thin and the enormous ventricles can be seen.

the orbits to give a grossly prominent forehead. Papilloedema is not present. There may be associated congenital deformities, especially spina bifida. The cortex of the brain is extensively thinned and the ventricles may become enormous (Fig. 10.3). In such cases mental deterioration is naturally severe.

In some infants with congenital hydrocephalus, natural arrest occurs, presumably as a result of recanalisation of the subarachnoid spaces. In the remainder there is steady progression with inevitable increasing brain damage and high mortality unless treatment is instituted.

Treatment

In congenital hydrocephalus of the progressive variety, a Spitz-Holter shunt is inserted (Fig. 10.4). This is an ingenious plastic tube which is passed from the lateral ventricle through a burr-hole

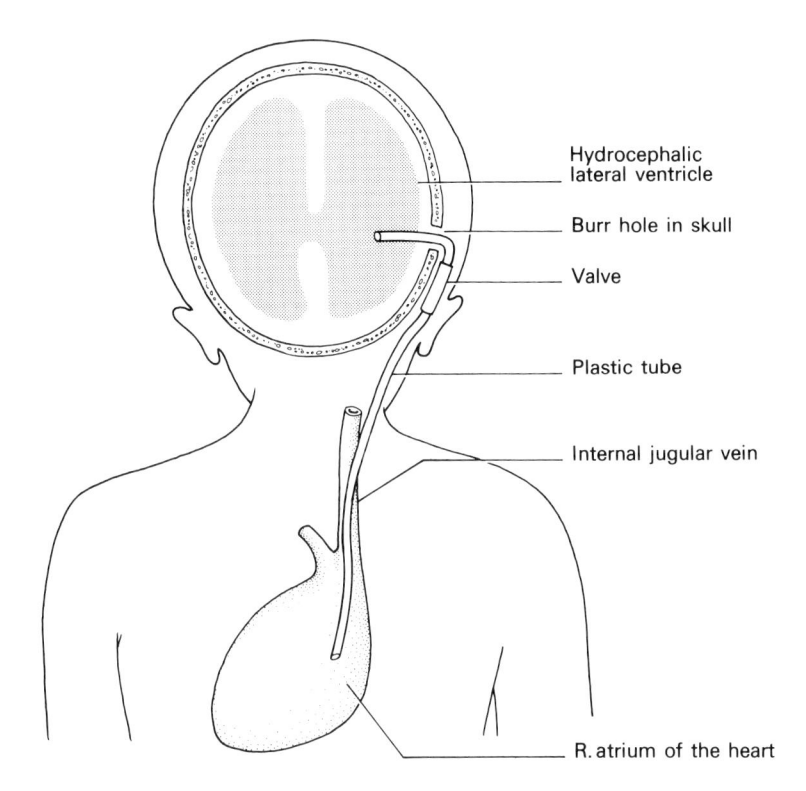

Fig. 10.4. Diagram of a Spitz-Holter valve, which shunts CSF from the dilated lateral ventricle into the right atrium. The valve prevents reflux of blood along the tube. (The child is viewed from behind).

to beneath the scalp, where it connects with a one-way valve. From this, the tube continues into the neck where it is threaded along the internal jugular vein into the right atrium of the heart. The valve mechanism allows C.S.F. above a set pressure to pass into the blood stream without allowing reflux of blood into the subarachnoid space.

One great risk of this operation is of infection of the catheter with resultant septicaemia; this may make removal of the shunt imperative.

In obstructive hydrocephalus direct removal of the cause of the occlusion is obviously the treatment of choice. Where this is impossible, the block may be short circuited by the *Torkildsen operation* of ventriculo-cisternotomy, in which a plastic tube is threaded into the lateral ventricle through a burr hole and then carried down into the cisterna magna through a cerebella exposure (Fig. 10.5).

SPACE OCCUPYING LESIONS

Space occupying lesions within the skull may be:
1. A haematoma following trauma (see page 155).
2. Cerebral abscess.

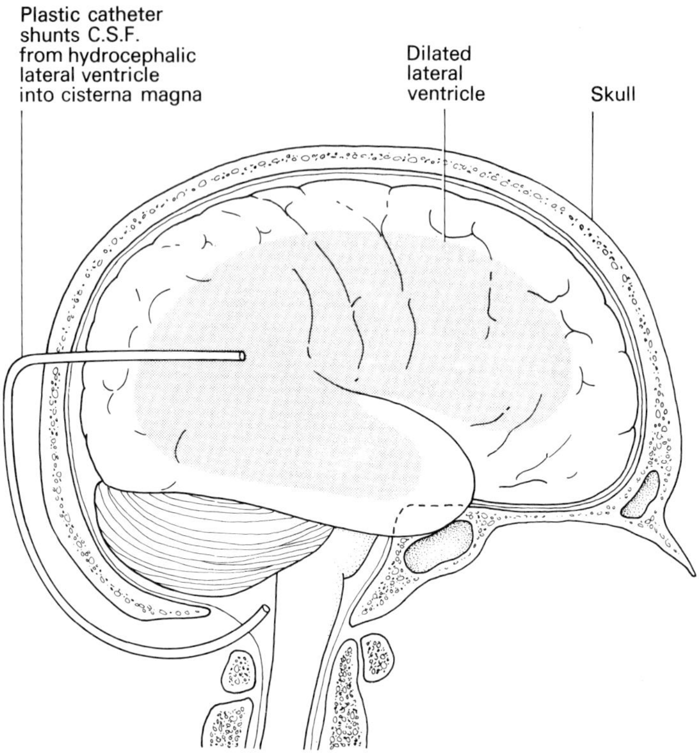

Fig. 10.5. Ventriculo-cisternotomy for obstructive hydrocephalus (Torkildsen operation).

3. An intracranial tumour—today by far the commonest cause. Other causes are rare in this country, although from time to time curiosities such as hydatid cyst or a syphilitic gumma are encountered.

Clinical features

A space-occupying lesion may produce raised intracranial pressure and/or localising signs in the central nervous system.

Raised intra-cranial pressure

A mass within the skull produces raised intracranial pressure, partly by its actual presence within the enclosed space of the cranium, partly by surrounding oedema, and sometimes by impeding the circulation CSF with the production of hydrocephalus (See page 133. If the rise in pressure within the skull is slowly progressive, the following features may be found:

1. *Headache*. This is severe and is often present when the patient wakes from his sleep; it is aggravated by straining or coughing.
2. *Vomiting*, which typically is often without preceding nausea.
3. *Papilloedema*—the raised pressure produces swelling of the optic disc of the fundus seen through an ophthalmoscope. This may be accompanied by blurring of vision and may even progress to blindness.
4. *Mental deterioration*—the patient may undergo a marked personality deterioration, become demented, or drowsy and eventually lapses into coma.

Localising signs

Localising signs will depend on the situation of the tumour. Severe personality change suggests frontal lobe involvement, spastic hemiplegia points to involvement of the internal capsule and defects in the visual field indicate pressure on the optic pathway, whereas cerebellar lesions are associated with inco-ordination, dizziness and often nystagmus (a flickering of the eyes on lateral deviation).

CEREBRAL ABSCESS

There are three common causes of brain abscess:
1. *A penetrating wound* of the skull, which allows direct access of bacteria into the brain.
2. *Direct spread* from an infection of the middle ear, the mastoid, or the frontal nasal sinus.
3. *Blood-borne spread*, especially from a lung infection (e.g. lung abscess or bronchiectasis).

Clinical features

The patient may present with features of the underlying cause, for example, a mastoid infection or a penetrating brain wound, followed by evidence of the development of an intracranial space-occupying lesion. During the early stages there may be marked toxaemia, fever and meningeal irritation. However, once the abscess is walled off, the general manifestations of infection may not be evident and the features we have already listed—headache, vomiting, papilloedema and mental deterioration—may dominate the picture.

Accurate localization of the abscess may require special investigations, including an electro-encephalogram, gamma scan, and cerebral angiography.

Treatment

Once the abscess is localised it should be aspirated by means of a brain needle passed through a burr hole. The pus is replaced with antibiotic together with a radio-opaque solution, which enables subsequent X-ray studies to be made (Fig. 10.6). The aspirations may require to be repeated and systemic antibiotics are given depending on the bacteriology report on the pus.

Occasionally the abscess fails to respond to aspiration, and its capsule must then be excised surgically.

INTRACRANIAL TUMOURS

It is a fascinating fact that the only cells in the human body that never give rise to tumours are the nerve cells of the C.N.S. This is because although all other tissues are constantly being replaced at a greater or lesser speed throughout life, no new brain cells form once our basic quota is established in fetal life—a thought that can give rise to a great deal of interesting philosophical discussion. Primary intracranial tumours can therefore only develop from the supporting framework of connective tissue cells (neruroglia) or from the numerous structures which surround the brain—the meninges, cranial nerves, the pituitary and pineal glands, blood vessels and the skull. Added to this it is important to remember that secondary deposits in the brain are very common. In specialised neurosurgical units they account for only about 15% of the cases seen, but many patients dying of widespread metastases have intracranial deposits and these do not usually come under specialist neurological care.

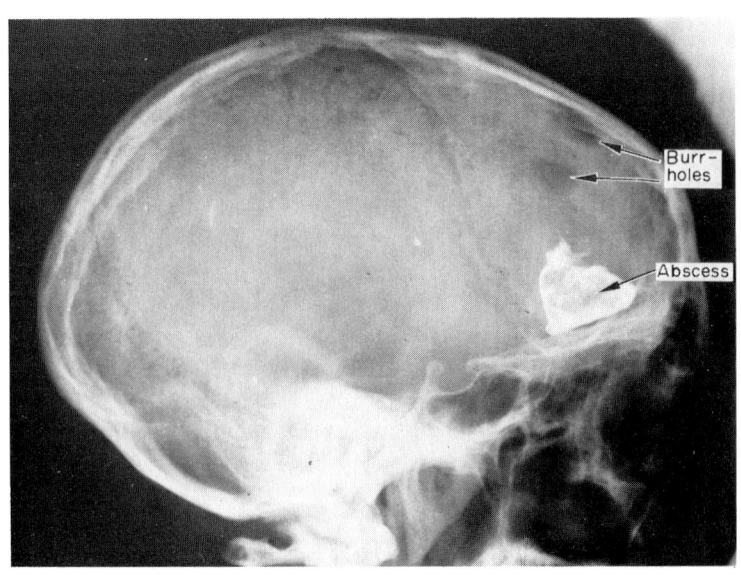

Fig. 10.6. Cerebral abscess shown by injection of radio-opaque dye following aspiration of the pus through a burr-hole.

The incidence of the various intracranial tumours encountered at a neurosurgical unit is approximately:

> Glioma—45%
> Meningioma—15%
> Metastases—15%
> Acoustic Tumours—5%
> Pituitary Tumours—5%
> All others—15%

Gliomas

The gliomas arise from the neuroglial supporting cells and are responsible for about 45% of intracerebral tumours (Fig. 10.7). They are classified according to the principal cell component and details of this highly complex field of neuropathology can be obtained in larger text books than this. The tumours vary considerably in their histological differentiation and invasiveness from highly anaplastic and rapidly destructive tumours to relatively benign, cystic, slowly growing lesions.

Meningioma

These account for 15% of intracranial tumours and arise from the dura mater, to which they are almost invariably attached. Typically they occur in middle-aged patients. The majority are slowly growing and do not invade the brain tissue, but involve it only by expansion

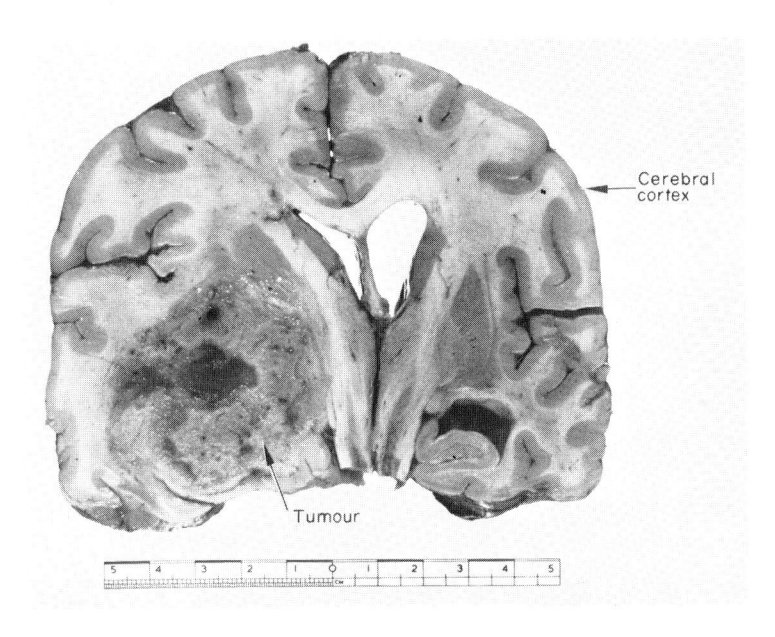

Fig. 10.7. A highly malignant glioma. Note the compression and displacement of the lateral ventricle by the tumour.

and pressure, so that they may eventually become buried in the brain. The tumour may invade the overlying skull producing a hyperostosis which may occasionally be enormous.

Acoustic tumours

Cranial nerve tumours arise from the cells of the nerve sheaths. The great majority arise from the 8th cranial nerve (the auditory nerve) and this accounts for 5% of intracranial tumours. It is usually found in adult patients.

As the acoustic tumour enlarges it stretches the adjacent cranial nerves, especially the 5th (trigeminal) and 7th (facial), as well as pressing on the neighbouring cerebellum and the brain stem. Initially, damage to the auditory nerve itself produces unilateral nerve deafness with giddiness and ringing in the ear (tinnitus). Pressure on the 5th and 7th nerves produces facial numbness and facial paralysis respectively, while compression of the cerebellum results in nystagmus and motor inco-ordination. Eventually features of raised intracranial pressure become evident.

Pituitary tumours

These account for about 5% of intracranial tumours. They have two special features—their endocrine disturbances and their relationship to the optic chiasma.

Pituitary tumours are classified by the staining reaction of their cells into chromophobe adenomas, whose cells are non-granular, eosinophilic tumours, whose cells have granules which stain with eosin, and basophilic tumours whose cell granules stain with basic dyes.

Chromophobe adenoma is the commonest pituitary tumour. As it enlarges it compresses the optic chiasma, producing blindness in both temporal fields (Fig. 10.8). It is a non-secretory tumour which gradually destroys the normally functioning pituitary. In childhood there is arrest of growth and in adults there is loss of sex characteristics. As the tumour extends there may be involvement of the adjacent hypothalamus with diabetes insipidus and obesity.

Eosinophil adenoma secretes the pituitary growth hormones. If it occurs before puberty it induces gigantism. After puberty acromegaly results (Fig. 10.9).

Basophil adenoma is small, produces no pressure effects, but is associated with hyperplasia of the adrenal cortex and Cushing's syndrome (see page 385).

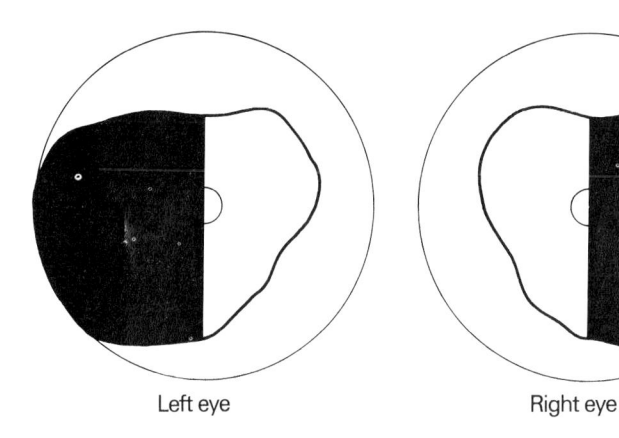

Fig. 10.8. Visual field chart in a patient with a pituitary tumour. Note the blindness in both temporal fields (bitemporal hemianopia), marked black on the chart.

Secondary tumours

Particular primary sites of origin are from carcinomas of the lung, breast and kidney. Small multiple deposits tend to be scattered through the brain, so that early features are personality change and confusion leading later to coma.

Special investigations

X-rays of the skull. Areas of calcification may be seen in 10% of tumours. The pineal gland is often calcified in adults and inspection of the films of the skull may show a shift of the pineal to one side, indicating a space-occupying lesion. Enlargement or erosion of the pituitary fossa suggests the presence of a pituitary tumour.

X-ray of the chest must always be performed to exclude a primary bronchogenic carcinoma, which is the commonest source of brain metastases.

Brain scan with radioactive isotopes is extremely important as a simple and painless method of obtaining a positive localising diagnosis (Fig. 10.10).

Air studies. Air may be introduced into the ventricles either through a burr-hole (*ventriculography*) or via a lumbar or cisternal puncture (*air encaphalography*). Deformity or displacement of the ventricles may outline a space-occupying tumour.

Cerebral angiography. An intracranial tumour may be localised by injecting radio opaque dye into the carotid artery. An abnormal vascular pattern may be seen in the tumour or the vessels may be seen to be displaced by the growth from their normal positions (Fig. 10.11).

Fig. 10.9. Acromegaly due to an eosinophil adenoma of the pituitary. Note the coarse enlarged features.

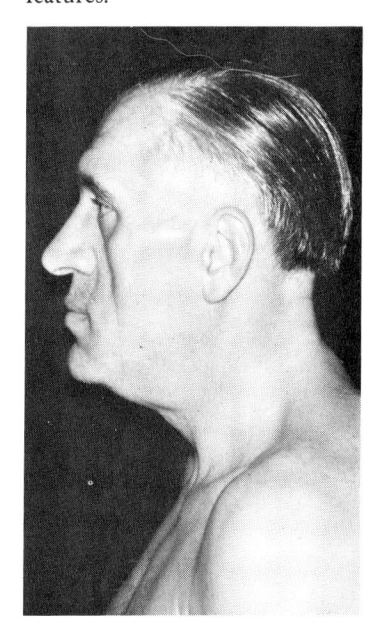

Fig. 10.10. Brain scan demonstrating a cerebral tumour, which shows as the relatively dense area.

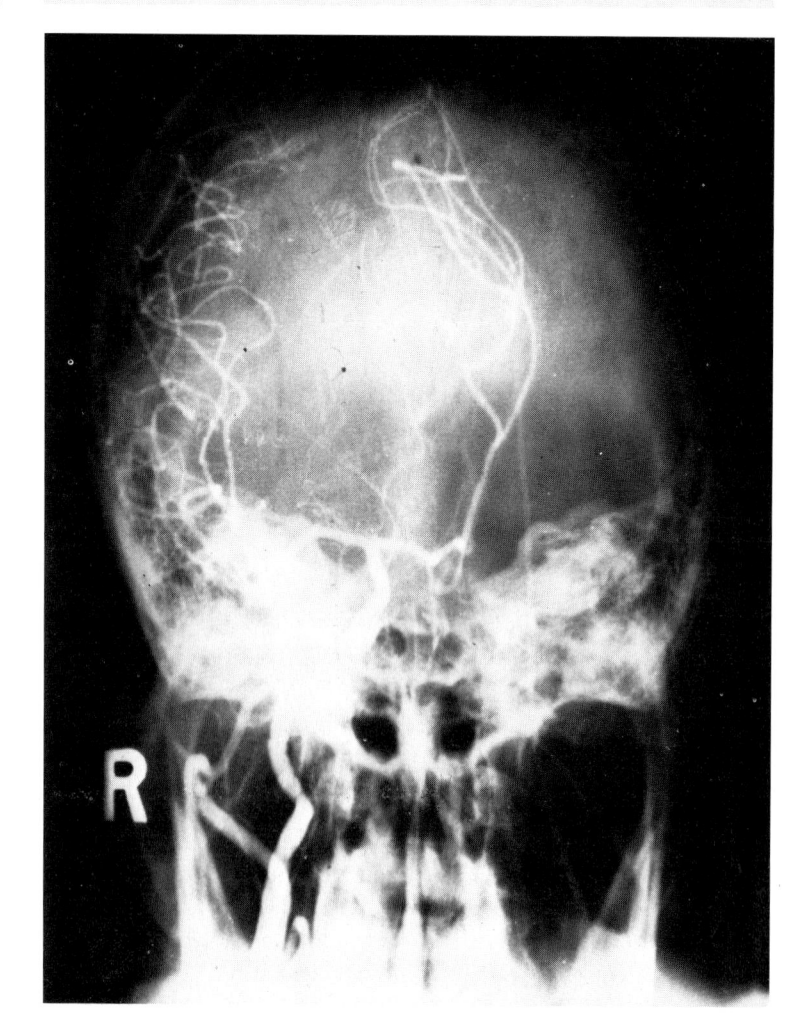

Fig. 10.11. A large right-sided cerebral tumour demonstrated by angiography. Note that the anterior cerebral artery, which should be in the mid-line, is displaced over to the left by the tumour mass.

Aspiration biopsy of the tumour may be performed through a burr hole.

Electro-encephalography (EEG) may give useful localising information in tumours of the cerebrum.

Treatment

Slowly growing encapsulated intracranial tumours are capable of surgical removal and these include many meningiomas, acoustic neuromas and pituitary tumours. Of the gliomas, only the well differentiated tumours are amenable to surgical removal. Malignant primary growths have an extremely poor prognosis and are treated by palliative radiotherapy after the diagnosis has been established by a biopsy.

INTRACRANIAL VASCULAR LESIONS

Aneurysms

The vast majority of intracranial aneurysms are congenital in origin, although occasionally they may be due to atherosclerosis or trauma. These congenital aneurysms are saccular ('berry aneurysm') which arise on the circle of Willis, the anastomotic communication between the internal carotid arteries and the vertebral arteries at the base of the brain. About 20% are multiple and the sexes are equally affected (see Fig. 8.3).

Clinical features

The importance of these aneurysms is that they are the commonest cause of spontaneous subarachnoid haemorrhage, but when they rupture they may also produce intracerebral or subdural bleeding. Rupture may occur at any age, but especially after 40; increasing atheromatous changes in the arteries and hypertension are probably precipitating factors.

The haemorrhage usually presents as a sudden severe headache with vomiting. The patient may become unconscious and the blood in the subarachnoid space causes severe cerebral irritation resembling meningitis (meningism). There may be neck retraction and the patient resists attempts to flex the neck. Lumbar puncture confirms the presence of blood in the CSF. If the blood is allowed to settle it will be noticed that the supernatant fluid is yellow in colour (*xanthochromic*) and by this means we can differentiate between a true subarachnoid haemorrhage and a 'bloody tap', produced by pricking a small blood vessel during the diagnostic lumbar puncture.

Haemorrhage from a ruptured aneurysm is serious and no less than a quarter of the patients die without recovering consciousness. Half the patients will bleed again within six weeks of the initial haemorrhage and the mortality in such cases is high. After six weeks the likelihood of recurrent haemorrhage becomes less, but it is still present.

Treatment

While the patient is in coma there is nothing to be done except careful nursing—exactly like the outline of treatment described for the nursing care of the unconscious head injury (page 146). If the patient recovers from the initial haemorrhage then cerebral angiography is performed to locate the site of the aneurysm and this should be carried out as soon as possible, preferably before the peak incidence of recurrent haemorrhage, which is after about 2 weeks.

If an aneurysm is demonstrated (Fig. 10.12) treatment comprises either direct or indirect surgery. In the direct attack the aneurysm is exposed via a craniotomy and is obliterated, either by excision, or by applying a silver clip to its base or to its supplying vessels, or by inducing thrombosis by wrapping it in a detached piece of muscle. The indirect approach comprises ligation of the common carotid artery in those instances where the aneurysm is supplied by the internal carotid artery, since diminution of the blood flow through the aneurysm encourages its thrombosis. About one third of the angiograms are negative and probably indicate that thrombosis has taken place spontaneously in a small aneurysm. Such cases are treated conservatively and the prognosis is good.

Angiomas

Developmental angiomatous malformations may occur in any part of the central nervous system, but particularly over the surface of the cerebral hemisphere. They may produce epilepsy, headaches, slowly progressive paralysis or may leak and result in subarachnoid haemorrhage. This is less catastrophic than in rupture of an aneurysm but accounts for about 10% of all examples of spontaneous subarachnoid bleeding.

The exact diagnosis and localisation is made by cerebral angiography.

In some cases excision of the angioma is possible and this should be carried out particularly if marked symptoms are present, or if

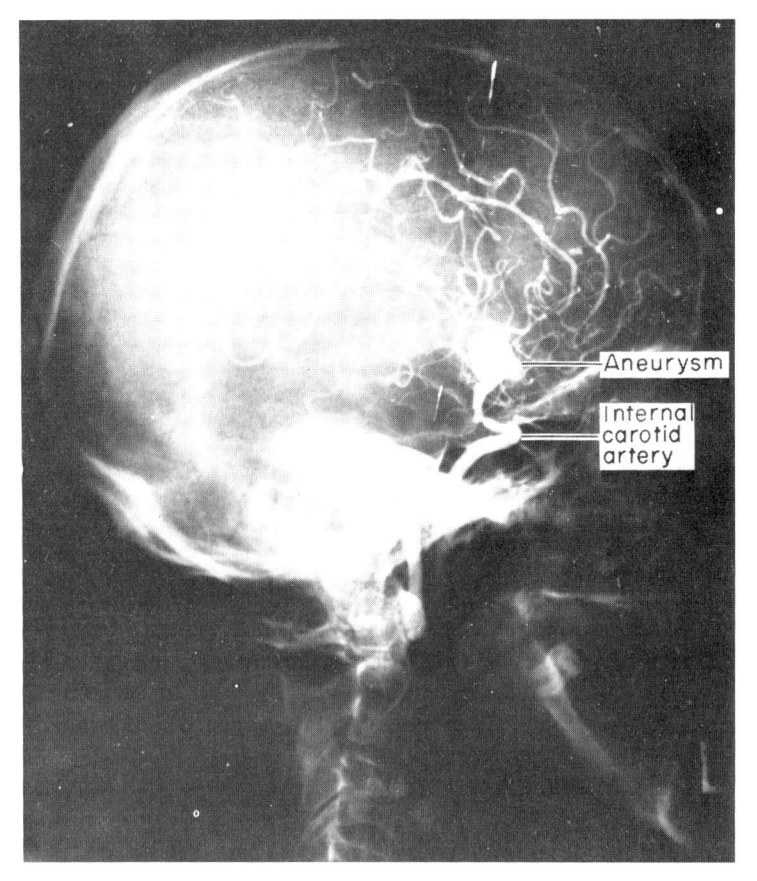

Fig. 10.12. A large cerebral aneurysm demonstrated by carotid angiography.

there has been preceding subarachnoid haemorrhage. In many cases, however, the angioma is too extensive or too deeply situated to make operation feasible.

HEAD INJURIES

One of the most serious responsibilities undertaken by a nurse is the care of a patient who has sustained a head injury. It is no exaggeration to say that his life depends upon her careful nursing and observation. Hippocrates, the father of medicine, wrote 'no head injury is so trivial that we can neglect it, nor so severe that there is no hope' and each year in this country patients die because what at first appears to be a trivial head injury is ignored, whereas others, rushed to theatre while being artificially ventilated or even undergoing cardiac massage, make a complete recovery. There is no mystique about head injuries and we hope to show, in this chapter, that their management is based on common sense.

The causes of coma

An everyday problem is the patient brought into Casualty unconscious. The following are the common causes to be considered:
1. Trauma to the brain.
2. Cerebral disease; for example, a stroke (the commonest), epilepsy, cerebral tumour, abscess or meningitis.
3. Drugs, especially the barbiturates and alcohol. For convenience, we can include carbon monoxide and coal gas poisoning in this group.
4. Diabetes—either hyperglycaemic or hypoglycaemic coma.
5. Uraemia—patients in advanced renal failure pass into coma.
6. Hepatic coma, the patient being deeply jaundiced and usually in the terminal stages of cirrhosis.
7. Profound toxaemia—for example in advanced peritonitis or septicaemia.
8. Hysteria.

The first four groups account for the great majority of emergency admissions. If there is any doubt about the cause of coma, blood should be taken for glucose, barbiturate and alcohol estimations.

It is usually easy enough to tell from witnesses that unconsciousness is due to trauma, but it is vitally important to remember that a drunk or an epileptic may have struck his head in falling so that his initial condition is complicated by a head injury. In contrast, a patient may have suffered a stroke, be seen to fall down and sustain what is, in fact, a trivial head injury which disguises the real cause of his coma being a serious intracerebral vascular accident.

The management of the unconscious head injury

This must be considered under three headings:
1. Nursing the unconscious patient.
2. Observation.
3. Indications for operative treatment.

The first two apply to every case but operative intervention is only needed in about 10% of head injuries. Although we consider these topics under separate headings, all three lines of management may be going on at one and the same time.

The nursing care of the unconscious patient

1. *The airway*

Without any doubt at all, the most important single factor in the care of the deeply unconscious patient, whatever the cause, is the maintenance of the airway. The patient in coma has lost his cough reflex and so cannot protect his respiratory passages from inhalation of vomit and blood; furthermore, the unconscious patient loses the ability we possess, even when asleep, of maintaining the tongue held forward so that it does not obstruct the laryngeal orifice. The patient must therefore be transported and nursed lying on one side with the body tilted head downwards ('the tonsil position'). This simple but absolutely vital manœuvre ensures that the tongue falls forwards and also that bronchial secretions or vomit drain from the mouth rather than being inhaled (Fig. 10.13). Suction may be required to remove excessive secretions or vomit from the pharynx. If the airway cannot be maintained satisfactorily by this technique, and this is particularly so when the presence of other injuries make it necessary for the patient to lie on his back (for example, associated fracture of the femur) then an endotracheal tube may be necessary (Fig. 10.14). If the patient remains unconscious, a tracheostomy using a cuffed tube may be required.

2. *Restlessness*

The unconscious head injury may be extremely restless. Morphia is contraindicated since this will depress respiration, disguise the level of coma and will also produce constriction of the pupils, which masks a valuable physical sign. Phenobarbitone or paraldehyde may be required for severe restlessness or epileptic fits. Judicious restraint, cot-sides and padding may be required to protect the patient from injuring himself. A cause of restlessness may be a distended bladder and often if the retention is relieved by means of a catheter the patient will calm down considerably.

3. *Feeding*

Many head injuries were allowed to die in the past due to dehydration and starvation. If it is obvious that the patient is going to

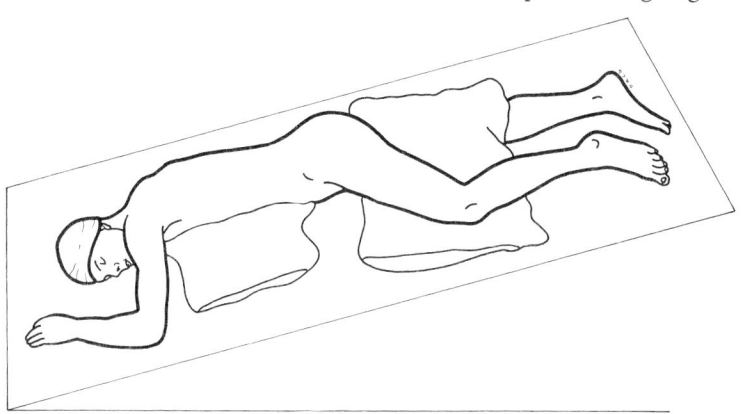

Fig. 10.13. The 'tonsil position' for transportation of an unconscious patient. Note the 'head down, feet up' inclination.

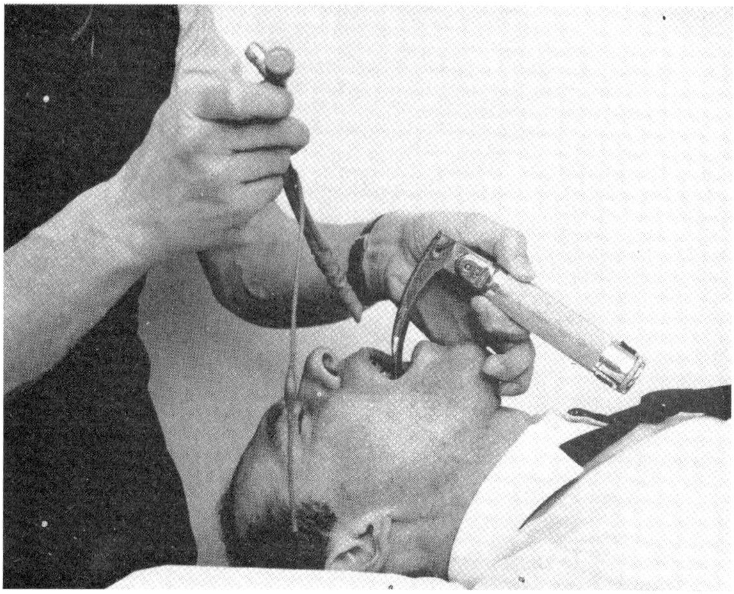

Fig. 10.14. Maintenance of an airway by means of the passage of an endotracheal tube.

remain unconscious and unable to swallow after 12 hours then a naso-gastric tube should be passed so that adequate fluid, electrolytes and calories can be provided. It is, of course, essential to ensure that the tube is lying correctly in the stomach since, if coiled in the oesophagus, there is the risk of regurgitation and inhalation into the respiratory passages.

4. *Skin and general nursing care*

A deeply unconscious patient is liable to bed sores; careful nursing attention is required for their prevention. Eye toilet to prevent exposure keratitis, frequent mouth hygiene and full range passive movement to all limbs to prevent contractures are all part of the nurse's heavy responsibilities.

5. *Sphincters*

The unconscious patient is frequently incontinent; the resultant excoriation of the skin makes him still more liable to pressure sores. The use of Paul's tubing on the penis, or of an indwelling catheter in the female patient, will help in the nursing care. Faecal impaction is quite common if the bowels are neglected; the unconscious patient usually requires regular enemas to clear the bowel, but digital disimpaction may be necessary.

Observations

The observations which must be carried out on an unconscious head injury fall into two groups.

The first is the complete clinical examination of the patient to determine whether or not other injuries are present. Following most accidents, the patient can tell us which parts of his body have been injured, but this is obviously not the case when he is in coma! An injury which has been sufficient to render a patient unconscious, a severe car crash for example, is likely to have produced damage elsewhere—it is surprising how common such gross things as fracture of the femur or a serious chest injury are overlooked in these cases and it is essential for the head injury patient to be checked over from head to toe.

Secondly, our observations are concentrated on looking for signs of deterioration in the patient which, for practical purposes, indicate that intracranial bleeding is taking place.

Three things can happen to head injury patients while under observation:

1. The great majority become lighter and recover completely.
2. A small proportion remain in relatively deep coma as a result of severe cerebral trauma and this state of affairs may persist for weeks or even months.
3. Another small proportion of patients pass into progressively deeper coma. This may be caused either by intracranial bleeding, with clot pressing on the brain, or oedema of the damaged cerebral tissues or, at a later stage, intracranial infection. The last is now fortunately rare except in some cases of penetrating compound fractures of the skull.

Since it is extremely difficult to differentiate between the progressive coma produced by intracranial haemorrhage (which requires urgent surgical intervention) and cerebral oedema, for practical purposes one may state that a patient with a closed head injury who becomes more deeply unconscious after the accident requires immediate surgery.

The repeated observations that are ordered for the unconscious head injury should not be regarded as a routine chore but as an essential process to detect that minority of patients who are developing the features of cerebral compression.

The observations fall into three groups which are, in order of importance:

1. The conscious level
2. The reaction of the pupils
3. The pulse, respiration and blood pressure.

In the early hours following a head injury these observations must be repeated at ten or fifteen minute intervals and plotted on a chart.

Conscious level

Vague terms such as comatose, semi-comatose, unconscious or stuperose should be avoided—they mean nothing when compared one to the other and are useless when charting changes in conscious level. Instead, we use the patient's responses to stimuli and these are very much the reactions of a person recovering from a deep anaesthesia. As the patient becomes progressively lighter, we can chart the following levels:

1. No response at all to painful stimulation—the deepest level of unconsciousness.
2. Incoordinated response to pain—for example, the patient moves all four limbs following a pin prick.
3. Coordinated response to pain—the patient is now light enough to push away the examiner's hand when pricked or pinched.
4. Response to simple commands—for example he now puts out his tongue when ordered to do so.
5. The patient is now able to talk but is disorientated and does not know his name, his whereabouts, the day or the time. Gradually he passes from this state to full orientation.

Any shift from a higher to a lower level in this scheme is highly significant of deepening coma and is undoubtedly the most valuable of all the observations that we can make.

Pupils

If a cerebral hemisphere is pressed upon by an enlarging blood clot, the third cranial nerve on that side becomes stretched and put out of action. Its paralysis results in dilatation of the corresponding pupil, since the third nerve transmits the nerve supply to the pupillary constrictor muscle. The pupil is also unable to respond to light. An important sign of acute cerebral compression is dilatation and loss of light reaction of the pupil on the same side as the cerebral compression. As compression continues, the third nerve on the opposite side becomes compressed and the opposite pupil, in turn, dilates and becomes fixed to light. Bilateral fixed dilated pupils in a patient with a head injury indicates great cerebral compression and the prognosis is now extremely grave (Fig. 10.15).

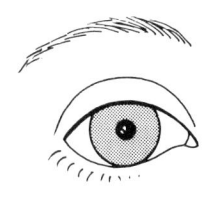

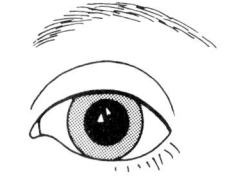

A At first the pupil is dilated on the affected side

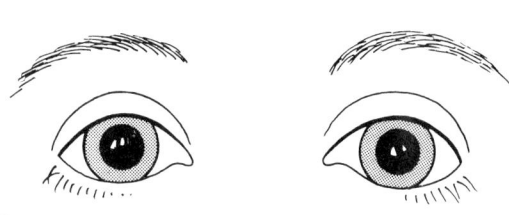

B Later stage, both pupils are dilated

Fig. 10.15. The pupil changes in acute cerebral compression.

Pulse, respiration and blood pressure

With increasing cerebral compression, the pulse progressively slows, the respirations become stertorous and the blood pressure rises. These changes usually go hand in glove with increasing coma and pupil dilatation.

Special investigations of the unconscious patient

We have already mentioned that if there is any doubt about the traumatic nature of the coma, blood should be sent to the laboratory for sugar, alcohol and barbiturate levels, as well as testing a specimen of urine for sugar.

High quality x-rays of the skull are obtained for evidence of fracture but it should be noted that an extensive fracture at the base of the skull may not show up at all on x-rays which demonstrate, for the most part, lesions of the skull vault (Fig. 10.16).

If the patient shows progressive deterioration in the first few hours after head injury we have noted that the diagnosis lies between intracranial bleeding and cerebral oedema. In a neurological unit, if there is time, the diagnosis may be greatly aided by a cerebral arteriogram which can demonstrate the site and size of any intracranial clot. If such facilities are not immediately available, the only safe procedure is rapid burr-hole exploration of the skull over the suspected site of the clot collection. If no clot is discovered, but oedema of the brain

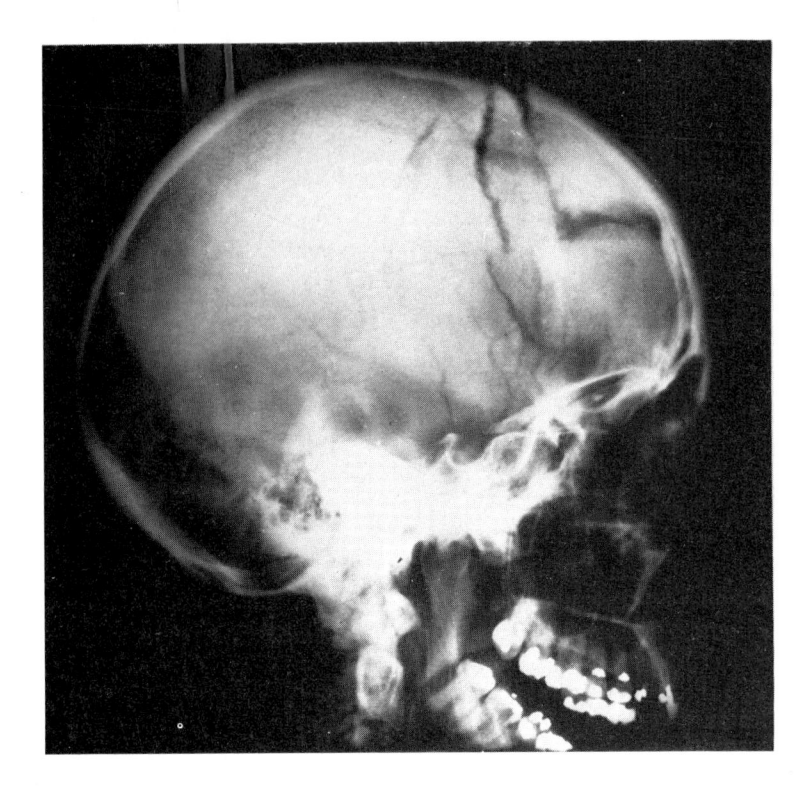

Fig. 10.16. An extensive fracture of the skull.

alone revealed, then a diagnosis of cerebral oedema is made. Intravenous mannitol may be used as an emergency temporary procedure to reduce oedema by its osmotic effect, but in severe cases hypothermia and controlled respiration are employed.

An important warning

Lumbar puncture should never be performed in an attempt to confirm the raised intracranial pressure. If the pressure in the spinal cerebrospinal fluid is reduced by removing fluid from the spinal dural sac, the high intracranial pressure may force the brain downwards through the foramen magnum (a phenomenon termed 'coning') and this may prove rapidly fatal.

Summary of indications for surgery in head injuries

We have mentioned that only about 10% of head injuries require surgical treatment. These cases comprise:
1. those with laceration of the scalp who will require excision and suture of the wound,

2. patients with compound fracture who, again, need surgical toilet, and
3. the patients with increasing coma who require burr-hole exploration for suspected intracranial bleeding.

Some patients may require later surgery for repair of skull defects, for plastic surgery in cases of deforming facial injuries, or for repair of lacerations of the dura with C.S.F. rhinorrhoea (see below).

FRACTURES OF THE SKULL

As with fractures of any bone, the most important sub-division is into closed and open or compound fractures. The fracture itself may be *fissured*, *comminuted* or *depressed* (Fig. 10.17).

The compound fracture may communicate to the exterior either

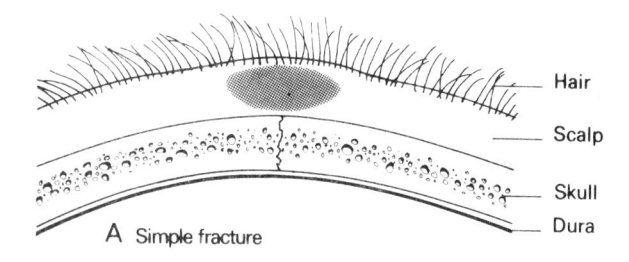

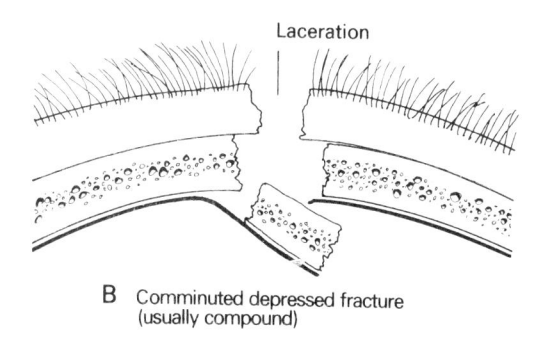

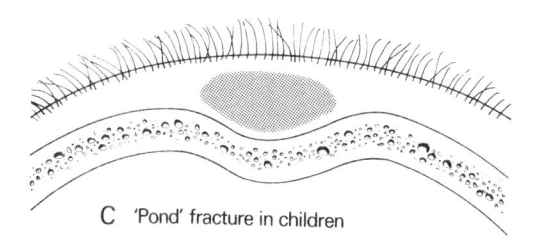

Fig. 10.17. Types of skull fracture.

by means of an external wound on the scalp or via the nasal or aural cavities.

Depressed fractures in adults are nearly always compound; it stands to reason that if the blow is severe enough to drive a fragment of the skull below its surrounds, it is also severe enough to tear through the overlying scalp. In children with their softer, more elastic bones, a 'pond' fracture may occur over which the skin remains intact and which rather resembles a dent in a table-tennis ball.

A compound fracture to the exterior is treated like any other compound fracture; the wound edges are narrowly excised, dead tissue, bone deprived of its periosteum and any pulped brain removed, the dura repaired if possible and the skin then sutured.

A special variety of compound fracture is where continuity to the exterior occurs through the nose or ear and is demonstrated by a discharge of cerebrospinal fluid through these orifices (C.S.F. rhinorrhoea or otorrhoea—the latter is far less common). In these instances a dural tear associated with a fracture of the skull base allows a ready pathway of infection along the nose or the ear to the meninges and brain. In such cases the patient is barrier nursed and placed on sulphadimidine, since the sulphonamides readily pass into the cerebrospinal fluid. If the leak persists then it may be necessary to repair the tear in the dura mater using a piece of fibrous deep fascia cut from the thigh.

Clinical accompaniments of skull fractures

Examination of the patient's head will often reveal features produced by the fracture of the skull itself or of injury to adjacent structures. There is frequently bruising, swelling and abrasions over the site of the blow and it is here that the fracture line is most likely to be placed. Fractures which involve the orbit are often accompanied by an orbital haematoma, in which the eyelids are swollen and bruised, the bruising being limited exactly to the orbital margin. The eyelids can be opened only with difficulty but then blood can be seen tracking beneath the conjunctiva. This is in contrast to the common 'black eye' due to a direct blow on the face, when bruising extends over the eyebrow and cheek and in which there is no blood beyond the conjunctiva. A haemorrhage may be seen, in these circumstances, in the conjunctiva itself, but this does not track posteriorly (Fig. 10.18).

Fractures of the base of the skull are frequently accompanied by bleeding from the nose or ear and we have already mentioned that occasionally cerebrospinal fluid or even pulped brain tissue may be seen to be escaping from either orifice.

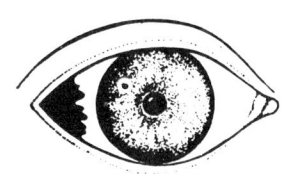

(A) SUBCONJUNCTIVAL HAEMORRHAGE
—NO POSTERIOR LIMIT

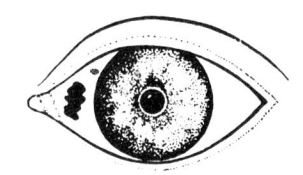

(B) CONJUNCTIVAL HAEMORRHAGE
—POSTERIOR LIMIT SEEN

Fig. 10.18. The differential diagnosis between subconjunctival (A) and conjunctival haemorrhage (B).

Cranial nerves may be injured if the fracture line passes across the foramina from which they emerge from the skull. Fractures involving the anterior part of the skull frequently damage the first cranial (olfactory) nerve and loss of smell (anosmia) is quite common following frontal injuries. The optic nerve may be torn with resultant blindness. The 7th (facial) nerve and 8th (auditory) nerve may be injured producing facial palsy and deafness. Any of the other cranial nerves may be involved but such injuries are relatively rare.

INTRACRANIAL HAEMORRHAGE

Following injury, haemorrhage may take place within the skull in a number of compartments (Fig. 10.19).

The extradural space lies between the dura mater and the skull. These two structures are usually firmly adherent to each other but may be stripped apart by haemorrhage.

The subdural space, between the brain and the dura.

The subarachnoid space, between the arachnoid and the brain.

Rarely haemorrhage occurs into the substance of the brain (*intracerebral*) and this may rupture into the ventricular system.

Extradural haemorrhage

This is sometimes badly named middle meningeal haemorrhage—a term that should not be used. It may indeed arise from a tear of the middle meningeal artery or vein, but an extradural collection of blood may also develop from a laceration of one of the other blood vessels running over the meninges, from the torn sagittal venous sinus or simply from blood oozing out of the bone marrow or stripped dura mater on either side of a fracture.

CLINICAL FEATURES

The typical story is of a relatively minor head injury which produces **temporary** concussion. The patient recovers from this (the 'lucid

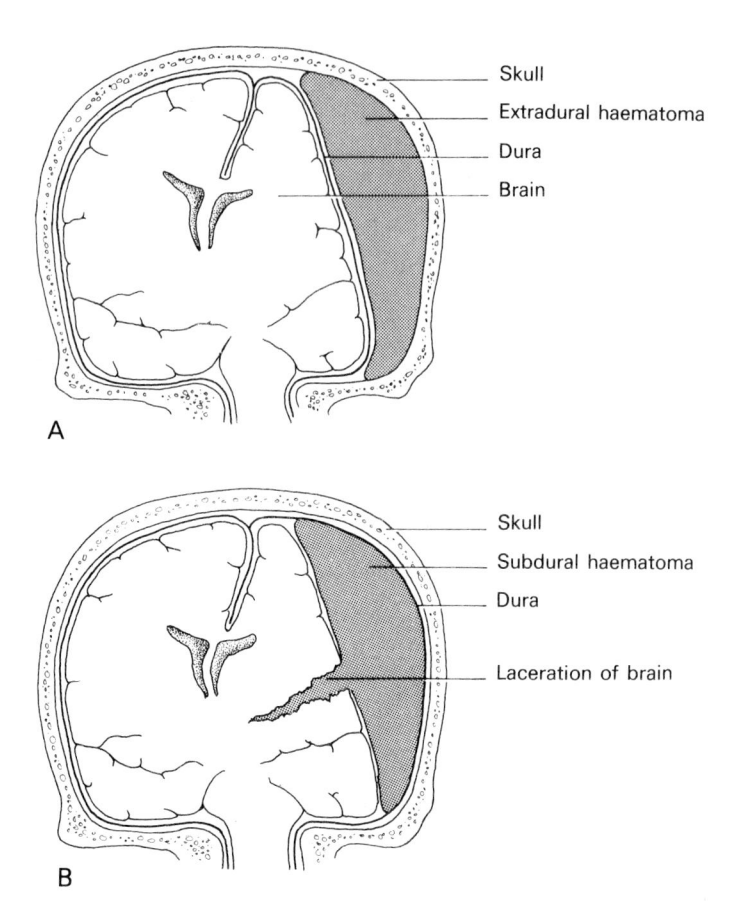

Fig. 10.19. Extradural haematoma (A) and subdural haematoma (B). The latter is associated with a severe brain laceration.

period') then, some hours later, develops headache and progresses to deeper and deeper coma due to cerebral compression produced by the extradural clot. Each year we read of tragedies in which someone has had too much to drink, falls down and hits his head, recovers enough to get home to bed and is found dead there in the morning, or the cricketer who is mildly concussed by a cricket ball, recovers enough to carry on with the game and dies that night. It is important to note, however, that this picture of recovery only accounts for about 50% of the cases. Often there is no lucid period and the patient progressively passes into deeper and deeper coma from the time of the initial injury.

The physical signs are those of rapidly increasing intracerebral pressure, which have already been discussed (page 149)—deepening coma, dilatation of the pupil on the affected side, a falling pulse rate, rise in blood pressure and stertorous respiration.

In addition, hemiplegia may develop on the side opposite to the lesion and occasionally Jacksonian fits occur. A boggy haematoma of the scalp usually overlies the site of the extradural haemorrhage; this is because some of the blood escapes through the fracture line into the subcutaneous tissues.

Skull x-rays may be very helpful; the haematoma is likely to be on the side of, and beneath, the fracture if one is present. In special neurosurgical centres, a carotid angiogram may accurately localise the position of the clot. Echo-encephalography has recently been introduced with great success to demonstrate shift of mid-line structures within the brain because of clot compression. This instrument works on the same principle as a depth-finder on a ship.

Treatment

An extradural haemorrhage is one of the few surgical emergencies where minutes really do matter both to prevent irreversible brain damage from taking place and to avert death as a result of compression of the respiratory centre in the medulla. The patient is taken immediately to the operating theatre, care being taken to maintain the airway, if necessary by an endotracheal tube and artificial ventilation. Under local anaesthetic a burr-hole is made over the suspected site of the clot by means of a drill (Fig. 10.20), the opening enlarged with nibbling forceps and the blood evacuated (Fig. 10.21). The source of bleeding on the dura is controlled either with silver Cushing clips, with diathermy or by under running the vessel with a

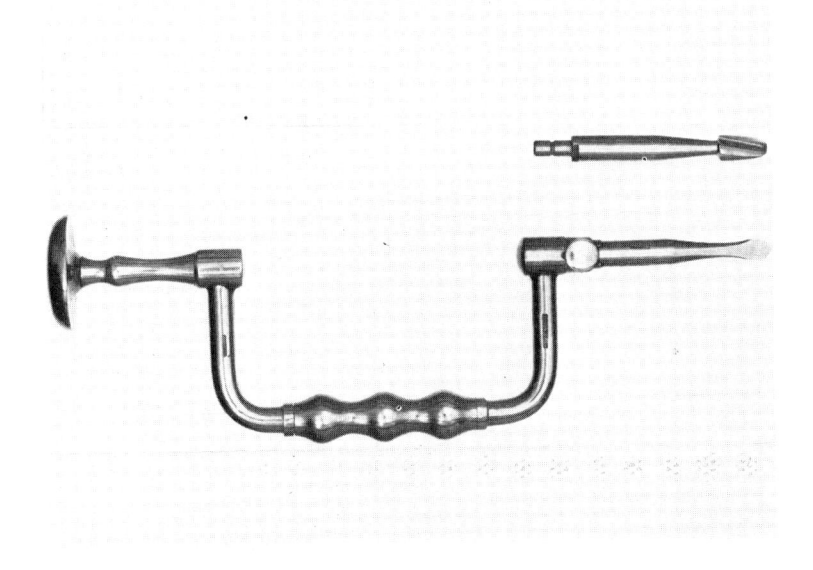

Fig. 10.20. A skull perforator with drill attachment.

Fig. 10.21. Evacuation of an extradural haematoma; the burr-hole opening has been enlarged with bone nibbling forceps. (The inset demonstrates the line of incision being infiltrated with local anaesthetic).

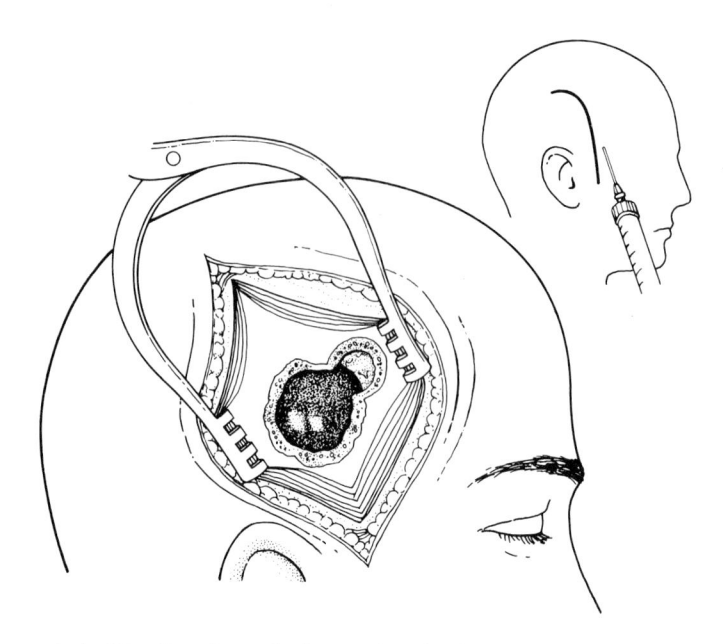

stitch. Bleeding from the bone edges is plugged by means of Horsley's wax.

If the patient is operated upon while he is still conscious the prognosis is good and the mortality rate is less than 5%. However, if the patient is in deep coma with fixed dilated pupils and not responding to painful stimulation, the mortality rate rises to about 75% and those that recover may well have residual brain damage.

Subdural haematoma

Collections of blood in the subdural space may be either acute or chronic.

ACUTE SUBDURAL HAEMATOMA

This results from bleeding into the subdural space from lacerated and pulped brain and is often part of a very severe head injury. The patient is frequently in deep coma from the moment of injury and his condition deteriorates still further.

Treatment

An inspection burr-hole is drilled in the temporal region just above the zygoma of the suspected side. The dura is seen to be bulging with underlying blood and the clot is released by incising the dura. The burr-hole is then enlarged by means of nibbling forceps, pulped brain is removed and bleeding controlled with clips and diathermy. If nothing is found on the suspected side, exploration should then be carried out contralaterally; indeed, it is not uncommon for the clot to be situated bilaterally.

CHRONIC SUBDURAL HAEMATOMA

This follows a fairly minor injury sustained perhaps weeks before and probably results from a small tear in a cerebral vein as it traverses the subdural space. Whenever the patient coughs or strains a little more blood extravasates to form an encapsulated haematoma.

Clinical features

The patient presents with what seems to be a rapidly developing intracerebral tumour. There is mental deterioration, headaches, vomiting and drowsiness which, untreated, eventually progress to coma. Examination of the optic fundi reveals papilloedema in about half the cases. The condition is often confused with an intra-cerebral tumour but a carotid angiogram demonstrates the outline of the clot.

Treatment

The clot is evacuated through burr-holes. Both sides of the skull must be explored because the condition is quite frequently bilateral.

SUBARACHNOID HAEMORRHAGE

Blood in the cerebro-spinal fluid after head injury occurs frequently and gives rise to the clinical picture of meningeal irritation. There is headache, neck stiffness and there may be a mild pyrexia. If there is any doubt about the diagnosis it can be confirmed by lumbar puncture, which reveals a blood-stained fluid. Treatment is by analgesics and bed rest until the severe headache has subsided, followed by rapid rehabilitation of the patient.

COMPLICATIONS OF HEAD INJURIES

We have already dealt with the following important complications of head injuries:
>Compound fracture
>Intracranial haemorrhage
>C.S.F. rhinorrhoea
>Cranial nerve palsies.

Other complications which require mention include meningitis, hyperpyrexia, post-traumatic neurosis and epilepsy.

MENINGITIS

Infection of the meninges may complicate a fracture of the skull which is compound either directly to the exterior or via a dural tear into the nasal or aural cavities. Confirmation of the diagnosis of meningitis is made by lumbar puncture and bacteriological examination of the fluid.

Treatment is appropriate chemotherapy, both systemically and into the spinal theca by means of lumbar puncture.

Occasionally, the infection of a penetrating wound of the brain may result in cerebral abscess (see page 137).

HYPERPYREXIA

Severe injury to the brain stem may result in prolonged unconsciousness, decerebrate rigidity with the legs held rigidly extended and the arms flexed to the sides (Fig. 10.22), pin-point pupils and, very dangerously, hyperpyrexia with a temperature rising up to 105° or more. This latter results from injury to the heat regulating centre and, unlike most fevers, there is no accompanying sweating.

Treatment requires most vigorous nursing care. All blankets are removed and the naked patient is treated with tepid sponging. If this proves ineffective, then crushed ice placed in polythene bags is applied over the trunk. Chlorpromazine may be useful to stop shivering since the latter will prevent cooling.

POST-TRAUMATIC NEUROSIS

This is not uncommon after a head injury. Unless reassured and rapidly rehabilitated a patient may easily be left to imagine that his brain has been irrevocably damaged and that he will never lead a normal life again.

Some idea of the severity of the injury is given by the period of amnesia, both the retrograde amnesia up to the time of the accident and the post-traumatic amnesia following injury. If this period amounts to only minutes or a few hours, the ultimate prognosis is good. Amnesia of several days or even weeks means that the chance of ultimate return to full mental function is much less.

Central nervous system

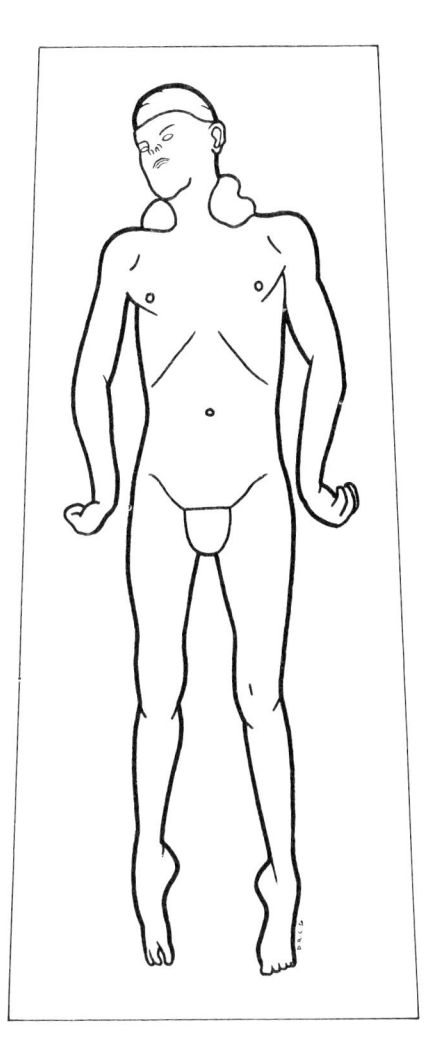

Fig. 10.22. Decerebrate rigidity in severe brain stem injury.

PERSISTENT EPILEPSY

This may especially complicate penetrating compound wounds with resultant scarring of the cerebral cortex. All such patients are given phenobarbitone for at least six months following injury. Established post-traumatic epilepsy is treated by means of anti-convulsant drugs (phenobarbitone, epanutin etc.); alcohol should be forbidden.

Chapter 11. Oesophagus, stomach and duodenum

Introduction

The alimentary canal extends from the lips to the anus. The mouth and pharynx are considered elsewhere and the rest of the alimentary canal will be taken in anatomical order from the oesophagus down.

Oesophagus

Anatomy

The oesophagus is a muscular tube which extends from the level of the cricoid cartilage, in the neck, to its junction with the stomach. In its entire length it is closely applied to the front of the bodies of the vertebrae. In the neck it is situated behind the trachea and it continues this relationship as it descends into the thorax in the posterior mediastinum (Fig. 11.1) until the trachea divides into the right and left main bronchi. It continues down behind the heart and pericardium, with the right and left vagus nerves closely applied to it, to enter the abdomen through the hiatus in the diaphragm. Just beneath the hiatus it enters the stomach at the cardia, the right vagus nerve becoming posterior and the left vagus nerve becoming anterior.

The oesophagus is lined by stratified squamous epithelium, which is both smooth and tough. At its upper end the muscle wall of the oesophagus is of the voluntary, striated kind, which allows the act of swallowing to be voluntarily initiated. This type of muscle gradually changes, until at the lower end the muscle is completely involuntary,

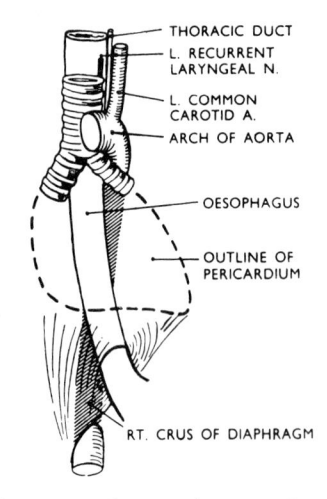

Fig. 11.1. The oesophagus and its anterior relations.

resulting in the automatic nature of the peristaltic wave that forces food and fluid into the stomach, even if the subject stands on his head.

Symptoms of oesophageal disease

1. *Dysphagia*—this term is used either to describe difficulty in swallowing or pain on swallowing. It always indicates that full investigation should be undertaken. Generally, with a progressive disease such as a cancer, the dysphagia will first cause a 'sticking' of solid foods. As it progresses, however, it results in difficulty in swallowing liquids.

2. *Regurgitation*—this occurs when saliva, food, or a mixture of the two, pool within the oesophagus. It is distinguished from vomiting by the fact that it frequently occurs soon after a meal; the ejected contents are slimy and contain food residue unstained by bile, alkaline to litmus paper, and recognisable as having been eaten with the previous meal.

A special form of regurgitation occurs with an oesophageal diverticulum. In this case the patient learns how to empty the diverticulum, or pouch, by external pressure on the neck, or by adopting a head-down position.

3. *Pain*—severe pain can arise from damage to the oesophageal lining or wall. Usually the pain is referred anteriorly to the neck, chest, or upper abdomen, according to the site of the injury. Occasionally, however, the pain is experienced in the back. Regurgitation of acid stomach contents produces inflammation in the oesophagus and this is experienced as a burning pain in the upper epigastrium or lower chest, a symptom commonly described as 'heartburn'.

4. *Chest complications.* A confusing and important symptom arises when dysphagia has progressed to the point when liquids cannot be swallowed. In this case saliva, constantly being produced, gradually fills up the oesophagus. During the daytime this will be regurgitated but, at night, when the patient is asleep, the saliva, together with other swallowed oesophageal contents, spills over into the trachea, resulting in an aspiration pneumonia. It is even possible for a young patient with achalasia of the cardia to present as an asthmatic. It is also quite common for newly born babies with oesophageal atresia to present as pneumonia for the same reason.

5. *Loss of Weight.* This results quite obviously from the fact that less food can be eaten and the total calorie intake falls below the level required to maintain the weight. Patients with long-standing severe

dysphagia can lose a considerable amount of weight and their primary oesophageal disease becomes eclipsed by their state of starvation and dehydration.

Investigations

1. *X-ray*; a plain chest X-ray will occasionally reveal a dilated or tortuous oesophagus, visible as a shadow behind the heart (usually achalasia).

The mainstay of X-ray diagnosis, however, is *the barium swallow*. The patient swallows a barium sulphate mixture while the radiologist observes the act on a television monitor actuated from an image intensifier. This is an extremely sensitive test as it allows the surface of the mucosa to be examined minutely and the shape and movement of the oesophagus can also be observed. The degree of accuracy of this investigation exceeds 90%, and it is unusual for even very small abnormalities of the mucosa to be missed.

2. *Oesophagoscopy*—Complementary with barium swallow is the direct inspection of the oesophagus. This has become much safer and easier of recent years with the development of the flexible fibre-optic, fibre-light, oesophagoscopes. With these instruments it is possible to see the mucosa very clearly and to take biopsies of any suspicious lesion. Oesophagoscopy must always be performed in every case of dysphagia, even if the X-rays do not reveal any abnormality. When a flexible oesophagoscope is used, it is possible to carry out this investigation without general anaesthetic, the patient usually only requiring a small intravenous dose of diazepam (Valium).

3. *General*—Patients who have been receiving a fluid diet for a long time may be anaemic and therefore a haemoglobin and full blood count should be carried out. If there has been dysphagia to liquids as well, blood urea and electrolytes should also be estimated.

Fig. 11.2. The usual form of oesophageal atresia. The upper end of the oesophagus terminates blindly; the lower end communicates with the trachea at the level of the 4th thoracic vertebra.

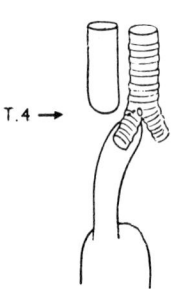

CONGENITAL ABNORMALITIES

The only common abnormality is *atresia*. This may be associated either with an abnormal connection from the narrow upper end of the oesophagus with the trachea or with a similar fistulous communication from the lower end of the oesophagus to the trachea or occasionally with both (Fig. 11.2). It has been estimated to occur in only 1 in 2,500 live births. When it does occur it is often associated with other congenital anomalies such as ventricular septal defect of the heart and other intestinal atresias.

The main danger of this condition in a baby who is otherwise normal is that the condition will not be diagnosed before aspiration pneumonia has occurred.

Clinical features

Presentation is by regurgitation of saliva and swallowed fluid with consequent choking and cyanosis as the baby is given its first feeds. When the condition is suspected a soft rubber catheter should be passed through the mouth and instead of slipping into the stomach will become obstructed at the level of the atresia.

Special investigations

X-ray contrast should not be introduced as this always finds its way into the lungs. Plain X-ray of the abdomen may show complete absence of intestinal gas shadows if there is no connection with the trachea or if gas shadows are present this indicates the presence of a distal tracheo-oesophageal fistula.

Differential diagnosis is from any pharyngeal or oral abnormality such as a cleft palate resulting in a feeding problem, or cerebral damage during birth.

Treatment

Once diagnosis has been made the baby should be transferred to a unit specialising in this kind of work where, providing the general condition is satisfactory, primary anastomosis between the two ends of the oesophagus via a thoracotomy is possible in a high number of cases. If the ends of the oesophagus will not meet, a cervical oesophagostomy is performed to allow saliva to escape, thus preventing the development of inhalation pneumonia. In order to feed the baby a gastrostomy has to be performed at the same time. Subsequently, when the infant has gained weight and is approximately one year old, oesophageal reconstruction by means of colonic interposition is carried out.

It is extremely important, when looking after these infants, to ensure that they are fed normally, first by bottle and then by spoon, even though the food is immediately ejected from the oesophagostomy.

SWALLOWED FOREIGN BODIES.

Children may swallow a coin such as a ten pence piece which then becomes stuck either half way down the oesophagus or somewhere near its lower end. The history is usually all that is required to make the diagnosis and a chest X-ray confirms it (Fig. 11.3, see also Fig. 20.46).

Treatment comprises oesophagoscopy under a general anaesthetic, which allows forceps extraction of the foreign body.

Adults with foreign bodies stuck in the oesophagus fall into two categories. In the first the foreign body is sharp, often a fish bone or sometimes a rabbit bone which has become swallowed and which has imbedded itself in the mucosa preventing its further passage into the stomach.

Many such objects are not radio-opaque but the diagnosis may be confirmed by a barium swallow examination.

Extraction is through an oesophagoscope, which may require considerable dexterity when the object is large, sharp and irregular. Numerous cases are recorded in which the foreign body has not been extracted and has then worked its way through the wall of the oesophagus, resulting in a perforation and peri-oesophageal abscess or, worse still, penetration of the aorta with a massive and fatal haemorrhage.

The second category in adults is when swallowed material cannot negotiate the oesophagus because of a pre-existing abnormality such as a stricture from either a malignant growth or peptic oesophagitis.

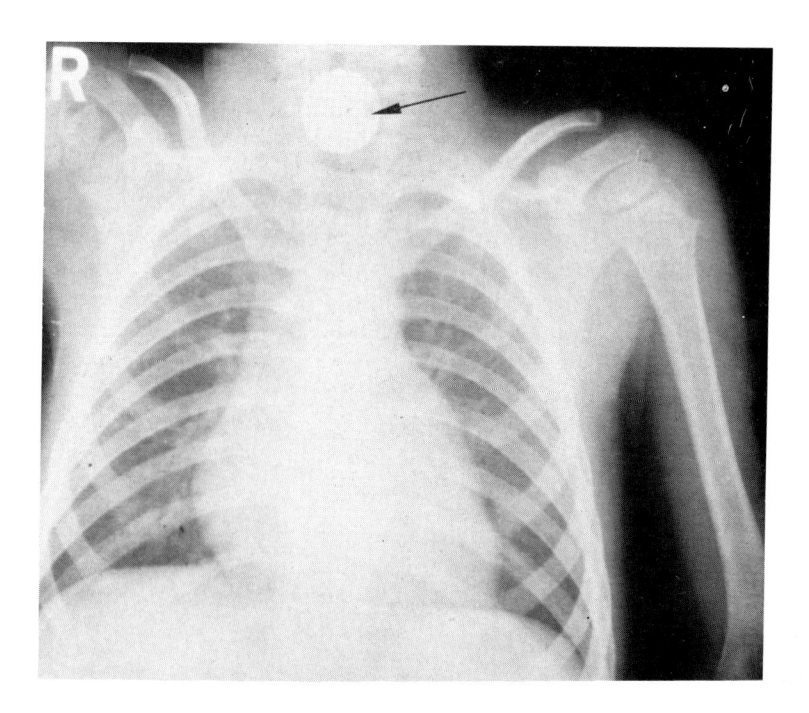

Fig. 11.3. X-ray of the chest of a child showing an opaque foreign body (an old-fashioned penny) lodged in the upper oesophagus.

Once again, these patients require full investigation by barium swallow and oesophagoscopy. Following this, treatment will be required to correct the basic abnormality of the oesophageal wall.

OESOPHAGEAL WEB

This is a narrowing of the upper end of the oesophagus which occurs in middle-aged women in association with iron-deficient anaemia and is given the name of the Plummer-Vinson or Patterson-Kelly syndrome. This syndrome may develop into a post-cricoid carcinoma, that is a carcinoma of the upper end of the oesophagus.

Treatment of this condition is aimed at the treatment of the iron deficiency by oral iron and requires frequent checks to detect possible development of a carcinoma.

OESOPHAGEAL (PHARYNGEAL) POUCH

See page 477.

ACHALASIA OF THE CARDIA

Achalasia of the cardia is a condition in which the normal peristaltic wave of the oesophagus, which occurs as food material is being swallowed, is not transmitted at the lower end of the oesophagus.

Clinical features

It is slightly more common in women than men, the onset tends to be insidious and patients may not even notice that they have had difficulty in swallowing for a considerable number of years. Generally the patients are underweight and aged between 35 and 50 years. As onset is so insidious, advanced malnutrition may occur. Sometimes the oesophagus becomes full of food and fluid debris, and when the patient becomes recumbent at night some of this material is aspirated into the lungs, so that he or she may present with pneumonia.

Special investigations

A chest X-ray may reveal a mediastinal mass produced by the grossly distended oesophagus.

A barium swallow clinches the diagnosis. The dilated, tortuous oesophagus is outlined, usually half full of retained food and fluid.

At its lower end it tapers into a short narrow segment that drains into the stomach (Fig. 11.4).

Oesophagoscopy is like going down a tunnel the bottom of which contains a puddle of food debris.

Treatment

Some patients may respond to regular dilatation of the lower end of the oesophagus or to one or more forcible stretches by means of a balloon introduced through an oesophagoscope. Most surgeons in this country prefer to carry out *Heller's Operation*, in which the thickened muscle wall of the lower end of the oesophagus (approached through a left thoracotomy), is split down to the mucosa. Most patients respond dramatically to this procedure (Fig. 11.5).

HIATUS HERNIA

In the normal person gastric juice cannot pass from the stomach up into the oesophagus because of a number of mechanisms, which include the physiological sphincter at the lower end of the oesophagus, the angle between the oesophagus and the stomach, the positive intra-abdominal pressure which tends to keep the oesophagus shut and the muscle fibres of the diaphragm which are wrapped around the lower end of the oesophagus, particularly from the right crus. In a considerable number of patients, especially females, with advancing years and increasing obesity, the oesophageal hiatus in the diaphragm becomes unusually wide, allowing the oesophago-gastric junction, sometimes together with part of the fundus of the stomach, to pass into the chest. The precise anatomical relationship between the oesophago-gastric junction and the hiatus allows hiatus herniae to be classified as follows (Fig. 11.6).

1. *Sliding hiatus hernia*—in this type the oesophago-gastric junction passes into the chest.
2. *Rolling hiatus hernia*—in which the oesophago-gastric junction remains in the abdomen but the fundus of the stomach passes into the chest.

Clinical features

The most common symptom to be associated with a hiatus hernia is produced by gastro-oesophageal reflux, resulting in a peptic oesophagitis. This is experienced as heartburn, a burning pain which is situated retrosternally and which is relieved by alkalis and an upright posture. Regurgitation of recently eaten food mixed with

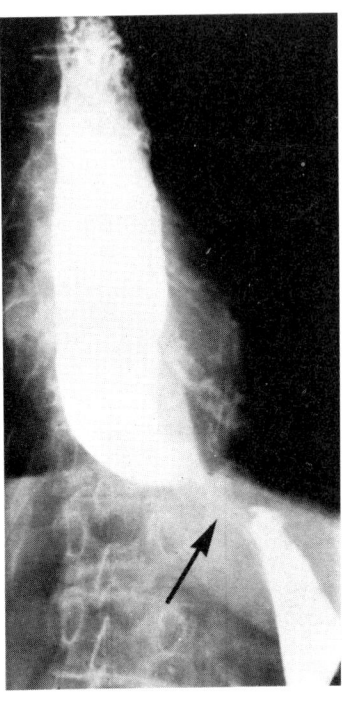

Fig. 11.4. Barium swallow in achalasia. Note the grossly dilated oesophagus above the narrow terminal segment (arrowed).

gastric juice commonly occurs when the patient bends forwards. Such common tasks as gardening and housework, which involves bending over, result in this reflux.

In the case of a rolling hiatus hernia it is quite possible for a significant portion of the stomach to enter the chest with the result that the stomach assumes an upside-down position (*a gastric volvulus*). In these patients acute symptoms may be precipitated by a heavy meal when the patient feels nausea and makes attempts at vomiting but without oesophageal regurgitation being able to occur. It is also common for these patients to have a competent oesophageal sphincter with no gastro-oesophageal reflux.

Complications

Continued peptic oesophagitis at the lower end of the oesophagus may result in *stricture formation* with progressive dysphagia. The inflamed mucosa may bleed, either acutely (haematemesis) or insidiously with the development of an iron-deficiency anaemia.

Special investigations

A Barium swallow and meal will delineate the hernia, although it may be necessary to tip the patient head-down in order to demon-

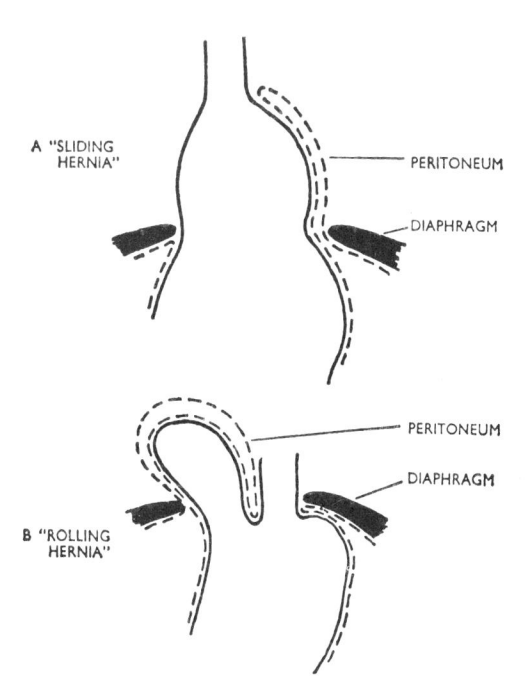

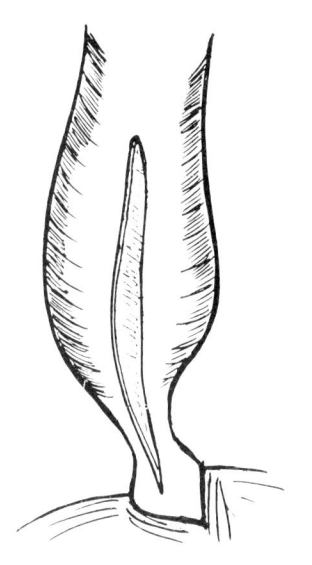

Fig. 11.5. Heller's operation. The muscle of the lower oesophagus is split down to the mucosa (compare Ramstedt's operation, Fig. 11.11).

Fig. 11.6. (A) A sliding hiatus hernia. (B) A rolling hiatus hernia. In the first, the stomach and lower oesophagus slide into the chest through the enlarged oesophageal hiatus; in the second the stomach rolls upwards through the hiatus alongside the lower oesophagus.

strate this (Fig. 11.7). Reflux will be shown by barium regurgitating into the oesophagus from the stomach and any associated stricture will also be revealed.

Oesophagoscopy may be necessary, particularly when the radiologist cannot be certain whether a stricture in these circumstances is benign or due to a co-existent carcinoma, a not infrequent situation.

Treatment

1. *Conservative*

Very many of the patients who complain of the symptoms of a hiatus hernia are overweight and the first line of treatment in such subjects will therefore be aimed at weight reduction with consequent lowering of the intra-abdominal pressure. An upright posture will aid in the maintenance of gastro-oesophageal continence, thus minimising oesophagitis. To this end patients are advised to raise the head of the bed slightly and to avoid stooping and bending positions.

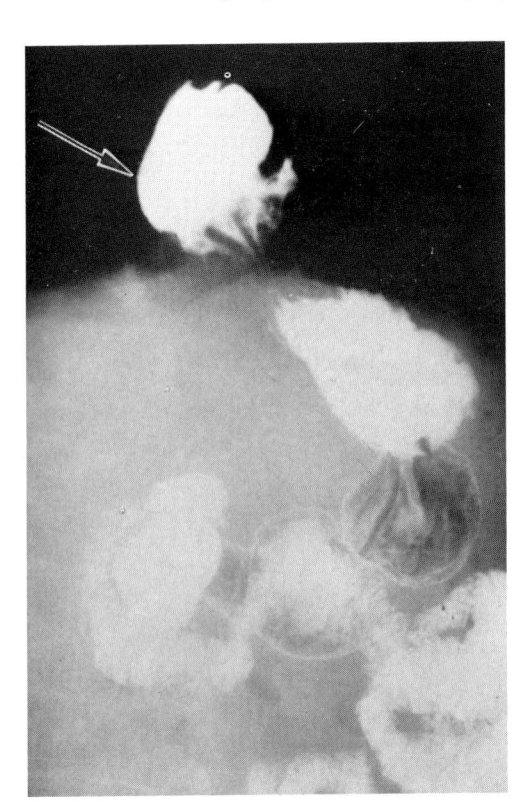

Fig. 11.7. Barium meal showing a sliding hiatus hernia. Note the large pouch of stomach above the diaphragm (arrowed).

The acid and peptic activity at the lower end of the oesophagus is then reduced to a minimum with non-absorbable alkalis, for example aluminium hydroxide or magnesium trisilicate.

These measures are successful in removing the symptoms due to a hiatus hernia in the majority of patients. It is even possible to arrest the progress and in a number of patients reverse the development of a peptic stricture. However there are some patients in whom these measures are not effective and who require surgery.

2. *Surgical treatment*

Numerous operations have been described for the repair of a hiatus hernia. The fact that so many procedures are available to the surgeon clearly indicates that none of them is entirely satisfactory. Allison has advocated the repair of the oesophageal ligaments using an approach through the chest. Belsey also uses an approach through the chest in which the oesophagus is firmly stitched to the underside of the diaphragm, the oesophago-gastric angle is restored and the diaphragmatic ligaments are repaired. Other surgeons employ an abdominal approach, pointing out that the virtue of this method is that an abdominal exploration can be carried out at the same time which permits the exclusion or treatment of other pathology producing similar symptoms, for example those associated with the presence of non-opaque gall stones. The hiatal procedure in this case comprises repair of the hiatus itself by means of several silk or nylon sutures through the crura of the diaphragm which may be combined with a fundoplication, carried out by wrapping the fundus of the stomach up around the lower end of the oesophagus.

A stricture of the oesophagus due to reflux may respond to conservative medical therapy or, if not too severe, may dilate up once the hiatus hernia is repaired and further reflux prevented. A severe stricture, however, may require dilatation via an oesophagoscope or surgical resection.

OESOPHAGEAL CARCINOMA

Pathology

The most common primary tumour of the oesophagus is the squamous cell carcinoma. It is more common in men than in women and in this country usually occurs in the age range from 50 to 70. There is a striking and curious racial and geographical distribution in that it is extremely common in the Bantu in Southern Africa. It is also common in Eastern races, particularly the Japanese. The most common site in the oesophagus to be affected is the lower one third. Rarely adenocarcinomas are found at the lower end of the oesophagus, arising either from islands of columnar epithelium which exist in the oesophagus near its junction with the stomach or from the epithelium of the stomach itself, the tumour then spreading up the oesophagus.

Non-epithelial tumours are also found, the most common of these is the leiomyoma which is the benign, or the leiomyosarcoma which is the malignant form of this smooth muscle tumour. Other tumours such as lymphosarcoma and secondary malignant tumours are rare.

Clinical features

The commonest symptom by far is difficulty in swallowing (*dysphagia*). At first this is for solids only but as the tumour grows the difficulty extends to liquids. Associated with this is a progressive loss of weight. There may be positive occult blood in the faeces, with anaemia. If dysphagia is complete there may be the symptoms and signs of aspiration pneumonia. It is common for patients who have progressed to this extent to complain of 'sialorrhoea' which is the production and expectoration of large volumes of saliva. Sometimes the tumour spreads to the cervical lymph nodes.

Special investigations

As with all oesophageal conditions, the diagnosis is by means of preliminary barium swallow followed by oesophagoscopy and biopsy (Fig. 11.8).

Treatment

If the patient is dehydrated and cachectic on admission, it is first necessary to improve his nutritional state. Often if food debris is cleared from the oesophagus by gentle lavage or at oesophagoscopy, he will then be able to swallow liquids such as milk and Complan to which vitamins can be added. If not, a plastic nasogastric tube may be threaded through the malignant stricture. Only if these simple measures fail is a feeding gastrostomy required in order to prepare the patient for further treatment.

If investigation reveals the carcinoma to be limited and in the lower third of the oesophagus, resection of the tumour is carried out using a thoraco-abdominal approach, either as one continuous incision from the abdomen into the left chest or as two incisions, one in the midline of the abdomen and the second at the level of the

Fig. 11.8. Barium swallow in carcinoma of the oesophagus. This is demonstrated by the narrow stricture in the mid-oesophagus (arrowed).

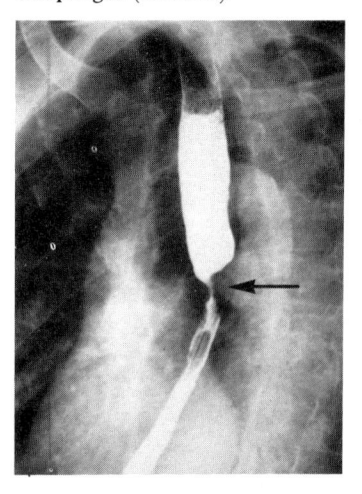

right fifth rib. The tumour is completely excised and the upper end of the oesophagus is joined to the fundus of the stomach, which is mobilised and brought into the chest. This always results in division of the vagus nerves and a pyloroplasty has therefore to be added.

In tumours of the middle third of the oesophagus resection is again the procedure of choice although technically this is much more difficult as the line of the anastomosis between the oesophagus and the stomach comes to lie above the arch of the aorta or is fashioned in the neck.

Tumours of the upper third of the oesophagus and post-cricoid carcinomas are usually treated by radiotherapy.

A tumour that has extended into tissues around the oesophagus thus preventing resection can be palliated by passing a tube such as the Mousseau-Barbin or Celestin tube (see Fig. 5.8) through it, to enable the patient to swallow food until extension of the carcinoma produces the inevitable death of the patient.

After intubation all food must be sieved and has to be followed by a drink to remove food debris from the lumen of the tube; it is found an advantage to use some form of effervescent fluid such as lemonade or soda water.

Unfortunately the long term results after resection of oesophageal carcinomas are not good and under 5% of patients are alive and free from tumour five years after the operation.

Stomach

Anatomy

The stomach (Fig. 11.9) is divided into a fundus, body, antrum and pylorus. The lines of division between these parts of the stomach are ill defined but nevertheless serve as useful descriptive terms. There is an extremely important functional difference between the fundus and the body, on one hand, and the antrum on the other and this relates to the type of cells found in the mucosa. Acid is only secreted in the body and fundus of the stomach. No acid is secreted from the antrum and it is from here that mucosal cells termed 'G-cells' produce the hormone *gastrin*. It is not possible by external inspection to distinguish between the body and the antrum.

The whole of the gastrointestinal tract is lined by an inner circular and outer longitudinal coat of involuntary muscle, but in the case of the stomach these are arranged in loops which permit considerable distension of the organ as it fills with food, allowing it

Fig. 11.9. The stomach and its subdivisions.

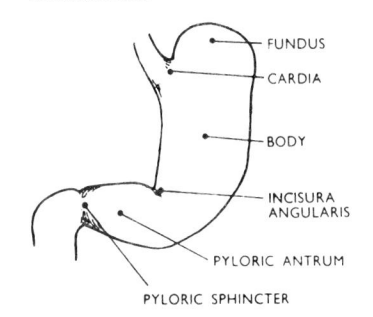

to fulfil its function as a reservoir. The muscle of the antrum is thicker than that in the body. The antrum undergoes vigorous, segmenting contraction with the result that food is broken down and converted to gastric chyme so that the process of digestion can continue rapidly in the intestine.

The pylorus is marked by a small vein which passes over its anterior surface, the 'pyloric vein of Mayo'. At operation the pylorus can be felt as a definite ring which will admit the tip of one finger. The precise function of the pylorus is still in some doubt. It does not seem to be concerned with the regulation of gastric emptying so much as in the prevention of duodeno-gastric reflux, although naturally if the pylorus is unable to expand sufficiently for any reason, such as scarring following duodenal ulceration, gastric emptying will be delayed.

The stomach is richly supplied with blood from the coeliac axis via the left and right gastric arteries and the left and right gastroepiploic arteries. The venous drainage follows the arteries and is to the portal vein; the ascending branch of the left gastric vein communicates with the azygos vein in the chest. These anastomotic channels in the lower oesophages and cardia become dilated in the condition of portal hypertension, a fact of considerable importance in the development of oesophageal varices. The lymphatic drainage tends to follow the venous drainage, there being lymph nodes along the lesser curve of the stomach with the lymphatics extending to the porta hepatis, and inferiorly along the greater curve of the stomach via the greater oemntum to the transverse mesocolon and the superior border of the pancreas. The nerve supply is from the vagus nerves (Fig. 11.10) and from the sympathetic nerves travelling with the arteries.

Gastric secretion

The cells lining the fundus and body of the stomach produce a complicated secretion which contains hydrochloric acid with inorganic ions, principally chloride, sodium and potassium, together with enzymes concerned with digestion, particularly pepsin, but also amylase and lipase in small quantities. The acid is produced from cells which can be readily identified on histological section called parietal cells. Thus the secretion from the body of the stomach is of a highly acid nature and the pH falls to the region of 1.5. In distinction to this is the secretion of the antrum, which is almost neutral. Antral cells produce gastrin, which is a hormone. This enters the bloodstream and when it recirculates and reaches the parietal cells it stimulates them to produce hydrochloric acid (HCl).

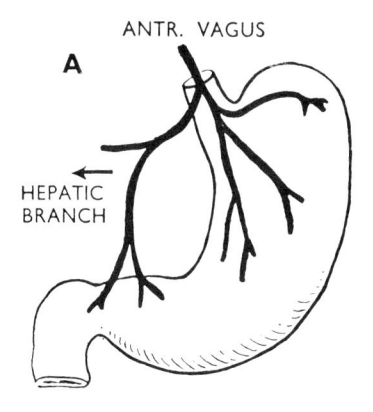

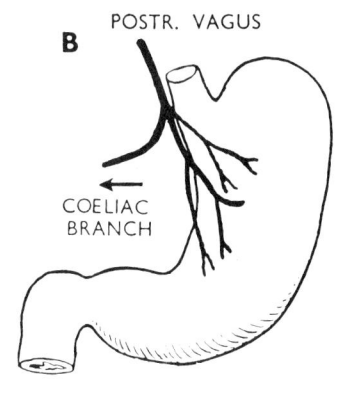

Fig. 11.10. The vagal supply to the stomach. (A) The anterior vagus; (B) the posterior vagus.

The stimuli to gastric juice production are:
1. *The psychic phase* of gastric secretion, that is the thought, sight or smell of food which results in the vagus nerve becoming active with consequent stimulation of both parietal cells and antral G-cells.
2. *Gastric phase of secretion*, which results from direct contact between the swallowed food and the stomach. Certain foods, particularly digested meat products, are powerful stimulators of the G-cells and result in the release of gastrin and an increased secretion of acid.

GASTRIC FUNCTION TESTS

The old term 'test meal' is misleading and should not be used. The amount of acid that the stomach can produce is measured by means of a gastric function test. In this the patient fasts for 12 hours overnight and a plastic tube is passed through either the nose or the mouth into the stomach. This is usually 45 cm from the incisors or 50 cm from the external nares. The juice is aspirated from the fasting stomach and usually only amounts to 25 ml, or so. The tube is then aspirated at a negative pressure of 5 cm of mercury for the next hour, the suction being broken every 10 minutes and 20 ml of air being blown down the tube to clear it of any plugs of mucus. This hour's secretion is termed the *basal hour* and is kept separate. The patient is now given an injection of Pentagastrin (which is a synthetic product composed of the terminal 5 peptides from the gastrin molecule, and is produced by I.C.I.) the dose being .02 micrograms/kg body weight administered intramuscularly. The secretion of the stomach is collected for the next 1 hour, as for the first hour, divided into separate 15 minute samples. The acid is measured by titration. The 'peak acid output' is calculated from the two highest 15 minute outputs in the hour expressed as milliequivalents of acid per hour. The average values for normal patients and those with duodenal and gastric ulcer are:

	Men	Women
Normal	25	17
DU	43	31
GU	22	15

Average peak acid output expressed as mEq H^+/hour to Pentagastrin stimulation

The insulin test

In this, the patient is prepared as above. A basal hour's secretion is collected and then an intravenous dose of insulin (0.2 units/Kg body weight) is given. The low blood sugar which results from the insulin produces reflex stimulation of the vagus nerve which in turn will produce secretion of acid by the stomach if its nerve supply is intact. This is therefore used as a test of completeness following the operation of vagotomy (see page 189).

CONGENITAL HYPERTROPHIC PYLORIC STENOSIS

Pathology

In this condition the pyloric muscle undergoes an intense hypertrophy to produce the characteristic 'pyloric tumour'. The aetiology of this condition is quite unknown.

Clinical features

80% occur in male infants, 50% are first-born and the condition may affect several children in the same family. Symptoms usually commence between 7 and 14 days after birth and it is extremely uncommon for a previously healthy infant to develop this condition after 12 weeks of age.

The child will take a feed of milk and then, after a few minutes, will return this with a massive and typically 'projectile' vomit. This is then followed by a period of screaming due to the baby's hunger and thirst. The vomit does not contain bile. There is failure to gain weight and, as a result of dehydration, the baby is constipated, the stools resembling the faecal pellets of a rabbit.

On examination the child may be obviously dehydrated and the dilated stomach may be visible in the upper abdomen. Careful palpation during a period when the child is not crying will reveal the hypertrophied pyloric sphincter as a palpable mass in the right upper abdomen.

Differential diagnosis is from gastro-enteritis, which is usually accompanied by diarrhoea, from the various forms of congenital intestinal obstruction, which usually commence within a day or two of birth and in which the vomit contains bile, and over-feeding, in which the child regurgitates the excess of each meal.

Treatment

If the child appears healthy, it may be submitted to operation soon after admission, but if there is dehydration, then a day or two must be spent in gastric lavage and fluid replacement, either by the subcutaneous or intravenous route, using half-strength saline.

Ramstedt's operation is usually carried out under a general anaesthetic through a transverse upper abdominal incision. The hypertrophied pylorus is delivered and the muscle fibres are divided down to the mucosa (Fig. 11.11). The infant is given glucose water 3 hours after the operation and this is followed by 3-hourly milk feeds, which are steadily increased in amount. Results are excellent and the mortality extremely low.

Medical treatment is used only when the diagnosis is in doubt and should not be persisted with for more than two days if symptoms

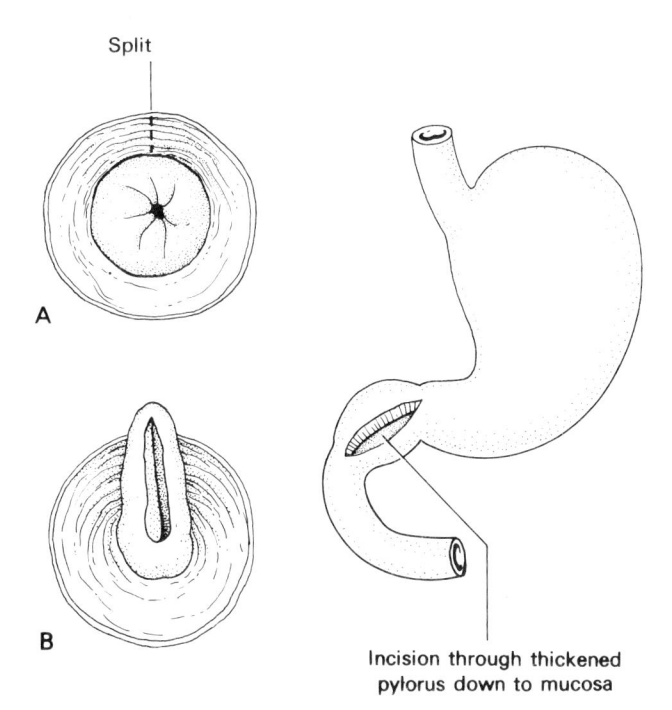

Fig. 11.11. Ramstedt's operation. The thickened muscle at the pylorus is split down to the mucosa. The inset diagrams show the pathology and the operative procedure in transverse section.

continue. It comprises gastric lavage together with the use of the antispasmodic agent Eumidrine (atropine methyl nitrate) given 15 minutes before each feed.

GASTRIC ULCER

Pathology

Gastric ulcer is usually situated on the lesser curve of the stomach in its distal two-thirds down to and including the pylorus. An ulcer anywhere else in the stomach must be considered to be malignant until proved otherwise. The aetiology of this condition, in spite of much research, remains uncertain (Fig. 11.12).

Clinical features

Gastric ulcer occurs three times more commonly in men than in women and in a very wide range of ages, but it is more common between 30 and 50 years. The principal complaint is of upper abdominal pain which is related to the taking of food and may be relieved by alkali medicines. Quite often the patient is wakened at

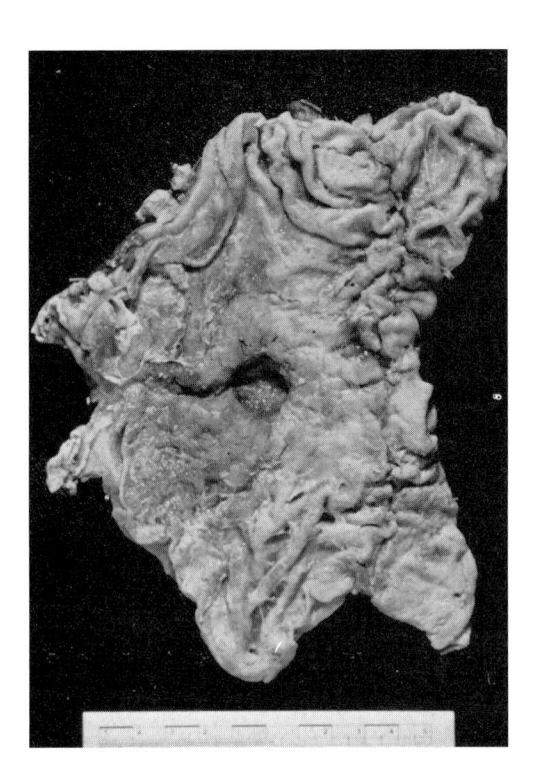

Fig. 11.12. Operation specimen of a gastric ulcer viewed from the mucosal aspect.

about 2 a.m. by pain. If the ulcer is penetrating into the pancreas posteriorly, pain may be experienced in addition in the region of the lower thoracic spine. The symptoms of duodenal and gastric ulceration are virtually indistinguishable.

Complications

These are:
1. Perforation into the general peritoneal cavity (see page 190).
2. Haemorrhage (see page 195).
3. Malignant change (rare).

Special investigations

Barium meal is the mainstay of the special investigations and yields a positive result in those patients with a gastric ulcer in over 90% of cases (Fig. 11.13). In some instances the ulcer may be overlooked, especially when it is high on the posterior lesser curve of the stomach. It may also sometimes be difficult to be certain whether or not the ulcer is benign or malignant.

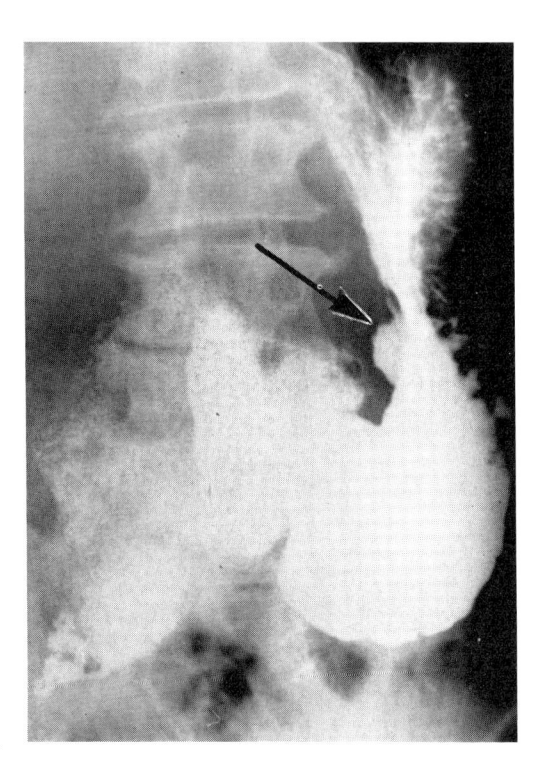

Fig. 11.13. Barium meal showing a large gastric ulcer on the lesser curve (arrowed).

Gastroscopy has become safer and more accurate with the recent development of fibre-optic instruments. The whole of the inside of the stomach can now be visualised and photographed as a permanent record, and a biopsy taken of the ulcer. (Fig. 11.14). A combination of barium meal and gastroscopy is highly accurate.

Treatment

The treatment of a gastric ulcer is medical in the first instance. Surgery is indicated if medical treatment fails, if complications supervene or if we cannot be certain that the ulcer is benign.

MEDICAL TREATMENT

Only three things are known to accelerate the rate of healing of a gastric ulcer and these are:
1. Bed rest
2. Carbenoxalone sodium (Biogastrone)
3. Abstinence from cigarette smoking.

Symptomatic relief is obtained by the taking of regular alkalis, for example Mist. magnesium trisilicate, together with a bland diet.

The difficulty with a medical regime is that it involves admitting the patient to hospital with consequent loss of earning and family disruption. A check barium meal and, if necessary, a gastroscopy, is carried out 6 weeks from the commencement of treatment to ensure that the ulcer has either completely disappeared or is at least

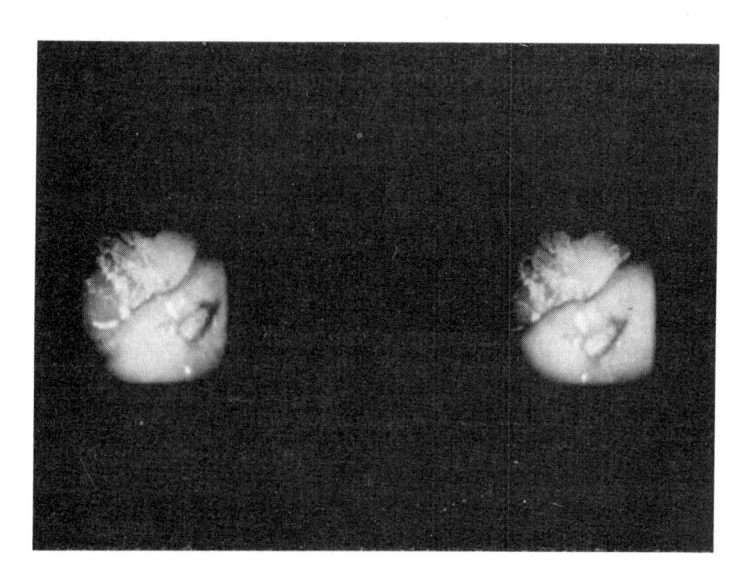

Fig. 11.14. A gastric ulcer photographed through the gastroscope.

healing. If not, the patient should be submitted to surgery if for no other reason than that malignant disease cannot be excluded.

SURGERY

The usual operative procedure is a Billroth I partial gastrectomy; this involves the removal of that part of the stomach which is liable to become ulcerated. The proximal remnant is joined to the duodenum (Fig. 11.15). The operative mortality for this procedure is under 1% and so is the recurrence rate. The result of this type of gastrectomy for a gastric ulcer is indeed so good that it is quite difficult to imagine how it can be improved.

Recently some surgeons have advocated vagotomy and pyloroplasty for gastric ulcer but the recurrence rate is so high that this is an unjustified procedure.

GASTRITIS

This is an inflammation of the stomach mucosa and can be due to a variety of causes:
1. Irritation due to certain foods such as curry.
2. Drugs—aspirin, cortisone, butazolidine and alcohol. (This group may produce acute gastric erosions).
3. Auto-immunity, e.g. pernicious anaemia.
4. Idiopathic

Clinical features

The usual symptom of gastritis is known to everyone, a feeling of discomfort in the epigastrium. It is often relieved by the taking of alkali together with avoidance of any causal factor.

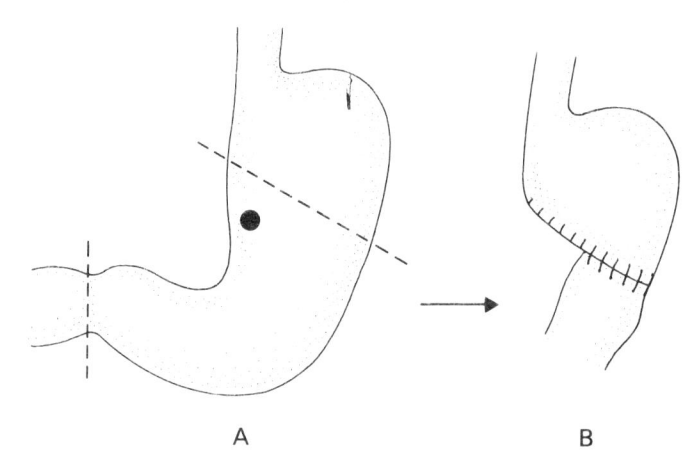

Fig. 11.15. The Billroth I gastrectomy: the gastric stump is anastomosed to the duodenum.

From the surgical point of view the drug and alcohol induced group is the most important since the acute erosions of the gastric mucosa that result are a common cause of gastric haemorrhage (see page 195).

TUMOURS OF THE STOMACH

The only common tumour to affect the stomach is the carcinoma which arises from its epithelium; other tumours are quite rare. These include the benign leiomyoma, the malignant leiomyosarcoma and lymphosarcoma, infiltration by Hodgkin's disease and rare invasion from adjacent tumours (pancreas or colon).

LEIOMYOMA

This arises from the muscle of the stomach wall, projects into the lumen of the stomach and becomes ulcerated at its apex, so that it may be an occasional cause of a brisk haematemesis. Rarely it undergoes malignant change to form a leiomyosarcoma.

LYMPHOSARCOMA

This rare tumour arises from lymphoid tissue in the wall of the stomach. It produces gross distortion and irregularity of the stomach and may fistulate into the colon. Spread takes place to the lymph nodes—first to those adjacent to the stomach and then widely to nodes in the neck, axillae and groins.

Treatment is by resection of the primary tumour, where possible, and radiotherapy to involved nodes.

CARCINOMA OF THE STOMACH

Pathology

This is an extremely common and important tumour. In this country it is headed in incidence only by cancer of the lung and large bowel in the male, and by carcinoma of the breast, uterus and large bowel in the female. Distribution is world-wide, although it is particularly frequent in some races, especially the Japanese. Any age may be involved, but it especially affects the age range 50–70. The incidence is raised in patients with pernicious anaemia and there is a definite link with subjects having blood group A, which suggests a genetic factor. Occasionally a gastric carcinoma arises in a previous chronic benign gastric ulcer.

About a quarter of stomach cancers arise in the pyloric region of the stomach. The remainder are distributed fairly evenly throughout the rest of the organ, or diffusely involve the whole of the stomach.

The tumour may take the form of a malignant ulcer with heaped overhanging edges (Fig. 11.16), or it may form a polypoid mass which proliferates into the stomach lumen, or it may widely infiltrate the submucous planes of the stomach which results in a thickened, contracted, organ with little if any superficial ulceration to which the title *'leather-bottle stomach'* is applied.

Spread of the tumour occurs locally through the wall of the stomach and adjacent organs (pancreas, abdominal wall, transverse colon) may be directly invaded. A gastro-colic fistula may develop.

Adjacent lymph nodes are commonly affected. Blood stream dissemination occurs via the portal vein to the liver and thence occasionally to the lungs and the skeleton. Seedlings of tumour may disseminate throughout the peritoneal cavity (transcoelomic spread) and this is characteristically accompanied by ascites.

Clinical features

Symptoms may be produced by the local effects of the tumour, by the secondaries, or by general features associated with malignant disease.

Local symptoms include epigastric pain, which may be indistinguishable from that produced by a chronic gastric ulcer. Vomiting is especially associated with a pyloric tumour producing gastric outlet obstruction and dysphagia (difficulty in swallowing) occurs in tumours at the cardio-oesophageal junction. Only occasionally does a carcinoma of the stomach present with either perforation or acute haemorrhage.

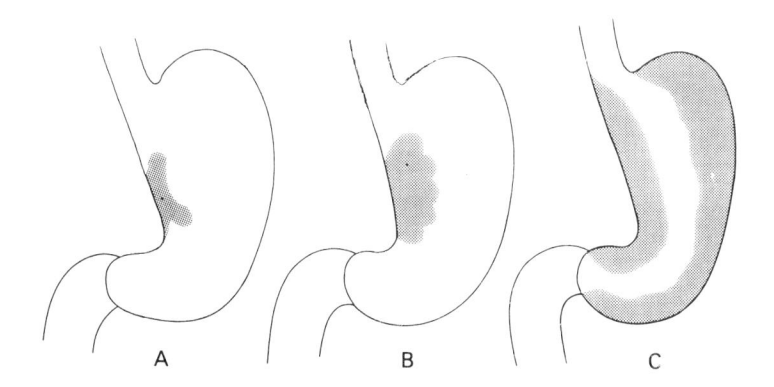

Fig. 11.16. The types of gastric cancer. (A) ulcer. (B) polypoid. (C) leather bottle stomach (linitis plastica).

Secondaries: the patient may first report with jaundice due to liver involvement or abdominal distention due to ascites.

General features: a frequent form of presentation are the general symptoms associated with malignant disease—anorexia, loss of weight and anaemia.

Clinical examination may reveal features which correspond to these three headings. There may be a mass to feel in the abdomen which is the tumour itself. An enlarged liver may be obvious, or the surgeon may detect ascites. Weight loss and anaemia may be obvious (see Fig. 5.7).

Special investigations

The barium meal is highly accurate; it may demonstrate an irregular stricture, a polypoid tumour, or an ulcer with raised edges (Fig. 11.17). Occasionally, however, the radiologist has considerable

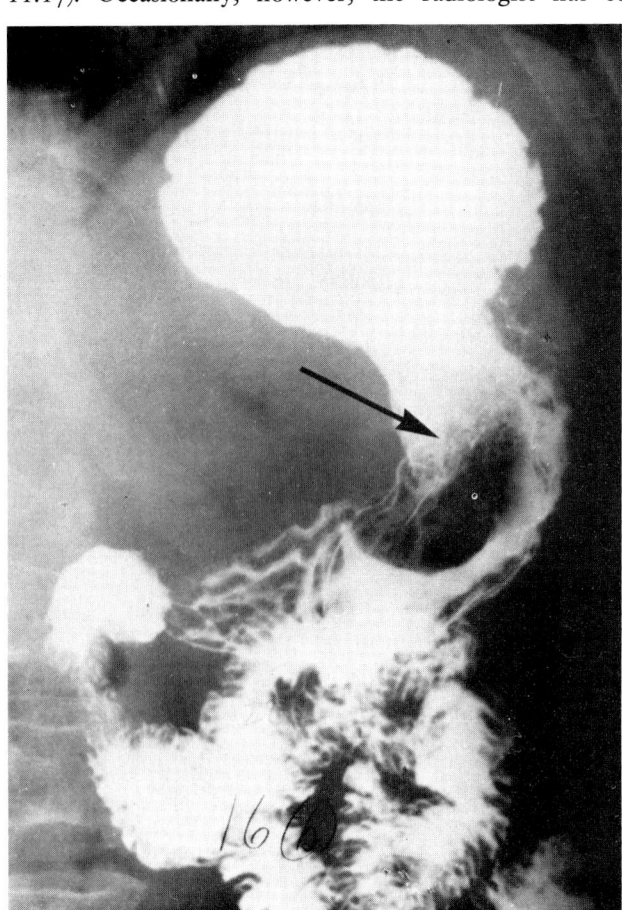

Fig. 11.17. Barium meal demonstrating a polypoid carcinoma of the stomach—note the filling defect (arrowed) projecting inwards from the lesser curvature of the stomach.

difficulty in distinguishing between a benign and malignant stomach ulcer. If necessary *gastroscopy* can then be performed using the fibre-optic instrument. The ulcer can then be directly visualized and a biopsy taken for microscopic examination.

Treatment

The only possible chance of cure for this condition is surgical removal, and this depends on early diagnosis. A tumour at the pylorus or antrum can be removed by partial gastrectomy in which the distal two-thirds of the stomach is removed, the duodenum closed, and a loop of the first part of the jejunum joined to the stomach (Polya gastectomy). If the tumour occupies the body of the stomach or the cardia, it may be necessary to carry out total gastrectomy, close the duodenum and anastomose the jejunum to the divided oesophagus (the Roux-en-Y anastomosis). These procedures are illustrated in Fig. 11.18.

If the tumour cannot be resected because of local invasiveness it may be possible to carry out a gastro-enterostomy to relieve obstruction of the pylorus or intubation by means of a plastic tube (see Fig. 5.8) may relieve the dysphagia of an advanced carcinoma at the cardia. Irradiation and cytotoxic therapy are of only limited value.

Prognosis

This depends on how extensive the tumour is at the time of surgery and on its microscopic nature; the more undifferentiated or anaplastic the tumour, the worse the prognosis is likely to be. The overall outlook is poor; only 5% of all patients presenting to hospital survive for 5 years. However, 20% of patients who undergo radical curative surgery are alive at the end of a five-year period.

Duodenum

Anatomy

The duodenum commences immediately after the pylorus and travels in a C-shape to join the jejunum at the duodeno-jejunal junction (Fig. 11.19). Enclosed within the concave border of the 'C' is the head of the pancreas. The common bile duct runs behind the first part of the duodenum and then, after traversing the posterior aspect of the head of the pancreas, enters the medial wall of the

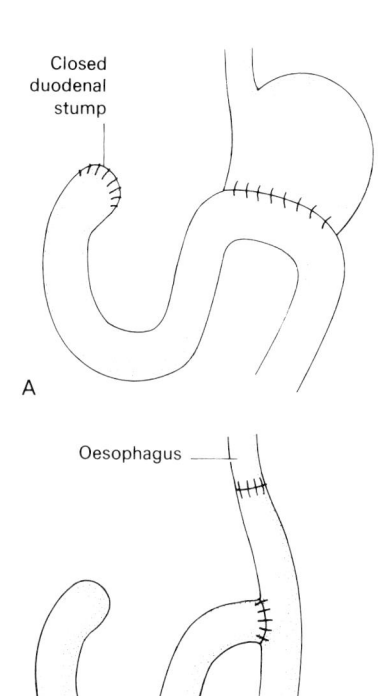

Fig. 11.18. Diagram of the Polya partial gastrectomy (A) and total gastrectomy (B). In the first, the duodenum has been closed and a loop of jejunum anastomosed to the gastric remnant. In the second, the duodenum has again been closed and Roux-loop of jejunum brought up and sutured to the oesophagus.

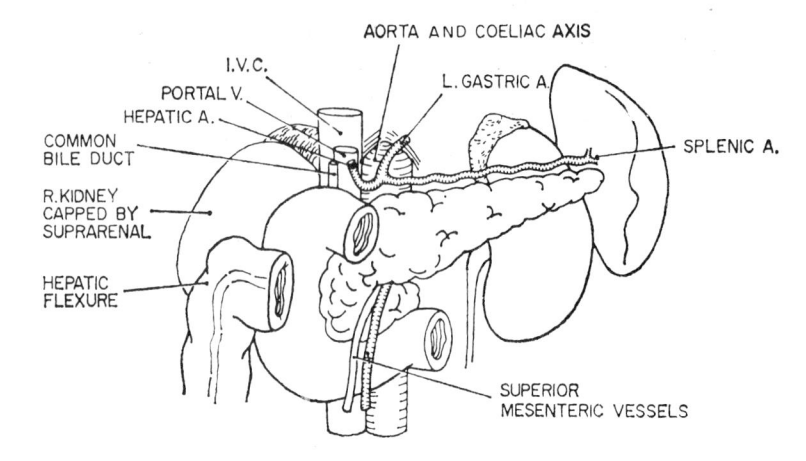

Fig. 11.19. The duodenum and its immediate relations.

second part of the duodenum. The pancreatic duct opens in conjunction with the termination of the common bile duct in one-third of subjects; in the remainder it opens as a separate, but closely related orifice guarded by the sphincter of Oddi.

Physiology

In addition to transmission of food from the stomach to the jejunum, the duodenum has several important special functions. It is here that gastric chyme is mixed with biliary and pancreatic secretion and the digestive process commences; fats commencing to break down into their constituent fatty acids and glycerol, proteins to amino-acids, and starches into sugars.

As soon as food comes into contact with the duodenum the hormones secretin and pancreozymin are secreted by the duodenal mucosa. These circulate in the blood stream to reach the pancreas and stimulate its secretion. Cholecystokinin is also liberated, and this hormone produces contraction of the gall bladder with expulsion of its contained bile into the duodenum. The duodenum is also responsible for the absorption of iron and possibly calcium and, for this reason, any operation that results in a by-pass of the duodenum may cause iron deficient anaemia.

DUODENAL ULCER

Pathology

In this condition an ulcer develops in the first part of the duodenum. It may be situated on the posterior or, less often, the anterior wall of the duodenum, and occasionally a giant ulcer will saddle across both walls. It is more common in men than women, in the ratio of 2:1. The peak age incidence is from 35–45, although ulcers may occur in children and in the elderly. It is three times more common in Scotland than in the south of England, although its incidence in the British Isles has been declining since 1955. The social class does not affect the incidence and different groups of workers are affected more or less equally. It is a common disease and approximately 400,000 men and 200,000 women were estimated to be suffering from this condition in 1968.

The cause of duodenal ulcer is unknown. One striking fact is that, on average, patients with this condition secrete an excess of gastric juice which contains more acid and pepsin than in normal subjects. On very rare occasions this hypersecretion of acid is due to the production of the hormone gastrin by a tumour of the islet cells of the pancreas (the Zollinger-Ellison syndrome). There is an increased incidence of duodenal ulceration in patients of blood group O.

It has been said that duodenal ulcer is due to worry and that it occurs in anxious individuals, but evidence to confirm or refute this theory is lacking.

In summary this condition occurs in patients who tend to secrete more acid from the stomach than normal, it is becoming less common, but the fundamental reason for both these observations remains unknown.

Clinical features

There is usually a characteristic history of epigastric pain which comes on anything up to two hours after meals and may wake the patient in the middle of the night. It is relieved by taking alkalis, milk, or food, although later in the disease these remedies become less effective. If the ulcer is situated posteriorly and erodes into the head of the pancreas, the pain may be experienced in the lower thoracic region of the spine, as well as in the epigastrium. Quite frequently there is a family history of the disease, especially in patients whose symptoms commence in their teens.

Examination usually reveals little apart from upper abdominal tenderness.

Special investigations

The *barium meal* is usually highly accurate in making the diagnosis. The ulcer crater itself may be visualized, or the scarring and deformity of the first part of the duodenum (Fig. 11.20).

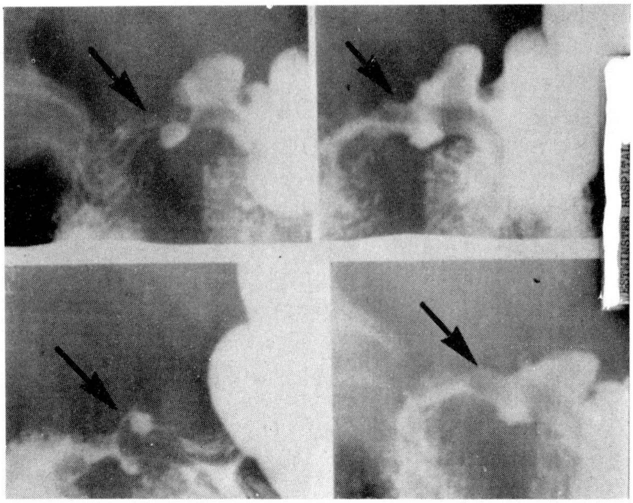

Fig. 11.20. Barium meal series demonstrating a duodenal ulcer (arrowed).

Gastroduodenoscopy has become an important adjunct in recent years and the flexible duodenoscope allows visualization of the mucosa of the duodenum.

Gastric function tests may be carried out to measure the amount of acid that the stomach is capable of secreting. A flexible nasogastric tube is passed into the stomach after an overnight 8 hour fast. The peak acid output (see page 175) is then measured after stimulation by pentagastrin.

A high peak acid output is useful corroborative evidence of duodenal ulcer, but, unfortunately, because of wide variability in this measurement, it cannot be taken as proof of diagnosis.

Treatment

Uncomplicated duodenal ulcers are treated medically in the first instance. Surgery is reserved for those patients who fail to respond adequately to medical therapy, or who are suffering from the complications of this disease.

MEDICAL TREATMENT

After the diagnosis of duodenal ulcer has been confirmed, the patient is advised to regulate his life so that he is able to take at least small quantities of food every two hours during the day. In addition to this, regular antacids are prescribed in the form of aluminium hydroxide tablets or magnesium trisilicate tablets to be sucked slowly after meals, or to be taken when symptoms occur. It may also be helpful to give the patient atropine-like preparations, for example, probanthine 15 mg t.d.s. which will be effective in reducing the gastric acid secretion.

There is no evidence that diet has any part to play in the treatment of chronic duodenal ulcer. In days that have now happily gone by, patients were advised to take a restricted diet which consisted of milk puddings, mashed potatoes, fish, and things that were considered to be soothing and non-irritating to the gastric lining. This approach has been shown to be without foundation and patients should merely be advised to avoid those things that they know will produce indigestion.

SURGICAL TREATMENT

The emergency surgical procedures which may be required in perforation and haemorrhage are considered in the appropriate sections below.

The principle underlying elective surgery for duodenal ulcer is that the ulcer will heal, provided that the high acid production of the stomach is abolished. This can be effected either by removing the bulk of the acid secreting area of the stomach, that is to say, its body and lesser curvature, by means of a Polya partial gastrectomy with closure of the duodenum and anastomosis of the gastric stump to the proximal jejunum, or else by dividing the vagus nerves. Since vagotomy not only abolishes the reflex phase of gastric secretion but also affects the emptying of the stomach, this must be accompanied by a gastric drainage procedure, either gastro-jejunostomy or a pyloroplasty, which is a plastic enlargement of the pylorus (Fig. 11.21).

The vagotomy may either be *truncal*, in which the two main trunks of the nerve are excised as these travel alongside the oesophagus through the hiatus in the diaphragm to the stomach, or *selective*, when only those fibres passing to the stomach itself are divided or *proximal gastric*, preserving the fibres to the antrum (Fig. 11.22).

Most surgeons in this country now perform vagotomy and pyloroplasty, but substitute a gastro-jejunostomy when gross disease of the duodenum makes the former procedure difficult. The operative mortality associated with vagotomy is under 0.5%. The recurrence rate is approximately 5%. Some patients may complain of bile vomiting after the operation and others of 'dumping', which is a feeling of weakness associated with sweating and palpitations following meals. Satisfactory results can be anticipated in between 85 and 90% of patients.

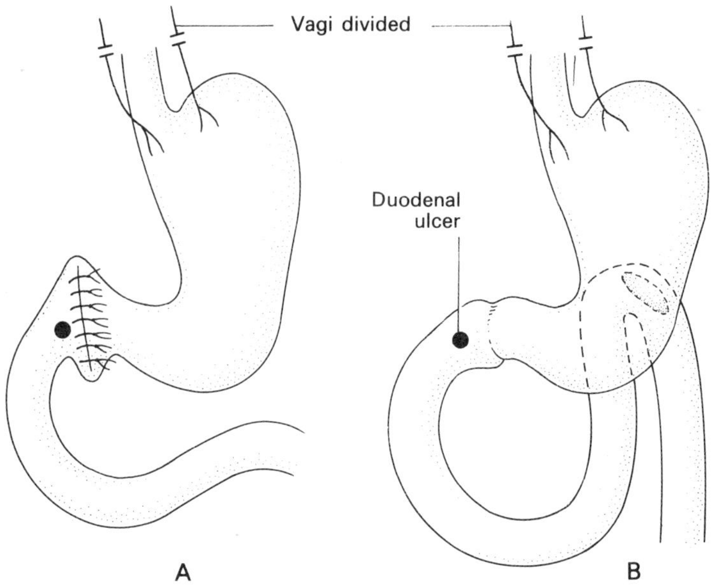

Fig. 11.21. Types of gastric drainage after vagotomy (A) pyloroplasty and (B) gastrojejunostomy.

Before submitting a patient with peptic ulcer to surgery he should be checked for four things:

1. The haemoglobin level; these patients have often been on a diet low in iron and may also have had occult bleeding.
2. The teeth; these often require dental treatment, since gross dental caries predisposes to postoperative parotitis and there is always the risk of dislodgement and inhalation of a loose and septic tooth during anaesthesia.
3. Vitamin C; peptic ulcer patients are often deficient in this vitamin because of their long use of a diet which lacks fruit and vegetables.
4. These patients are often heavy smokers with a chronic cough. Smoking is forbidden and intensive chest physiotherapy given in order to reduce the incidence and severity of postoperative pulmonary collapse.

PERFORATED PEPTIC ULCER

Pathology

Perforation complicates about 10% of all peptic ulcers. Of all perforations, 90% occur in duodenal ulcer, and 90% are in males, especially in the 25–50 year age group. Infants and the very elderly, however, are not immune. There is a high incidence of perforation in patients with peptic ulcer who are on heavy cortisone therapy, and

THE VAGOTOMIES

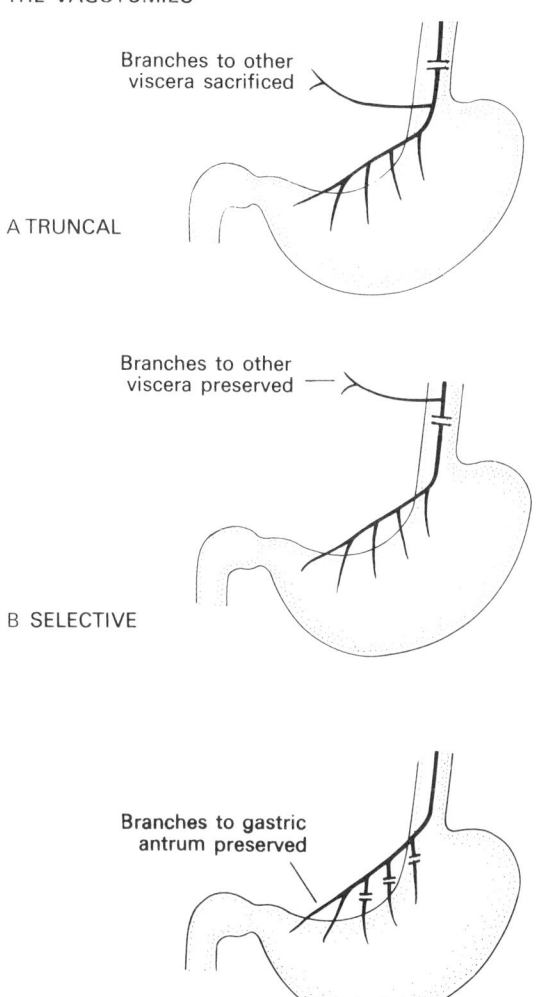

Fig. 11.22. (A) Truncal, (B) selective and (C) proximal gastric vagotomy.

in these the perforation may be relatively silent. Gastric carcinomas occasionally perforate.

Clinical Features

A previous history of peptic ulceration is often obtained, although this may be forgotten by the patient in his agony. Typically there is a sudden severe generalised abdominal pain. Irritation of the lower aspect of the diaphragm by gastric contents may be indicated by radiation of the pain to one or both shoulders, usually the right.

The pain is aggravated by movement and the patient lies rigidly still. There is nausea but only occasionally vomiting.

Examination reveals a patient in severe pain, cold and sweating, with rapid shallow respiration. However, in the early hours, there is no clinical evidence of true shock; the pulse is steady and the blood pressure normal. In the early stages also the temperature is either normal or a little depressed. The abdomen is retracted and when touched is as rigid as a board. On auscultation bowel sounds are absent.

In the delayed case, after 12 hours or more, the features of late peritonitis with paralytic ileus become manifest; the abdomen becomes distended, effortless vomiting occurs and the patient is extremely toxic and in shock.

X-ray of the abdomen with the patient erect may show free gas below the diaphragm in about 70% of cases (Fig. 11.23).

Treatment

The stomach is emptied by means of a nasogastric tube to diminish further leakage through the perforation, and is an essential pre-anaesthetic measure. Morphia is given to relieve pain and an intra-

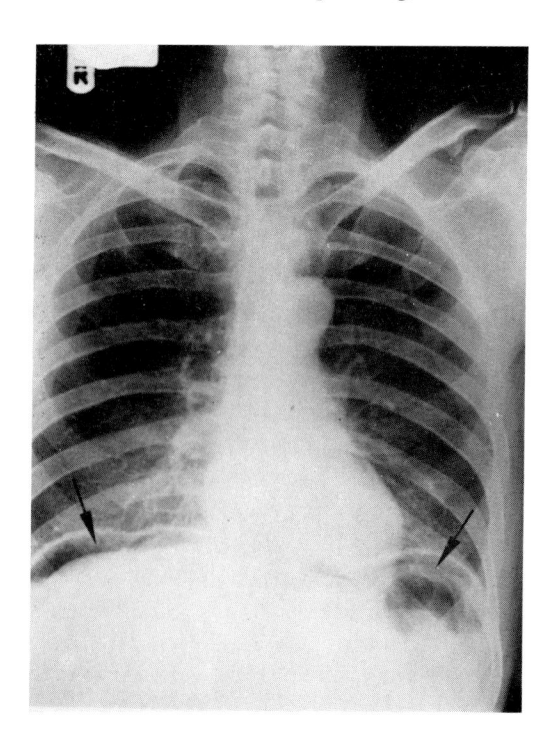

Fig. 11.23. A chest X-ray in a patient with perforated duodenal ulcer. Note that there is free air in the abdomen which is seen between the liver and the diaphragm on the right and between the fundus of the stomach and diaphragm on the left (arrowed).

venous drip commenced. Ampicillin is given to contend with the peritoneal infection. At operation the peritoneal cavity is sucked clear of all contaminating material and the perforation closed with three or four catgut sutures (Fig. 11.24). Provided undue delay has been avoided, prognosis is good but the mortality is high in patients who do not reach hospital until 12 hours or more from the perforation and this delay is particularly serious in elderly patients.

The late prognosis following perforation depends on whether or not the ulcer is chronic. If there is a previous history of ulceration, about 50% have further serious symptoms and usually come to later elective surgery. If the ulcer is acute with no previous history, this figure falls to 20%. A second subsequent perforation is not rare.

PYLORIC STENOSIS

By common usage, this term has come to include all conditions which result in obstruction to the outflow of the stomach, whether situated in the distal antrum, at the pylorus itself, or in the first part of the duodenum.

The common causes in the adult are scarring due to chronic duodenal ulcer, a benign peptic ulcer of the antrum, or a carcinoma of the pyloric end of the stomach.

Congenital pyloric stenosis in infants is considered on page 176.

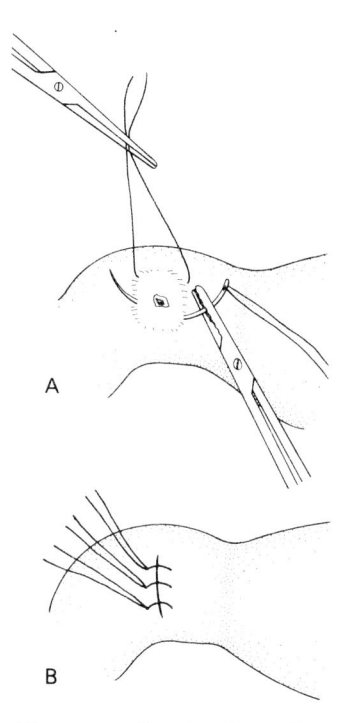

Fig. 11.24. Repair of a perforated duodenal ulcer by means of interrupted catgut sutures.

Clinical features

The cardinal symptom of pyloric stenosis, whatever the cause, is vomiting. This is characteristically profuse, free from bile, and may contain food eaten one or two days previously. If the obstruction is due to a stenosing duodenal ulcer there is usually a history of peptic ulceration which has been present for some years. However, if obstruction is due to a carcinoma of the pyloric end of the stomach, the history is usually much shorter, often only weeks or months in duration.

If vomiting persists, the patient's nutrition suffers and he loses weight. There may be dehydration and weakness due to loss of fluid and electrolytes.

On examination the patient may appear dehydrated and wasted. The abdomen may reveal the characteristic succussion splash which is elicited by gently shaking the patient from side to side and listening for the noise produced by the fluid and air contents splashing within the dilated stomach. Sir James Walton, a surgeon at the London Hospital, described three stages of pyloric stenosis:

1. 'the stomach that you can hear'; this is the succussion splash.
2. 'the stomach that you can see'; when a patient with advanced pyloric stenosis is observed, it is possible to see waves of gastric peristalsis which pass from left to right in the epigastrium.
3. 'the stomach that you can feel'; in this very marked case the wall of the stomach is so hypertrophied that it can be palpated through the abdominal muscles.

Investigations

1. *Gastric aspiration* yields a morning resting juice of over 100 ml. It may, in fact, amount to a litre or more of foul-smelling gastric contents containing stale food residue.
2. *Barium meal* shows dilatation of the stomach with a narrow outlet and considerable delay in emptying (Fig. 11.25). It may be difficult or impossible for the radiologist to be certain whether or not the obstruction is due to a benign peptic ulcer of the distal stomach or duodenum, or due to a carcinoma.
3. *Biochemical investigations.* Prolonged vomiting results in loss of

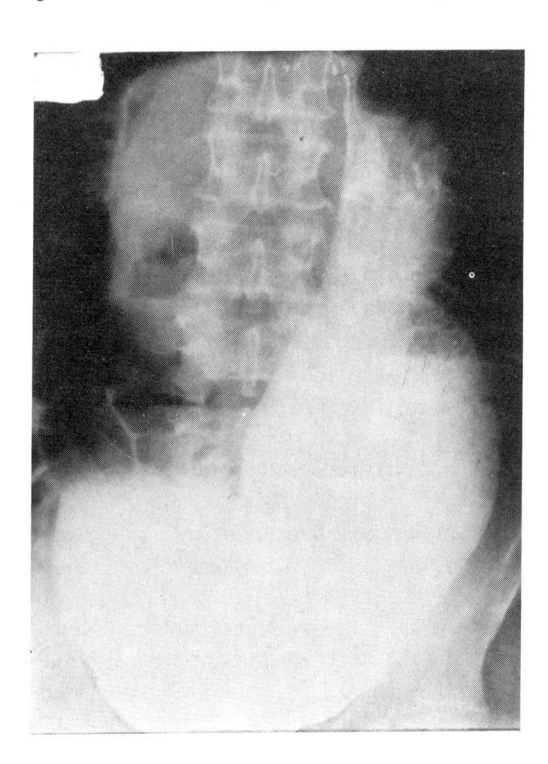

Fig. 11.25. Barium meal in pyloric stenosis due to a duodenal ulcer. The stomach is grossly dilated due to obstruction at its outlet.

water, hydrochloric acid and electrolytes. The loss of acid results in the condition of alkalosis so that the plasma bicarbonate is elevated. The serum chloride, sodium and potassium may be lowered. The blood urea may rise, partly as a result of dehydration and partly because of renal impairment secondary to the electrolyte disturbances.

Treatment

The treatment for established pyloric obstruction, whatever its cause, is invariably surgical. Before operation dehydration and electrolyte depletion are corrected by intravenous replacement of normal saline and of potassium. Daily gastric lavage is performed to remove the debris from the stomach and in addition this often restores function to the stomach and allows fluid absorption to take place by mouth. Vitamin C is given, since the patient with chronic duodenal ulcer is often deficient in ascorbic acid.

Surgical correction is carried out as soon as the patient's general condition is satisfactory, usually about 7 days after admission to hospital. If the obstruction is due to carcinoma of the stomach a partial gastrectomy of the Polya type is performed. A stenosing duodenal ulcer is best treated by vagotomy combined with gastro-jejunostomy.

GASTRO-INTESTINAL HAEMORRHAGE

Gastro-intestinal haemorrhage may comprise *haematemesis* (the vomiting of blood), *melaena* (the passage of altered black, tarry, blood per rectum) or a combination of the two. In this country the commonest single cause of this entity is duodenal ulcer. It is a common condition which complicates about 10% of all patients with peptic ulcer, and is also dangerous, bearing with it a mortality rate of about 10%.

The management of patients presenting with gastro-intestinal haemorrhage is threefold:
1. The assessment and replacement of the blood loss.
2. An attempt to diagnose the source of the bleeding.
3. The treatment and control of the source of bleeding.

Blood loss

Before doing anything else, it may be necessary to initiate a blood transfusion in a patient who is obviously shocked with pallor, sweating, a pulse rate above 100, and a blood pressure which has a systolic below 100 mm Hg. Every case is grouped on admission and blood made available by cross-matching even if this is not immediately required.

The source of bleeding

Bleeding may be from some local source or result from a general bleeding tendency, such as haemophilia or anticoagulant therapy.

It is useful to consider the possible local causes anatomically:

Oesophagus—oesophageal varices associated with portal hypertension or peptic oesophagitis associated with hiatus hernia.

Stomach—gastric ulcer, acute erosions (including those associated with aspirin, alcohol, butazolidine and cortisone), gastric tumours.

Duodenum—duodenal ulcer, and rarely erosion of the duodenum by a pancreatic tumour.

Intestine—tumours, Meckel's diverticulum.

About 85% of patients with acute gastrointestinal haemorrhage in this country have either a peptic ulcer or an erosion of the stomach or duodenum. About 5% of patients have oesophageal varices, and the remainder are accounted for by the other causes listed above.

Diagnosis is made on history, examination, and special investigations.

There may be a typical story of peptic ulceration and perhaps the patient has had a positive barium meal previously. Careful enquiry must be made about ingestion of drugs which may produce acute gastric erosion. A story of alcoholism or previous virus hepatitis may suggest cirrhosis with the development of oesophageal varices and an alcoholic debauch may also have precipitated acute gastric erosion.

Clinical examination is usually negative, apart from those features suggesting blood loss, but the presence of jaundice, an enlarged liver and spleen suggest oesophageal varices, secondary to cirrhosis.

If the bleeding settles, it may be possible to investigate the patient by means of a barium meal together with gastroduodenoscopy, but if the patient is bleeding actively, these are extremely difficult because of clot in the stomach.

Treatment

In the first instance this is medical. The patient is admitted to hospital and put to bed. He is reassured and reassurance is supplemented with morphia if he is restless. If shocked, as assessed by pallor, rapid pulse, and a low blood pressure, a blood transfusion is commenced and a careful shock chart instituted in every case. As soon as active bleeding ceases, milk is allowed by mouth in the form of regular hourly or two-hourly drinks, and as soon as possible the patient is transferred to a semi-solid gastric diet. Aluminium hydroxide gel 10 ml is prescribed every two hours by day and during waking hours at night. Since some of these patients have been shown to be deficient in vitamin C this should be given at the rate of 200 mg t.d.s. for five days and then continued at a dosage of 100 mg per day.

On this regime three out of four patients will settle down. In the remaining patients, bleeding either continues or recurs while under observation and it is in these that emergency surgery is obligatory. Unless operation is performed and the bleeding point controlled the patient will die of continued haemorrhage.

In such cases, the blood transfusion is continued and urgent preparation made for laparotomy. At operation the source of bleeding is found and controlled. This usually takes the form of a gastrectomy for a chronic gastric ulcer and either a gastrectomy or a vagotomy with pyloroplasty and undersewing of the bleeding ulcer for duodenal ulceration. In cases of acute erosion it may be possible to undersew the bleeding vessel after opening the stomach (gastrostomy).

In the patients who are treated medically and who settle down, careful assessment is made in the convalescent period. If the presence of a chronic duodenal or gastric is established, then surgery is usually advised as an elective procedure since once a chronic ulcer has bled subsequent haemorrhages are likely to occur.

The management of haemorrhage from oesophageal varices

This is considered on page 290.

Chapter 12. The intestine

The small intestine

Anatomy

The upper half of the small intestine is termed the jejunum and the lower half the ileum. There is no obvious junction between the two parts, and it is not possible to tell exactly where one ends and the other begins. However, at operation, the jejunum has a thicker wall and only one arterial arcade, whereas the ileum has a much thinner wall and a double arterial arcade (Fig. 12.1). The small intestine is richly supplied with blood vessels, the arterial source being derived exclusively from the superior mesenteric artery. If this vessel is occluded, the small intestine will inevitably undergo necrosis. The veins from the small intestine drain into the superior mesenteric vein which, after joining the splenic vein, becomes the portal vein. Thus all the blood from the small intestine passes directly through the liver.

The mucosa of the jejunum is thrown up into folds or *villi* which have the effect of producing a very large surface area of mucosa for the absorption of food material. When the surface of the mucosa is examined at operation it has a velvety appearance due to the villi, in addition to which the mucosa is folded on itself, producing a series of ridges which run around the wall of the intestine, the valvulae conniventes.

Fig. 12.1. The simple arterial arcades of the jejunum (A) compared with the complex arcades of the ileum (B).

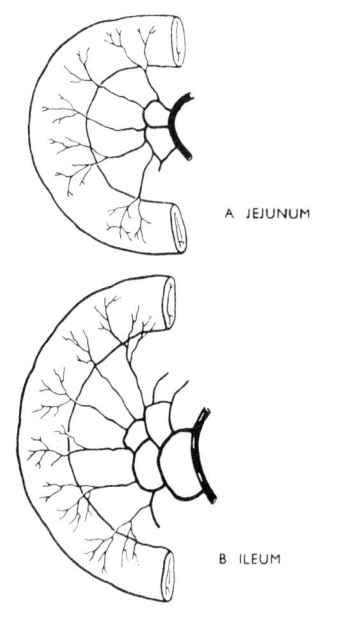

Physiology

As might be expected from the anatomical distinctions described above, the jejunum is responsible for the absorption of the majority of foodstuffs. The transmission of the contents however are quite rapid, and barium if ingested with a meal is seen to enter the ileum after only 30 to 60 minutes. In distinction to this, the ileum slows down the transit of its contents and this is the reason that patients who lose significant sections of the terminal ileum tend to develop the symptoms of intestinal hurry, which include diarrhoea. The ileum is responsible for the absorption of water and in addition has some special functions for the absorption of certain substances. The first of these is Vitamin B_{12}, bound to intrinsic factor, which is absorbed by the terminal 100 cm of ileum. The second is conjugated bile salts which have been secreted into the duodenum, have played their part in the digestion of fat and are then re-absorbed so that they can re-circulate in the so-called entero-hepatic circulation for the digestion of more fat.

MECKEL'S DIVERTICULUM

Pathology

Meckel's diverticulum is a pouch which is found on the ante-mesenteric border of the terminal ileum and is a remnant of the vitello-intestinal tract. This duct in the fetus communicates with the yolksac and protrudes through the gap in the anterior abdominal wall which later becomes the umbilicus. Normally, the duct closes just prior to birth, but in some people the small blind remnant persists (Fig. 12.2). As an aid to memory the 'rule of 2's' has been formulated; and this is that Meckel's diverticulum occurs in 2% of the population, 2 feet from the ileo-caecal valve and is on average 2 inches long. Obviously this is merely a useful approximation. It occurs equally in both men and women.

Section of the Meckel's diverticulum reveals that there are all layers of the bowel wall present and the mucosa is generally similar to normal ileal mucosa. In a few cases, however, ectopic gastric mucosa is found which is capable of secreting hydrochloric acid.

Fig. 12.2. A Meckel's diverticulum.

Clinical features

The vast majority of Meckel's diverticula do not give rise to any symptoms, and either are never found or are incidental observations at autopsy. A few cases of Meckel's diverticulitis occur, however, when the diverticulum becomes inflamed in an exactly similar way to the appendix in appendicitis. The symptomatology is indistinguishable from that of appendicitis, being initially central abdominal pain, later shifting to the right iliac fossa, associated with anorexia and vomiting.

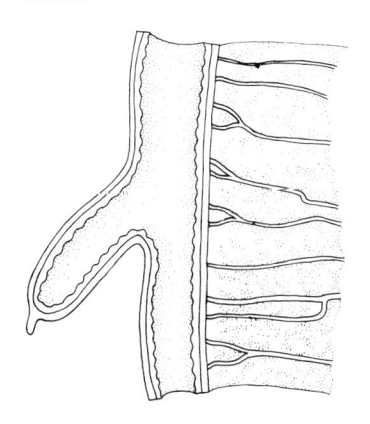

Another fortunately rare complication is the presence of ectopic gastric mucosa which secretes acid and which results in the formation of a peptic ulcer in the diverticulum. This may give rise to pain, which is always extremely difficult to diagnose, but more important than this is that it may give rise to bleeding with melaena, especially in children.

Occasionally the apex of the diverticulum is attached by an adhesion to the region of the umbilicus and intestinal obstruction by volvulus has been described.

Treatment

If the Meckel's diverticulum is found during an operation for some other definite pathology and if it has a wide opening into the bowel and is not too long it should be left alone. If, however, it is long with a narrow neck or is found during laparotomy for previously unexplained abdominal pain, it should be removed. It should also be removed if it is inflamed or shows any other pathological change.

SPECIFIC INFECTIONS

Enteritis is a condition that is known to all of us at one time or another. Perhaps the most common cause, although this has never been proved for certain, is a virus. Often symptoms of enteritis accompany or follow symptoms of an upper respiratory tract infection and in this case it is assumed that the virus is capable of attacking a variety of epithelial surfaces. Other specific infections include the staphylococcus which has multiplied in prepared meats which have been allowed to stand in unsuitable warm conditions. In this case the symptoms may be produced either by the staphylococcus itself or by a toxin which the staphylococcus produces.

Typhoid is fortunately rare in this country and exists as a number of different types, depending on the precise infecting organism. In the most severe types of salmonella typhi infections the lymphoid patches of the small bowel become involved and eventually ulcerate through the mucosa. If the infection is unchecked, rupture of the small intestine can occur, with the development of a virulent and usually fatal peritonitis.

Cholera, due to infection by the vibrio cholerae, is usually not seen in this country except in patients brought here by means of air travel.

Tuberculosis, usually caused by the bovine mycobacterium, is still common in India. It affects usually the terminal ileum just as it enters the caecum and has been termed ileo-caecal tuberculosis. Ulceration of the terminal ileum is produced and if the infection is controlled at this stage it very commonly results in stricturing of the bowel.

Generally the contents of the small bowel are sterile, except when any surgical procedure or any disease process results in an alteration either of the anatomy or of the pH relationships within the intestine. For example, after gastrectomy the gastric contents have a higher pH value than normal, less gastric acid being secreted with a consequent reduction in the bacterial filter that normal gastric acid exerts. In this case the small bowel becomes colonised with colonic bacteria. Similarly, when the terminal ileum is damaged or has to be resected and reimplanted in the colon, it is quite common for bacteria to colonise the lower part of the small bowel. In this type of situation the bacteria within the intestine may produce little or no inflammatory response although sometimes they interfere with the absorption of certain metabolites by, for example, deconjugating bile salts and thus rendering them non-absorbable.

Clinical features

The symptomatology of small bowel inflammation includes central abdominal pain, which is ill-localised and often associated with small bowel colic, together with malaise, nausea, vomiting and diarrhoea.

Treatment

This naturally depends on the specific cause. In order to make an accurate diagnosis culture of faeces is essential and when the specific infecting organism has been isolated appropriate antibiotic therapy is given. As was pointed out above, however, most cases of enteritis do not yield a specific organism and resolve spontaneously without specific treatment.

Symptomatic treatment includes rapid replacement of water, sodium and potassium if the patient has become dehydrated by virtue of diarrhoea and vomiting. In the case of cholera, the rehydration assumes massive proportions and many litres of fluid are given both orally and intravenously as this condition produces death by dehydration and not by any other effect of the organism. In less severe forms, diarrhoea can be minimised by giving tablets of Lomotil, codeine or mist. kaolin et morph. 15 ml every 2 hours until the diarrhoea is controlled. If there is associated nausea, one of the anti-emetics will produce considerable symptomatic relief; a useful preparation is trifluroperazine (Stelazine) 2–5 mg t.d.s.

CROHN'S DISEASE

Pathology

Many different names have been applied to this condition but that of Crohn's disease is preferred since it affects not only the terminal ileum but also the colon, rectum and anus, and rarely the mouth, the oesophagus, the stomach and the duodenum.

It was originally described by Crohn, Ginsberg and Oppenheimer in 1932, and the most typical manifestation is of an inflammatory disorder which affects the terminal ileum, but, as has been pointed out above, any part of the alimentary tract may be involved. The terminal ileum alone is the most frequently involved part of the gut, accounting for about 50% of all cases, but it seems that the colonic manifestation of the disease is becoming more common and now forms about 20% of the total.

When the condition is seen at operation, the affected bowel is found to be intensely inflamed, with considerable oedema and thickening of the mesentery. The mesenteric lymph nodes are also enlarged and inflamed (Fig. 12.3). Characteristically the inflammation exists in a fairly short segment of ileum, (10–20 cm), there is then a segment of ileum which is normal followed by a second inflamed segment. This has given rise to the term 'skip' lesions. There may be ulceration of the intestine, although this is by no means always present.

The histological appearance of Crohn's disease is extremely variable but centres in most cases on the existence of clusters of lymphocytes arranged round giant cells, that is cells containing more than one nucleus. This is the sort of histological picture which is also seen in tuberculosis and it is not surprising therefore that for many years this condition was confused with this. However, in the case of Crohn's disease tubercle bacilli are never found.

Many different theories have been advanced as to the cause of the condition but the origin is still unknown. It affects both men and women equally, the incidence rising to a peak between the ages of 20 and 30, being rare under the age of 10. Beyond the age of 30 the incidence flattens out and the disease occurs at all ages beyond this. From experience in the United States of America it is found to be more common in Jews and less common in Negroes than in the

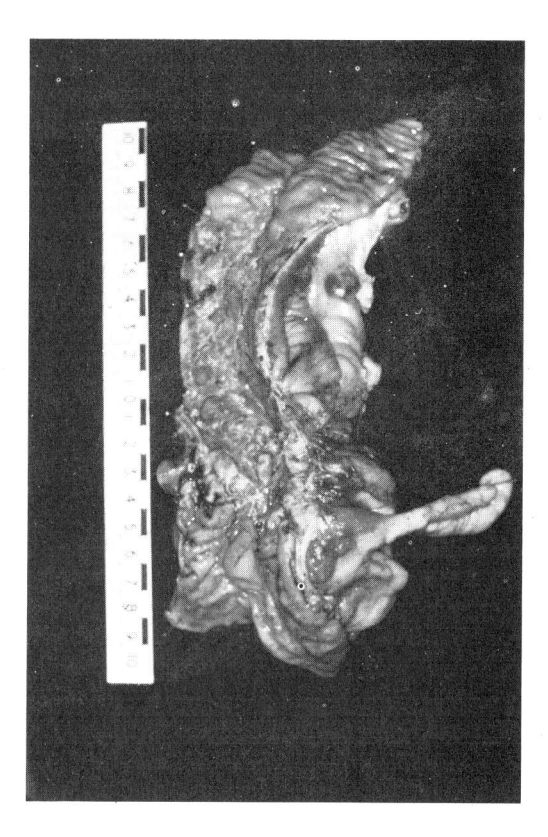

Fig. 12.3. Crohn's disease of the intestine. Note the gross thickening of the bowel wall.

general white population. It appears that the incidence of the condition is increasing.

Clinical features

The symptomatology of a patient with Crohn's disease of the terminal ileum is variable and depends upon the degree of activity. In its most minor form it may only produce some discomfort in the right iliac fossa, though possibly with slight diarrhoea. As the disease progresses, pain becomes a more prominent feature and it is possible for stenosis of the ileum to occur, with consequent intestinal obstruction. The symptoms then become typical of the latter condition, namely abdominal pain, abdominal distension, vomiting and absolute constipation.

One of the features of Crohn's disease of the small intestine is malabsorption. In young people, stature, weight and general body configuration may be significantly below normal. One of the food factors which may be specifically involved is Vitamin B_{12}, since this is absorbed from the terminal ileum and over 50% of cases of Crohn's disease involve just this part of the intestine.

Special investigations

Diagnosis is by means of barium meal and follow-through so that the column of barium is observed on the X-ray image intensifier screen as it passes through the small bowel. Two forms of Crohn's X-ray changes are recognized. The first of these is the non-stenotic type, in which oedematous mucosa and alteration of the normal mucosal pattern is seen. The second type is the stenotic phase in which, as the name implies, a narrowed section of ileum is found, (Fig. 12.4). Often more than one segment of the bowel is involved

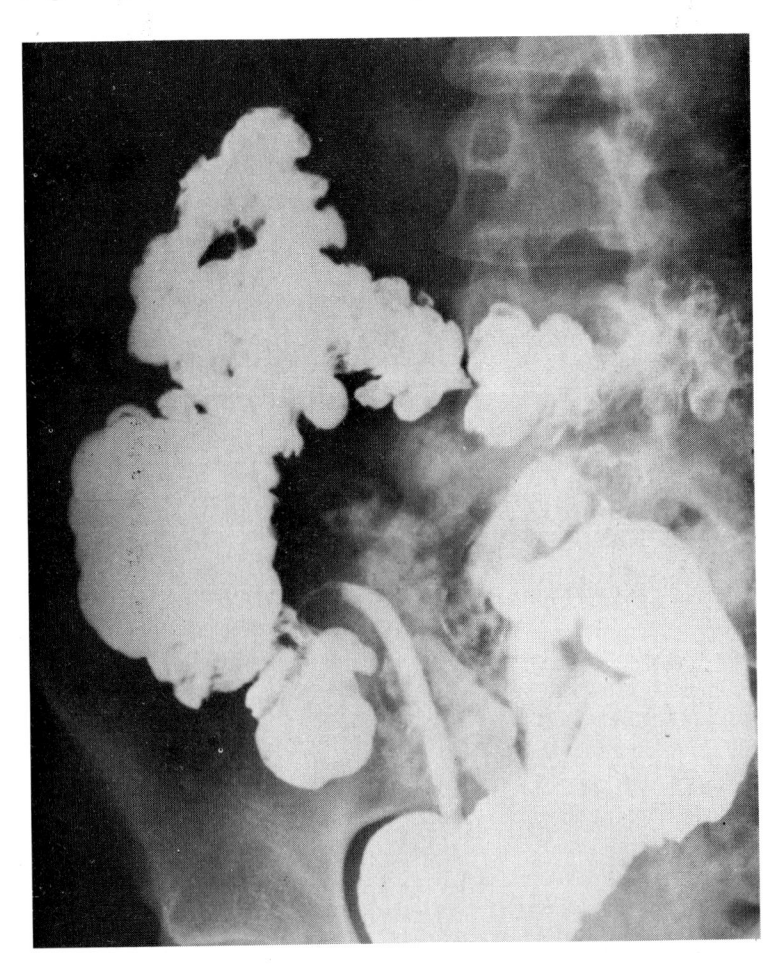

Fig. 12.4. The X-ray appearance in Crohn's disease. Note the narrow segment which gives the 'string sign' where the terminal ileum enters the caecum.

with normal ileum between, giving the so-called 'skip' area. The narrowed segment of ileum often gives the appearance of a thin column of barium, in some cases looking like a piece of string—the 'string' sign. The X-ray appearances of Crohn's disease in the rest of the intestinal tract are those of an ulcerating inflammatory condition. Considerable confusion can exist in differentiating between Crohn's colitis and ulcerative colitis, although in many cases experienced radiologists are able to distinguish one from the other. There do remain a few cases, however, in which in spite of X-rays and even biopsy the distinction between these two conditions in the colon cannot be made.

Treatment

No specific treatment exists for this condition. The implication of this is that treatment should be directed at symptoms and should not be undertaken merely for X-ray or other structural changes. Diarrhoea can be controlled using codeine phosphate 30 mg, diphenoxylate (Lomotil) 5 mg or mist. kaolin et morph. 15 ml three to four times daily. These drugs should be taken at a frequency controlled by the patient simply to control the diarrhoea. Occasionally the involvement of the ileum has resulted in the non-absorption of bile salts and this has been responsible for diarrhoea. In these cases cholestyramine, an ion-exchange resin, may abolish diarrhoea which hitherto has been intractable. This can be taken as a sachet up to 30 g daily although as little as 2 g may be effective. Steatorrhoea, that is the excretion of excessive quantities of fat (above 7 g per 24 hours), is controlled by limiting fat intake to approximately 40 g per day.

Symptoms of intestinal obstruction should be treated with great caution and do not usually require urgent surgical relief. In such a case water and electrolyte balance is maintained by an intravenous drip and the stomach is kept empty by means of a nasogastric tube; in many cases the symptoms will subside.

Prednisone is frequently used. This has the effect of being anti-inflammatory, immunosuppressive and in addition it improves the mood of the patient and stimulates the appetite. It is used when there is evidence of considerable activity of the disease, for example when there is fever or tachycardia, for systemic complications such as uveitis and arthritis, when there is extensive intestinal involvement, when multiple previous resections have been carried out or when there is early disease in a young patient. It should not be used when there is chronic stenosis of the intestine, a fistula either between loops of intestine or from intestine to the abdominal wall, when there is uncontrolled sepsis or an abdominal mass. The initial dosage is high, e.g. prednisone 40–60 mg per day, rapidly reducing to a maintenance level 5–15 mg daily after two weeks or so.

One of the interesting recent developments, the evidence for which is now beginning to accumulate, is that when a remission in the disease is produced by steroids this may be maintained by the use of immuno-suppressive therapy. In this case Imuran is given in a dose varying between 50 and 100 mg per day controlled by initially frequent white cell counts, every third day or so, and then being continued in the long term. It must be realised that immuno-suppressive therapy is difficult to maintain and is attended by the significant dangers of uncontrolled infection and possibly, in the long term, the development of carcinoma of various tissues. It may be justified, however, by virtue of the fact that Crohn's disease is an extremely serious condition which may result in the death of the patient.

Surgery is frequently required for this condition when there is a persistent intestinal obstruction or fistula formation. In a patient who has not had previous surgery the affected portion of the intestine should be completely excised, a method of treatment obviously only applicable if a relatively short segment is involved. Discussion has existed in the past as to whether the diseased segment should be excised or by-passed, but it would seem that results of excision are better than those for simple by-pass. Unfortunately, long term results of surgery are not entirely satisfactory because of recurrence of the disease and in a series of patients investigated in Leeds 10 years after primary surgery, 40% had required a second operation. In addition, the early postoperative mortality is high, being between 3 and 5%, this being due to a combination of infective complications and fluid and electrolyte imbalance. However, the long term outlook is better after surgery than after medical treatment alone and proponents of this form of therapy point to the fact that following surgery over 70% of persons are in good general health compared with under 20% before surgery has been carried out.

VASCULAR DISEASE OF THE INTESTINE

Obstruction to either the artery or the vein which supplies a segment of intestine will result in gangrene. Arterial occlusion may occur either as a result of an embolus or thrombosis due to degenerative arterial disease. Venous thrombosis occurs, but is rarer, and the cause is more difficult to determine.

In a case of vascular gangrene of the intestine laparotomy is required with resection of the affected portion of the intestine and reconstitution by end-to-end-anastomosis. Occasionally embolectomy or removal of the thrombus may restore circulation to all or part of the infarcted intestine. The patients who develop this condition usually have generalised arterial degenerative disease which results in a poor general outlook from resection.

TUMOURS OF THE SMALL INTESTINE

One of the many mysteries of tumour formation is the rarity of growths from beyond the pylorus to the ileo-caecal valve, in spite of their great frequency in the stomach and large intestine.

The epithelium may give rise to a benign adenoma or malignant adenocarcinoma. It is also a site for the carcinoid tumour which is considered below. The walls of the small intestine may give rise to benign or malignant tumours of its plain muscle (leiomyoma and leiomyosarcoma respectively), and its lymphoid tissue may be the site of a lymphosarcoma. Secondary invasion may occur directly from adjacent stomach or colon or by metastases from, for example, the breast.

Tumours of the small intestine may present with intestinal bleeding, obstruction, intussusception or volvulus and treatment, where possible, is by resection.

THE CARCINOID SYNDROME

Carcinoid tumours occur most commonly in the appendix, but may be found anywhere in the alimentary tract, and occasionally in the lung. The tumour arises from cells which take up special silver stains and which occur in the crypts of the intestinal mucosa. The tumour is very slowly growing, and those of the appendix are relatively benign. However, those arising in the small intestine and large bowel spread eventually to the regional lymph nodes and the liver.

Where there is an extensive mass of tumour, symptoms are produced because of the serotonin (5 hydroxy-tryptamine or 5 HT) which is secreted by the carcinoid cells.

Clinical features

The carcinoid syndrome comprises any of the following features:
1. An abdominal mass or an enlarged liver produced by the tumour itself or by its secondaries.
2. Flushing with attacks of cyanosis.
3. Diarrhoea with noisy bowel sounds (borborygmi).
4. Bronchospasm.
5. Pulmonary stenosis.

The diagnosis is confirmed by estimating the breakdown product of 5 HT which is 5 hydroxyindole acetic acid (5-HIAA), which can be readily estimated and whose level is considerably raised in this syndrome.

Treatment

This comprises resection of the tumour in early cases. Local deposits in the liver are also occasionally amenable to surgical excision. Even if widespread deposits are present, the tumour is slowly growing and the patient may survive for many years.

SMALL INTESTINAL OBSTRUCTION

This may be divided into adynamic and dynamic.

ADYNAMIC OBSTRUCTION

This is due to the loss of propulsive power of the small intestine and is termed 'paralytic ileus'. This inevitably follows laparotomy and also occurs when any form of irritation to the peritoneum occurs, such as peritonitis. It is also encountered in patients with extensive retroperitoneal haemorrhage such as may occur in fractures of the lumbar spine.

Clinical features

In the postoperative case, the patient has no more pain than would be expected from his laparotomy wound. The abdomen is distended, generally rather tender, and silent on auscultation. There may be nausea or vomiting and no flatus is passed.

Treatment

The treatment of this condition is that of its underlying cause in many instances (see peritonitis below). However, one of the important effects of paralytic ileus is that the intestine is not only unable to move, but also unable to absorb fluid, which therefore pools within its dilated loops. In order to maintain the patient in satisfactory general condition, intravenous saline will be required, together with supplements of up to 80mEq of potassium per 24 hours. A strict fluid chart is obligatory. A naso-gastric tube is passed in order to keep the stomach empty. This prevents vomiting and the possibility of aspiration of gastric contents.

If the ileus is very prolonged, that is for more than three or four days, intravenous feeding with amino acids, fructose and fat should be given in order to maintain nutrition.

DYNAMIC OBSTRUCTION

Dynamic obstruction occurs when there is some mechanical block along the length of the bowel.

Classification

Whenever one considers obstruction of a tube anywhere in the body this should be classified into:
1. Causes in the lumen
2. Causes in the wall
3. Causes outside the wall (Fig. 12.5)

Applying this classification to obstruction of the small intestine, we have:

1. *Causes within the lumen*—these are rather unusual, but may result from the presence of an inspissated mass of food, particularly fruit pith or vegetable material. Occasionally a gall stone enters the small intestine via a fistula between the gall bladder and the duodenum; if sufficiently large it may impact in the bowel producing a *gall stone ileus*.

2. *In the wall*—congenital atresia, Crohn's disease, tumours, etc.

3. *Outside the wall*—This is the commonest type of obstruction of the small intestine and may be due to a strangulated hernia, volvulus, intussusception or intraperitoneal adhesions or bands.

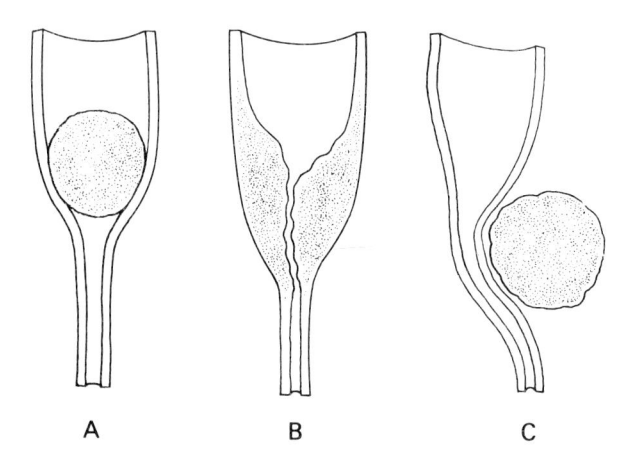

Fig. 12.5. Any tube in the body may be obstructed by causes in the lumen (A), causes in the wall (B) and causes outside the wall (C).

Pathology

Simple obstruction occurs when the bowel is occluded without damage to its blood supply; in *strangulation obstruction*, the blood supply of the involved intestine is cut off, and unrelieved, gangrene of the involved segment will take place.

When the intestine is obstructed by a simple occlusion, the intestine above the obstruction becomes dilated, partly with gas (most of which is swallowed air) and partly by fluids secreted by the stomach, intestinal wall, liver and pancreas. There is increased peristalsis in an attempt to overcome the obstruction. As the bowel distends, the blood supply to the tensely distended gut wall becomes impaired and in extreme cases there may be mucosal ulceration and eventually perforation. Perforation may also occur from the pressure of a band or the edge of the hernia neck on the bowel wall producing local ischaemia.

In strangulation obstruction the situation is even more serious since the ischaemic bowel is unable to contain its bacteria and their toxins within its lumen so that a transudation of organisms into the peritoneal cavity rapidly takes place, with secondary peritonitis. Unrelieved strangulation is followed by gangrene of the ischaemic bowel with perforation (Fig. 12.6).

The lethal effects of intestinal obstruction result from fluid and electrolyte loss due to the copious vomiting and exudation into the bowel lumen, protein loss into the gut and toxaemia due to the migration of toxins and bacteria either through the intact but ischaemic bowel wall or through an actual perforation.

Clinical features

The cardinal symptoms of intestinal obstruction are four in number:
1. Colicky pain
2. Distension
3. Absolute constipation (for flatus as well as for faeces)
4. Vomiting

These features can easily be deduced from the pathology described above. The *colicky pain* results from the increased peristalsis in the obstructed gut, and is usually the first symptom. The *distension* results from progressive dilatation of the gut above the site of occlusion by gas and fluid. The *absolute constipation* is produced by the blockage of the bowel. However, a partial or chronic obstruction may be accompanied by the passage of small amounts of flatus and even in complete obstruction the patient may pass one or two normal stools as the lower bowel empties after the onset of the obstruction. *Vomiting* usually occurs early when the obstruction is high in the intestine,

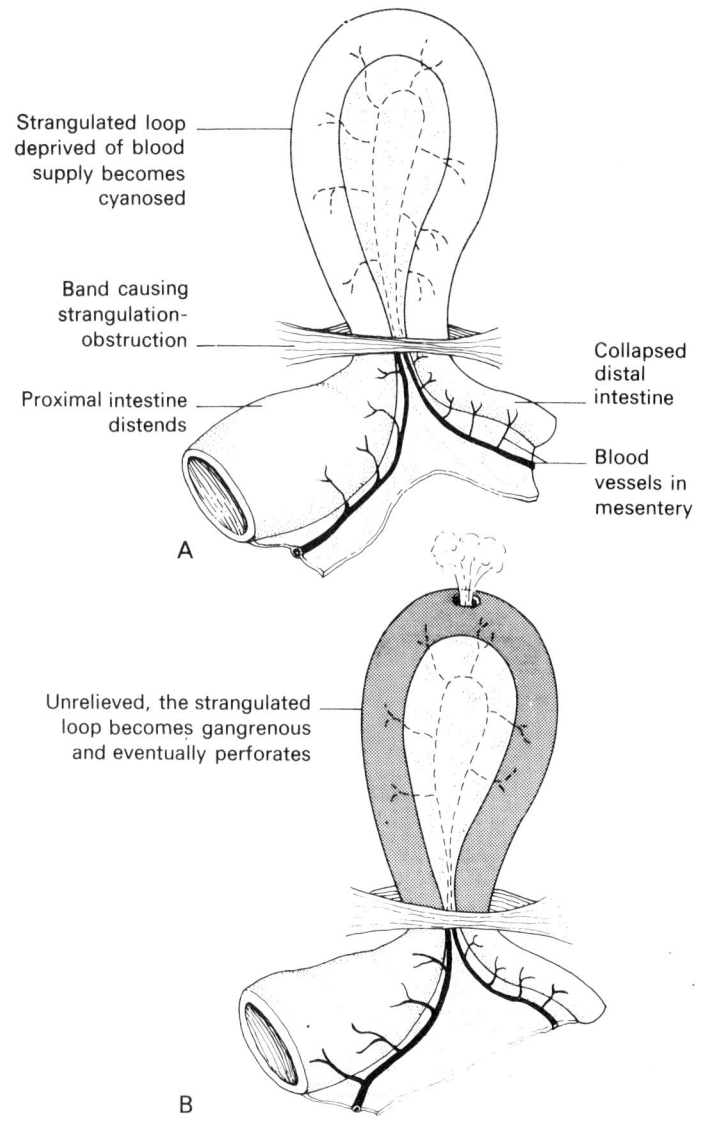

Fig. 12.6. Unrelieved strangulation obstruction (A) results in gangrene of the affected segment and eventually perforation (B).

but is late or even entirely absent in chronic or large bowel obstruction. In the late stages the vomiting becomes faeculent due to bacterial decomposition of the stagnant contents of the gut.

On examination the patient may be obviously dehydrated, he is in pain and may be rolling about with colic. The pulse is usually elevated but the temperature frequently is normal. The abdomen is distended, visible peristalsis may be present and noisy bowel sounds are heard on listening to the abdomen. It is important to look carefully for two features; the presence of a strangulated external hernia, which will make the diagnosis easy, and the presence of an abdominal scar. Intestinal obstruction in the presence of this evidence of a previous operation immediately suggests either adhesions or a band as the cause.

Special investigations

Plain x-rays of the abdomen are valuable in the diagnosis of intestinal obstruction. Dilated loops of small intestine can be seen when the patient is in the supine position. When the patient is X-rayed in the standing position, the gas floats to the top of the fluid within the dilated loops and appears as multiple fluid levels (Fig. 12.7).

Treatment

All cases of dynamic intestinal obstruction require laparotomy. It is essential, before this is carried out, to resuscitate the patient. Blood is taken for estimation of haemoglobin, urea and electrolytes as well as for the grouping and cross-matching of blood. A nasogastric tube is passed so that the stomach can be maintained empty. An intravenous drip of saline is commenced to replace the losses the patient has

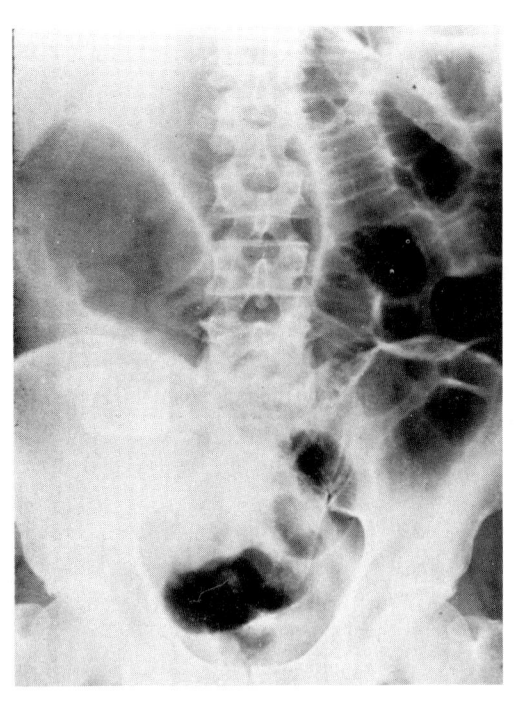

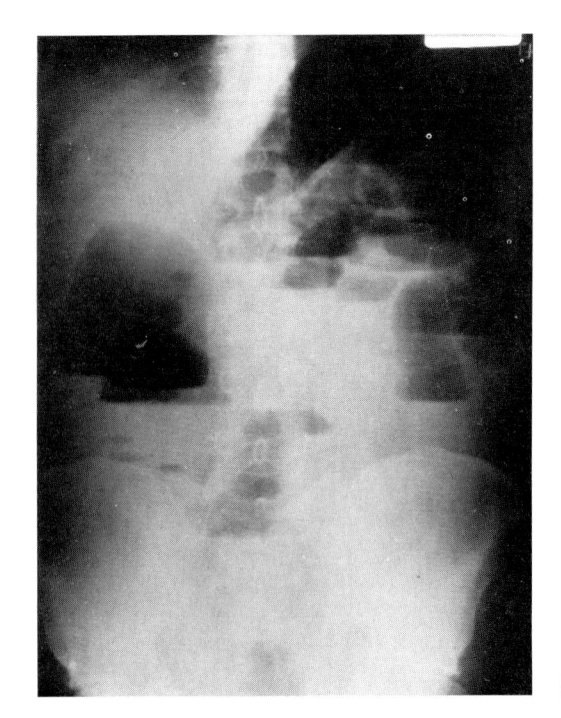

Fig. 12.7. X-rays of the abdomen in a case of intestinal obstruction due to post-operative adhesions. (A) supine position; the dilated loops of small intestine are visualised. (B) in the standing position multiple fluid levels are seen.

suffered by virtue of vomiting and loss of fluid into the dilated intestine and to maintain the patient during the time fluids can not be absorbed normally through the small bowel. It is an important rule that the only person who can give an analgesic to the patient is the surgeon who makes the decision whether to operate or not. If analgesics are given too early in the process of diagnosis and treatment there is the danger that all pain will be removed and the true diagnosis will be missed with resulting delay in effective treatment.

When the patient is fully resuscitated, rehydrated and has a normal blood pressure (the pulse rate usually takes some time before it falls to normal levels) and is passing urine, then and only then is laparotomy performed. At laparotomy the small intestine will be found to be dilated proximal to the obstruction, that distal to the obstruction is collapsed. If the obstruction is of long standing, the wall of the proximal intestine will be oedematous and soft. The dilated proximal intestine is decompressed by means of a long sucker (a Savage decompressor) and the obstructing agent is removed, or if this is not possible, for example in some cases of secondary carcinoma, it is by-passed. If the intestine is strangulated, the necrotic section of the intestine is resected and continuity is restored by end-to-end anastomosis.

There are some cases in which it is not possible to tell whether the intestine is necrotic or not. In this situation the segment in question is wrapped in warm, moist packs and is left for 10 minutes or so. Its viability or otherwise is then assessed on the basis of pulsation of the vessels in the mesentery, colour of intestinal wall and the presence of intestinal movement. If in doubt, and a massive length of small intestine is involved, it is quite permissible to return the intestine to the peritoneal cavity and to re-inspect it at a second laparotomy 24 hours later. Fortunately this circumstance is extremely rare.

Postoperatively a long continued paralytic ileus is the rule. During this period fluid will be lost into the paralysed intestine, via the urine and by insensible losses through the skin and in expired air, which are often increased by virtue of postoperative pyrexia. It is extremely important, therefore, to keep up with the additional fluid losses and there is a tendency for patients to be dehydrated after operation because too rigid a policy of fluid restriction is adopted. It is likely that in the first 24 hours after operation an adult male patient will require between 5 and 6 litres of fluid to maintain his normal fluid balance and provide additional water for urinary output in excess of one litre. In the second postoperative day less fluid volume is required, in the region of 3 to 5 litres, depending upon circumstances.

When the paralytic ileus recovers, fluid within the lumen of the intestine is absorbed and excreted in the urine and this is found to result in a diuresis. It is interesting that when this diuresis occurs, and the paralytic ileus recovers with the passage of flatus, patients seem to have turned a corner in the process of recovery, their comfort and well-being are then rapidly improved.

OBSTRUCTION OF THE SMALL INTESTINE IN CHILDREN

A number of important conditions produce obstruction of the small intestine in infants and children. These include congenital intestinal atresia, volvulus neonatorum, meconium ileus and intussusception. Neonatal obstruction of the large bowel due to Hirschsprung's disease and ano-rectal atresias are dealt with in the section on rectum.

Continuous vomiting in the newborn may be due to intracranial injury, infection, or intestinal obstruction. If the vomit contains bile, this indicates, almost without exception, that intestinal obstruction is present. In addition to vomiting there may be constipation, abdominal distention and visible peristalsis.

A plain X-ray of the abdomen is invaluable in demonstrating the distended loops of intestine with fluid levels.

CONGENITAL ATRESIA

This may be a septum across the small intestine which may be complete or partial, or a complete gap (Fig. 12.8); multiple segments may be involved.

Treatment

This comprises resection of the stricture and end to end anastomosis, but the operation is difficult and the mortality high.

VOLVULUS NEONATORUM

Occasionally the normally wide attachment of the small bowel mesentery to the posterior abdominal wall is defective and this allows torsion, or volvulus, of the whole of the small intestine together with the right side of the large bowel (Fig. 12.9). Untreated, the whole of this segment of intestine becomes gangrenous. There may in addition be a congenital band which passes from the large bowel across the duodenum (Ladd's band) and which may produce secondary obstruction of the duodenum.

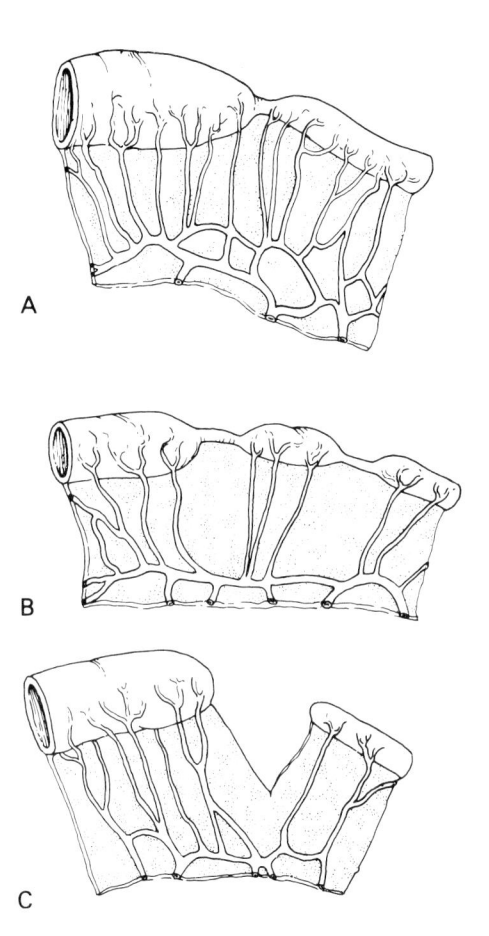

Fig. 12.8. Varieties of congenital atresia of the small intestine.

Treatment

Comprises untwisting the volvulus, dividing the transduodenal band and attaching the abnormally mobile ascending colon to the lateral abdominal wall.

MECONIUM ILEUS

This is a manifestation of mucoviscidosis, which is a generalised defect of mucus secretion of the intestine, the bronchial tree and the pancreas (*fibrocystic pancreatic disease*). Because of the loss of intestinal mucus and a blockage of pancreatic ducts with loss of tryptic digestion, the lower ileum of the new born babe is blocked with sticky, thick meconium (Fig. 12.10). The X-rays of the abdomen

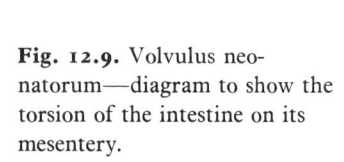

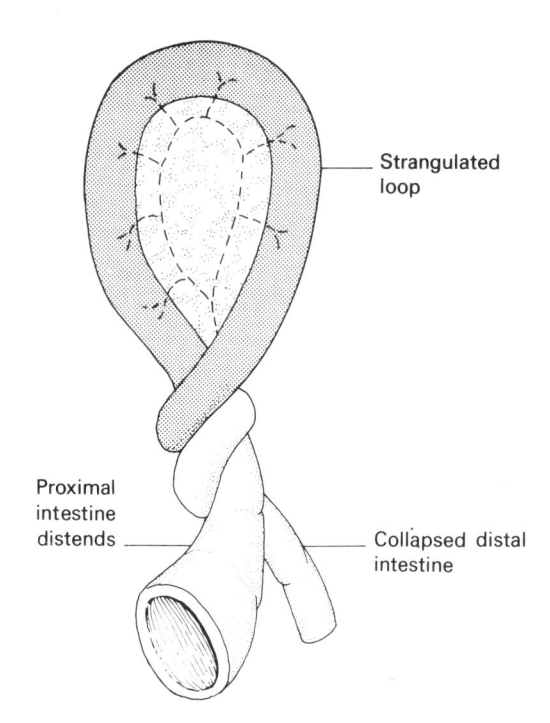

Fig. 12.9. Volvulus neonatorum—diagram to show the torsion of the intestine on its mesentery.

are characteristic. In addition to the distended coils of bowel, a typical mottled 'ground glass' appearance of meconium can be seen within the abdominal cavity.

Treatment

The inspissated meconium may require removal by lavage through a small incision in the intestine. Occasionally the impacted segment of small intestine may show areas of gangrene from pressure necrosis and requires resection. Postoperatively the infant is given pancreatic extract by mouth to replace the deficient trypsin.

Prognosis is poor, and because of lack of mucus secretion in the bronchi, recurrent chest infection is almost inevitable.

INTUSSUSCEPTION

Intussusception is the invagination of one portion of the gut into the lumen of the immediately adjoining bowel (Fig. 12.11).

Aetiology

95% of cases occur in infants or young children where there is usually no obvious cause. The mesenteric lymph nodes in these cases are

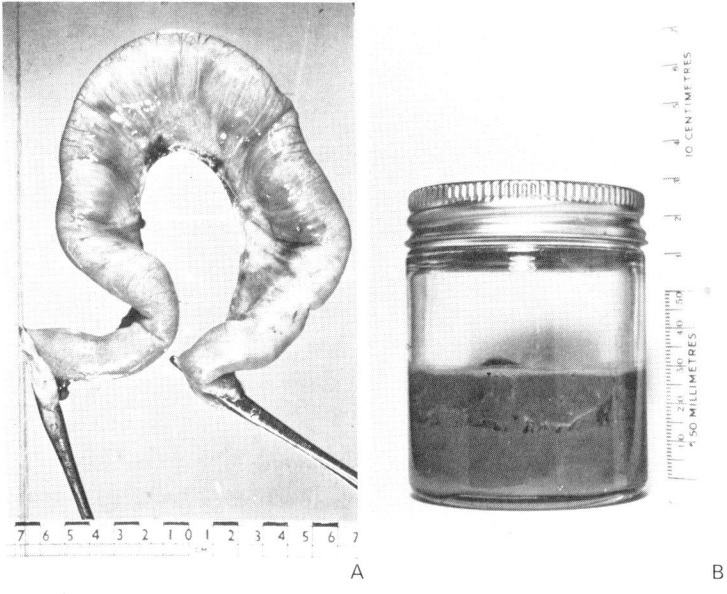

Fig. 12.10. Meconium ileus. (A) This segment of small intestine was so impacted with meconium that it required resection. (B) The sticky meconium from the bowel lumen.

usually enlarged and it has been suggested that the lymphoid tissue in the bowel wall becomes swollen due to a virus infection. In adults and in some children a polyp, a tumour, or an inverted Meckel's diverticulum may form the apex of the intussusception.

The inner layer of the intussusception has its blood supply cut off by the direct pressure of the outer layer, as well as by stretching of its supplying mesentery so that, if left untreated, gangrene is inevitable.

Most cases affect the ileo-caecal region so that the small intestine protrudes into the ascending colon.

Clinical features in infants

Usually previously healthy children are affected aged between 3 and 12 months; boys twice as often as girls.

The history is of spasms of abdominal colic typified by screaming and pallor. There is vomiting and a mixture of blood and slime ('red currant jelly') is passed per rectum. A sausage-shaped mass may be felt on abdominal palpation.

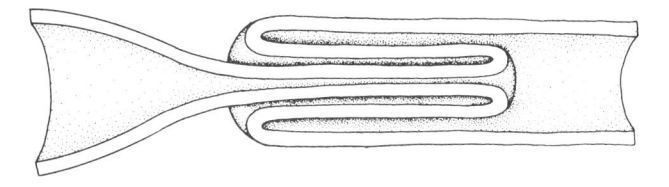

Fig. 12.11. Diagram of an intussusception.

Treatment

In most centres operative treatment is employed. The intussusception is reduced at laparotomy or, if gangrene has already taken place in a late case, resection or short circuit may be necessary.

It is sometimes possible to reduce the intussusception by running barium into the rectum in the X-ray department. The pressure of the head of the barium reduces the intussusception and X-rays are taken to confirm that this has taken place.

The appendix

Anatomy

The appendix arises from the caecum about one inch below the ileo-caecal valve. It is a diverticulum that varies in length from about $1\frac{1}{2}$ to 9 inches. Its position is extremely variable, more so than any other organ. Most commonly it lies behind the caecum, but it may hang down into the pelvis or pass in front or behind the terminal ileum (Fig. 12.12). The mesentery of the appendix carries the blood supply to this organ along the appendicular artery, a branch of the ileo-colic artery (Fig. 12.13). This represents the entire vascular supply of the appendix and if any of its branches are thrombosed secondary to acute infection of the appendix, then gangrene and subsequent perforation are inevitable.

ACUTE APPENDICITIS

This is the commonest abdominal emergency, and it is estimated to affect 1 in 6 of the British population. However, it is only found in civilised communities or in primitive peoples who have been unwise enough to change to Western diet.

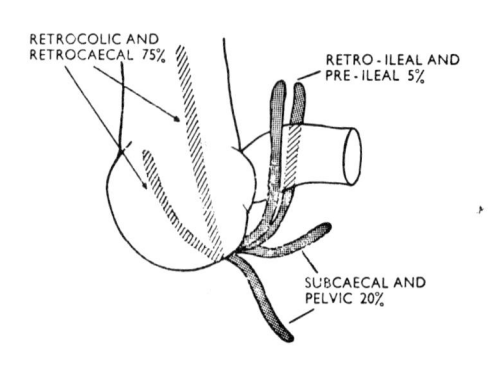

Fig. 12.12. The positions in which the appendix may lie, together with their approximate incidence.

Pathology

Acute appendicitis usually occurs when the appendix is obstructed. This may be due to a pellet of faecal material (faecolith), a kink from inflammatory adhesions, or enlargement of the lymph collections in its wall secondary to a catarrhal inflammation of its mucosa. Since the appendix of the infant is wide-mouthed and well drained, and since the lumen of the appendix is almost obliterated in old age, appendicitis in the two extremes of life is relatively rare. The obstructed appendix acts as a closed loop; bacteria proliferate in its lumen and invade the appendix wall, which is damaged by pressure necrosis. Thrombosis of its supplying blood vessels then results in gangrene and perforation (Fig. 12.14).

The acutely inflamed appendix may resolve, but, if so, a further attack can usually be expected, so that it is not uncommon for a patient to admit to one or more previous milder episodes of pain. More often the inflamed appendix undergoes gangrene and then perforates, either with a general peritonitis, or with the formation of a localised appendix abscess.

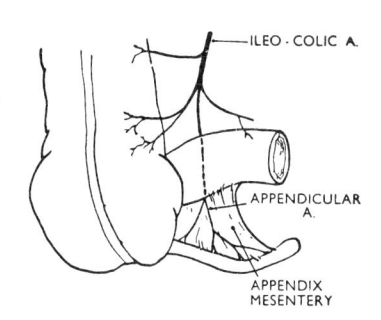

Fig. 12.13. The blood supply of the appendix.

Clinical features

A typical attack of acute appendicitis commences as a central abdominal colic which shifts after approximately 6 hours to the right

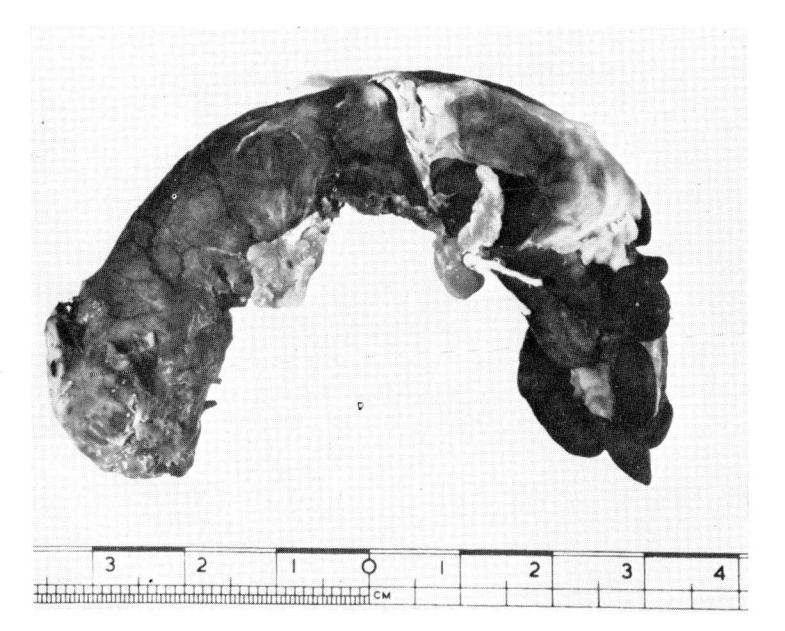

Fig. 12.14. A perforated gangrenous appendix removed at operation.

lower abdomen. The central abdominal pain is visceral in origin; the shift of pain is due to involvement of the sensitive peritoneum lining the abdominal wall which is irritated by the inflammatory process. Nausea and vomiting are usually present, so that Murphy described as a diagnostic sequence: central abdominal pain, followed by vomiting, followed by a shift of the pain to the right iliac fossa.

With perforation of the appendix there may be a temporary remission of pain, but this is followed by a more severe and generalised pain with profuse vomiting as general peritonitis develops.

On examination, the temperature and pulse are usually raised. The patient is flushed and is in obvious pain. The tongue is coated and the breath is foul. Examination of the abdomen reveals localised tenderness in the region of the inflamed appendix. There is usually guarding of the abdominal muscles over this site.

In late cases with generalised peritonitis the abdomen becomes diffusely tender and rigid, bowel sounds are absent, and the patient is obviously very ill.

Special investigations are of little value in making the diagnosis though they may have been needed to exclude other possibilities. The white cell count is usually raised with a polymorph leucocytosis. X-rays of the abdomen have no truly diagnostic features.

Differential diagnosis

Although the diagnosis of appendicitis is frequently quite straightforward, it may be a great mimic of other diseases, and these should be considered systematically:

1. *Other intra-abdominal conditions.* These include perforated peptic ulcer, acute cholecystitis, acute intestinal obstruction, gastroenteritis, acute Crohn's disease and acute diverticulitis of the colon.
2. *Urinary tract.* Renal colic and acute pyelonephritis. The urine must be tested for blood and pus cells in every case of acute abdominal pain.
3. *The chest.* Basal pneumonia and pleurisy may give referred abdominal pain, which may be surprisingly difficult to differentiate, especially in children.
4. *Central nervous system.* The pain which precedes the eruption of herpes zoster (shingles) affecting the 11th and 12th thoracic segments and the irritation of these posterior nerve roots in spinal disease may give referred pain to the lower abdomen.
5. *Gynaecological causes.* The commonest pitfalls are acute salpingitis, ruptured ovarian cyst and ruptured ectopic pregnancy. It is useful to consider that 'every lady is pregnant until proved otherwise'!

Treatment

Treatment of acute appendicitis is appendicectomy unless an appendix mass has formed without evidence of general peritonitis (see below) or in those rare circumstances where operation would be difficult or impossible, for example in a small boat at sea, or in a mountain hut in a blizzard. Here reliance must be placed on the hope that the attack will resolve or that a local abscess will form rather than on one's surgical skill using a razor blade and a bent spoon.

If at operation the appendix is found to have become gangrenous, or perforated with general peritonitis, then, in addition to removing the appendix, antibiotic therapy is commenced and here ampicillin is the first drug of choice. If there is considerable local infection a drain is inserted in the wound.

THE APPENDIX MASS

It is not rare for a patient to present with a history of several days of abdominal pain, by which time a localised mass has developed in the right iliac fossa. In these circumstances the inflamed appendix has become walled off by adhesions to adjacent organs and immediate surgery in such circumstances may simply spread the infection through the peritoneal cavity.

Treatment

At first this should be conservative. The mass is outlined on the skin with a marking pencil (Fig. 12.15). The patient is put to bed on a fluid diet and his general condition, together with temperature and

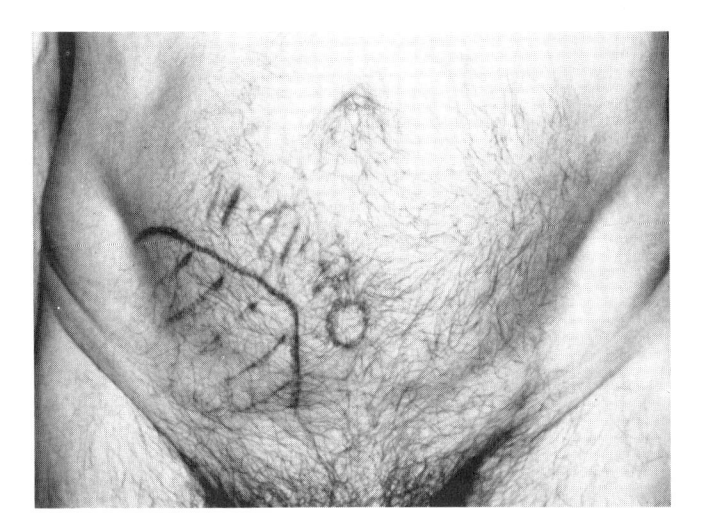

Fig. 12.15. The outline of an appendix abscess marked on the skin.

pulse are carefully observed. Antibiotics are *not* prescribed since these may simply produce a chronic inflammatory mass, which is honeycombed with abscess cavities, a condition that has received the nickname 'antibioticoma'. On this treatment 3 out of 4 cases resolve, the temperature settles and the mass subsides. In the remainder, the mass enlarges and the temperature persists. Under these circumstances the abscess requires surgical drainage.

After the mass has resolved (whether under conservative treatment or following drainage) then appendicectomy is carried out after an interval of 2 or 3 months when the inflammatory condition has settled completely. Unless appendicectomy is performed, there is a considerable risk of a further attack of acute appendicitis.

PERITONITIS

Perforation of the acutely inflamed appendix is the commonest cause of peritonitis in this country. This is a convenient point, therefore, to consider this subject in detail.

Aetiology

Peritonitis can be defined as inflammation of the peritoneal cavity. Bacteria may enter this space by four portals:
1. *From the exterior*—a penetrating wound of the abdominal wall, or by infection introduced at laparotomy.
2. *From intra-abdominal viscera*—either from perforation (for example perforated duodenal ulcer, perforated appendicitis, or rupture of the intestine from trauma), gangrene of a viscus (e.g. acute cholecystitis or infarction of the intestine), or postoperative leakage of an intestinal anastomosis.
3. *Via the bloodstream*—as part of a septicaemia, a rare source of infection today.
4. *Via the female genital tract*—following acute salpingitis or puerperal infection (inflammation of the genital canal during childbirth). Approximately 40% of all cases of peritonitis are due to acute appendicitis, 20% result from postoperative complications, and 20% are due to perforated peptic ulcers.

Clinical features

Peritonitis inevitably follows some precipitating lesion which itself may have definite clinical features. For example, the onset may be an attack of acute appendicitis, or a perforated duodenal ulcer, or abdominal trauma, each with its appropriate symptoms and signs.

In the early hours, peritonitis is characterized by a generalized severe pain. The patient wishes to lie still because any movement aggravates his agony. Irritation of the lower aspect of the diaphragm may be accompanied by pain which is referred to the shoulder tip. Vomiting is frequent. The temperature is usually elevated and the pulse rises progressively. Examination at this time shows a seriously ill patient with localised or generalised tenderness of the abdomen, depending on the extent of the peritonitis. The abdominal wall is held rigidly and rebound tenderness is present. The abdomen is silent on stethoscopic examination.

In advanced cases, the abdomen becomes distended, signs of free fluid are present, the patient becomes increasingly toxic with a rapid, feeble pulse. Vomiting becomes faeculant and the patient is obviously shocked with moist, cold and cyanosed skin.

Treatment

Specific causes of peritonitis may require specific therapy. These are dealt with in their appropriate sections. The general principles of treatment are as follows:
1. *Relieve pain* by means of morphia.
2. *Gastric aspiration* by means of a naso-gastric tube; this reduces the risk of inhalation of vomit and prevents further abdominal distention by removing swallowed air.
3. *Fluid and electrolyte replacement* by intravenous therapy. Blood may be required in the presence of shock.
4. *Antibiotic therapy.* Ampicillin is the usual first drug of choice, but therapy is guided where possible by checking the sensitivity of the responsible organisms.
5. *Surgery* is indicated if the source of infection can be removed or closed. For example, a perforated peptic uler is sutured, a gangrenous perforated appendix removed and ruptured gut resected or repaired.

Conservative treatment is indicated where the infection has been localised (e.g. an appendix mass), or where the primary focus is irremovable as in pancreatitis, or post-partum infection, where the patient is moribund, or where there is a lack of surgical facilities, as on board ship. Here reliance must be placed on intravenous therapy, gastric aspiration, and antibiotics.

Any localised collection of pus requires drainage and later surgery may be required for the evacuation of residual abcesses. Following peritonitis, pus may collect in the subphrenic spaces or in the pelvis.

SUBPHRENIC ABSCESS

Pus may collect between the diaphragm and the liver or immediately below the liver on either the right or left side; indeed rarely they are bilateral.

About one third follow perforated appendicitis, one third from perforations of peptic ulcer, and a sixth from abdominal operations.

Clinical features

Subphrenic infection usually follows a general peritonitis after 10 days to 3 weeks, although if antibiotics have been given, an abscess may be disguised and may only become obvious weeks or even months after the original episode. Often there are no localizing symptoms, but the patient merely presents with a swinging pyrexia, malaise, nausea, loss of weight and anaemia. There may, however, be localising features of pain in the upper abdomen, the lower chest, or referred to the shoulder, and there may be swelling or tenderness in the upper abdomen or lower chest.

Special investigations

The white cell count is raised to the region of 15,000 to 20,000, with a relative increase in polymorphs.
Screening of the chest is the vital investigation which reveals an abnormality in nearly all cases. The signs are elevation of the diaphragm on the affected side, diminished or absent mobility of the diaphragm, a pleural effusion, and/or collapse of the lung base on the affected side, and gas together with a fluid level below the diaphragm (Fig. 12.16).

Treatment

If there is no gas and free fluid on X-ray, an early case may respond to antibiotic therapy, but if there is clinical or X-ray evidence of a localised abscess or if resolution fails to occur on antibiotic therapy, then surgical drainage is indicated.

PELVIC ABSCESS

A pelvic abscess may follow any general peritonitis, but it is particularly common after acute appendicits (75%), or after gynaecological infections. In the male the abscess lies between the bladder and the

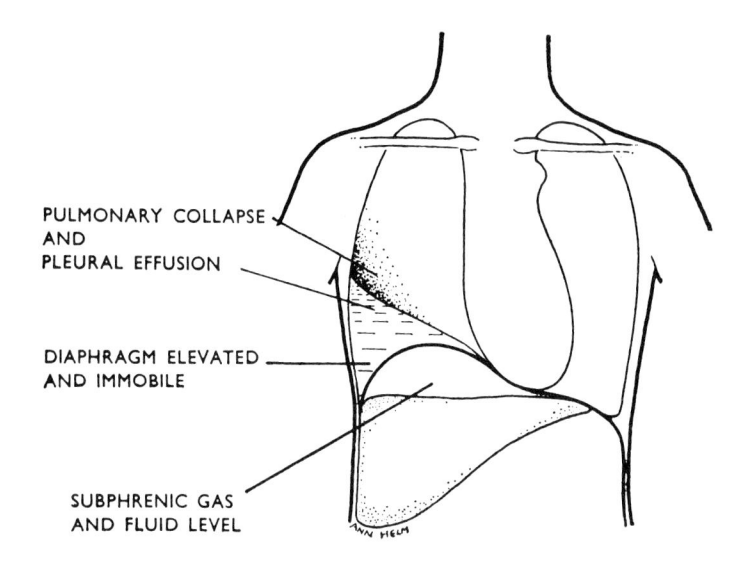

Fig. 12.16. Diagram of the X-ray appearances of a right subphrenic abscess. The diaphragm is raised (and fixed on screening), a fluid level is present beneath it and there is a pleural effusion with compression and collapse of the lung base.

rectum, in the female between the uterus and posterior fornix of the vagina anteriorly, and the rectum posteriorly (pouch of Douglas).

Left untreated the abscess may burst into the rectum or vagina, or may discharge onto the abdominal wall, particularly if there has been a previous abdominal laparotomy incision at the time of the original episode of peritonitis. Occasionally the abscess may rupture into the peritoneal cavity.

Clinical features

1. General—swinging pyrexia, toxaemia, weight loss with leucocytosis.
2. Local—diarrhoea, mucous discharge per rectum, the presence of a mass felt on rectal or vaginal examination, which is occasionally large enough to be palpated abdominally.

Treatment

An early pelvic cellulitis may respond rapidly to a short course of chemotherapy, but there is the risk that the prolonged antibiotic treatment of an unresolved infection may produce a chronic inflammatory mass studded with small abscess cavities in the pelvis. It is safer, therefore, where there is an established pelvic abscess, to withhold chemotherapy and await pointing into the vagina or rectum through which surgical drainage can be carried out. Very often even this is not required since firm pressure by the finger in the rectum may be followed by rupture of the abscess through the rectal wall.

The colon

Anatomy

The colon is a bulky muscular tube which extends from the caecum in the right iliac fossa via the ascending colon, the hepatic flexure, the transverse colon, the splenic flexure, the descending colon and the pelvic (sigmoid) colon to terminate in the rectum, which commences opposite the centre of the third piece of the sacrum and which empties to the exterior via the anal canal (Fig. 12.17).

The junction between the ileum and caecum is protected by the ileocaecal valve. This is a thickening of the circular muscle of the terminal ileum which exerts some regulation of the emptying of ileal contents, and prevents reflux from the caecum. Just beneath the ileocaecal junction is attached the appendix.

The characteristic appearance of the colon is due to two main features in the arrangement of the muscle coat. The first of these is the regular pouching of the colon into 'haustra' and the second is the condensation of the outer longitudinal muscle into three separate bands known as the *taenia coli*.

Fig. 12.17. The colon and its blood supply.

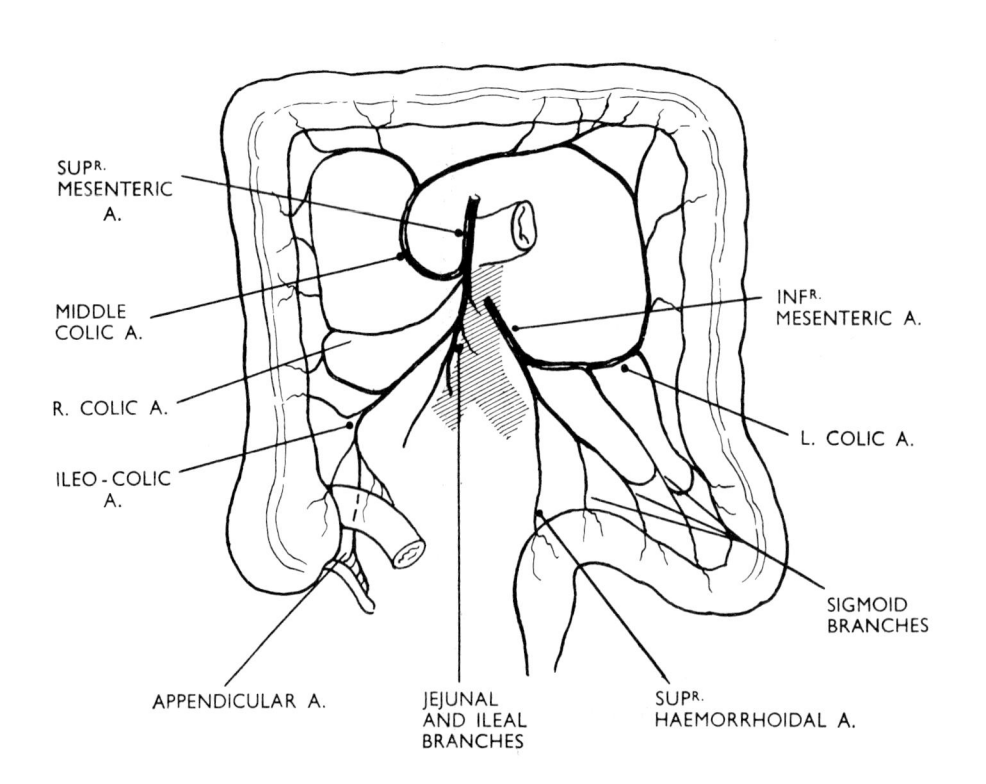

The taenia coli become a continuous coat over the surface of the appendix and distally over the rectum. The ascending colon and the descending colon are retroperitoneal in situation; the transverse colon however is an intra-peritoneal structure, its blood supply being carried to it along the transverse mesocolon. Hanging from the under surface of the transverse colon is the fatty sheet, the greater omentum, which, above the colon, becomes attached to the greater curve of the stomach. The pelvic colon is also intra-peritoneal and also has a mesocolon.

The blood supply of the caecum, the right side of the colon and the transverse colon is derived from the superior mesenteric artery via the ileo-colic, right colic and middle colic branches. The descending and pelvic colon, together with the upper part of the rectum, are supplied with blood from the inferior mesenteric artery, which arises from the front of the aorta just above its bifurcation. The venous drainage of the colon passes to the portal vein. The lymphatic drainage follows the venous drainage and lymph nodes are found at the edge of the colonic wall and alongside the aorta.

As with the whole of the intestine, the nerve supply is both from the sympathetic and parasympathetic nervous systems. The sympathetic nerves are carried to the wall of the intestine both from the retro-peritoneal plexuses and with blood vessels. The parasympathetic supply is derived for the right side of the colon and half of the transverse colon from the vagus nerve and for the left side of the colon from the parasympathetic sacral outflow.

Considering the function of the colon, its wall is surprisingly thin. This has the effect that it is extremely distensible. The mucosa appears on inspection to be pale pink in colour with a shiny, smooth surface. When viewing the normal mucosa through a sigmoidoscope it is possible to distinguish individual blood vessels running beneath its surface.

The colon acts as a reservoir. Water is reabsorbed so that liquid ileal contents are converted into solid faeces.

Contraction of the colon and a desire to defaecate result when the wall becomes distended or with the gastro-colic reflex which follows taking a meal.

Apart from these normal causes of colonic contraction, certain drugs, including Senokot, castor oil and phenolphthalein, have a similar action.

ULCERATIVE COLITIS

Ulcerative colitis is a disease of the colon and rectum of unknown cause. Among many suggestions as to its aetiology are psychosomatic factors, an allergy or auto-immune disease.

Pathology

Females are more commonly affected than males. Although the disease may occur at any age, the peak incidence is between 20 and 40 years. In the majority of cases the condition affects the rectum first, but later spreads to involve the whole of the colon. Initially there is oedema and reddening of the mucosa. This is followed by bleeding from the inflamed mucosa when it is touched ('contact bleeding'), then ulceration (Fig. 12.18.). Eventually the wall of the colon becomes oedematous and fibrotic so that it is rigid with loss of its normal haustrations.

Clinical features

The patient complains of profuse diarrhoea, which contains blood, mucus and pus. There may be accompanying cramp-like abdominal pains. There may be an acute onset of fulminating disease accompanied by fever, toxaemia, severe bleeding and the risk of perforation. More often attacks are less severe and intermittent, or the patient may pass into a stage of chronic active disease.

Investigations

Sigmoidoscopy reveals oedema of the mucosa with contact bleeding in the early mild cases, proceeding to granularity of the mucosa and then frank ulceration, with pus and blood in the bowel lumen. Biopsy will give confirming histological evidence of the diagnosis.

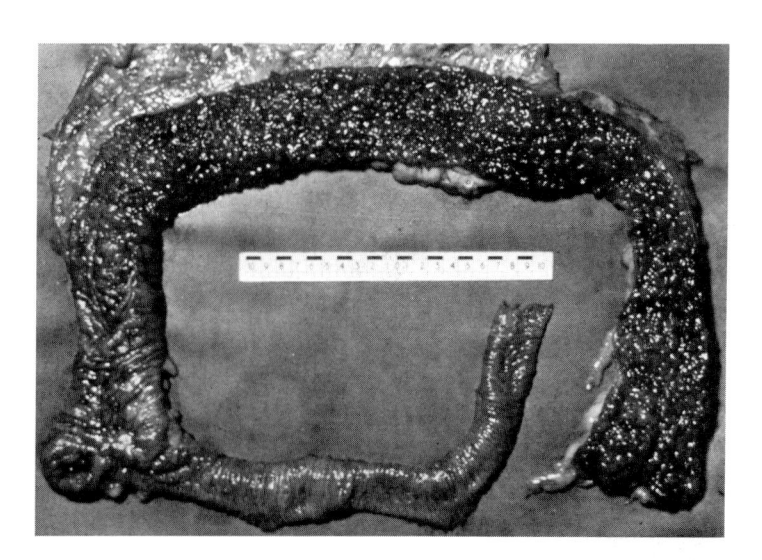

Fig. 12.18. Ulcerative colitis. The specimen removed at operation has been opened to demonstrate the diffuse ulceration of the mucosa.

A barium enema shows ragged ulceration and in the chronic case the fibrosis and loss of haustration produces the typical appearances of the 'drainpipe' colon (Fig. 12.19.).

Stool examination reveals pus and blood but no specific organism can be grown.

Differential diagnosis must be made from other causes of diarrhoea especially those due to specific infecting organisms producing amoebic or bacillary dysentery. This is particularly true in patients who are, or have been, domiciled overseas. Carcinoma of the colon and Crohn's disease of the large bowel are also important differential diagnoses.

Complications

These may be either local or general.

Local complications are perforation of the colon, haemorrhage, which may either be acute or chronic with progressive anaemia, stricture formation, peri-anal infection, fistula-in-ano, and malignant change. Patients with ulcerative colitis, particularly those with long standing disease, are at far greater risk of developing carcinoma of the large bowel than normal individuals.

General complications are toxaemia, loss of weight, anaemia, arthritis, iritis, ulceration of the legs and abscesses of the skin, which may break down into ulcers (pyoderma gangrenosa).

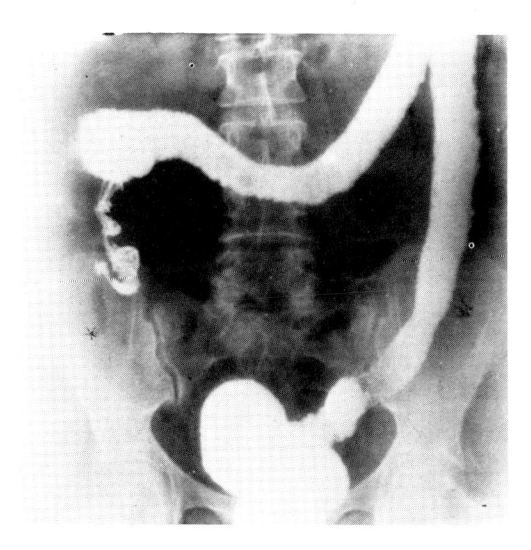

Fig. 12.19. Barium enema in advanced ulcerative colitis to show the typical 'drain pipe' appearance of colon and fine ulceration of the mucosa.

Treatment

Initially this is medical in the uncomplicated case, but surgery is required when medical treatment fails or if complications supervene.

1. *Medical treatment*

A high protein diet is prescribed with vitamin supplements and iron. Blood transfusion is given if the patient is severely anaemic. If there has been severe depletion of fluids and electrolytes due to profuse diarrhoea, this must be corrected by an intravenous drip. In many cases the acute attack may be brought under control by a combination of steroids given systemically and also as retention enemas. Sulphasalazine (salazopyrine), which is a sulphonomide/salicilate compound, is also of value. Diarrhoea may be controlled with codeine or isogel.

2. *Surgical treatment*

Surgery is required in a fulminating attack of colitis which does not rapidly respond to conservative measures, particularly where there is any suspicion that the bowel may have perforated. Local complications, including severe haemorrhage, stricture, or any question of malignant change, or the development of any general complications also make surgery obligatory. Operation is also advised where the patient is in chronic ill health due to repeated episodes of the disease or continued colitis.

The only certain cure for ulcerative colitis in our present state of ignorance about its aetiology is total excision of the colon, rectum and anal canal, with permanent ileostomy. In some patients it is possible to resect the colon and then to anastomose the ileum to the rectum (colectomy with ileo-rectal anastomosis). This has the clear advantage of preservation of the rectum and anus, although, because of the loss of most of the reservoir capacity of the large bowel, the patient usually experiences frequency of defaecation in the region of 3–7 bowel actions daily. The surgery is also technically more difficult with a greater number of postoperative complications. With the rectum left in place there is also the risk of later development of a carcinoma in the stump.

At present the choice of operation depends on a careful assessment of the individual patient; the presence of gross disease of the rectum obviously makes its preservation hazardous, but a patient may well wish to take any risk in order to preserve the anal sphincter. If an ileostomy is necessary, the patient must be reassured that a full and active life can be lead, thanks to the development of modern adhesive ileostomy appliances (Fig. 12.20). It is useful to introduce him preoperatively to a patient who has already well adapted to the ileostomy life.

ISCHAEMIC COLITIS

This condition has been recognised quite recently and results from a defective blood supply to the region of the splenic flexure of the colon. It is at this point that an anastomosis occurs between the arterial supply of the colon from the superior mesenteric and inferior mesenteric arteries (see Fig. 12.17). The lesion is found in old people with generalised atherosclerosis.

Gross ischaemia may result in frank gangrene of the bowel, but more often there is mucosal ulceration and fibrotic narrowing of the affected segment.

The diagnosis is confirmed by barium enema X-ray which reveals a short segment of irregularity with narrowing in the splenic flexure region.

The majority of patients recover without permanent damage to the colon, but stricture formation may require resection and, of course, gangrene of the bowel precipitates emergency surgery.

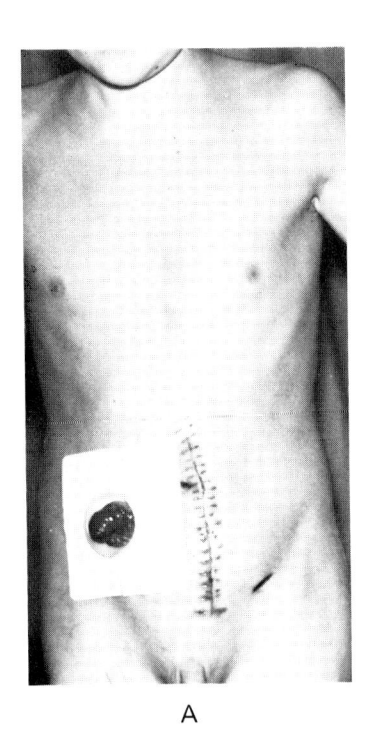

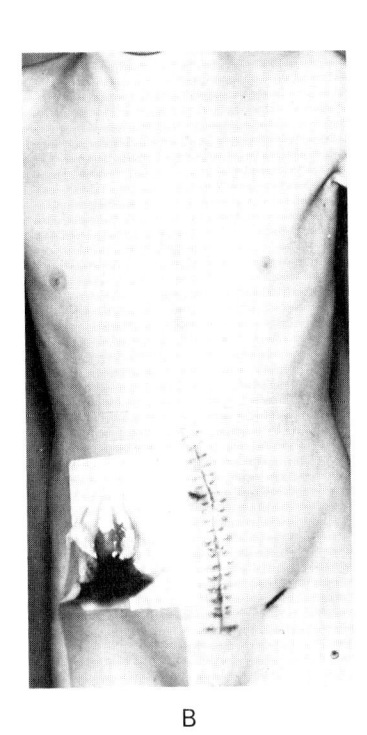

Fig. 12.20. An adhesive ileostomy appliance, (A) without and (B) with bag.

Pathology

A diverticulum is a small pouch of mucosa pouting through the muscular wall of the colon, rather like the inner tube of a bicycle tyre bursting through the outer casing. Diverticula are found most commonly in the pelvic colon and become increasingly rare in passing from the left to the right side of the large intestine. They are unusual before the age of 40, but in the elderly they are found in about 30% of all post mortems. Sex distribution is roughly equal. Although the exact cause of diverticula is not known, they are associated with hypertrophy of the muscle of the colon wall, which undergoes contraction and produces out-pouchings at the sites of potential weakness in the muscle wall, which correspond to the points of entry of the supplying vessels to the bowel. (Fig. 12.21). Although colonic diverticula are so common in Western civilised communities they are extremely rare among primitive peoples, and it may be that the modern refined low roughage diet may be responsible for the muscle thickening which is the primary lesion in this condition.

Complications

The majority of patients with diverticula of the colon are symptomless, and this condition is termed *'diverticulosis'*. Some patients have symptoms produced by the thickening of the colonic wall (Fig. 12.22) and this is termed *chronic diverticular disease*. A diverti-

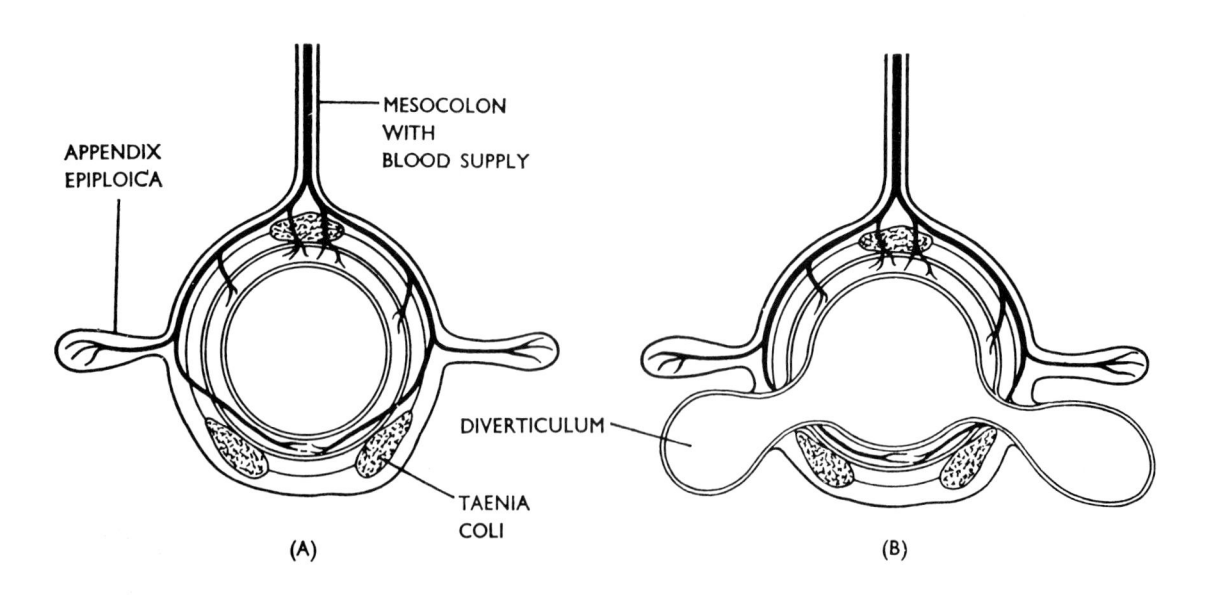

Fig. 12.21. The relationship of diverticula of the colon to the penetrating blood vessels. (A) normal colon, (B) colon with diverticula.

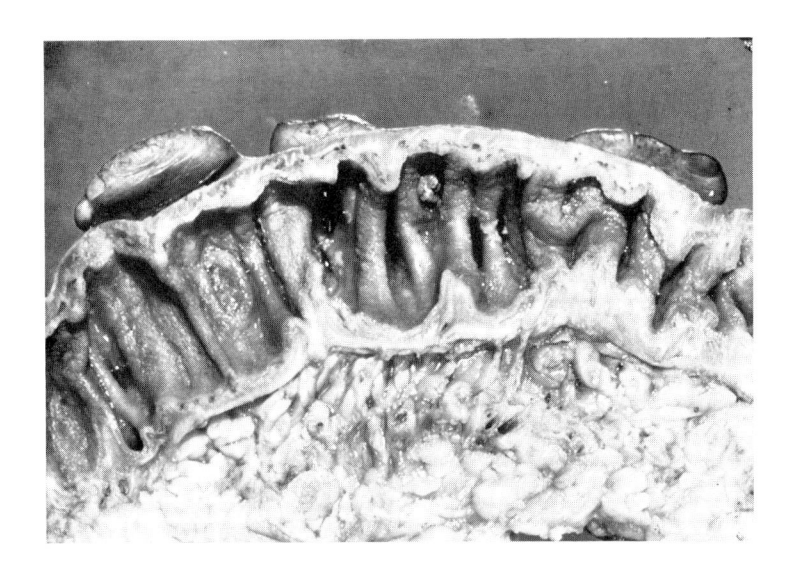

Fig. 12.22. The thickening of the colon wall in chronic diverticular disease. Note the mouths of the diverticula.

culum may become acutely inflamed (*acute diverticulitis*) and this may:
1. Perforate
    (a) into the general peritoneal cavity.
    (b) with the formation of a localised abscess.
    (c) into adjacent structures, particularly bladder, small intestine or vagina.
2. Produce chronic infection with inflammatory fibrosis.

Another occasional complication of diverticula of the colon is haemorrhage as a result of erosion of a vessel at the neck of a diverticulum.

Clinical features

Chronic diverticular disease exactly mimics the local clinical features of carcinoma of the left side of the colon. There may be diarrhoea alternating with constipation which progresses to large bowel obstruction, accompanied by vomiting, distension, colicky abdominal pain, and absolute constipation. There may be episodes of pain in the left lower abdomen and the passage of muscus or bright red blood per rectum. Examination reveals tenderness in the left iliac fossa and there may be a thickened mass to feel in the region of the pelvic colon.

More unusual presentations are:
1. A sudden severe rectal haemorrhage.
2. A fistula into the bladder with passage of faeces and gas bubbles (pneumaturia) in the urine.

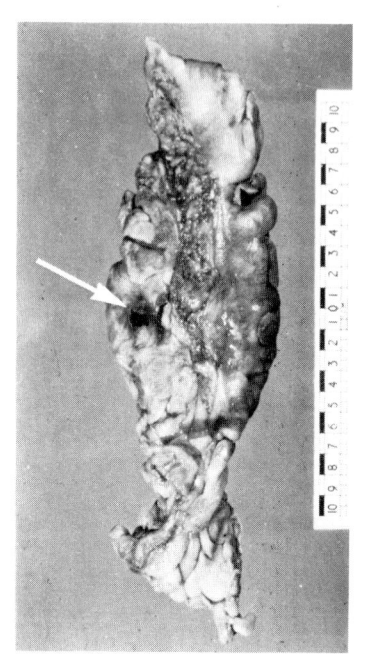

Fig. 12.23. A post-mortem specimen of a perforated acute diverticulitis (the perforation is arrowed).

Acute diverticulitis is well nicknamed 'left-sided appendicitis'. There is an acute onset of central abdominal pain which shifts to the left iliac fossa and which is accompanied by fever, vomiting and local tenderness and guarding. A vague mass may be felt in the left iliac fossa. Perforation into the general peritoneal cavity (Fig. 12.23) produces the signs of general peritonitis. If the infection is localized, a pericolic abscess forms which is comparable to an appendix abscess but is situated on the left side. There is a tender mass, an associated swinging pyrexia and a raised white cell count.

Investigations

Sigmoidoscopy. If the affected segment is low in the colon there may be an oedematous block to the passage of the instrument.

A barium enema demonstrates diverticula as globular out-pouchings (Fig. 12.24). Diverticular disease is characterised by stricture formation which may closely mimic a carcinoma.

Differential diagnosis

It may be very difficult to differentiate even at operation between chronic diverticular disease and a carcinoma of the colon, and indeed these two common conditions not infrequently co-exist.

Treatment

Acute diverticulitis is managed conservatively. The patient is put to bed, placed on ampicillin and given a fluid diet. The great majority settle on this regime.

A pericolic abscess is treated conservatively in a similar way to an appendix abscess. If the abscess enlarges, drainage is indicated. This is often followed by the formation of a faecal fistula and is therefore best combined with a transverse colostomy.

General peritonitis from rupture of an acutely inflamed diverticulum is a dangerous condition. Laparotomy is performed, the perforation repaired, or the affected section of colon resected and a defunctioning colostomy fashioned. Full antibiotic therapy is given.

Acute obstruction due to diverticulitis requires laparotomy to establish the diagnosis and a transverse colostomy to relieve the obstruction. Following this emergency procedure, elective resection can be carried out and the colostomy subsequently closed.

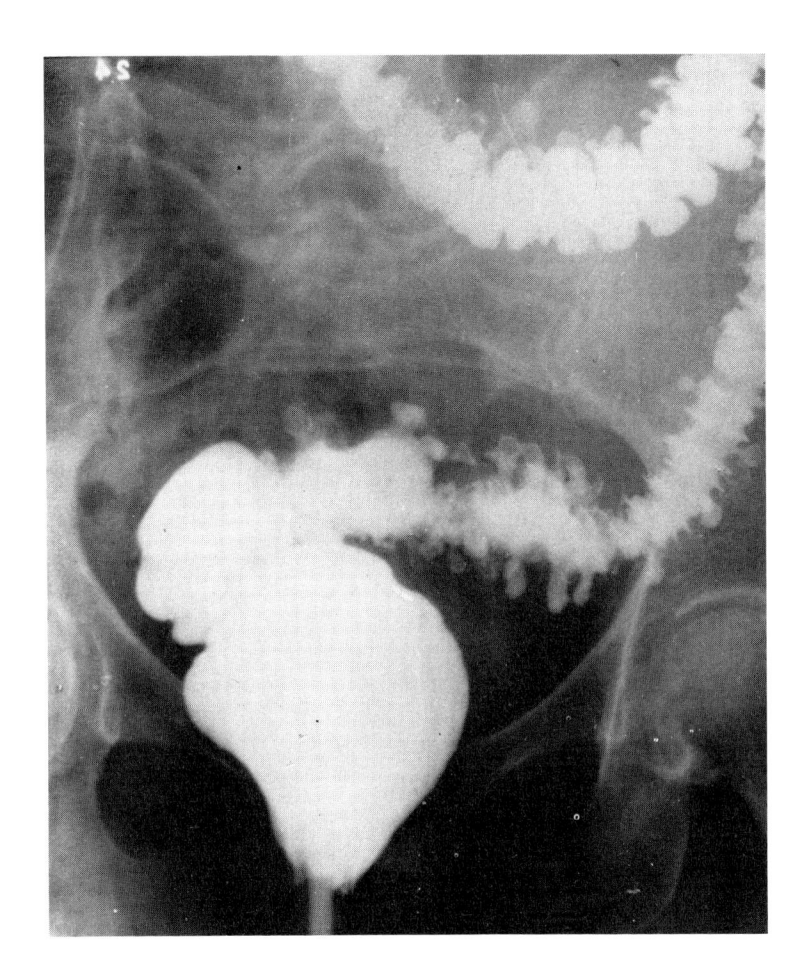

Fig. 12.24. A barium enema demonstrating extensive diverticulosis of the sigmoid colon.

Chronic diverticular disease If the diagnosis is made with considerable certainty and the symptoms are mild, the patient is treated conservatively. The bowels are regulated by means of Milpar or some other lubricant laxative. A high roughage diet is prescribed which contains plenty of fruit and vegetables to ensure normal bowel actions. If, however, symptoms are severe, or if carcinoma cannot be excluded, then laparotomy and resection of the affected segment of colon is performed.

Recently a new form of operation has been used which involves splitting of the thickened muscle of the colon down to the mucosa, a procedure that is termed myotomy. It resembles, in principle, the splitting of the thickened muscle in Heller's operation for achalasia of the cardia (see page 167) and Ramstedt's operation for congenital pyloric hypertrophy (see page 176). The exact place of this operation is as yet not certain.

VOLVULUS OF THE COLON

Definition

Volvulus is a twisting of a loop of bowel around its mesenteric axis (Fig. 12.9). This results in a combination of obstruction and occlusion of the main vessels at the base of the involved mesentery. Most commonly it affects the pelvic colon, or the caecum or the small intestine, but volvulus of the gall bladder or stomach may also occur.

SIGMOID VOLVULUS

This condition is relatively rare in Great Britain, but is much more common among primitive black African negroes and also occurs quite frequently in Russia and Scandinavia. This may be associated with areas where a high bulk diet is eaten.

Clinical features

There is a sudden onset of colicky abdominal pain with characteristic gross and rapid abdominal distension.

A plain X-ray of the abdomen shows an enormously dilated loop of bowel (Fig. 12.25). If left untreated the strangulated colon undergoes gangrene and perforates so that the patient dies from peritonitis.

Treatment

If the patient is seen early, a rectal tube is passed through a sigmoidoscope. This often untwists the volvulus and is accompanied by the passage of vast amounts of flatus. If this method fails, laparotomy is required. The volvulus is untwisted and the bowel decompressed via a rectal tube threaded upwards from the anus. Subsequently an elective resection of the redundant sigmoid loop is carried out in order to prevent recurrent torsion.

If gangrene has occurred, the affected segment is excised and the two open ends brought out as a double-barrelled colostomy which is later closed.

VOLVULUS OF THE CAECUM

This is usually associated with a congenital defect in the peritoneal attachment of the caecum so that instead of it being tethered to the posterior wall, the caecum and ascending colon have a persistent mesentery which allows torsion to occur.

Clinically there is an acute onset of pain in the right side of the

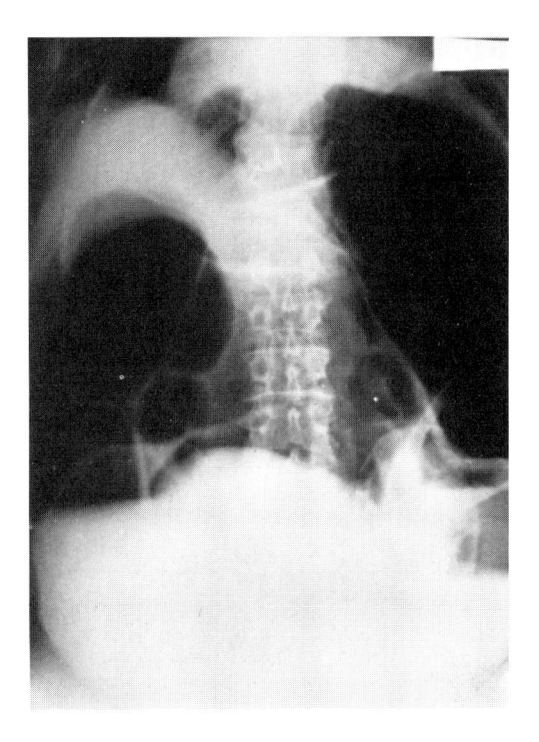

Fig. 12.25. X-ray of the abdomen in volvulus of the sigmoid. Note the enormous dilated loop of colon.

abdomen accompanied by rapid abdominal distension. X-ray shows a grossly dilated loop of intestine on the right side.

Treatment

Laparotomy is performed and the volvulus untwisted. The distended gut is decompressed by means of a temporary caecostomy which also effectively fixes the caecum by means of adhesions and thus prevents further torsion.

TUMOURS OF THE COLON

Classification

Tumours of the large bowel may be benign or malignant. The benign lesions include the adenomatous polyp (which may be multiple) and the papilloma. These are important because undoubtedly some undergo malignant change.

Malignant tumours are the carcinoma, carcinoid tumour (see page 207) and lymphosarcoma, which originates in the lymphoid tissue in the wall of the colon. Secondary malignant tumours are rather rare, apart from those resulting from invasion from adjacent organs, e.g. stomach, bladder, uterus or ovary.

CARCINOMA OF THE COLON

Pathology

The large bowel is the second commonest site for cancer in the United Kingdom and is next in frequency only to cancer of the lung, (see Fig. 17.5). The tumour may occur at any age, although it particularly affects the 50 to 70 year group. Females are affected slightly more often than males, although the reverse is true in rectal cancer. The sigmoid colon is the commonest site in the colon itself although the rectum accounts for one-third of all the large bowel cancers.

Predisposing factors include pre-existing polyps, familial polyposis coli (an unusual disease characterized by innumerable polyps throughout the colon, which is inherited and which invariably proceeds to malignant change between about the twentieth and fortieth years of life), and ulcerative colitis (see page 227).

On the right side of the large bowel, the tumour usually takes the form of an ulcer with a raised everted edge or of a papilliferous growth, whereas on the left side of the colon the tumour typically grows around the circumference of the bowel to produce a stricture, which may also become ulcerated (Fig. 12.26).

Spread

The tumour spreads locally, first encircling the wall of the bowel, invading its coats and eventually involving adjacent viscera, including small intestine, stomach, duodenum, uterus and bladder; in the last case a vesico-colic fistula may result. Lymphatic spread passes to the regional lymph nodes and bloodstream spread occurs along tributaries of the portal vein to the liver. Deposits of malignant nodules may occur throughout the peritoneal cavity by transcoelomic spread; this is usually accompanied by malignant ascites.

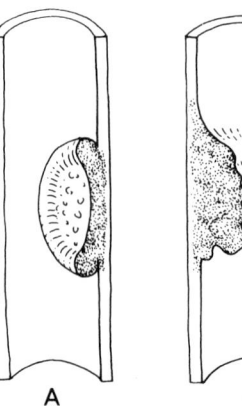

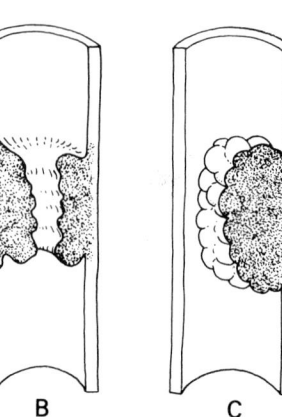

Fig. 12.26. Diagram of the types of carcinoma of the colon. (A) malignant ulcer, (B) stricture, (C) the proliferative 'cauliflower'

Clinical Features

The manifestations of carcinoma of the colon can be divided, as with any tumour, into those produced by the tumour itself, those caused by the presence of secondaries and those resulting from the general effects of the tumour.

Local Effects; the most common symptom is a change in bowel habit. If the lesion has ulcerated, it may give rise to bleeding which may appear as recognisable red blood in the stool or, if the ulcer is on the right side of the colon, the blood may be dark and altered. In other instances the blood loss is occult; continuous small loss may result in a severe iron-deficient anaemia, which may indeed be the presenting feature. Cancers on the left side of the colon tend to be constricting growths and moreover the contained stool is solid; therefore obstructive features predominate with colicky abdominal pain, distension and constipation which may eventually become absolute (i.e. the patient is unable to pass even flatus).

Secondary Deposits; the patient may present with jaundice, hepatomegaly or abdominal distension due to ascites.

The general effects of malignant disease include anaemia, anorexia and loss of weight.

Clinical examination may reveal a palpable mass, felt either abdominally or per rectum, evidence of intestinal obstruction, evidence of secondary spread (enlargement of the liver, jaundice, ascites) or clinical evidence of anaemia or loss of weight, both of which are suggestive of malignant disease.

Special investigations

A barium enema is a most helpful investigation. This is extremely accurate when carried out by an experienced radiologist. The tumour is demonstrated either as a stricture or as a filling defect projecting into the lumen of the bowel (Fig. 12.27). Even minute lesions, 2 or 3 mm. in diameter, may be demonstrated by the 'double contrast' technique in which the colon is coated with barium sulphate suspension and is then distended with air. It is important for the bowel to be carefully prepared before X-ray by means of aperients and an enema, since a false positive X-ray may result from the presence of faecal material in the bowel lumen.

Sigmoidoscopy will reveal tumours up to the recto-sigmoid region and allow positive evidence by biopsy to be obtained. Even if the tumour is not reached directly, the presence of blood or slime trickling down from higher in the bowel is strongly suspicious of malignant disease.

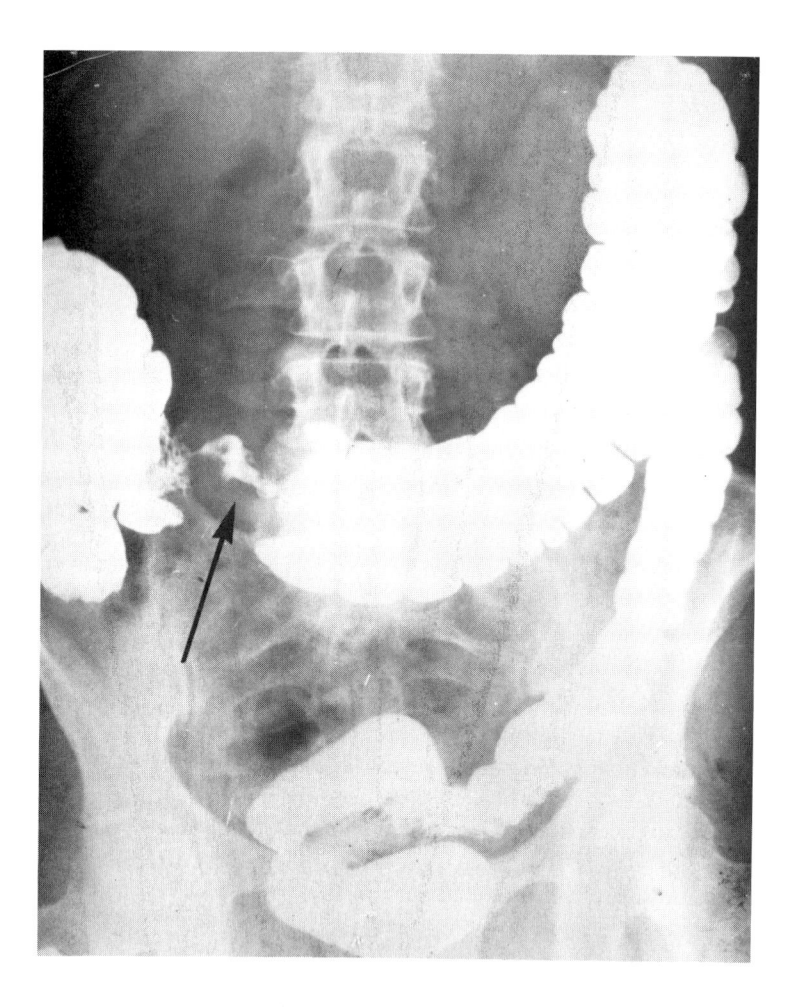

Fig. 12.27. Barium enema demonstrating a carcinomatous stricture in the transverse colon (arrowed).

Colonoscopy using the flexible colonoscope enables a more extensive direct examination of the colonic mucosa, although it is technically difficult to examine the whole of the colon round to the ileo-caecal valve.

Treatment

The treatment for a carcinoma of the colon is surgical excision. In the elective case, preliminary preparation of the colon is essential and this takes about 5 days (see page 26). The patient is given a low residue diet, which for the 24 hours prior to operation consists of fluids only. In addition, an aperient such as magnesium sulphate is given and the colon is cleared from below by means of an enema 2 days before operation and a further washout one day before operation. By these means, all faecal residue is removed from the colon.

Most surgeons give a non-absorbable antibiotic neomycin and pthallylsulphathazole) during this period to sterilise the bowel lumen as much as possible.

The operation that is carried out is a hemicolectomy; for a caecal carcinoma this is a right hemicolectomy, for a transverse colon carcinoma a transverse hemi-colectomy, and for a carcinoma of the descending colon or pelvic colon a left hemicolectomy (Fig. 12.28).

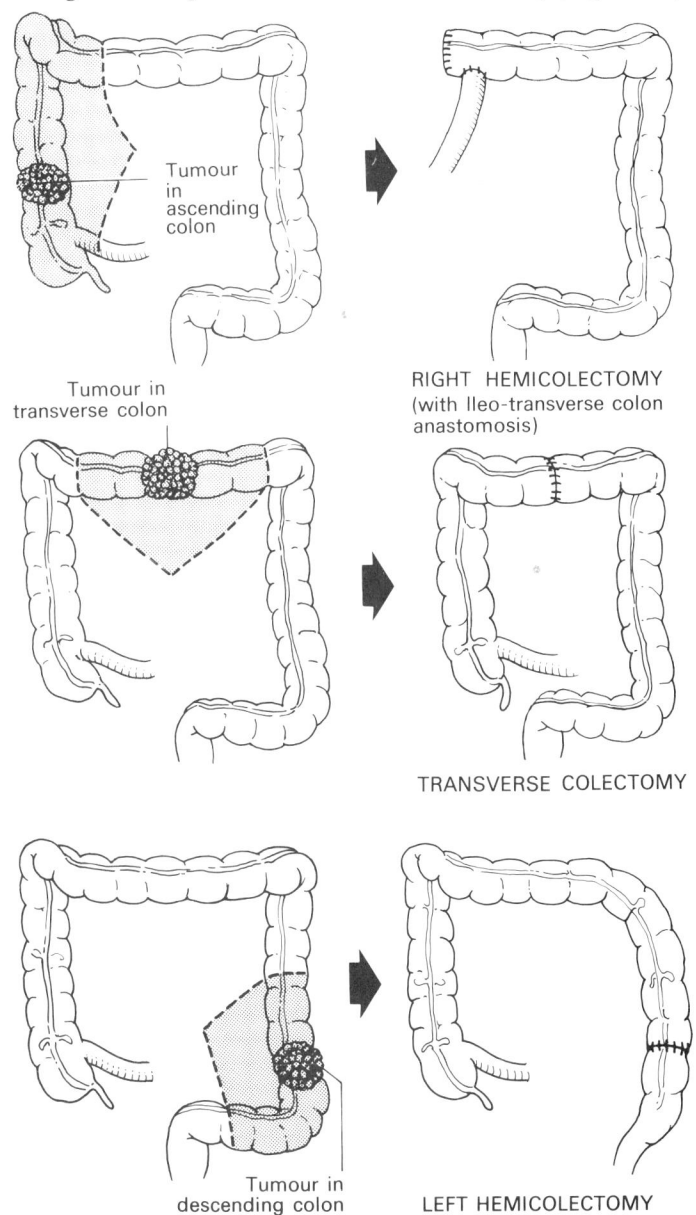

Fig. 12.28. The types of partial colectomy.

An end to end anastomosis is performed and if there is any technical difficulty in performing this anastomosis or if the suture line encroaches on the rectum, a protecting side colostomy is performed proximal to the anastomosis.

If the patient has any degree of obstruction due to the carcinoma it is essential to perform a preliminary colostomy. This allows the colon to deflate to its normal dimension and the faecal residue held up by the carcinoma to be evacuated. The second stage of the procedure then involves the hemicolectomy. The third and final stage is the closure of the colostomy.

If there is any evidence of spread of the disease beyond the confines of the resected specimen of colon, cytotoxic agents such as 5-Fluorouracil administered at weekly intervals intravenously have been found to be of use in checking the continuing growth of the carcinoma.

COLOSTOMY

A colostomy is an artificial opening between the colon and the skin of the abdominal wall. When it is fashioned in the operating theatre the mucosa of the colon is stitched to the cut edge of the skin in the opening in the abdominal wall that has been made to receive it. Flatus and faeces are then discharged through this opening on to the surface of the abdomen, where they are collected into a plastic or rubber bag.

There are a number of different types of colostomy which are carried out for a variety of different reasons (Fig. 12.29).

1. *Terminal colostomy.* This is formed when the divided end of the colon is brought out to the surface of the left iliac fossa following abdominoperineal excision of the rectum. This is obviously a permanent state of affairs.

2. *Side colostomy* is formed when the anterior wall of the colon is sutured to the abdominal wall, a small side hole being made in the colon. This is used in two main situations. The first of these is when the distal colon is obstructed, for example by a carcinoma. Relief of the obstruction in this way will prevent further dilation of the proximal intestine and relieve pain and vomiting. The second indication is to 'protect' an anastomosis in order to ensure that it is not placed under any pressure and that if a leak does occur it remains small and localised. For example, when anterior resection of the rectum is carried out the descending colon is joined to the rectum quite low down in the pelvis. This anastomosis is not only technically quite

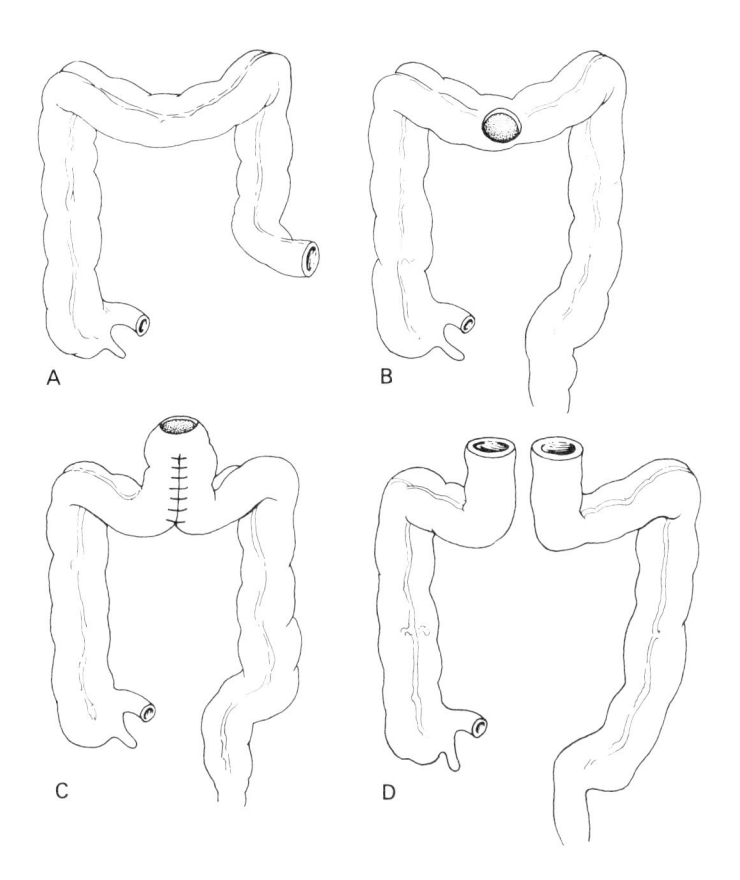

Fig. 12.29. The types of colostomy. (A) terminal, (B) side, (C) loop, (D) defunctioning.

difficult but also has a reputation for leaking as it has been estimated that this will occur in up to one-third of these cases.

3. *Loop colostomy* is performed when a loop of the colon, usually the transverse colon, is exteriorised and passed over a glass rod. This is used for similar cases to the side colostomy but suffers the disadvantage of being bulky and relatively difficult to manage. However, it is easy to carry out and almost completely defunctions the distal bowel, at least for the first few days after operation. The glass rod is withdrawn after 5 to 7 days and the exteriorised colon falls back into the abdomen with the exception of the muco-cutaneous junction. The end result of this manoeuvre is a side colostomy.

4. *Defunctioning colostomy*, (Devine Colostomy) It is sometimes necessary to ensure that *no* faeces pass into the distal colon. In this case the colon is transected, and the two ends, proximal and distal, are brought out through separate openings in the abdominal wall.

5. *Double barrelled colostomy*, (Paul-Mikulicz Operation) This is an

old fashioned procedure for the removal of an obstructing carcinoma of the pelvic colon. The loop of the pelvic colon, with the tumour at its apex, is exteriorised from the abdomen and after the peritoneal cavity has been closed and the colon fixed to the surface of the skin, the loop with its contained carcinoma is excised. The two ends of the colon then discharge on to the surface of the skin, rather like the barrels of a double-barrelled shotgun. This operation is no longer performed for cancer because the excision of the carcinoma is inadequate as it does not include the regional lymph nodes. It is still used in cases of gangrene or perforation of the transverse or pelvic colon, for example gunshot wounds, and in gangrenous volvulus of the pelvic colon.

Colostomy care

Broadly speaking the care of a colostomy falls into one of two categories. The first of these employs the 'wash-out' technique. Each morning the patient washes out the colon with water, using a special syringe and nozzle, until no more faecal material can be obtained. Providing that the diet has been well controlled the colon will not discharge any more of its contents for the rest of that day and the stoma merely requires a small dry dressing held in place by a suitable pad and plastic tape or a belt. The second method is to allow the colon to assume a normal rhythm in which it will usually discharge faeces once, twice or three times per day. In this case a suitable receptacle in the form of a disposable plastic bag has to be applied to the surface of the abdominal wall. These plastic bags may be held in place by a belt and a ring protected by plastic foam. An example of this type of appliance is the Schacht device, which is useful for a temporary colostomy fashioned for the relief of obstruction which will be closed a week or two after its formation (Fig. 12.30). A more appropriate appliance for longer-term use is a flange which is stuck to the surface of the skin by adhesive. In this case the disposable plastic bags are attached to the flange either by more adhesive or by being slipped over a specially designed ring. An example of this type of apparatus is the Translet appliance (Fig. 12.31).

There must be almost as many different detailed methods of colostomy care as there are patients with colostomies. One of the first things to convey to a patient faced with this enormous alteration in the pattern of his or her life is to emphasise that near normal activity can be carried out. There need be no interruption in the social, recreational, sexual or domestic life of the patient. The patients can swim, meet their friends, marry and have children in

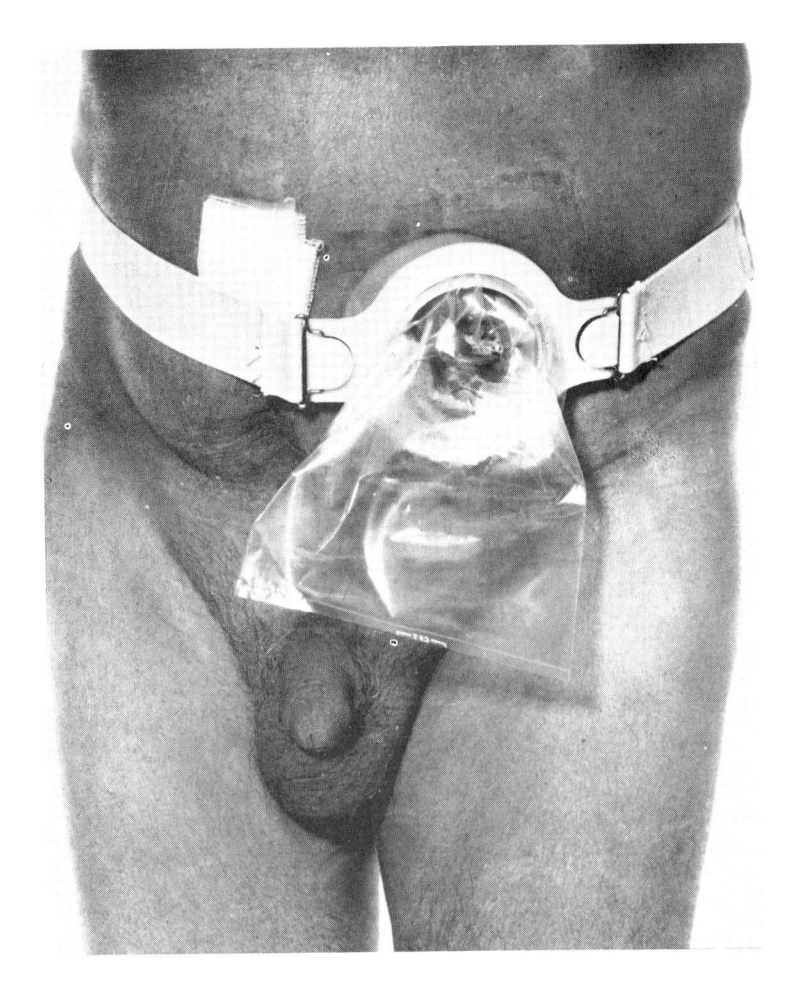

Fig. 12.30. The Schacht colostomy appliance.

spite of what may be initially regarded as a totally disastrous alteration of anatomy.

It is probably wrong to advocate one method of colostomy care to the exclusion of all others. Many intelligent patients prefer to washout their colostomies each morning and thereby to be free of the difficulties of bag changing during working hours. For less intelligent patients the wash-out method can have some dangers because if the nozzle of the syringe is introduced into the colostomy in the wrong direction or with too much force it is possible to pump a large volume of 'wash-out' water through a tear in the wall of the colon into the peritoneal cavity. For these patients therefore, some sort of adhesive flange is more appropriate.

Diet is found to be extremely important. Increase in roughage will often produce colostomy diarrhoea which, as may be imagined, is

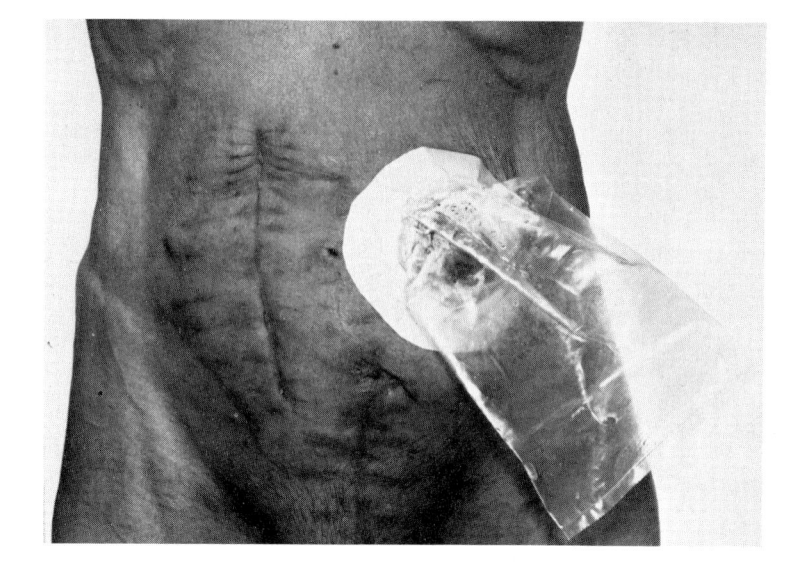

Fig. 12.31. The Translet colostomy appliance.

much more difficult to cope with than in the normal person. Onions and certain other pungent foods may result in an unpleasant odour which is difficult to control. Most patients learn very quickly how to regulate their diet so as to avoid these complications.

The rectum and anal canal

Anatomy

The rectum is continuous with the pelvic (sigmoid) colon opposite the middle of the third piece of the sacrum and is 5 inches long (Fig. 12.32). It is supplied with blood from 3 haemorrhoidal arteries, the upper one being derived from the inferior mesenteric artery, the middle and lower ones from the internal iliac arteries.

The veins follow the arteries and the submucosa of the rectum is therefore a point of junction between the portal and systemic venous systems. The nerve supply is from the lumbar sympathetic and the sacral part of the parasympathetic outflow. The sensations that the rectum is capable of initiating are those of distension together with the ability to distinguish between flatus and faeces. Pain may also be experienced but this is deep seated and ill localised—a visceral type of pain.

The *anal canal* is $1\frac{1}{2}$ inches long and terminates at the anal orifice. Its lower half is lined by a squamous epithelium, unlike the columnar mucosa that lines the rest of the intestine. This lower part of the anal

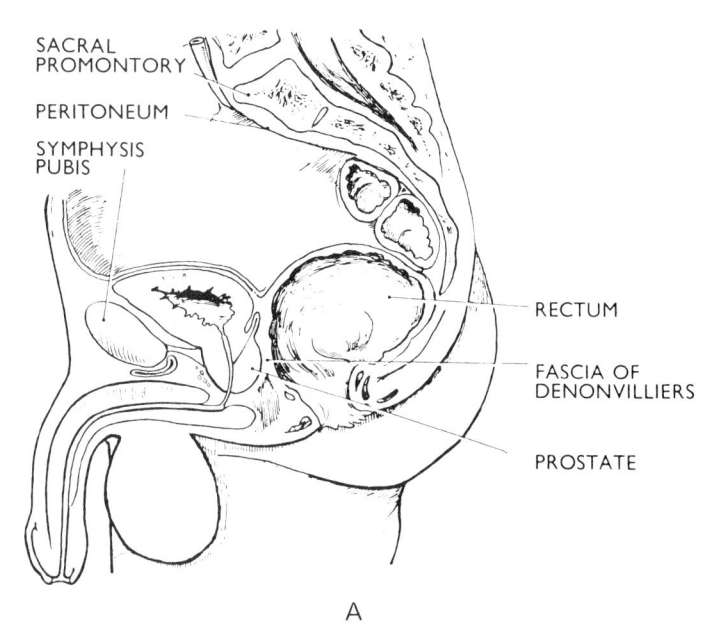

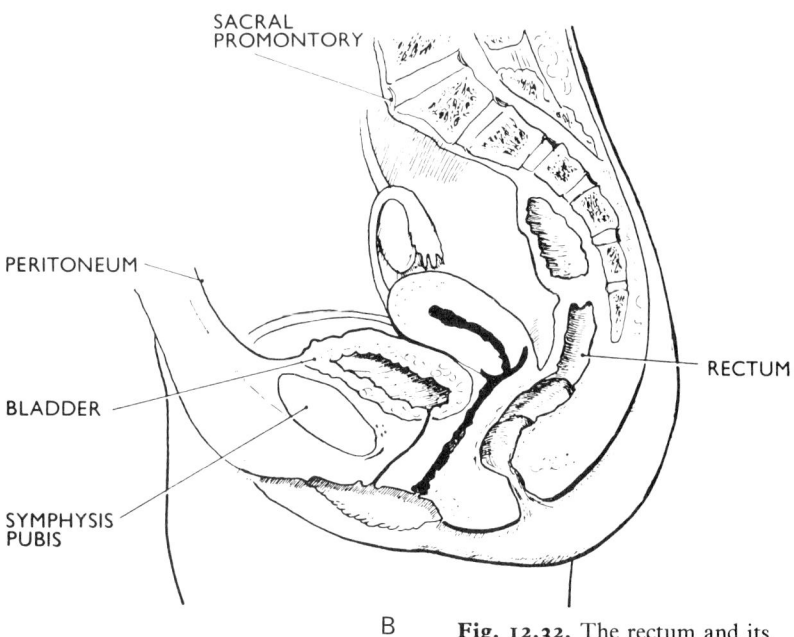

Fig. 12.32. The rectum and its related viscera (A) in the male and (B) in the female.

canal receives innervation from the inferior haemorrhoidal nerve which subserves normal cutaneous sensation; the lower canal is therefore extremely sensitive to the prick of a needle, whereas injection of a haemorrhoid, by inserting a hypodermic needle into the mucosa of the upper part of the anal canal, is almost painless.

ANO-RECTAL ATRESIA

The anal canal is formed in the embryo by a junction between the distal extremity of the hind gut and an invagination of the epithelium between the buttocks termed the proctodaeum. This accounts for the upper part of the canal becoming lined with an intestinal mucosa and the lower part being covered with squamous epithelium. If the septum between the two structures fails to break down then the condition of atresia results (Fig. 12.33). Any degree of severity of this condition may occur, from imperforate anus, made up of a thin septum, to complete absence of the anal canal and rectum. About half the infants with atresia have an associated fistula, which in the female passes into the vagina and in the male into the bladder or urethra.

Clinical features

The anus may be entirely absent or represented by a dimple or by a blind canal. Of course the infant is unable to pass any meconium, although this escapes either through the vagina or through the urethra if there is an associated fistula.

The extent of the defect is judged by X-raying the child, held

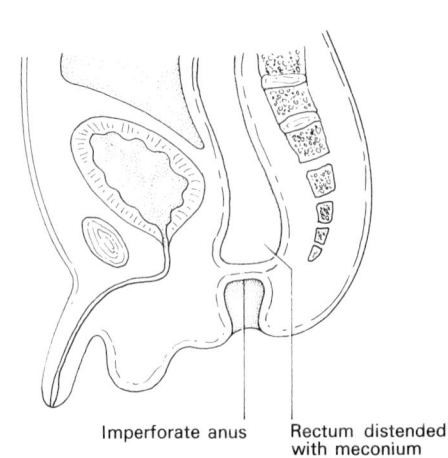

Fig. 12.33. Atresia of the anal canal.

Imperforate anus   Rectum distended with meconium

upside down, with a metal marker at the site of the anus. The distance between the gas bubble in the lowere bowel and the marker can then be measured.

Treatment

If the septum is thin it can be divided with suture of the edges of the defect of the skin. However, if there is an extensive gap between the blind end and the anal verge, a colostomy is made and a later attempt at a reconstructive operation is carried out when the child is about 2 years of age. If a vaginal fistula is present then surgery is not urgent, since the bowel decompresses through the vagina and elective surgery can be performed when the girl is older.

HIRSCHSPRUNG'S DISEASE

Pathology

This condition, which also receives the term congenital megacolon, is produced by faulty development of the parasympathetic nerve supply of the lower bowel. It is characterised by the absence of nerve cells in the rectum; this aganglionic segment sometimes extends into the lower colon and rarely affects the whole of the large bowel. The involved segment is spastic and the colon proximal to this becomes grossly distended (Fig. 12.34).

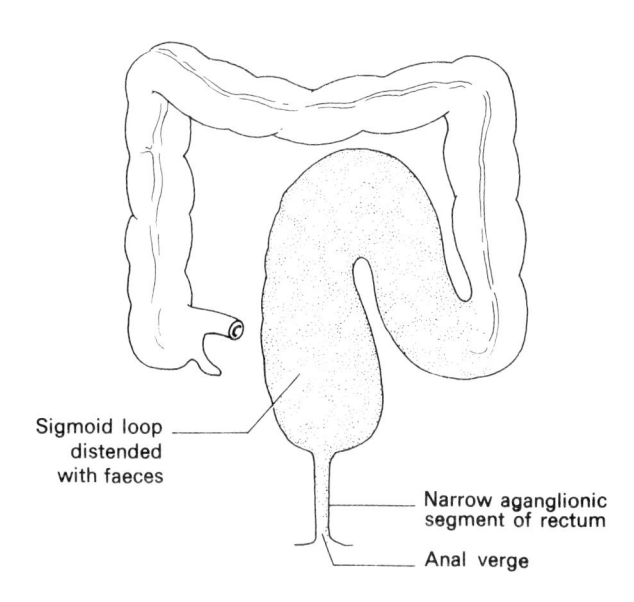

Fig. 12.34. Hirschsprung's disease.

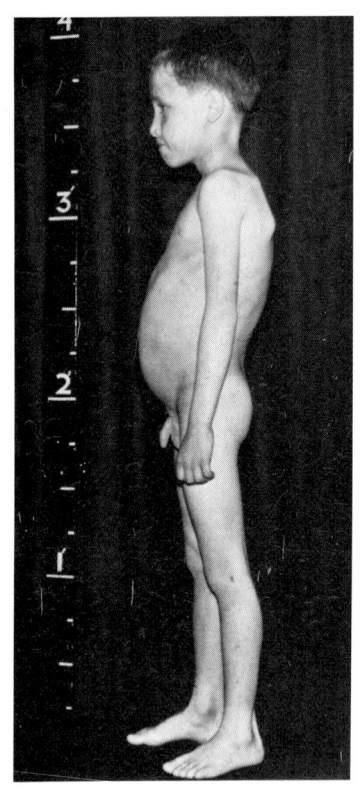

Fig. 12.35. A child with Hirschsprung's disease; note the gross distension of the abdomen.

Clinical features

The majority of patients are male. In severe cases, obstructive symptoms commence in the first few days of life with gross abdominal distension; death results unless urgent treatment is instituted. Less marked examples present with extraordinarily stubborn constipation in infancy and these children survive into adult life with gross abdominal distension and stunted growth (Fig. 12.35).

Examination of the rectum reveals a narrow empty canal above which faecal impaction may be felt.

Special investigations

A barium enema demonstrates a characteristic narrow rectal segment, above which the colon is dilated and full of faeces.

Biopsy of the rectal wall shows characteristic complete absence of ganglion nerve cells.

Treatment

If the child is obstructed in the neo-natal period, a colostomy is performed. Elective surgery is carried out between the first and second year of life. The aganglionic segment is resected and an abdominoperineal pull-through anastomosis is carried out between the normal colon and the anal canal. It is important at the time of operation to carry out frozen section histological examination to ensure that the resection is taken back into healthy colon which contains normal nerve ganglion cells.

PILES (HAEMORRHOIDS)

The name 'piles' literally means 'lumps'. Piles are extremely common and comprise the mucosa of the anal canal covering dilated submucous veins.

Piles are classified according to their size into first, second and third degree. First degree piles do not prolapse through the anus and can only be seen on proctoscopy. Second degree piles prolapse through the anus on defaecation but return spontaneously. Third degree piles prolapse through the anal verge and are so large that they can only be returned digitally, (Fig. 12.36).

Clinical features

The most common symptom to be associated with piles is the passage of bright red blood per rectum on defaecation, usually without pain.

Characteristically the bleeding is quite profuse, splashing into the lavatory pan. If bleeding continues unchecked the patient may become anaemic. The other symptoms associated with piles are those of prolapse, which in the case of third degree piles can be extremely troublesome, and pruritus (itching).

It is essential that all patients who complain of bleeding per rectum shall be fully examined. Included in this examination must be sigmoidoscopy and proctoscopy. A sigmoidoscope is 30 cm in length and it is possible to see the whole of the anal canal, rectum and the terminal part of the pelvic colon (Fig. 12.37). Proctoscopy provides a better means of inspection of the terminal part of the rectum and anal canal specifically in the pile bearing area. The main point of the examination which is carried out on these patients is to exclude a cancer of the rectum which may present with exactly similar symptoms, that is painless bleeding of bright red blood per rectum.

The most serious complication is *prolapse with strangulation*. In this case, because of anal spasm the blood supply is cut off and the piles become gangrenous (Fig. 12.38). This is an intensely painful condition as the blood within the piles thromboses and the thrombotic process extends to the peri-anal tissues to produce a characteristic ring of oedema around the anus. The treatment of this condition is to admit the patient to hospital and, if the strangulation is not of long standing, to carry out an emergency haemorrhoidectomy. In

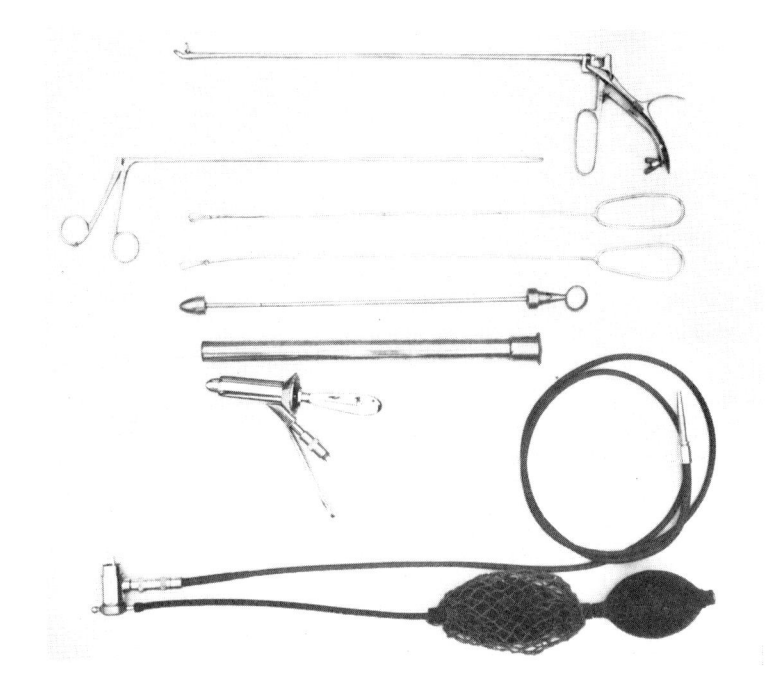

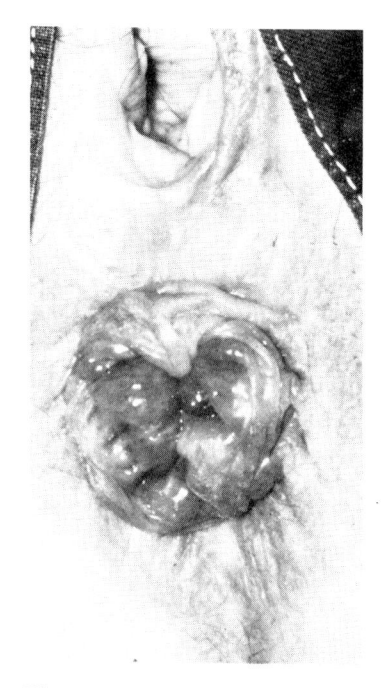

Fig. 12.36. Prolapsing piles.

Fig. 12.37. Proctoscope, sigmoidoscope, and accessories.

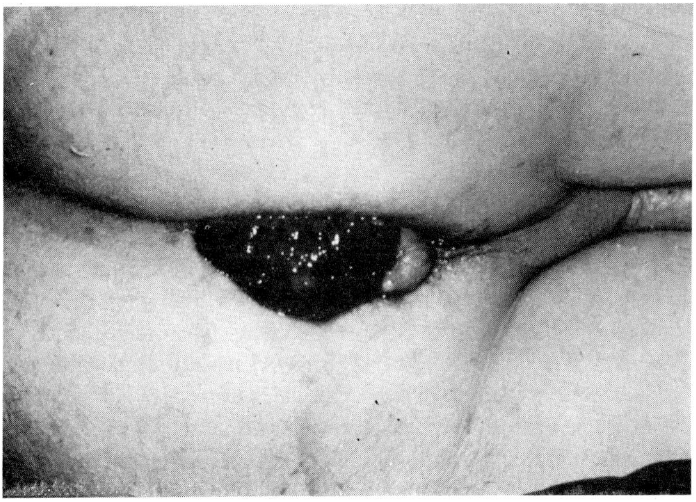

Fig. 12.38. Strangulated piles. The prolapsed mucosa has become gangrenous.

later cases, with a good deal of infection, conservative treatment is indicated. The patient is put to bed, the foot of which is raised, and a cool compress of lotio plumbi is applied to the anus. Only fluids are allowed so as to reduce the bulk of the stools and on this regime the condition rapidly settles. As the piles have undergone gangrene, often an 'auto-haemorrhoidectomy' has been carried out. But if significant piles remain then haemorrhoidectomy is required 3 months after the episode of strangulation.

Treatment

The treatment of internal piles depends upon their size. First and second degree can be treated by injection. In this case 5% Phenol in Almond Oil is injected beneath the anal canal mucosa and around, but not into, the dilated veins (Fig. 12.39). This procedure is painless and can be carried out quite quickly in the Out-Patient Department. It is usually necessary to repeat these injections on 2 separate occasions separated by intervals of 2 weeks.

If the piles are third degree the operation of haemorrhoidectomy is required. After the colon has been emptied by one or more enemas the patient is given a general anaesthetic, the piles are excised and each pedicle firmly transfixed and ligated with thread. A great deal has been said about how much agony is experienced after this operation, but in fact many people do not seem to experience great pain. One of the principal sources of discomfort post-operatively is the development of an impacted stool in the rectum. If this is allowed to happen the patient very often has to have a general anaesthetic for

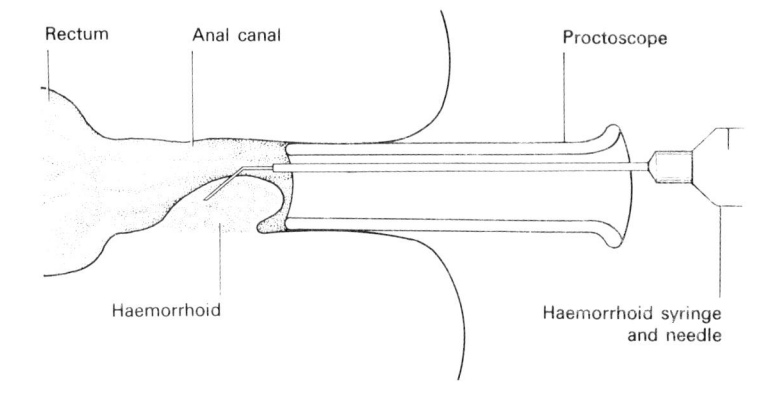

Fig. 12.39. The injection treatment of piles.

it to be removed. In order to prevent this series of events, Normacol is given, commencing before the operation and continuing as soon as possible post-operatively. If the patient has not defaecated within 24 hours he is given a dose of Senokot and with this combined therapy success is usually achieved by the end of the second day.

One important complication that can occur following haemorrhoidectomy is that of a secondary haemorrhage due to the infection of one of the ligated pedicles, which takes place about 7 to 10 days postoperatively. In this case quite large quantities of blood may be lost, occasionally requiring replacement by transfusion. It may be necessary to pack the anal canal in order to control the bleeding. It is for this reason that patients after this procedure should remain in hospital until approximately the tenth post-operative day.

PERI-ANAL HAEMATOMA

This lesion, (also termed 'thrombosed external pile') is produced by rupture of a tributary of the inferior haemorrhoidal vein in the peri-anal skin. Unlike internal piles, it is covered by squamous epithelium supplied by cutaneous nerve endings and is therefore extremely painful. The onset is acute, with sudden pain, and the appearance of a tense, dark blue, cherry-sized lump at the anal verge (Fig. 12.40).

Treatment

The treatment is quite simple and can be carried out in the Out-Patient Department. With the patient in the left lateral position a small quantity of 1% lignocaine gel is smeared over the surface of the pile. After two minutes 2 to 3 ml of 1% lignocaine solution is in-

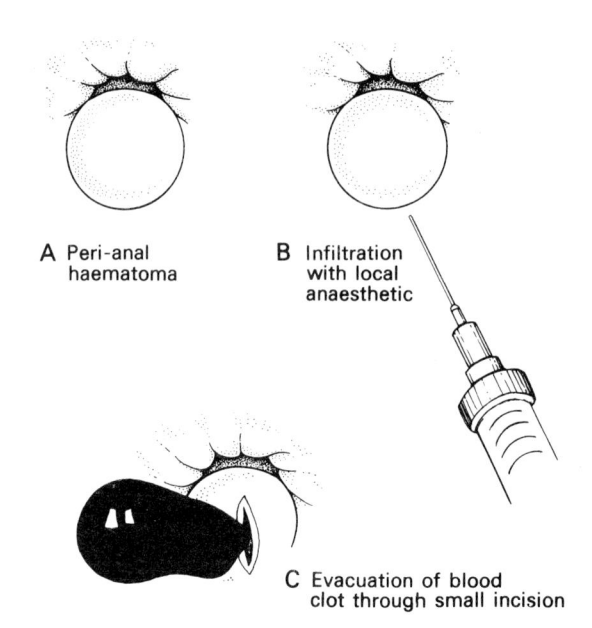

Fig. 12.40. A perianal haematoma and its surgical treatment.

A Peri-anal haematoma

B Infiltration with local anaesthetic

C Evacuation of blood clot through small incision

jected beneath the surface of the skin overlying the haematoma through a fine needle. When the skin is anaesthetised it is incised with a scalpel and the clot is evacuated, with immediate relief of pain. The cavity that is left after the clot has been evacuated is simply left to drain and it usually heals within a week to 10 days.

FISSURE IN ANO

A fissure in ano is a crack in the anal skin and is associated with intense anal pain and spasm of the anal sphincter. In 90% of cases it is in the midline posteriorly. Ten per cent of the patients have a fissure in the mid-line anteriorly and the greater proportion of these patients are women. The story is characteristic, with the pain starting on defaecation. The patient often notices a small quantity of blood on the surface of the stool. When the anal region is examined the external end of the fissure has a small oedematous tag of skin associated with it; this is the so called 'sentinel pile' (Fig. 12.41).

Complete examination of the anal canal is usually impossible because of severe pain, which prevents even gentle digital examination.

Fissures may be divided into one of two types: the acute anal fissure and the chronic anal fissure which has often been present for months or sometimes years.

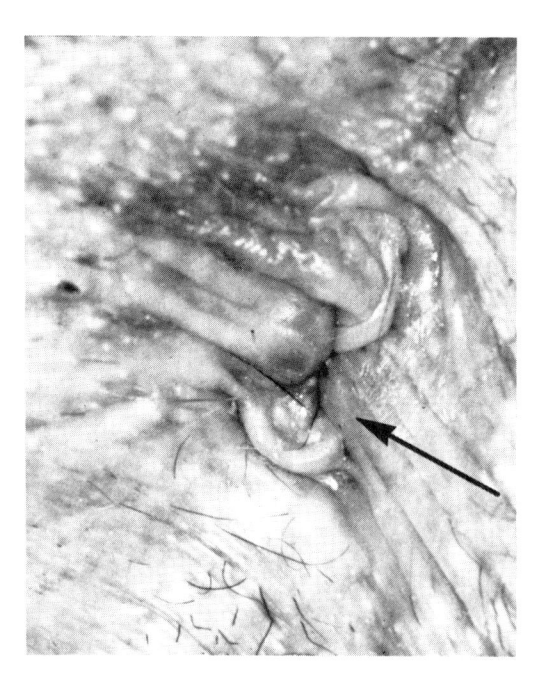

Fig. 12.41. Fissure in ano with sentinel pile (arrowed).

Because of the severe pain associated with this condition it may be necessary to admit the patient for an examination under a general anaesthetic. This is important to exclude a neoplasm of the rectum or anal canal.

Treatment

In some cases it is possible to treat an acute anal fissure conservatively. The stool is made soft by the use of Normacol granules which have the added advantage of preventing constipation. In addition, an anal dilator may be used daily, lubricated with 1% lignocaine gel, but care has to be exercised in the use of all local anaesthetic preparations for the peri-anal region because of the tendency for 'sensitization' to occur. When this happens the peri-anal skin becomes sore and inflamed and a vicious circle is set up. That is, in order to relieve the soreness, more lignocaine gel is applied by the patient when this is the very agent which is producing the inflammation.

In the case of a chronic anal fissure a variety of operative procedures have been described. The most effective treatment is to dilate the anus moderately under general anaesthetic, followed by simple excision of the fissure. Obviously this will convert what is a small fissure into a large wound in the anal canal. The reason that this is effective is that the edges of the wound are 'freshened' and have a normal blood supply which allows healing to occur. It is important that the excised tissue from the edges and base of the fissure should be submitted to histological examination because occasionally fissures are one of the complications of Crohn's disease of the rectum and colon.

There is unfortunately a tendency for fissures to recur because the anal skin of these patients is thin, dry and abnormal. It is quite definitely not to the patient's advantage to take large quantities of an aperient of any type in an attempt to reduce the bulk of the stool and increase the frequency of the bowel action. Some patients develop phobic anxiety in relation to their bowel habit and consume enormous quantities of liquid paraffin to achieve what they consider to be a satisfactory bowel action. If the stool is maintained in a liquid state, the dilating action of the normal stool is lost and the end result is a narrow, inadequate and thoroughly unsatisfactory anal canal. It should be realised that the normal frequency of defaecation varies from 3 bowel actions per day at one extreme to one bowel action every 3 days at the other, and within these limits the patients should be encouraged not to feel anxiety about minor variations or irregularity of frequency. There is no doubt that the best regulation of bowel habit is achieved by adjustment of food and, generally speaking, a diet containing a reasonable amount of bulk in the form of fruit and vegetables is the ideal.

PRURITUS ANI

This is the term given to the intensely uncomfortable symptom of anal and perianal itching. As may be imagined it causes acute social embarrassment and misery. It may be associated with thread worms (which are more common in children but also may occur in adults), diabetes mellitus, or any condition that results in damp perianal skin, e.g. prolapsed piles. In the majority of patients, however, no obvious cause can be found.

Examination of the anus reveals a red, sore area of moist skin which may be more or less excoriated depending upon the amount of scratching it has been submitted to. Sigmoidoscopy is usually negative, although in some cases there may be associated distal proctitis.

Treatment

It is extraordinary how often patients with this symptom do not pay even the most rudimentary attention to their personal hygiene. They should be advised to bathe the anus following each act of defaecation with warm water and ordinary toilet soap, making sure that all soap is then rinsed from the skin. The skin should then be gently dried with a soft towel and sometimes a little talcum powder will be soothing. In many cases this is the only treatment that is required. As an adjunct to the important hygienic care of the anus a small quantity of topical steroid cream will rapidly effect relief. One of the cheapest and yet the most effective applications is 1% hydrocortisone cream. If there is a co-existant proctitis this may be treated either by suppositories containing prednisilone (Predsol) or by a foam steroid applicator (Proctofoam) which has the effect of applying a small quantity of betamethasone cream to the terminal mucosa of the rectum, anal canal and the perianal skin all at the same time.

This regime is always effective, certainly as long as steroid cream is being applied. Often when this is gradually withdrawn after one or two weeks the pruritus recurs. In this case steroids are used again and again withdrawn until the condition resolves.

One important detail that has to be sought in the history is the use by the patient of antiseptics. Many people feel that in order to control the inevitable 'infection' around the anus a strong antiseptic should be used. All such local applications must be stopped because they may be *producing* pruritis. Another potent cause of pruritis is the application of topical analgesic, for example cinchocaine or lignocaine.

PERI-ANAL ABSCESSES

The soft tissues around the lower rectum and anal canal are a common site for abscess formation. These may be:

1. *Subcutaneous*—resulting from infection of a hair follicle or a sweat gland adjacent to the anal verge.
2. *Ischio-rectal*—involving the space bounded by the lower rectum, the levator ani muscle, the ischium and the peri-anal skin, as a result of infection spreading from the small anal glands within the anal canal.
3. *Submucous*—as a result of infection of a fissure or laceration of the anal canal.
4. *Pelvi-rectal*—as a result of spread from a pelvic abcess; fortunately this is rare (Fig. 12.42).

Clinical features

The patient complains of pain adjacent to the anus. On inspection a tender mass is found which is hot and over which the skin is reddened. A deeply placed abscess in the ischio-rectal region may be quite difficult to diagnose in its early stages but on gentle palpation of the skin of the buttock and on careful rectal examination an indurated, tender swelling may be found.

Naturally, a severe local infection is also accompanied by the general features of pyrexia and malaise.

Left untreated, the abscess may rupture into the anal canal and also on to the peri-anal skin with the formation of a fistula-in-ano.

Treatment

As with abscesses in any situation, the treatment is incision and drainage as soon as possible. The cavity is kept open with a wick of ribbon gauze soaked in Eusol and is allowed to heal from below upwards.

FISTULA IN ANO

A *fistula* is an abnormal communication between two epithelial surfaces, for example between a hollow viscus and the surface of the body or between two hollow viscera. A *sinus* is a granulating track leading from the source of infection to a surface.

The term fistula in ano is loosely applied to both fistulae and sinuses in relation to the anal canal. The great majority result from

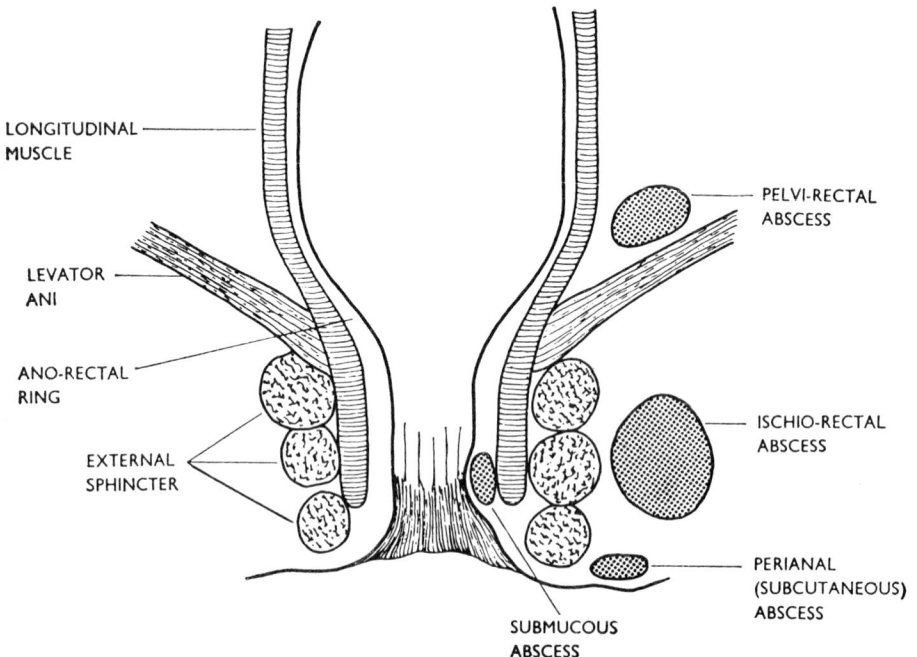

Fig. 12.42. The types of peri-anal abscesses.

an initial abscess forming in one of the anal glands which then ruptures into the lumen of the anal canal and onto the peri-anal skin. Much more rarely, fistula in ano may be associated with tuberculosis, Crohn's disease, ulcerative colitis or carcinoma of the rectum.

Subcutaneous and submucous fistulae are superficial tracks which result from rupture respectively of subcutaneous and submucous abscesses. Anal fistulae have their tracks passing through the external anal sphincter. Most of these are at a low level but some are higher and open in close relationship to the junction between the anal canal and rectum. Ano-rectal fistulae which extend above the ano-rectal junction are fortunately rare.

Clinical features

There is usually a story of an initial perianal abscess which discharges. Following this, there may be recurrent episodes of peri-anal infection with persistent discharge of pus or even faecal material. Examination reveals the external opening of a fistula (Fig. 12.43).

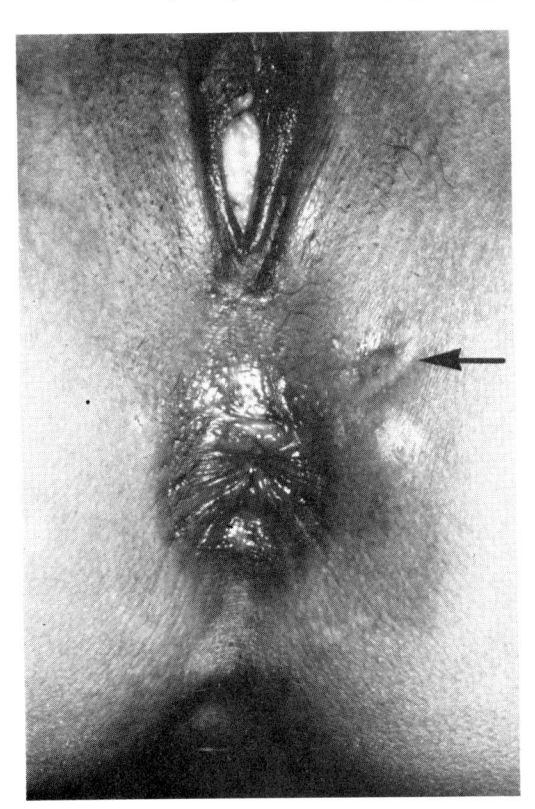

Fig. 12.43. The external opening of a fistula in ano to the left side of the anal verge (arrowed).

The internal opening may be felt on rectal examination but probing of the track is painful and should be deferred until the patient is anaesthetised.

Treatment

Once established, a fistula will not heal spontaneously and surgical cure is necessary. The patient is anaesthetised and placed in the lithotomy position. A director is passed along the track of the fistula, which is then excised (Fig. 12.44). A biopsy of the wall of the track is taken to exclude any of the associated conditions mentioned above. A Vaseline gauze dressing is then applied. The wound that results requires careful daily dressing until it has healed by granulation tissue from its base to the surface.

A high fistula, which extends above the anal sphincter, presents a very considerable problem of management, because damage to the sphincter carries with it the risk of faecal incontinence. It may be possible to excise the fistula completely by 'coring' it out but there is a risk of recurrence following this procedure.

ANAL WARTS

In the same way that infective warts occur on the fingers of young adults, so may these troublesome eruptions be implanted in the anal skin, usually by scratching. Occasionally they may develop to a

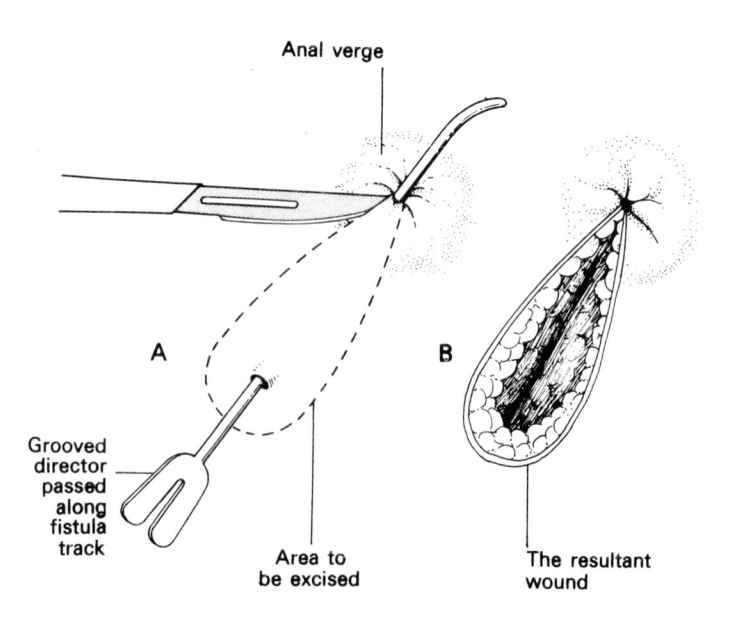

Fig. 12.44. Excision of a fistula in ano.

horrifying degree so that when the anal area is inspected the anus itself is lost beneath an abundant collection of warts (Fig. 12.45). The symptoms are those of anal discomfort, itching and pain on defaecation.

Treatment

Treatment is either by the local application of Podophyllin or by destruction by diathermy coagulation. Considerable care has to be exercised in the use of Podophyllin as it is extremely toxic and if spilt on the surface of the skin, will result in the formation of a blister with actual skin destruction or at the least an area of unpleasant and painful inflammation. The Podophyllin is applied carefully on the tip of an orange stick and the surrounding skin is protected by being smeared with Vaseline. Unless considerable care is exercised it is possible for the buttocks to come into contact with each other and with the treated warts, resulting in a widespread burn of the opposing buttocks.

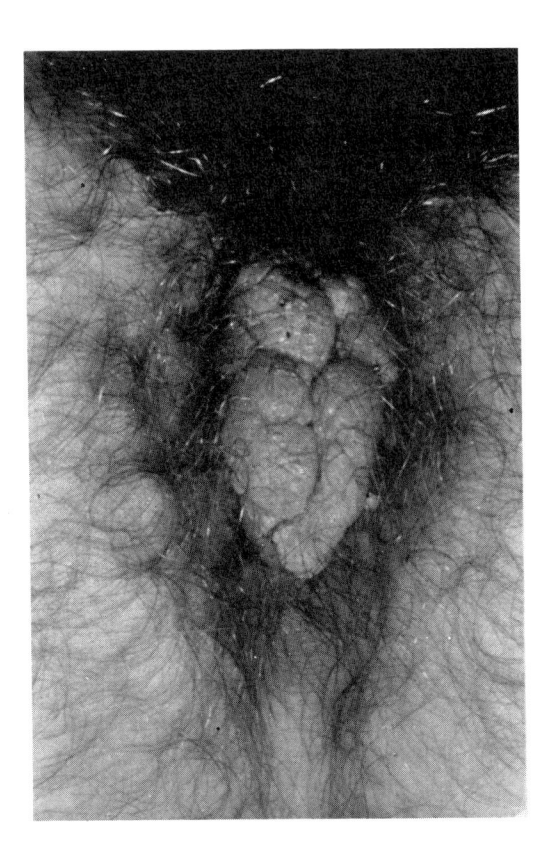

Fig. 12.45. Anal warts.

Coagulation of the warts requires a general anaesthetic, but it is to be preferred to the Podophyllin method when the warts are extensive.

ANAL SKIN TAGS

These small folds of skin at the anal margin are extremely common in both men and women of an older age group. They are presumably due to past episodes of peri-anal haematoma. They have little significance apart from the fact that they have to be distinguished from anal condylomata, which are large waxy skin tags associated with ano-rectal gonorrhoea. Usually anal skin tags require no treatment although some patients demand their excision.

PROLAPSE OF THE RECTUM

In this condition the mucosa of the rectum prolapses through the anal canal. As the condition progresses the anus becomes more dilated, allowing more mucosa and eventually the whole rectal wall to be everted through the sphincter (Fig. 12.46).

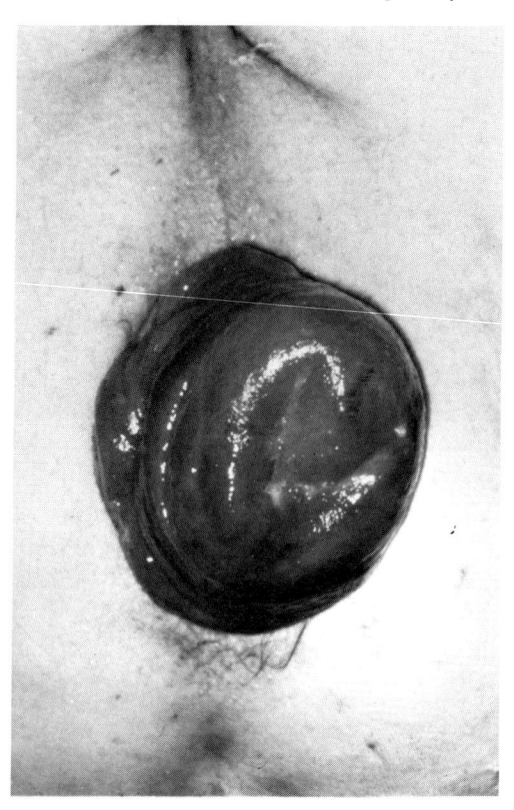

Fig. 12.46. A complete rectal prolapse.

Clinical features

A mucosal prolapse results in a feeling of discomfort, partial loss of continence with the escape of flatus and a persistent peri-anal dampness. As the prolapse becomes more complete, continence is lost and faeces are discharged without the patient realising it. It is possible for several inches or even a foot of the rectum and pelvic colon to protrude from the anus.

This condition is always associated with a lax or non-existent anal sphincter without which the patient is unable to exert any voluntary control. When the examining finger is placed in the anal canal and the patient is asked to contract the anal sphincter, very often no movement occurs. It is a condition which is more common in women than in men. It is also usually associated with an atrophic muscular pelvic floor and a non-existent peri-anal body, (that is the knot of fibro-muscular tissue that exists between the anus and the vagina).

Treatment

Treatment has in the past been unsatisfactory, with the result that a large number of operations have been described. The most satisfactory procedure at the present time is the polyvinyl sponge wrap of the rectum. This is carried out as a lower abdominal operation in which a sheet of polyvinyl sponge is wrapped around the rectum after having been sutured to the front of the sacrum. This procedure is effective because of the fibrous tissue which the plastic material stimulates, so sticking the rectum back into place.

In very old people or in those who are unfit for a major abdominal operation a Thiersch wire or braided nylon suture may be placed beneath the peri-anal skin to restrict the diameter of the anus so that the prolapse cannot occur. This is a useful, but far from ideal, procedure.

CARCINOMA OF THE RECTUM

Pathology

The rectum is the most common site in the large bowel to be affected by carcinoma. Other tumours are also found, such as carcinoid and lymphosarcoma, but these are relatively rare. Carcinoma of the rectum occurs more commonly in men than in women and the peak age incidence is over 55. The tumour is usually an ulcer which is hard to the touch and which has a raised, rolled and everted edge (Fig. 12.47). Occasionally the carcinoma is proliferative and has a heaped-up appearance with a cauliflower-like shape. Another rare variant is a carcinoma that does not produce ulceration of the mucosa

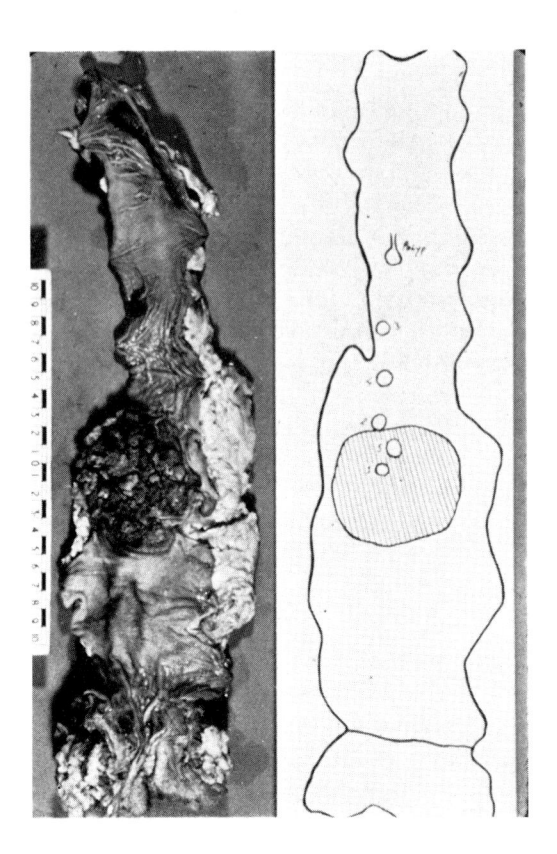

Fig. 12.47. Specimen of carcinoma of the rectum, removed by abdomino-perineal excision.

but infiltrates widely round the rectum, producing a stricture. In these cases diagnosis is very difficult because even quite adequate biopsies, by normal standards, do not reveal the typical carcinoma cells.

Clinical features

Unfortunately, most early carcinomas of the rectum are relatively free of symptoms. The most common method of presentation is by bright red bleeding per rectum. This is noticed on defaecation only and is not associated with pain, but slime may accompany the bleeding as the result of mucous discharge from the surface of the tumour. If stenosis of the rectum occurs there will be an alteration in bowel habit and some patients notice that the calibre of the faeces is altered. Although usually constipation occurs, if a considerable degree of obstruction exists it is sometimes possible for mucus and liquid faeces to leak around the faecal residue, and trickle through the narrow segment of rectum ('spurious diarrhoea'). Finally, as with carcinomas anywhere, presentation may be by the finding of distant metastases producing for example, jaundice, ascites or hepatomegaly.

When a patient presents in the Out Patients Department with a history of rectal bleeding he must be fully examined and this must include rectal examination and sigmoidoscopy. Carcinomas of the rectum are only missed when this examination is omitted. The diagnosis is confirmed when a biopsy of the suspicious area provides the typical microscopic appearance.

Treatment

The treatment of a carcinoma of the rectum depends on the situation and extent of the tumour. If it is more than 11 cm from the anal verge it may be possible to resect the carcinoma and the adjacent rectum, with a clear margin below the tumour and to re-anastomose the pelvic colon to the cut end of the rectum. This operation is termed *anterior resection of the rectum* since it is carried out through the abdomen. After the anastomosis has been finished a proximal colostomy is fashioned to protect it. After the anastomosis has healed, in approximately 10 to 14 days, the colostomy may be closed.

If the carcinoma is below 11 cm from the anal verge the rectum has to be completely excised. This procedure is usually carried out by two surgeons, one working from the perineum and the other from the abdomen and is termed *abdomino-perineal excision of the rectum* (Fig. 12.48). Naturally, when this operation is performed a terminal left iliac colostomy is required as a permanent stoma. At

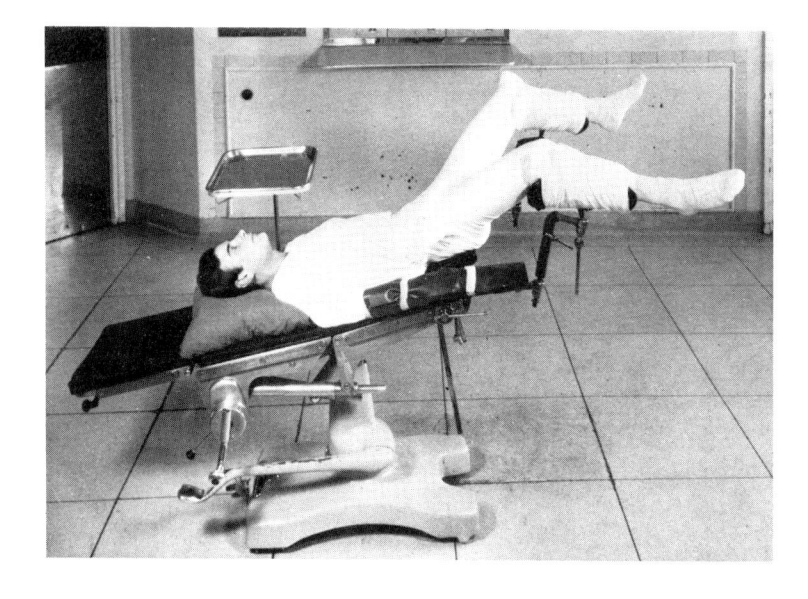

Fig. 12.48. Position of the patient for abdomino-perineal excision of the rectum.

first this may seem a disaster, but it has the virtue of a very high cure rate. More than this, patients who have permanent colostomies quickly learn that they are able to carry on a life that is very close to normal.

Prognosis

Prognosis following these operations depends to a large extent on the staging of the tumour. This has been defined by Duke's classification into four categories (Fig. 12.49). A is a tumour of the mucosa only, B: the tumour involves the full thickness of the rectal wall. C: the tumour involves the pararectal lymph nodes and D: distant metastases. The result of an abdomino-perineal excision of the rectum for a Duke's A carcinoma is 95% five year cure rate. Duke's B is not quite so satisfactory, the cure rate being in the region of 60%. Duke's C is much less satisfactory and the cure rate falls to 25%. It is rare for D cases to have more than an extremely limited prognosis. Most tumours are found to be in the B category.

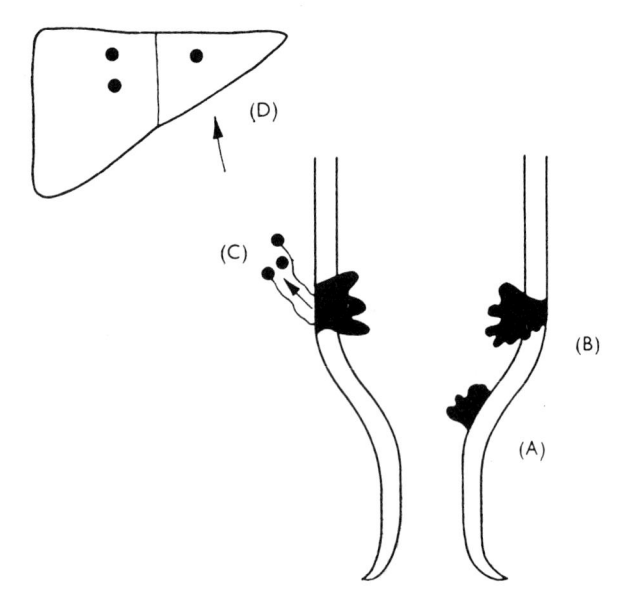

Fig. 12.49. Duke's classification of tumours of the large bowel. (A) confined to bowel wall, (B) penetrating wall, (C) involving regional lymph nodes, (D) distant spread.

Chapter 13. Hernia

General considerations

A hernia is defined as 'a protrusion of a viscus or part of a viscus through its covering into an abnormal situation'. Most hernias occur as an out-pouching of the peritoneal cavity and therefore have a sac of peritoneum. A diagram of a typical hernia is given in Fig. 13.1 and the following parts can be described:

1. *The sac*—this is made up of the walls of the hernia and, in the case of abdominal hernias, it is formed by peritoneum.
2. *The fundus*—the distal extremity of the sac.
3. *The neck*—the orifice in the body wall through which the hernia protrudes.
4. *The contents*—the viscus or viscera contained within the sac.

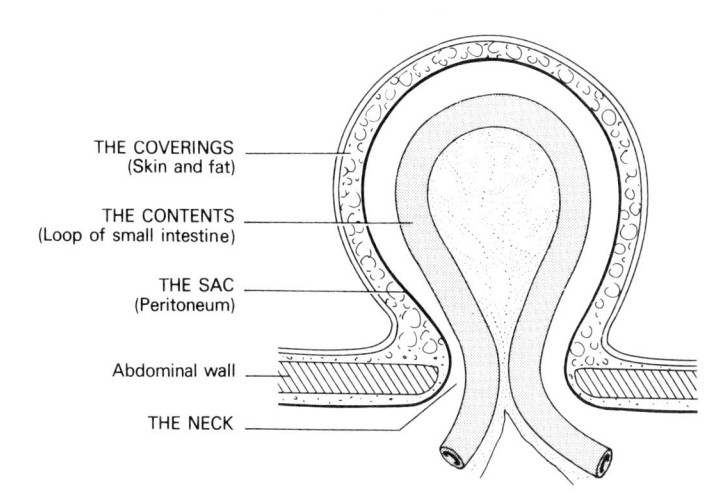

Fig. 13.1. The composition of a typical hernia.

Hernias can occur almost anywhere in the body. For example, after a compound fracture of the skull a portion of the skull vault may be missing; this enables the underlying brain to herniate through the defect in the bone (*cerebral hernia*); or the upper end of the stomach may herniate through an enlarged oesophageal hiatus (*hiatus hernia*). The commonest hernias are those which occur through the abdominal wall and these, in order of frequency, are:
1. Inguinal
2. Incisional
3. Femoral
4. Umbilical
5. Ventral and epigastric

The rest of this chapter will deal only with these abdominal hernias, but mention of other types of hernia will occur elsewhere in this book.

Aetiology of abdominal hernias

Hernias occur at a site of weakness in the abdominal wall. This weakness may be *congenital*, for example, an out-pouching of peritoneum down into the scrotum occurs in the fetus, along which the testicle descends. This processus vaginalis normally obliterates, but it may persist and give rise to a congenital inguinal hernia. Occasionally the umbilicus fails to close completely at birth and this is the aetiology of congenital umbilical hernia. The abdominal wall is also potentially weakened at sites of penetration of structures through it; particularly at the inguinal canal, which allows the spermatic cord to pass obliquely through the lower abdominal muscles into the scrotum, and also at the femoral canal, which is a point of weakness where the femoral vessels emerge into the thigh. The abdominal wall may be weakened following surgical incision, by poor healing either as a result of an infection, haematoma formation or poor operative technique, with subsequent formation of an incisional hernia.

In addition to these primary factors, the formation of a hernia may be aggravated by anything which produces an increase in intra-abdominal pressure—a chronic cough, constipation, pregnancy, urinary obstruction or distension of the abdomen with ascites—or by any factor which weakens the abdominal muscles, for example, gross obesity or muscle wasting in cachexia.

Varieties of abdominal hernias

An abdominal hernia at any site may be:
1. Reducible

2. Irreducible
3. Strangulated

The contents of a *reducible hernia* can be returned completely into the peritoneal cavity, either when the patient lies down, or else by gentle manipulation. A hernia becomes *irreducible* usually because of adhesions of its contents to the inner wall of the sac, or sometimes as a result of adhesions of contents to each other to form a mass greater in size than the neck of the sac. Occasionally inspissated faecal material within the loops of the bowel inside the hernia sac prevents reduction.

When *strangulation* occurs, the contents of the hernia are constricted by the neck of the sac to such a degree that circulation is cut off. In addition there is intestinal obstruction, with distension of the intestine above the site of the strangulation and, worse still, unless the constricting ring is relieved, gangrene of the strangulated contents of the hernia is inevitable. If gut is involved, perforation of the gangrenous loop will eventually occur into the sac. These three varieties of hernia are illustrated in Fig. 13.2.

It is obvious that the narrower the neck of the hernia, the more dangerous it is, since it is more likely to strangulate. A very large hernia with a wide neck is thus much less dangerous to the patient than a much smaller hernia with a narrow orifice (Fig. 13.3). It must be emphasised that the main reason for operating on a patient's hernia is not just to remove an unsightly bulge, but to prevent this risk of strangulation. Fifty years ago, about half the cases of intestinal obstruction in this country were due to strangulated hernias, but now that most patients are sensible enough to report when they notice a hernia and have the lesion repaired electively, the incidence of intestinal obstruction due to this cause is progressively falling. However, among less sophisticated communities, for example in Africa, strangulated hernia remains one of the commonest emergencies and heads the list of causes of intestinal obstruction in these parts of the world.

Clinical features

A *reducible hernia* presents as a lump which may disappear on lying down and which is usually not painful, although it may cause some discomfort.

An *irreducible hernia* is one that cannot be made to disappear but which is painless and gives rise to no other symptoms.

In *strangulated hernia* the patient complains of severe pain and symptoms of intestinal obstruction soon appear—vomiting, distension

Chapter 13

A REDUCIBLE HERNIA

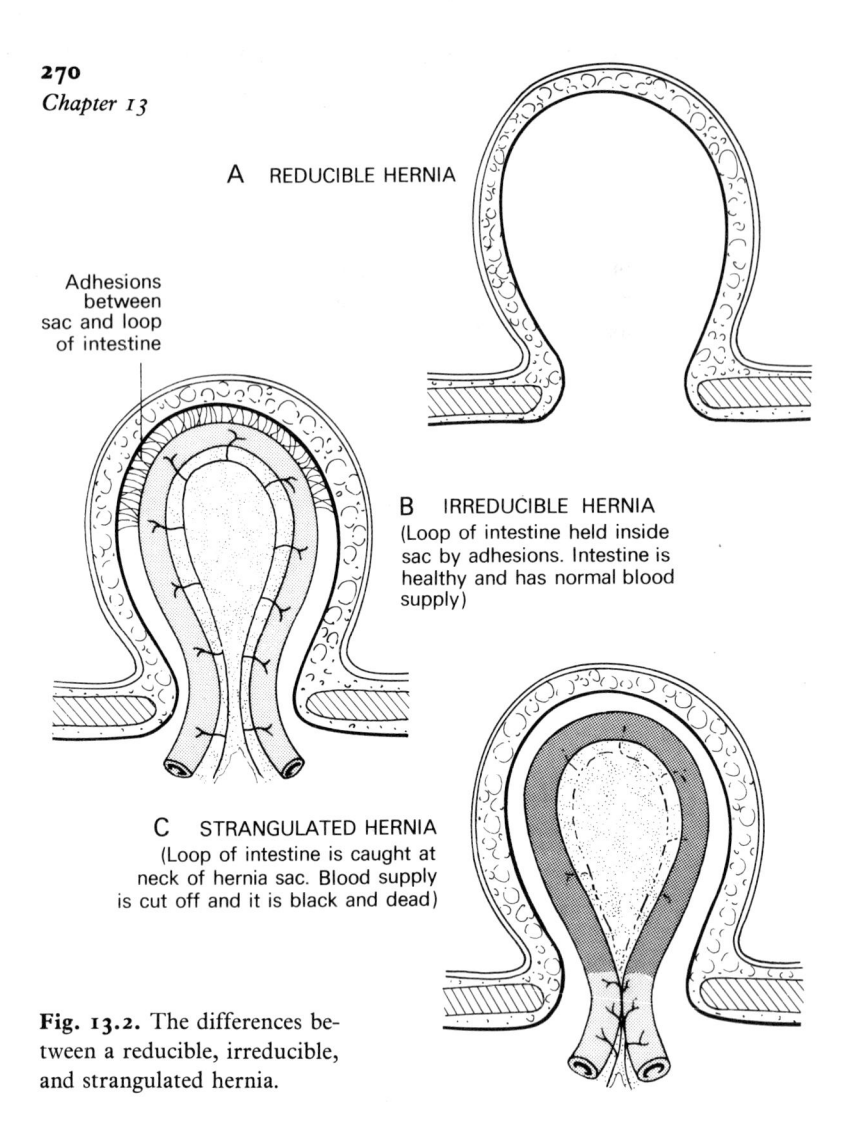

Adhesions between sac and loop of intestine

B IRREDUCIBLE HERNIA
(Loop of intestine held inside sac by adhesions. Intestine is healthy and has normal blood supply)

C STRANGULATED HERNIA
(Loop of intestine is caught at neck of hernia sac. Blood supply is cut off and it is black and dead)

Fig. 13.2. The differences between a reducible, irreducible, and strangulated hernia.

and absolute constipation. Examination will show a tender, tense hernia which cannot be reduced. The overlying skin becomes inflamed and oedematous and there are the signs of intestinal obstruction, with abdominal distension, tenderness and noisy bowel sounds. The features of obstruction are absent and pain is less marked when omentum rather than intestine is contained within the sac.

The three common types of hernia to strangulate are indirect inguinal, femoral and umbilical. Direct inguinal hernia, incisional and ventral hernias do so only rarely.

Hernia

INGUINAL HERNIA

It has been estimated that 5% of the population of Great Britain have an inguinal hernia and that its repair accounts for about 10% of general surgical operations. 60% are right sided, 20% are left sided and 20% bilateral. Inguinal hernia comprises about 80% of all external hernias in the general population and the proportion of male to female is approximately 10 to 1. This is explained quite simply by the fact that the spermatic cord in the male, by its very size, produces a far greater weakness of the inguinal canal than the corresponding narrow round ligament in the female.

Anatomy (Fig. 13.4)

The inguinal canal is the oblique passage, $1\frac{1}{2}''$ long, which is taken through the lower abdominal wall by the testis and spermatic cord in the male and by the round ligament in the female. It lies immediately above the groin and passes downwards and medially from the internal inguinal ring to the external inguinal ring. The internal ring represents the point at which the spermatic cord (or round ligament) pushes through the inner aspect of the anterior abdominal wall and the external ring is the defect in the external oblique fascia through which it emerges.

An inguinal hernia may be classified as *indirect* when it enters the internal inguinal ring, traverse the canal and, if large enough, emerge through the external ring and descend into the scrotum (Fig. 13.5),

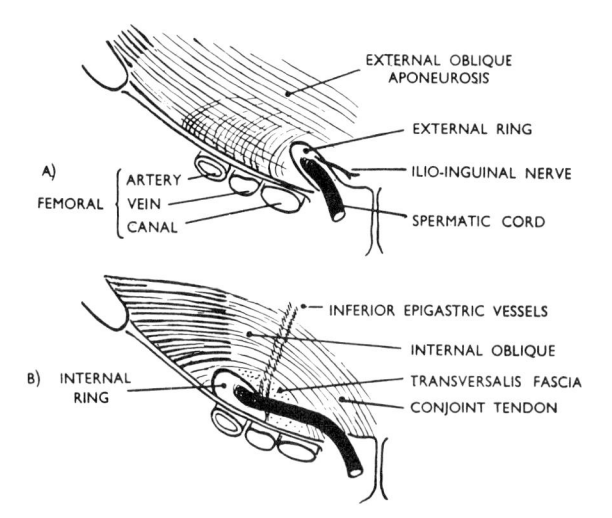

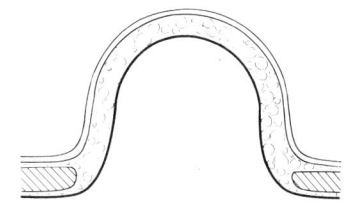

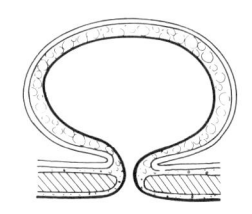

Fig. 13.3. A hernia with a wide neck (A) is at less risk of strangulation than one whose neck is narrow (B).

Fig. 13.4. The anatomy of the inguinal canal. (A) With the surrounding aponeuroses in place. (B) with the aponeurosis of the external oblique removed.

or *direct* when it pushes through the posterior wall of the inguinal canal.

Indirect hernias may be *congenital*, due to the persistence of the *processus vaginalis*, which is the projection of peritoneum along which the testis descends into the scrotum in fetal life. These congenital hernias present at or soon after birth or arise in adolescence. The *acquired* variety may occur at any age in adult life and here the sac is formed by an evagination of the abdominal peritoneum. Some authorities maintain that indirect hernias at all ages represent congenitally formed sacs. The *direct hernia*, in contrast, is always acquired and therefore is usually seen in middle-aged or elderly patients. The difference between an indirect and a direct hernia is not just in the realms of exotic anatomy; a direct hernia has a large orifice and strangulation is consequently rare. In contrast, the internal inguinal ring is frequently narrow, so that the indirect hernia has a distinct tendency to strangulate.

Treatment

The treatment of inguinal hernia in infants and children comprises *herniotomy*, which is simple removal of the peritoneal sac. There is no optimum time for operating on the infant's hernia and surgery should be carried out as soon as possible after diagnosis has been made, since strangulation is not at all uncommon. In adults, surgery is usually advised; this comprises excision of the sac together with repair of the weakened inguinal canal and narrowing of the internal inguinal ring. A large variety of operations are employed, but particularly popular in this country is the nylon darn repair in which monofilament nylon is used to reinforce the posterior wall of the inguinal canal (Fig. 13.6).

A truss should only be prescribed for patients who are in very poor general health but even in such cases a painful hernia which threatens strangulation is much better repaired as an elective procedure, if necessary under a local anaesthetic, rather than as an emergency when strangulation has supervened.

If strangulation occurs, then, of course, emergency surgery is obligatory. A naso-gastric tube is passed, intravenous replacement of fluid and electrolytes commenced and the patient prepared as rapidly as possible for operation. The sac is opened and the constriction (which is usually at the neck of the hernia or at the external ring) is divided. It is now essential to assess the viability of the contents of the sac. If this is solely omentum, this can be excised if there is any doubt at all concerning viability. In the case of stran-

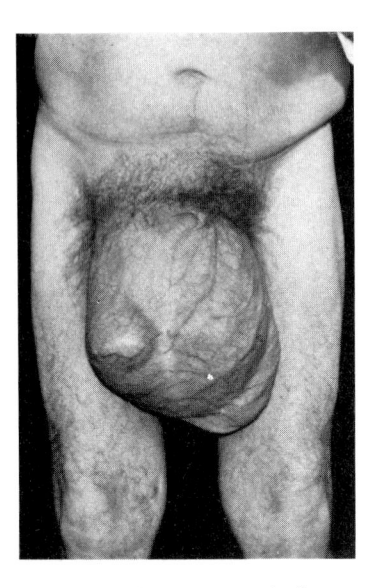

Fig. 13.5. An enormous indirect inguinal hernia which has descended into the scrotum.

Fig. 13.6. Nylon darn repair of an inguinal hernia. The sac is transfixed and excised (A), followed by repair of the posterior wall of the inguinal canal (B). The spermatic cord is retracted by the sling.

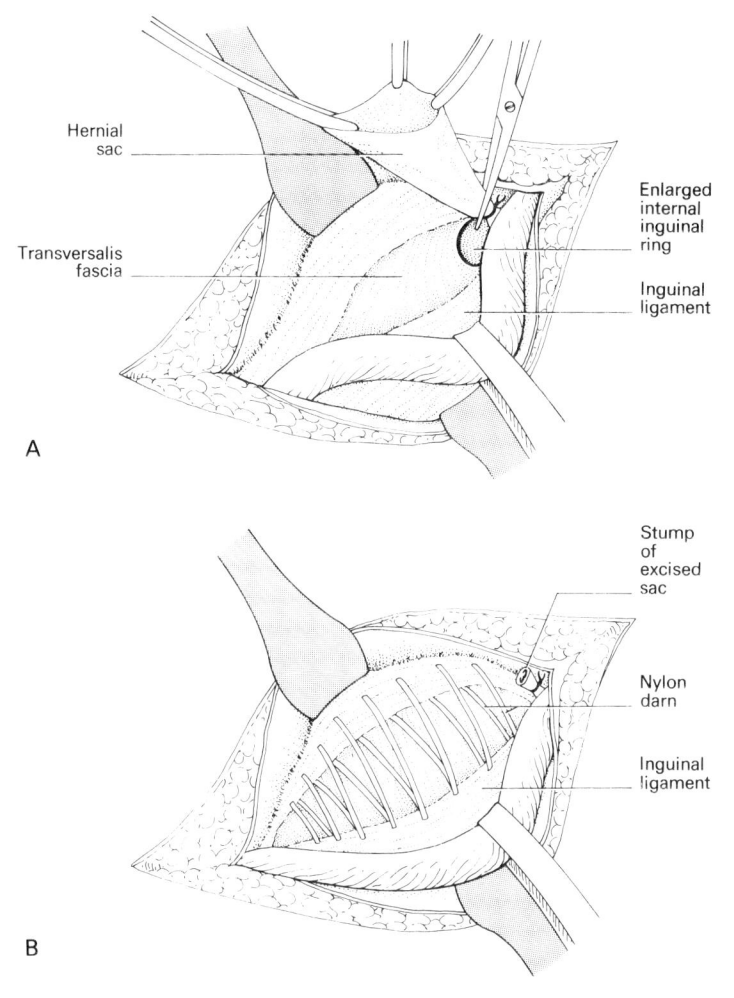

gulated intestine, it is quite easy to identify perfectly healthy gut, which rapidly regains its normal colour, has a glistening covering peritoneum and has normal pulsation in its mesentery. Obviously non-viable intestine is green or black, oedematous, has lost its normal sheen and may be covered with fibrin flakes. The vessels in the mesentery supplying it are pulseless. If there is any doubt, the strangulated loop is wrapped in a warm saline pack and observed again after five or ten minutes. If there is still any doubt at all it is safer to resect the affected loop than to risk returning it into the peritoneal cavity where it may subsequently necrose completely and perforate. The healthy bowel is then reduced, the sac excised and a nylon darn repair is carried out.

FEMORAL HERNIA

Anatomy (Fig. 13.7)

A femoral hernia traverses the femoral canal. This is a gap that just admits the tip of the little finger and which lies at the medial extremity of the fascial tube, termed the femoral sheath, which contains the femoral artery and vein. The canal lies immediately medial to the femoral vein and presumably exists to allow considerable distension of the vein on exercise of the leg. It is filled by a plug of fat and contains a small lymph node. The neck of the canal is narrow and has a particularly sharp rigid medial border; for this reason irreducibility and strangulation are extremely common in hernias at this site.

Clinical features

Femoral hernias occur more commonly in females than in males because of the wider female pelvis which renders the canal larger in women than in men. The hernia is never due to a congenital sac

Fig. 13.7. The anatomy of the femoral canal.

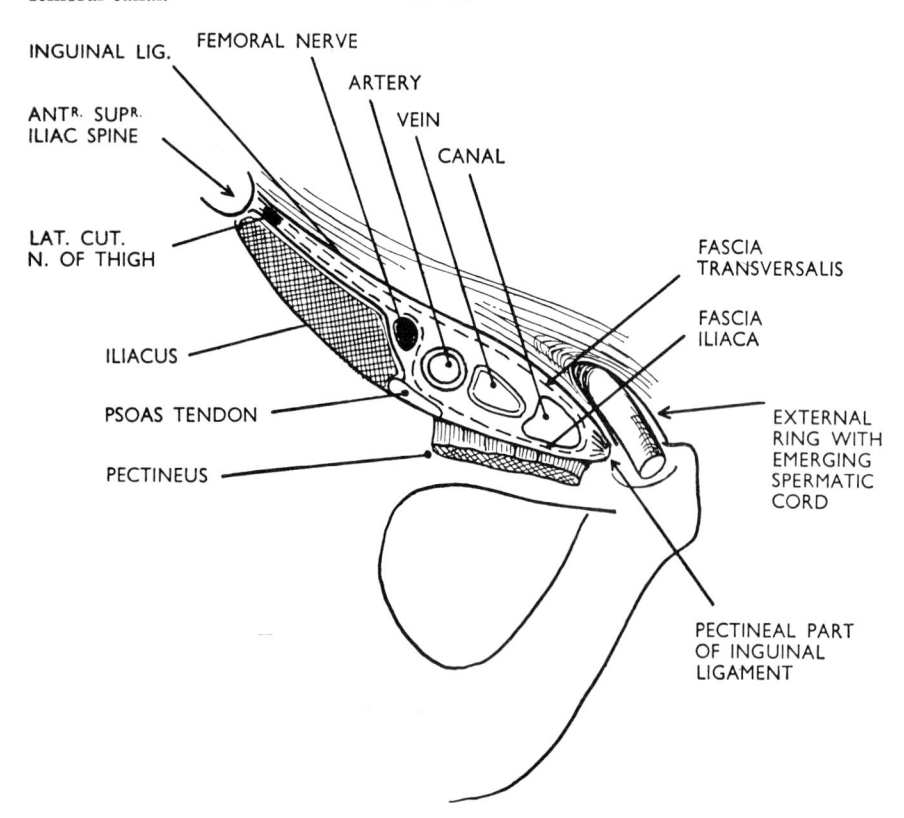

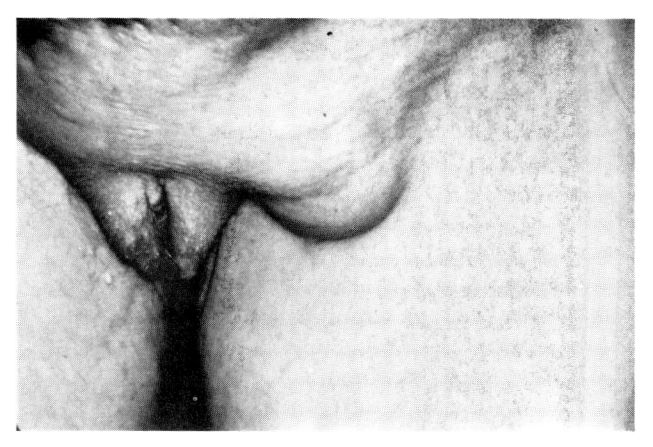

Fig. 13.8. An irreducible left femoral hernia in an elderly female.

but is invariably acquired. Cases rarely occur in children but are usually seen in the middle-aged and elderly (Fig. 13.8). The patient presents because of the lump in the groin. If strangulation occurs, the lump becomes tense and tender, and if bowel is incorporated in the contents of the hernia, features of intestinal obstruction supervene. It is surprising how often an old lady is unaware of the fact that she has a femoral hernia and she may present with intestinal obstruction without having noticed the irreducible lump in the groin; this must always be looked for specifically in such cases.

An interesting variety of strangulated femoral hernia is the *Richter's hernia*; here only a part of the wall of the small intestine is caught up and strangulated by the femoral ring. Because the lumen of the bowel is not completely encroached upon, symptoms of intestinal obstruction do not occur, although the knuckle of bowel may become completely necrotic and even perforate into the hernial sac (Fig. 13.9).

Treatment

All femoral hernias should be repaired because of this great danger of strangulation; the sac is excised and the femoral canal closed by sutures. If the patient presents with a strangulated hernia, treatment is carried out just as described above in the case of strangulated inguinal hernia.

Fig. 13.9. A Richter's hernia. Note that only a part of the wall of the gut is involved.

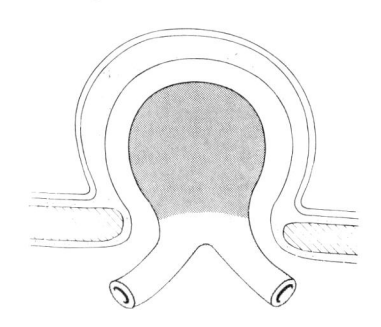

UMBILICAL HERNIA

Congenital umbilical hernia

Normally at birth there is complete closure of the umbilical scar; if this is defective, the baby presents with a reducible bulge at the umbilicus. This is especially common in Negro children. The vast majority close spontaneously during the first year of life, but should the hernia persist after the child is two years old, then surgical repair should be carried out. The parents of a newborn infant with an umbilical hernia should be reassured that most disappear over the next few months without treatment. Strapping the hernia with adhesive is not required and may only give the baby a sensitivity rash, but from time to time it is necessary to carry out this procedure or provide a rubber truss simply to allay parental anxiety.

Exomphalos

This is a rare condition in which the baby is born with the intestine prolapsed through a translucent sac which protrudes through a defective anterior abdominal wall. Untreated this may rupture with fatal peritonitis.

Treatment comprises immediate surgical repair.

Acquired umbilical hernia

This is a common rupture which is found especially in obese multiparous women (Fig. 13.10). It occurs above or just below the umbil-

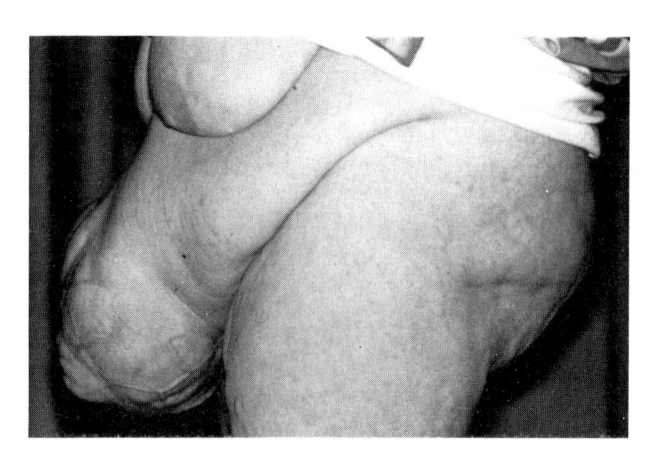

Fig. 13.10. A large umbilical hernia.

icus and is more accurately termed a para-umbilical hernia. The neck is narrow, and, like a femoral hernia, it is particularly liable to become irreducible or strangulated.

Treatment comprises excision of the sac and repair of the defect by overlapping the edges of the rectus sheath (Mayo operation, Fig. 13.11).

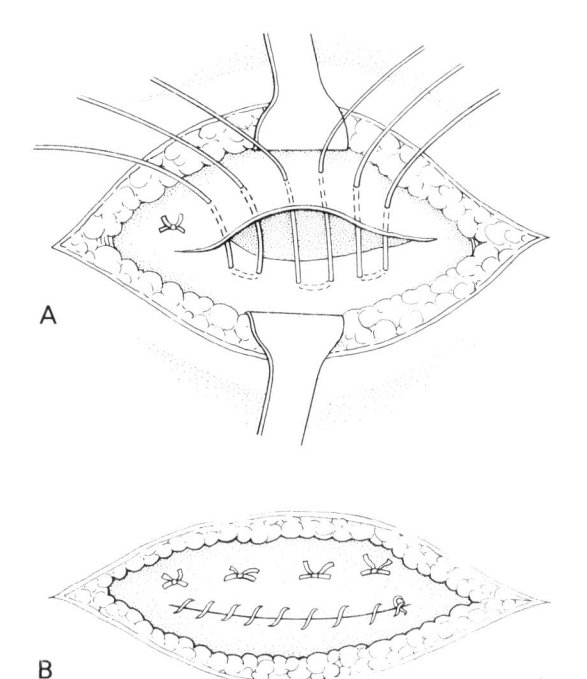

Fig. 13.11. Mayo repair of an umbilical hernia, using interrupted nylon sutures to overlap the rectus sheath.

EPIGASTRIC AND VENTRAL HERNIAS

An epigastric hernia is a small protrusion in the mid line of the upper abdomen which occurs through a defect in the linea alba, the dense fascial septum which passes from the xiphoid to the pubis, and which is especially wide in the upper abdomen.

The defect is small and usually only contains some extra peritoneal fat, but it is often surprisingly uncomfortable. Occasionally

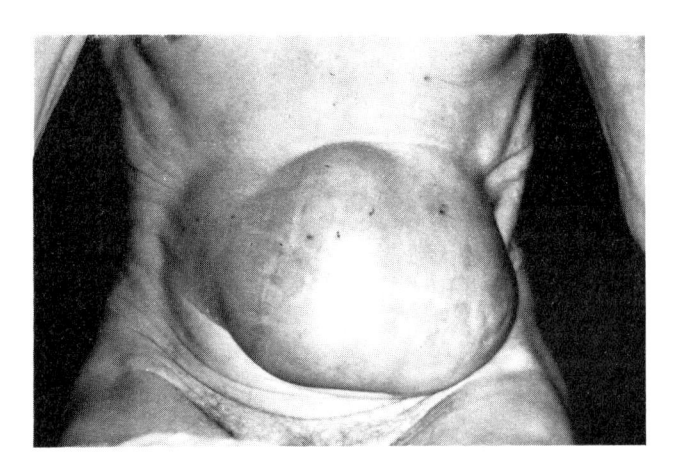

Fig. 13.12. An incisional hernia. Note the transverse scar of a laparotomy performed many years previously.

a long gap occurs in the linea alba, producing a more extensive midline bulge which is termed a *ventral hernia*.

Treatment comprises suture of the defect.

INCISIONAL HERNIA

An incisional hernia occurs through a defect in the scar of a previous abdominal operation (Fig. 13.12). There is usually a wide neck and strangulation is consequently rare.

Treatment. If the general condition of the patient is good, the hernia is repaired by resuturing the layers of the abdominal wall. If operation is considered inadvisable, an abdominal belt is prescribed.

Chapter 14. Liver, gall bladder, spleen and pancreas

ANATOMY OF THE LIVER AND BILIARY TRACT

The liver, which is the largest single organ in the body, is situated in the upper abdomen, closely applied to the under surface of the diaphragm. It is divided into a right and left lobe by its peritoneal attachments and by the structures which enter the porta hepatis. It is enclosed by a capsule (Glisson's capsule) and outside this by peritoneum. It is suspended from the diaphragm by folds of peritoneum known as 'peritoneal ligaments', that which runs anteroposteriorly being termed the *falciform ligament* and at right-angles to this there are left and right triangular ligaments suspending the right and left lobes (Fig. 14.1).

The liver is supplied by blood from two distinct sources. The first of these is the *hepatic artery* derived from the coeliac axis and the second is the *portal vein*, which drains blood from the spleen, the stomach and the small and large intestine. Blood drains from the liver via *hepatic veins*, two or three in number, which are short and wide and pass straight into the inferior vena cava. The bile is drained from the liver by the bile ducts. There is a *left* and *right hepatic duct* draining the respective lobes of the liver which join at the porta hepatis to form the *common hepatic duct*. This passes out of the liver to the right of the hepatic artery and in front of the portal vein and is joined after two to five centimetres by the *cystic duct*. At this point the bile duct is called the *common bile duct* which is naturally divided into three parts. The first of these parts is superior to the duodenum, the second part runs behind the first part of the duodenum and the third part runs behind the head of the pancreas terminating at the

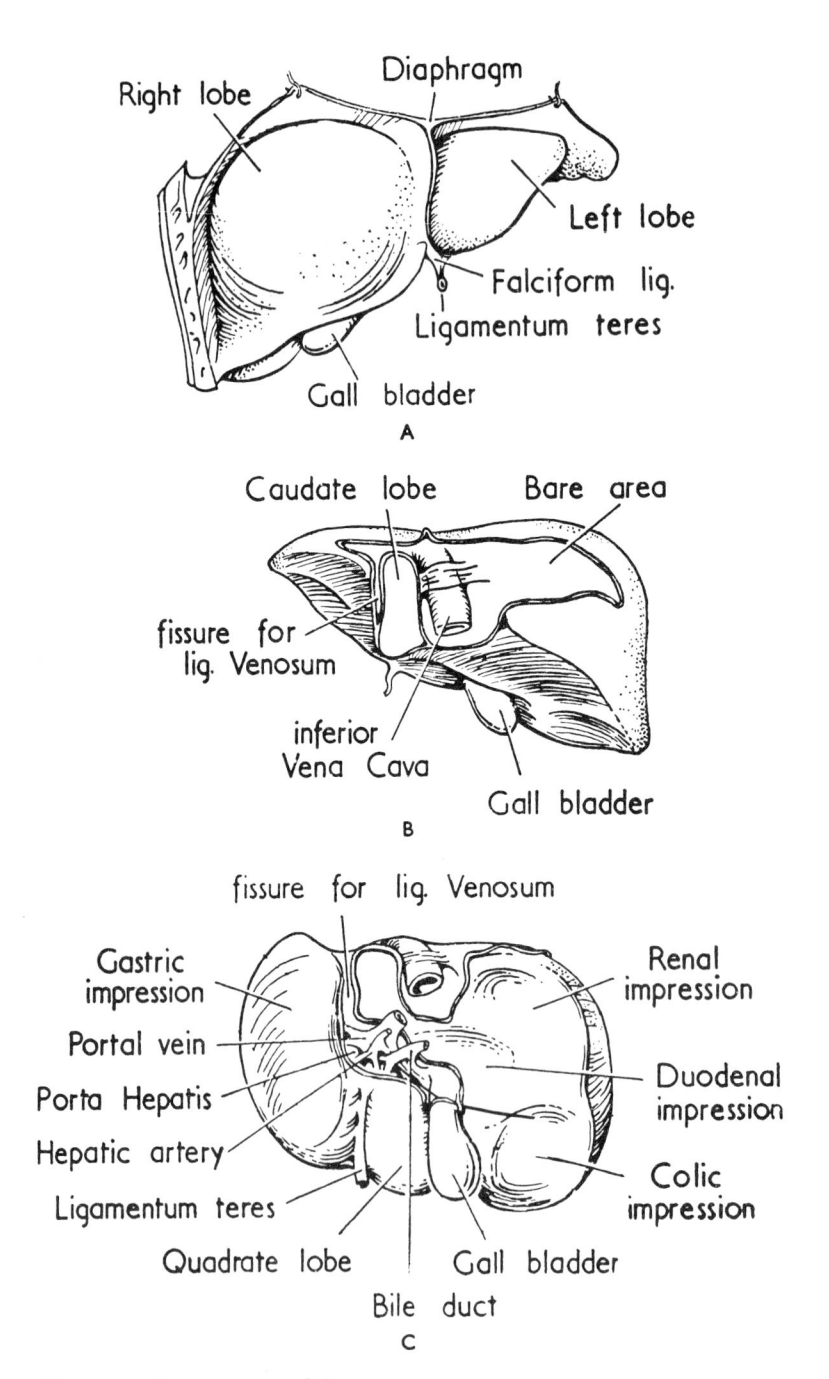

Fig. 14.1. The anatomy of the liver.

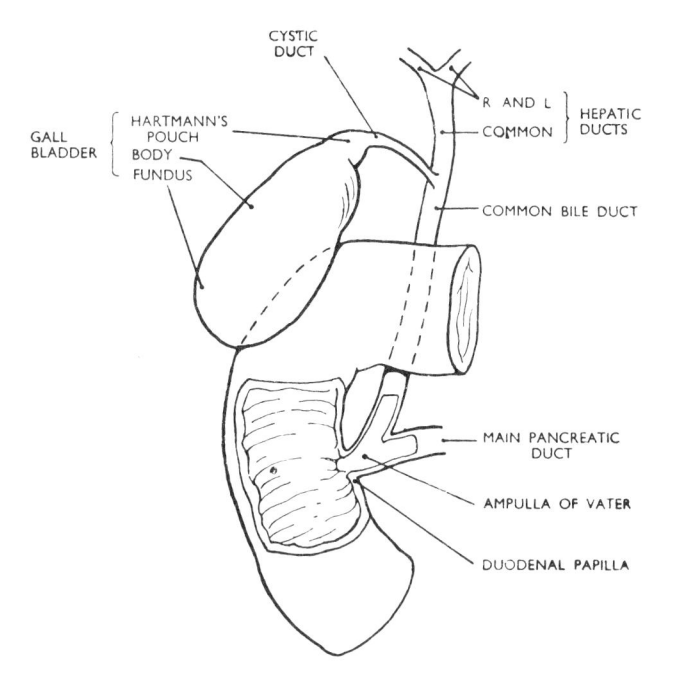

Fig. 14.2. The gall bladder and its duct system.

ampulla of Vater, where the bile duct enters the medial aspect of the second part of the duodenum (Fig. 14.2).

The gall bladder is a thin walled sac which in life appears a bluish colour. Its duct, the cystic duct, joins the common hepatic duct.

The microscopic anatomy of the liver comprises a series of lobules, each having a central vein, which drains ultimately into the hepatic vein. The lobule is surrounded and separated from other lobules by the portal tracts, each of which contains terminal radicles of the hepatic artery and portal vein together with the fine commencing radicles of the bile ducts, the bile canaliculi. Thus blood filters from the hepatic artery and portal vein at the periphery of the hepatic lobule to the central vein through the hepatic capillaries, and the products of hepatic cell metabolism pass to the periphery of the lobule and enter the bile canaliculi. The capillaries along which the blood passes within the lobule are richly supplied with phagocytic cells which are capable of removing particulate matter, such as bacteria, from the blood stream. This arrangement of a dual blood supply ensures first that a ready supply of highly oxygenated blood is available to the hepatic cell which has a high metabolic rate, second that there is an intimate contact between the liver cell and the substances which have just been absorbed from the intestine and which are being carried into the body via the portal blood stream.

Physiology

The liver is responsible for a number of functions:

1. *Secretion of bile*

Bile contains water, inorganic ions (including sodium, bicarbonate, potassium and chloride and calcium) together with cholesterol in a micellar solution, conjugated bile salts, bile pigments from which the characteristic greenish colour derives, certain lipoproteins and enzymes such as alkaline phosphatase.

In addition to this list, some breakdown products of, for example, hormones and drugs must be added.

2. *Storage*

The liver stores a considerable quantity of carbohydrate in the form of glycogen which is available for conversion to glucose should a source of energy be required. In addition, vitamin B_{12} and vitamin K are stored in the liver.

3. *Protein synthesis*

The liver is responsible for the synthesis of albumen and in conditions of impaired liver function the plasma albumen will be reduced. Vitamin K is converted in the liver to prothrombin, one of the factors concerned with the coagulation of blood.

4. *Protein breakdown*

Proteins which have no further function within the body are broken down to urea, which is excreted by the kidney.

5. *Detoxification*

Substances such as the oestrogenic hormones are rendered inactive by being combined (conjugated) with molecules such as taurine and glycine before being excreted.

JAUNDICE

Jaundice occurs when the level of bilirubin in the blood is such that the tissues, particularly the whites of the eyes, look yellow. The normal range of bilirubin is from 0.2 to 0.5 mg/100 ml of blood and in most people yellowness of the sclerae will become evident when the level rises to 2 mg/100 ml of blood. There are three main groups of causes of jaundice:

1. *Pre-hepatic*

This is due to an increased production of bilirubin.

2. *Hepatic*

This type is usually due to damage to the liver cells by infection by toxic substances, by tumours or, in rare cases, it may be due to an hereditary abnormality of enzyme systems within the liver cell.

3. *Post-hepatic*

It is the post-hepatic jaundice with which surgeons are involved because in this case there is obstruction to either the common hepatic or the common bile duct preventing the passage of bile into the intestine. Post-hepatic jaundice can be further subclassified into:

(a) *Obstruction within the lumen of the bile duct*, for example gall stones, the commonest of all causes of post-hepatic or obstructive jaundice or, very rarely, parasites which include ascaris lumbricoides.

(b) *Obstruction due to an abnormality of the wall of the duct*, for example by accidental surgical division, congenital obliteration of the bile duct or carcinoma of the bile duct.

(c) *Compression of the bile duct* or invasion of it from outside, for example by carcinoma of the head of the pancreas, tumours in the lymph nodes in the porta hepatis, or acute and chronic pancreatitis.

It is important that surgeons should be aware of all types of jaundice so that the post-hepatic, obstructive jaundice can be distinguished from the other types of jaundice.

General features of obstructive jaundice

The major and minor bile ducts become dilated and if the liver is examined under the microscope plugs of bile may be seen in the bile canaliculi. Apart from this the architecture of the liver is usually normal, although longstanding obstruction may result in hepatic enlargement and the development of biliary cirrhosis. If infection of the static bile occurs, the process of hepatic cell damage is greatly accelerated; this condition is known as *cholangitis*.

The serum bilirubin rises and may reach extremely high levels. The patient appears yellow, later becoming a deep orange yellow, occasionally with a green tinge as the jaundice progresses. Since bilirubin is bound to protein, the superficial parts of the body with a high protein content appear to be more yellow than other parts and this is the explanation of the obvious yellow colour of the sclerae which persists for some time even after the relief of the obstruction. The urine is dark and contains an excess of bilirubin which will result in a positive reaction when tested with a labstix. If the urine is shaken it will be abnormally frothy. Flowers of sulphur sprinkled on the surface of urine in a jar will sink to the bottom whereas in the normal urine they remain floating on the surface. If the obstruction to the bile duct is complete the faeces are pale and clay-coloured.

One of the characteristic symptoms of obstructive jaundice is severe cutaneous itching (*pruritus*) and patients with this condition commonly have scratch marks over the legs, arms and abdomen.

Examination of the patient, apart from the obvious icterus, may reveal a palpable gall bladder. The Law of Courvoisier states that 'in the jaundiced patient, a palpable gall bladder indicates that jaundice is not due to stone.' The reason for this law is that if gall stones are present in the gall bladder, the wall of the gall bladder will become so thickened that it cannot dilate (Fig. 14.3). In practice in this country the most common cause of obstructive jaundice with a palpable gall bladder is a carcinoma of the pancreas.

By consideration of the history, the clinical state of the patient on examination and the biochemistry, it is usually possible to decide whether the patient is suffering from pre, or post-hepatic jaundice. Cholestatic jaundice does however cause some confusion. This is an hepatic-type of jaundice with an equivocal biochemical picture suggestive of post-hepatic jaundice. It is due to certain drugs which include methyl-testosterone, chlorpromazine, trifluoroperazine, thiouracil and chlorpropramide. The important point to make is

Fig. 14.3. Courvoiser's law. Obstructive jaundice due to a stone is usually associated with a small contracted gall bladder (A). Therefore 'in the presence of jaundice a palpable gall bladder indicates that the obstruction is probably due to some other cause—the commonest being carcinoma of the pancreas' (B). Exceptions are a palpable gall bladder produced by one stone impacted in the neck of the gall bladder resulting in a mucocele of the gall bladder and another in the common duct causing obstruction (C), which is very rare, or much more commonly, the gall bladder is distended when explored at operation but is clinically impalpable (D).

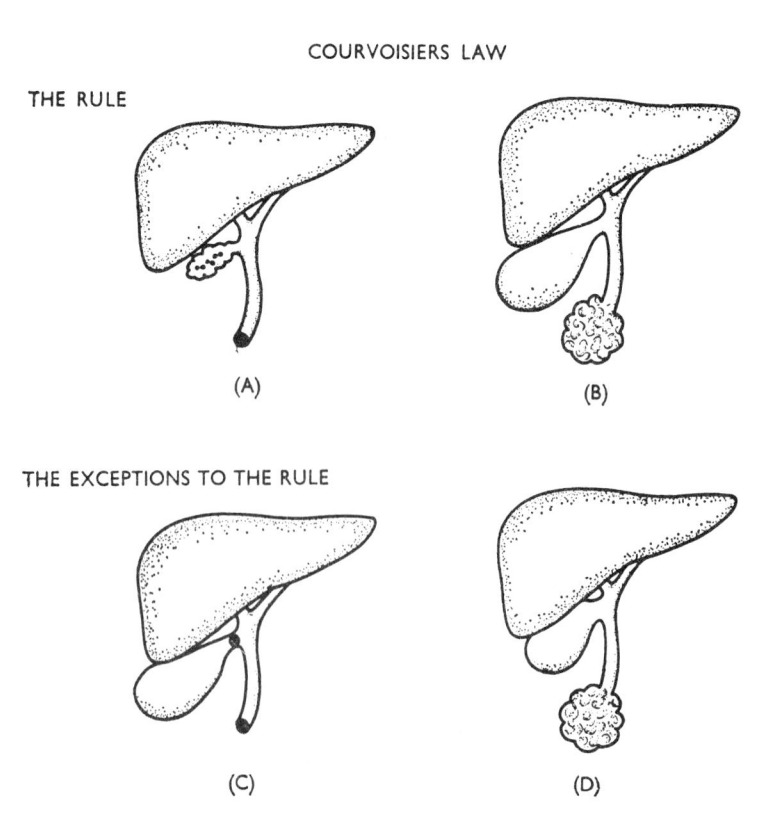

COURVOISIERS LAW

THE RULE

(A)   (B)

THE EXCEPTIONS TO THE RULE

(C)   (D)

that in any jaundiced patient, a full history of previous drug ingestion must be obtained.

Occasionally it is imperative to know exactly the level of obstruction in a jaundiced patient, when cholecystography (either oral or intravenous) is not possible, in which case *percutaneous transhepatic cholangiography* may be employed. A needle is inserted into the liver substance through the skin under local anaesthetic. The needle is gradually withdrawn until the tip slides back into one of the dilated intra-hepatic bile ducts and this is recognised by the ability to withdraw bile from the needle. X-ray contrast medium (25% Hypaque) is now injected and X-rays are taken. This is an investigation which is attended by some complications (especially haemorrhage) and should only be carried out just prior to operation (Fig. 14.4).

Surgery in jaundice

In all cases of post-hepatic jaundice the obstructing agent must be removed or the patient will ultimately die of liver failure. The patient is admitted to hospital and the depth of the jaundice is measured from day to day. If the jaundice is lessening, the patient is treated conservatively until the bilirubin has fallen to normal levels when the obstructing agent can be removed electively. If the bilirubin rises, surgical intervention will be required to prevent liver damage.

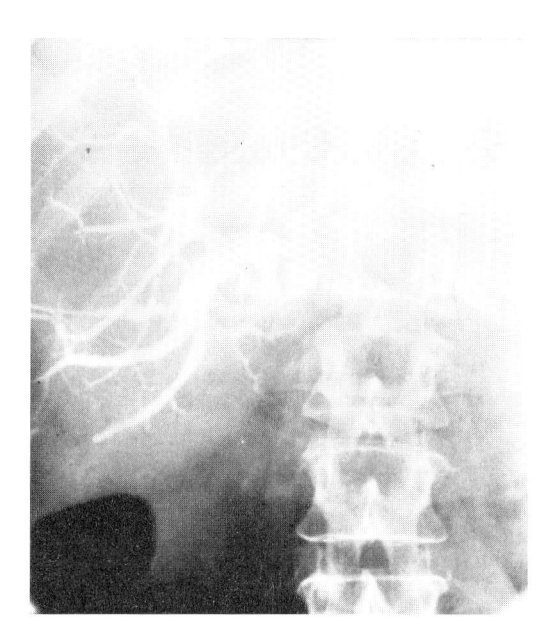

Fig. 14.4. Percutaneous transhepatic cholangiogram is obstructive jaundice. The patient has a complete stricture of the common hepatic duct due to injury at a previous cholecystectomy. Note the grossly dilated biliary radicles.

Careful pre-operative preparation is essential. As has been mentioned previously, these patients do not absorb fat and therefore they do not absorb fat soluble vitamins. One of these is vitamin K and failure to absorb it will ultimately result in lowered plasma prothrombin levels with the result that the patient has a blood coagulation defect. This is readily corrected by giving injections of vitamin K (for example Konakion) 10 mg intramuscularly per day. Before surgery is embarked upon, the prothrombin level must be checked and found to be normal. Another problem that exists in these patients is the sensitivity of the kidney to reduced blood flow. Whereas in a normal patient the kidney is quite able to function in spite of considerable operative trauma, the kidneys of a patient with obstructive jaundice are affected by shortlived and mild episodes of hypotension which result in renal tubular necrosis, the so-called hepato–renal syndrome. To protect the patient against this complication it is necessary to ensure that an active diuresis is occurring before, during and for 48 hours after the operation. To this end the patient is catheterised and an intravenous infusion of 10% mannitol is started. Mannitol is a sugar which is excreted unchanged in the urine and therefore carries water with it by virtue of its osmotic pressure. If the kidneys have already failed, however, it will act as a plasma expander and if too much is infused the patient will go into congestive cardiac failure. For this reason a preliminary test dose of 100 ml is infused on the night prior to operation and the urinary output is checked and should rise in the hour after the infusion to a level of 1 ml per minute. Providing this condition is fulfilled, the 10% mannitol infusion is commenced an hour prior to the operation at the rate of one litre per 24 hours and is continued throughout the operation and for 48 hours post-operatively.

The extra-hepatic biliary apparatus can be approached either through an upper right paramedian incision or a right subcostal (Kocher) incision (Fig. 14.5). The surgery from this point depends upon the precise cause of the obstructive jaundice. In general terms

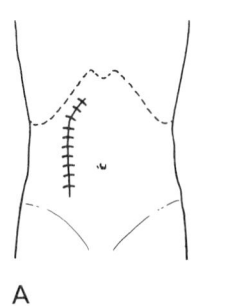

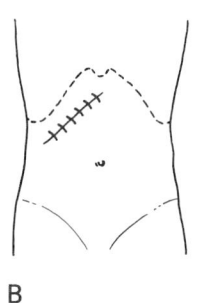

Fig. 14.5. The incision used in biliary surgery (A) upper right paramedian, (B) right subcostal Kocher incision.

the obstruction may either be removed, as is the case with gall stones which are extracted through an incision made in the dilated common bile duct, or the obstruction may be by-passed when, for example it is due to advanced irremovable carcinoma of the head of the pancreas. In this latter case by-pass may be achieved by anastomosing the gall bladder to a loop of jejunum (Fig. 14.6).

Whenever the common bile duct is opened, a T-tube is inserted into it at the end of the procedure. The reason for this is that oedema at the site of the operation may result in a temporary block to the passage of bile from the liver to the intestine. A T-tube within the common bile duct allows free drainage to the exterior and thereby prevents leakage through the sutures in the duct into the peritoneal cavity. It should be remembered that the bile is normally sterile and that the connection between the T-tube and the bile-collecting apparatus should not be broken except under sterile conditions. Also it is a good general rule that if a foreign body is left in the patient, some form of chemotherapeutic cover should be used; we use ampicillin, at first intravenously and then orally, until the T-tube is removed. Since it is undesirable for large quantities of bile to be lost from the patient the T-tube is clamped for progressively longer periods starting on the fifth post-operative day. This not only ensures that bile has to pass into the intestine, but also serves as a test of patency of the bile duct. On the fifth post-operative day the tube is clamped for one hour and providing there is no abdominal pain, the next day it is clamped on two occasions for two hours. Again, as long as there is no reaction on the seventh it is

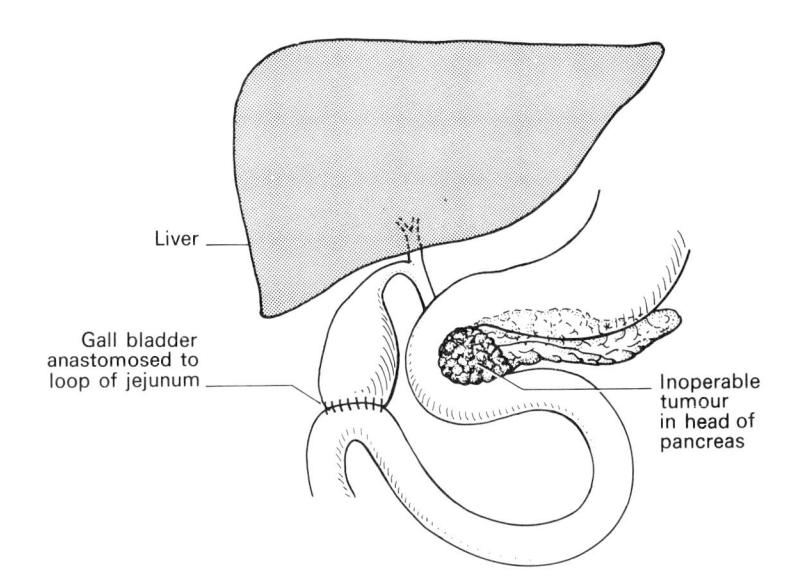

Fig. 14.6. Cholecyst-jejunostomy to by-pass an inoperable carcinoma of the pancreas which is producing obstructive jaundice.

clamped on three occasions for three hours and on subsequent days it is permanently clamped. On approximately the tenth day the patency of the bile duct is checked by means of cholangiography. Radio-opaque dye is injected down the T-tube and X-rays are taken of the abdomen at the same time (Fig. 14.7). Providing there is no residual obstruction to the common bile duct, the T-tube, which is made of soft latex rubber, can be removed by simple traction. The small puncture wound in the abdominal wall will leak bile from between a half and one and a half hours only. In addition to the drainage of the common bile duct, a corrugated plastic drain is inserted to the region of the operation via a stab incision well to the lateral side of the main operative incision. Providing only small quantities of bile and haemoserous fluid are draining, this drain is shortened on the second post-operative day and removed on the third post-operative day.

ENLARGEMENTS OF THE LIVER

The main groups of causes of enlargement of the liver are:
(a) Polycystic disease, a rare congenital condition.
(b) Inflammatory—infective hepatitis, homologous serum hepatitis, leptospirosis and actinomycosis.

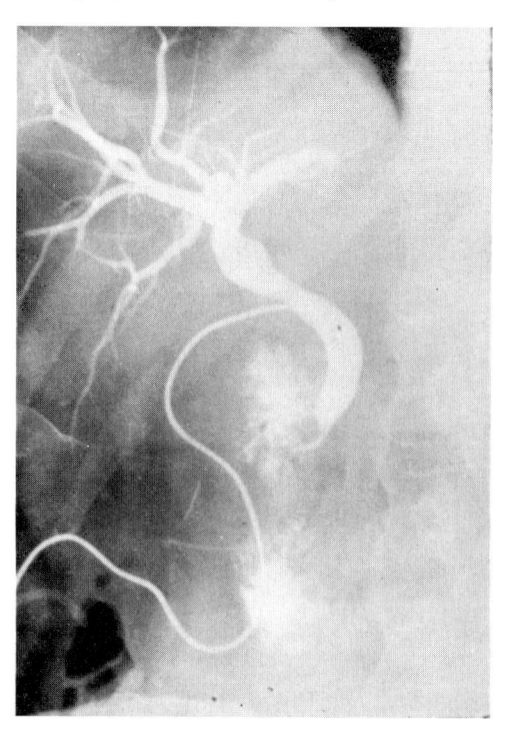

Fig. 14.7. A normal T-tube cholangiogram. The bile ducts are of normal size, no stones are visualised and the dye is seen to enter the duodenum.

(c) *Parasites*—amoebic hepatitis and hydatid disease.
(d) *Neoplasm*—primary carcinoma of the liver and secondary carcinoma.
(e) *Cirrhosis*—portal, biliary, cardiac and haemochromatosis.
(f) *The reticuloses*—Hodgkin's disease, lymphosarcoma and leukaemia.
(g) *Blood diseases*—polycythaemia.
(h) *Metabolic*—amyloid, glycogen storage disease.

TRAUMA TO THE LIVER

Bleeding from this source may be massive and complicate the picture in multiple injuries if the patient is shocked and the peritoneal cavity contains blood.

If an isolated part of the liver is damaged, for example the left lobe, the most effective method of treatment is to remove it. If there are, however, general lacerations this will not be possible and haemorrhage will be controlled either by packing or by large gently placed sutures holding the fragile tissues loosely together. Partial hepatectomy is occasionally necessary where trauma is extensive.

CIRRHOSIS

Aetiology

This condition is characterised by a progressive infiltration of the liver by fibrous tissue with destruction of hepatic cells. There are a number of causes which include:
(a) *Portal*—this occurs in alcoholics, as a result of nutritional deficiency particularly protein deficiency, and following severe hepatitis. However it frequently may occur in the absence of any of these conditions and be idiopathic.
(b) *Biliary*—due to longstanding and unrelieved extra-hepatic bile duct obstruction or primary, of unknown cause, found in women between the ages of 40 and 50 (Hanot's cirrhosis).
(c) *Cardiac*—due to congestive cardiac failure.
(d) Cirrhosis may also occur in *haemochromatosis* due to the deposition of iron.

Clinical features

As the condition progresses from whatever cause more and more hepatic cells are destroyed. Eventually this will lead to hepatic failure. The time span from the commencement to the hepatic failure is usually of the order of several years and other effects of the condition therefore become obvious before death from liver failure occurs. One of these effects is an increase of the pressure of the blood in the portal vein—*portal hypertension*. There is also an increased incidence of chronic duodenal ulcer.

Apart from acute haemorrhage, the clinical picture of a patient with cirrhosis is one of steadily deteriorating liver function and on examination the liver is often palpable together with the spleen which also becomes enlarged. The skin of these patients occasionally contains large deposits of melanin which gives them an overall brown appearance. Also in the skin may be seen small angiomas—spider naevi—generally on the upper trunk, arms and face. If there is considerable loss of hepatic function an erythema of the thenar and hypothenar eminences may be seen. This is known as 'liver palm.'

If a patient is in incipient liver failure, the most common symptom is a loss of cerebral function with disorientation and inability to perform fine movements of the hands.

Portal hypertension

The pressure of the blood in the portal vein in a normal person is between 5 and 10 cm of water, this may rise to as high as 30 cm of water in patients with cirrhosis. The reason for the increased pressure is an intra-hepatic block to the flow of blood from the portal vein to the inferior vena cava. The reduced blood flow has two main effects, the first of which is an accelerated rate of damage to the liver and the second is the development of a collateral venous circulation. There are several potential sites at which portal blood can drain into the systemic veins. These are around the oesophagus and stomach, along the normally obliterated umbilical vein, in the region of the rectal venous plexus, and from veins associated with the ascending and descending colon. These collateral veins become greatly dilated and engorged with blood and those in the region of the oesophagus bulge into the lumen of the oesophagus, resulting in *oesophageal varices*. Bleeding from oesophageal varices is one of the causes of haematemesis and a not infrequent cause of death in these patients.

Treatment

1. *Conservative*

When a patient presents with bleeding from oesophageal varices, emergency treatment consists of blood replacement and, if necessary, the passing of a Sengstaken tube (Fig. 14.8) which has an arrangement of two balloons so that one balloon retains the tube in the

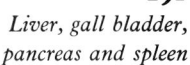

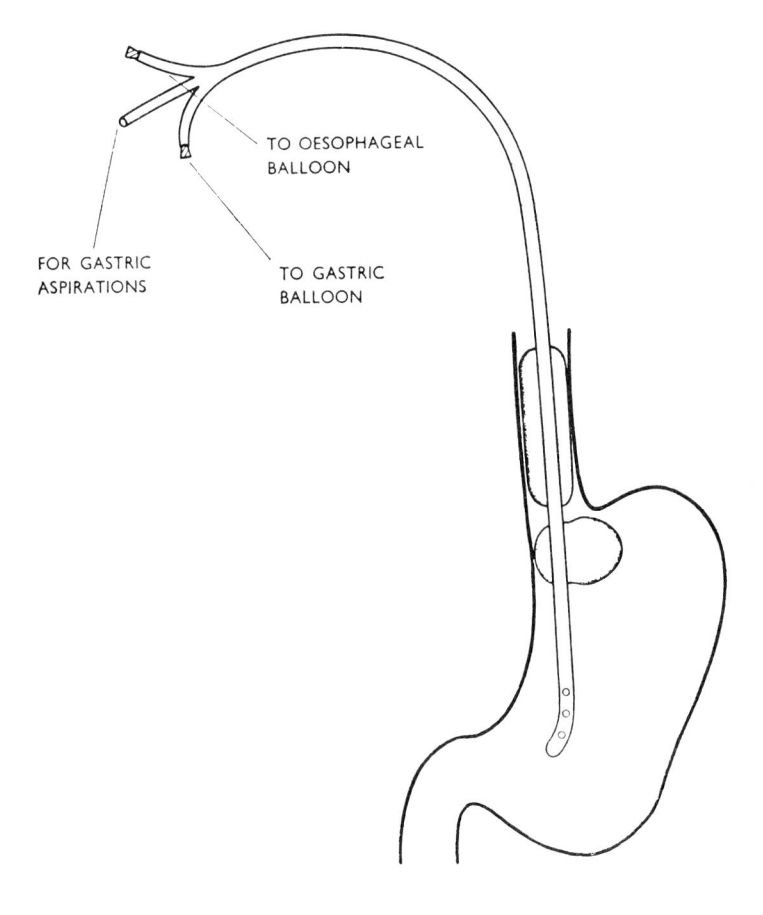

Fig. 14.8. The Sengstaken tube. Balloons in the oesophagus and in the cardia of the stomach compress the bleeding varices. The gastric tube can be used either for aspirating the stomach or for feeding purposes.

stomach while a second balloon presses against the oesophageal varices in the oesophagus and so occludes them. The lumen of the tube protrudes into the stomach and thus allows evacuation of any clot or secretion. Unfortunately, the tube can only be left in place for approximately 24 hours, otherwise oesophageal damage will occur. Other methods of treatment include giving intravenous Vasopressin which reduces the flow of blood into the splanchnic circulation.

In a patient with even a minor degree of liver failure an acute haemorrhage will tend to worsen the condition because blood, when it is passed into the bowel, will be digested and the products of digestion overload the liver's ability to deal with them. In this case the method of treatment is to evacuate the large bowel, where the incompletely digested products of the blood are fermenting, by means of an enema and to administer an oral non-absorbed antibiotic such as neomycin 1g 6 hourly.

2. Surgical

Emergency operations sometimes have to be carried out on these patients and the procedures which are required are either an oesophageal transection, in which the bleeding veins are ligated via a thoracotomy, or a high gastric transection which achieves the same object. Both these operations are attended by a significant mortality (10%) and morbidity and further, the results tend not to be permanent. The most permanent operative procedure, although one which is difficult and dangerous to perform when the patient is actually bleeding or soon after a major haemorrhage, is the diversion of portal blood to the systemic circulation, for example by means of a porto-caval anastomosis. In this procedure the side of the portal vein is joined to the side of the inferior vena cava in the region of the foramen of Winslow (Fig. 14.9).

GALL STONES

Initially at least gall stones form in the gall bladder. There are three main types (Fig. 14.10):
1. Cholesterol stones.
2. Pigment stones.
3. Mixed cholesterol, pigment and calcium phosphate stones.

Methods of formation

Cholesterol, which is a lipid, is excreted in the bile. Bile is an aqueous solution and in the normal person there exists a physico-chemical mechanism whereby the cholesterol is dissolved by means of Nature's detergents—the bile salts, together with phospho-lipids. If anything

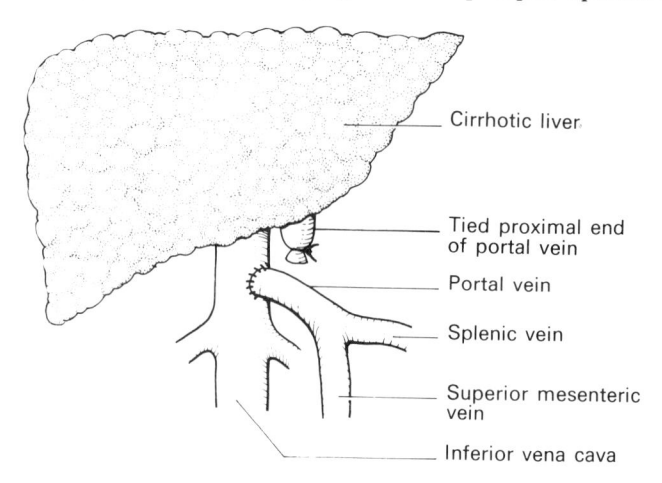

Fig. 14.9. An end-to-side porto-caval anastomosis between the portal vein and the side of the inferior vena cava. This decompresses the high pressure within the portal system.

MIXED

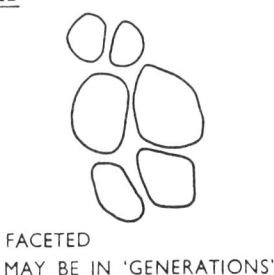

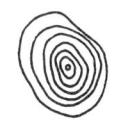

FACETED
MAY BE IN 'GENERATIONS'

CUT SURFACE—
CONCENTRIC RINGS

CHOLESTEROL

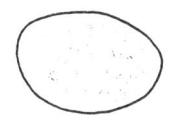

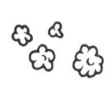

'SOLITAIRE'
OR CLUSTERS OF 'MULBERRIES'

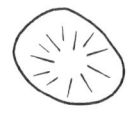

CUT SURFACE—
RADIATING CRYSTALS

PIGMENT

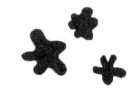

MULTIPLE, SMALL,
BLACK AND BRITTLE

CUT SURFACE —
AMORPHOUS

Fig. 14.10. The varieties of gall stones.

Liver, gall bladder, pancreas and spleen

occurs to disturb the normal relationship between these three substances, cholesterol is deposited in a crystalline form. The gall bladder is responsible for concentrating the bile by absorbing water and it is therefore in this situation that the cholesterol concentration rises and precipitation of crystals is most likely to occur. Once crystals of cholesterol have been deposited more cholesterol attaches to the nucleus and a cholesterol stone is formed.

Once the gall bladder comes to contain cholesterol stones there is the ever present risk of infection occurring within it. If the bile in the gall bladder does become infected, calcium and phosphate is deposited on the surface of the cholesterol stone together with bile pigments, and a mixed stone results.

In conditions in which there is an increased production of bilirubin, for example, any of the haemolytic jaundices such as hereditary spherocytosis (acholuric jaundice) the concentration of the pigment in the bile rises and pigment stones are formed in much the same way as are cholesterol stones.

Clinical features

Gall stones may be present within the gall bladder and cause no symptoms whatsoever.

If symptoms are experienced whilst the stones are in the gall bladder and in the absence of infection, these are usually described as being 'flatulent dyspepsia'. Pain may be experienced almost anywhere in the abdomen, but is commonly in the right hypochondrium and it may radiate through to the back at the lower pole of the right shoulder blade. The abdominal discomfort is generally aggravated by eating, particularly fatty food.

Cholecystitis

If the contents of the gall bladder become infected, the condition of cholecystitis will occur. In this the patient experiences severe pain in the right hypochondrium associated with a tachycardia and fever. There is often a preceding history of flatulent dyspepsia and fat intolerance. There may be associated vomiting, anorexia and malaise. There is commonly a family history of gall stones.

When the patient is examined a well localised area of tenderness is found at the point where the lateral edge of the rectus muscle passes over the right costal margin. If this region is palpated as the patient breathes in, pain is experienced as the inflamed gall bladder moves down and touches the examining hand. This is Murphy's sign of acute cholecystitis.

Gall stone ileus

One rare complication of gall stones is the development of a fistula between the gall bladder and the duodenum. This most commonly occurs when there is a large 'solitaire' stone in the gall bladder which ulcerates through its wall. Occasionally very large stones find their way into the duodenum by this route, and are too big to pass through the ileocaecal valve, resulting in the condition known as gall stone ileus, which is in reality an obstruction of the small bowel.

Carcinoma of the gall bladder

A further unusual complication of gall stones is the development of a carcinoma of the gall bladder. This is a rare tumour but when it occurs it is universally fatal except when the gall bladder is removed by good fortune with an extremely early carcinoma within it.

Pancreatitis

About 30% of patients with this condition have associated gall stones.

Special investigations

Plain X-ray of the abdomen will not reveal the presence of cholesterol stones as cholesterol is radiolucent. Similarly pigment stones will not be shown by plain X-ray. Mixed stones, however, have a characteristic 'ring shadow' appearance (Fig. 14.11).

The mainstay of diagnosis is the cholecystogram in which the patient swallows tablets which contain an iodine compound which is excreted in the bile. Providing the patient is not jaundiced the dye passes with the bile into the gall bladder where it is concentrated and when X-rays are taken an outline of the gall bladder will be seen (Fig. 14.12). In approximately 40% of these investigations it is also possible to see the outline of the major extra-hepatic ducts as well. Stones may be seen within the gall bladder or bile ducts as filling

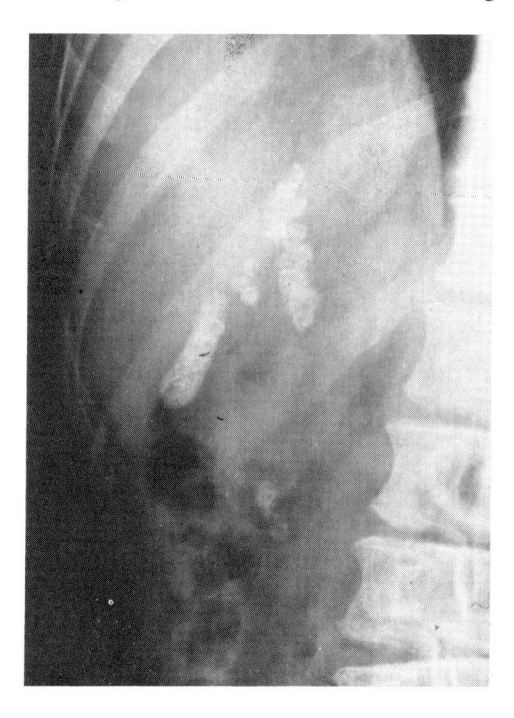

Fig. 14.11. Plain X-ray of the abdomen of a deeply jaundiced patient demonstrating multiple gall stones in the gall bladder and common bile duct.

Fig. 14.12. Normal cholecystogram (A) before (B) after a fatty meal. The fat has made the gall bladder contract, thus emptying its contents into the duodenum.

Fig. 14.13. Cholecystogram demonstrating multiple stones within the gall bladder. These appear as filling defects outlined by the radio-opaque dye within the gall bladder.

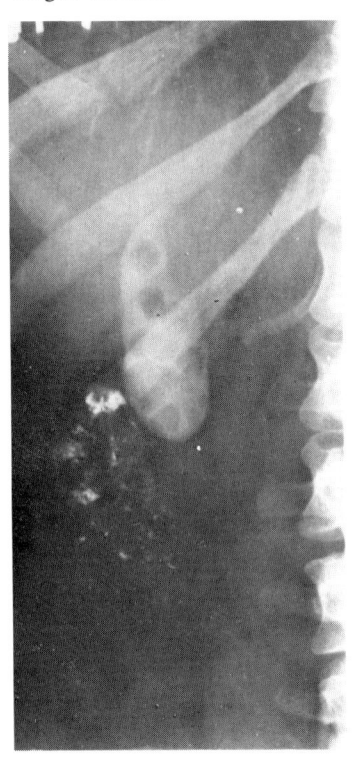

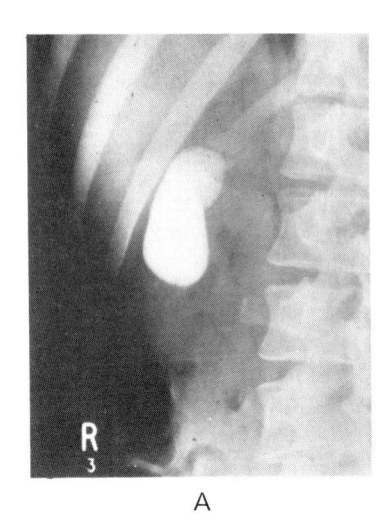

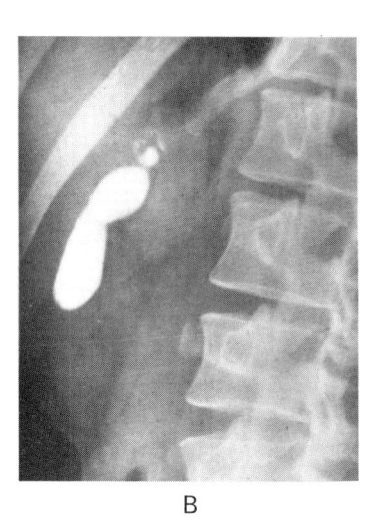

defects (Fig. 14.13) and the diameter of the bile duct can often be judged. If significant obstruction has occurred, the common bile duct will be wider than the upper limit of normal which is 10 millimetres. Once the gall bladder has been visualised it is possible to give the patient a meal containing fat when a normal gall bladder will contract. If the contrast within the gall bladder is of inadequate concernation, an intravenous cholangiogram can be carried out in which a large quantity of dye is injected intravenously. This should not be done in the jaundiced patient as renal and more hepatic damage may result.

Treatment

Patients with acute cholecystitis are treated at first expectantly. They are put to bed and if vomiting has been severe and they are dehydrated an intravenous infusion is set up to correct and maintain their fluid and electrolyte balance. Antibiotics are given, the one of choice being ampicillin, 500 mg orally 6 hourly. Pulse rate and temperature are measured at hourly intervals and the abdomen is frequently examined to ensure that the inflammatory process which is occurring in the gall bladder is not spreading to the rest of the peritoneum. The danger with cholecystitis is that part of the wall of the gall bladder may necrose with release of infected bile into the peritoneal cavity and the development of generalised peritonitis. This occurrence is rare, but if in spite of bed rest and the treatment mentioned above the pulse rate and temperature do not rapidly settle, operation will be required. If the attack of cholecystitis has been present for some days it is not possible to carry out an emergency cholecystectomy and external drainage of the gall bladder with removal of the stones from the gall bladder will have to be performed—*cholecystostomy*. This can be a life-saving operation and may be performed even on the aged and infirm who are weakened by their cholecystitis. A small incision is made in the abdomen over the inflamed gall bladder, the gall bladder is opened and the stones within it removed and pus and bile is sucked out. The opening in the gall bladder is then sutured to the parietal peritoneum around a drain which protrudes through the abdominal wall. Since the major cause of the inflammation has been removed the patient's condition will rapidly improve.

It will be necessary when the inflammation has completely settled for the gall bladder to be removed. This usually will be three months after the acute attack of cholecystitis. Should the patient follow the more usual course and the attack of acute cholecystitis subsides over the period of 24 to 48 hours, cholecystectomy will be required three months later. These patients' gall bladders never return to normal and since the complications of stones in the gall bladder, that is obstructive jaundice, are so severe, cholecystectomy should be insisted on in every case. Indeed if gall stones are discovered by accident in a patient with only few symptoms, cholecystectomy is the safest course.

Cholecystectomy is performed through a right upper paramedian or right Kocher incision. Before the gall bladder is removed an operative cholangiogram is performed. In this a tube is placed in the cystic duct and radio-opaque dye injected down it (Fig. 14.14). If stones are shown in the common bile duct, these are removed and the duct drained by means of a T-tube (see page 287).

Fig. 14.14. Operative cholangiogram. There is a stone at the lower end of the common bile duct although dye can be seen entering the duodenum and refluxing into the pancreatic duct. (A) The stone was removed via an incision in the common bile duct which was then drained by means of a T-tube. (B)

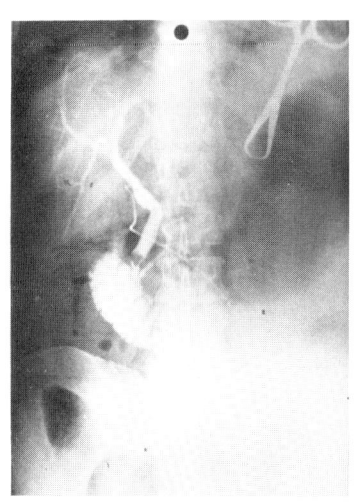

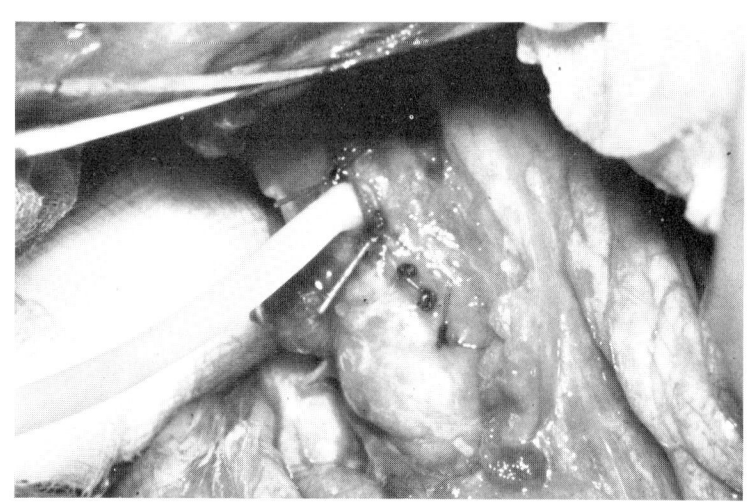

A

B

The spleen

Anatomy

The spleen (Fig. 14.15) is situated in the upper left abdomen. Blood is supplied to the hilum by the splenic artery, which is one of the major vessels coming from the coeliac axis. A smaller but important supply is derived from the short gastric arteries from the fundus of the stomach. The splenic vein passes to the right along the superior border of the pancreas to join the superior mesenteric

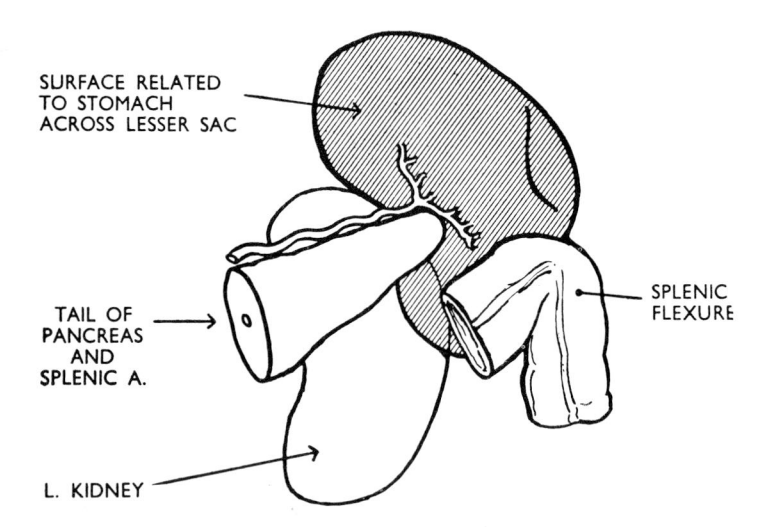

Fig. 14.15. The spleen and its immediate relations.

Fig. 14.16. The portal venous system.

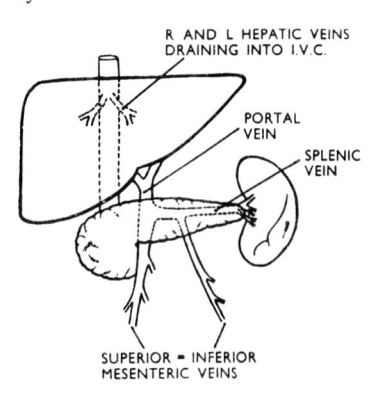

vein, the confluence becoming the portal vein (Fig. 14.16), which then passes to the hilum of the liver. Blood from the splenic artery becomes diffused within the splenic tissue, which has the characteristic structure of a sponge. There are numerous macrophage cells lining the sinuses within the spleen and these are capable of ingesting red cells, particularly at the end of their life. The spleen is thus the organ which is principally responsible for controlling the length of life of the red cell which, in the normal, is from 100–120 days.

The spleen has to enlarge by about $2\frac{1}{2}$ times before it can be palpable. One of the characteristic features of a palpable spleen is that it moves from beneath the left costal margin in the direction of the right iliac fossa on deep inspiration as it is pushed down by the descending dome of the diaphragm. If it enlarges sufficiently it may be possible to palpate the notch on the lower edge of the enlarging organ.

Conditions for which splenectomy is required

1. *Ruptured spleen—immediate*

A not uncommon injury in road traffic accidents or other cases of abdominal trauma is rupture of the spleen. When this occurs the only safe treatment is rapid splenectomy otherwise the patient runs considerable risk of death from haemorrhage. When a patient has fracture of the left 10th, 11th or 12th ribs, those caring for him should be suspicious of splenic rupture.

The operation is carried out via a left subcostal or upper midline incision through which the spleen can readily be lifted forward into the light which permits separate ligation of the splenic artery and the vein.

2. *Ruptured spleen—delayed*

One of the difficulties of this subject is that the spleen may not actually rupture although there has been disruption of the splenic pulp to such an extent that an extensive haematoma forms beneath the splenic capsule. This haematoma increases in size in much the same way as a subdural haematoma increases in size, and a full-scale rupture of splenic tissue occurs some time from 2nd to 10th day after the original trauma. When a subcapsular haematoma is suspected, then immediate splenectomy is essential.

Very rarely spontaneous rupture of the spleen occurs in the complete absence of a history of abdominal trauma. This may follow an area of infarction of the splenic tissue, but is always sudden and calamitous. Usually the only diagnosis is one of massive intraperitoneal haemorrhage and immediate laparotomy has then to be carried out with subsequent removal of the spleen.

3. *Haematological disorders*

Several conditions may require splenectomy to remove the main source of erythrocyte destruction in those conditions where cells are unusually fragile. Notable amongst these are acholuric jaundice, primary thrombocytopenic purpura, acquired haemolytic anaemia, thalassemia and sickle cell anaemia. Occasionally splenectomy is also required for aplastic and myelosclerotic anaemia when the red cell destruction component of the blood picture is greatest.

4. *Tropical diseases*

Splenectomy may be indicated when the spleen becomes hugely enlarged in chronic malaria, Kala azar or schistosomiasis.

5. Neoplastic disease

Hodgkin's disease may require splenectomy for two distinct reasons. First, the spleen may be involved by Hodgkin's tissue and second splenectomy appears to exert a desirable influence on the regression of Hodgkin's disease. A third advantage is that when splenectomy is performed the abdominal cavity can be diligently searched for signs of disease, thus permitting accurate staging and allowing appropriate treatment to be carried out. Thus in a patient with Hodgkin's disease in the glands of the neck, the treatment of stage I, that is when the disease is localised to one group of glands, is different to the treatment of stage III when there is disease not only in the glands of the neck but also within the abdominal cavity. In the former case the glands will be completely excised or irradiated and in the latter case radiotherapy combined with cytotoxic drugs will be employed.

The pancreas

Anatomy

The pancreas is the best example of a mixed exocrine and endocrine gland. It is situated behind the peritoneum of the posterior abdominal wall and is a posterior relation of the stomach (Fig. 14.17). It is composed of the *head*, which fills the 'C'-shaped curve of the first, second and third parts of the duodenum. This is joined by a poorly defined *neck* to the *body* which extends across the posterior part of the abdomen, crossing in front of first the inferior vena cava and then the aorta at the level of the second lumbar vertebra. To the left of the vertebral column the body becomes the *tail* which

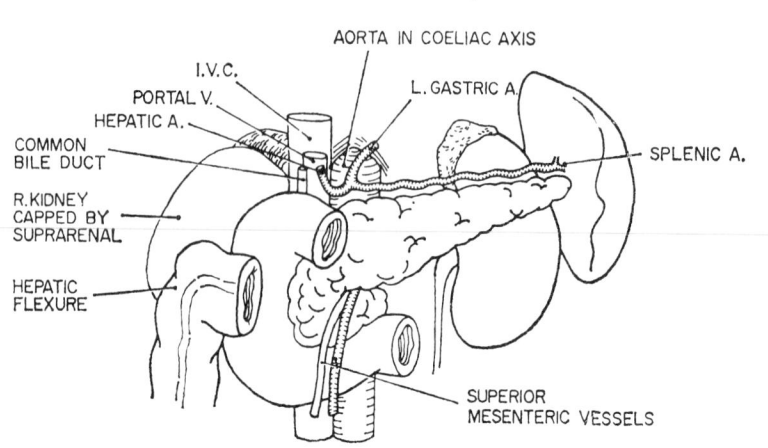

Fig. 14.17. The pancreas and its relations.

extends to the hilum of the spleen. An important posterior relationship of the head of the pancreas is the infraduodenal portion of the common bile duct, which runs in a groove before entering the medial aspect of the second part of the duodenum. In one third of patients the common bile duct is joined at its termination by the main pancreatic duct (the duct of Wirsung). Emerging from beneath the inferior border of the neck of the pancreas are the superior mesenteric vessels as they pass to the whole of the small intestine and to the ascending and transverse colon. Running along the superior border of the pancreas is the splenic artery and vein and these are both associated with a large number of lymph nodes. The superior mesenteric vein, which drains blood from the whole of the small intestine, passes upward behind the pancreas where it is joined by the splenic vein to become the portal vein.

The external appearance of the pancreas is of a lobular structure which reflects the microscopic anatomy. The lobules drain the exocrine secretion into a main duct which runs the whole length of the gland and which enters the duodenum just below the common bile duct at the ampulla of Vater (Fig. 14.18). There is in addition a smaller accessory duct which drains the superior part of the head of the pancreas (the duct of Santorini).

Microscopic examination of the gland reveals large clumps of cells that are quite distinct, these are the *'islets' of Langerhans*. They contain cells of several different types, the first of which are alpha cells which secrete glucagon. The second type of cell is the beta cell and these produce insulin. In certain disease processes other cells make their appearance, notably G-cells in the primary islet cell tumours responsible for the Zollinger-Ellison syndrome.

Physiology

1. *Exocrine pancreas*

The exocrine pancreas secretes a juice which passes into the second part of the duodenum and which is essential for normal digestion

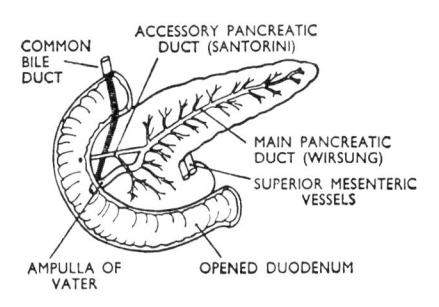

Fig. 14.18. The duodenum and pancreas dissected to show the pancreatic ducts and their orifices.

of carbohydrates, fats and proteins. The juice contains amylase, which hydrolyses polysaccharides, such as starch and glycogen, down to the disaccharide stage, lipase which acts on emulsified fat in the presence of bile salts resulting in the release of fatty acids and glycerol, and a group of proteolytic enzymes, including trypsin and chymotrypsin, which are responsible for breaking proteins down to their constituent molecules. As well as these enzymes, pancreatic juice is also rich in bicarbonate, and contains calcium, sodium, chloride and potassium.

The stimulus to secretion is threefold. First, there is a rich nerve supply derived from the vagus and sympathetic nerves which, when activated by food, results in a secretion of high bicarbonate content. Second, gastric chyme entering the duodenum causes the secretion of the hormone secretin which recirculates in the blood and stimulates the exocrine pancreas to produce juice also of high bicarbonate content. Thirdly, the duodenal chyme also results in the release of a second hormone, pancreomyzin, which results in the secretion of a juice rich in enzymes.

2. *Endocrine pancreas*

Insulin is elaborated in the beta cells and secreted into the blood stream in response to variation in the level of the blood glucose. It is responsible for maintaining the blood glucose within closely defined limits. For example, following a meal, glucose tends to rise as it is absorbed from the intestine and this results in secretion of insulin which facilitates the inclusion of glucose into cells and its utilisation in the metabolic processes. This has the secondary result that the blood glucose level falls. In diabetes mellitus insufficient insulin is secreted in response to hyperglycaemia. This has the effect that the blood sugar rises and continues to rise, and metabolic pathways dependent on glucose become starved of their basic requirements.

The alpha cells secrete glucagon which has the opposite effect on blood glucose to insulin. That is, it results in an increase in blood glucose levels, but the mechanism of this increase is ill understood. Although it is produced in purified form so that it can be injected into patients, at the present time it has very little clinical application.

Two main groups of diseases affect the pancreas—inflammation (pancreatitis) and tumours.

PANCREATITIS

Pathology

This condition exists in one of three forms:
1. *Acute pancreatitis*, which may be fulminating with total destruction of all pancreatic tissue.
2. *Relapsing pancreatitis*.
3. *Chronic pancreatitis*.

In the condition of acute pancreatitis there is an inflammatory reaction throughout the whole gland. There are a number of conditions which may precipitate this and they are as follows:
1. *Infections*—for example mumps.
2. *Mechanical*—by the impaction of a gall stone at the lower end of the common bile duct, producing obstruction of the pancreatic duct.
3. *Metabolic*—for example, alcoholism, hyperparathyroidism.
4. *Vascular*—polyarteritis nodosa.
5. *Toxic*—alcohol poisoning.
6. *Traumatic*—due to external trauma, for example that sustained in a road traffic accident.
7. *Other causes*—for example, pregnancy and Hodgkin's disease.

It must be admitted, however, that no aetiological factor can be determined in the majority of cases.

Clinical features

These depend on the extent of the inflammatory change within the gland. There may be upper abdominal pain, which characteristically radiates through to the centre of the midback. At first the abdominal pain is localised but as the process extends and the typical bloodstained exudate spreads into the general peritoneal cavity (this has been described as being like prune juice), so the pain becomes more generalised. Eventually the patient gives the appearance of someone suffering from peritonitis and this disease is an example of a chemical cause of this condition.

If the attack is a relatively minor one there may be some elevation of the pulse, the other vital signs being stable. As the severity of the attack increases, the pulse rate rises and eventually the blood pressure falls. The periphery of the patient becomes pale and he becomes shocked. This is partly due to the loss of fluid into the tissues around the pancreas, into the peritoneal cavity and into the intestine. Another factor, however, is the release of vaso-active substances from the inflamed pancreas itself which produce a shock-like state.

Special investigations

Serum Amylase The characteristic finding is an elevation of serum amylase, generally above 1000 Somogyi units; this is because amylase is released into the peritoneal cavity from the inflamed pancreas and is absorbed into the bloodstream. The problem here is that the elevation may be transient, occurring only at the beginning of the attack, or in the case of haemorrhagic pancreatitis in which the pancreas is destroyed, the amylase will not rise at all, due to the destruction of the cells normally producing it.

In severe attacks the *serum calcium* is depressed, and this has been used as an index of prognosis. The more the calcium falls the worse the outlook for survival of the patient.

The urea and electrolytes are commonly normal unless the patient has been shocked or vomiting for a significant length of time, in which case the urea may become raised, sodium and chloride being low.

X-ray of the abdomen may show separation of loops of intestine by intraperitoneal fluid. A 'sentinel loop' of jejunum may be seen, this is due to the jejunum adjacent to the pancreas becoming paralysed because of the inflammatory process producing a localised area of paralytic ileus. Similarly, a colon cut off sign may be seen in which the transverse colon becomes distended with gas for the same reason.

Treatment

1. *Acute pancreatitis*

There is no effective specific remedy for pancreatitis. Therefore the treatment is supportive, aimed at relieving the pain and maintaining a satisfactory circulation. The patient is put to bed and given pethidine 100 mg 4 hourly, by intramuscular injection. Small quantities of water are allowed to be drunk for comfort and a fine nasogastric tube is passed to keep the stomach empty by aspiration, at first every hour and later every four hours. In every case intravenous fluid therapy will be required. From this point the vigour of the supportive measures depend upon the degree of inflammation in the pancreas. In severe haemorrhagic pancreatitis the patient may well be shocked, in which case fluid replacement should be controlled by means of a central venous pressure catheter and kept to a positive value (between +3 and +8 cm of water) with the use of plasma expanders such as plasma itself if necessary.

Trasylol inhibits the activity of proteolytic enzymes and since these are liberated by the process of acute pancreatitis, this drug has been suggested as being useful in acute pancreatitis. Unfortunately, although they have been extensively employed there is no evidence that they are effective. Antibiotics are valueless and should not be given. Similarly, steroids exert no beneficial effect. Occasionally, if the calcium level in the blood has dropped to an extremely low level it will be necessary to give intravenous calcium gluconate, 10 mg very slowly, to relieve the symptoms of tetany.

2. *Chronic relapsing pancreatitis*

In this condition there are episodes of acute pancreatitis interspersed with an entirely asymptomatic period or with a low background 'grumbling' pain. When they occur, the acute episodes of pancreatitis should be treated as above.

3. *Chronic Pancreatitis*

This can exist in an entirely asymptomatic form in which a chance X-ray of the abdomen reveals extensive calcification throughout the whole pancreas. More commonly, however, it is associated with severe persistent abdominal pain. This condition has been said to result in some patients becoming drug addicts or alcoholics. However, the situation is usually that the chronic pancreatitis is initiated and maintained by the consumption of alcohol.

It is essential to exclude other disease within the abdominal cavity, particularly in the biliary tract, and if gall stones are demonstrated on cholecystography they should be removed surgically. The great lack in the investigation of the pancreas is an efficient test which shows the duct system. The pancreatic duct can now be demonstrated by catheterisation via a flexible gastroduodenoscope. This is an extremely useful technique but unfortunately cannot be successfully achieved in every case in which it is attempted. The only other method of demonstrating the main pancreatic duct is by operative pancreatography when at laparotomy a tube is inserted after the duodenum has been opened opposite the ampulla of Vater. This is clearly a major undertaking, but if by any of these means a localised constriction in the main pancreatic duct can be demonstrated, this should be relieved by surgery. Many other surgical procedures have been described for pancreatitis but the sad fact remains that most of them are not effective. The pain in this condition can be so severe that some surgeons have advocated total removal of the pancreas. This obviously should only be reserved for the very severe degrees of this condition, as the quality of life without the pancreas is considerably impaired due to the 'brittle' diabetes and digestive abnormality.

CARCINOMA OF THE PANCREAS

Pathology

This is a fairly common malignant tumour and may be situated anywhere throughout the gland. As the greatest portion of pancreatic tissue is situated in the head, this is where the tumours are most commonly found, although a quarter occur in the body and 15% in the tail of the gland. Men are affected twice as commonly as are women and the peak age incidence is from 55 to 65.

In cut surface appearance the tumour is hard, white and infiltrates the normal pancreatic tissue and its surrounding structures (Fig. 14.19). Microscopically the tumours may be of duct origin or arise from the secreting cells of the termination of the ducts (acinar in origin), undifferentiated or rarely, may be associated with cystic spaces, the so called cystadenocarcinoma.

Spread is by local infiltration, which may result in obstruction to the lower end of the common bile duct and the common pancreatic duct, involvement of the medial wall of the duodenum with ulceration of the mucosa and eventually obstruction of the third part of the duodenum.

Clinical features

Unfortunately it is extremely difficult to diagnose an early carcinoma of the pancreas, with the result that this is one of the malignant tumours that tends to present by virtue of local or distant spread.

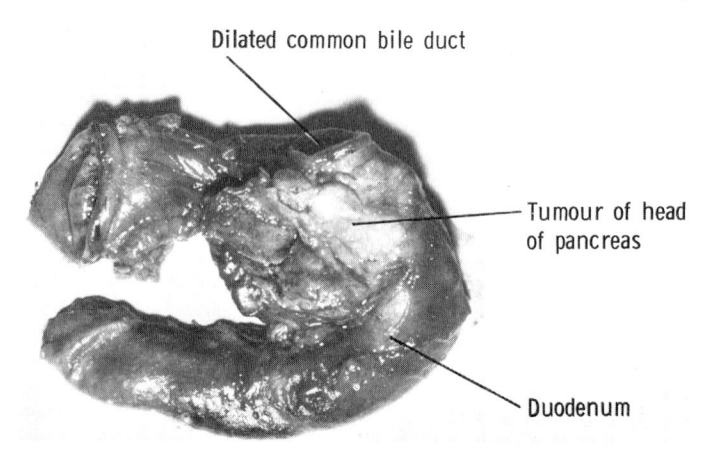

Fig. 14.19. Carcinoma of the head of the pancreas removed at a Whipple's operation together with the duodenum. (The specimen is viewed from the posterior aspect—note the dilated common bile duct).

Pain is a common feature and is usually experienced in the back, is ill-localised and of a deep seated type. Obstructive jaundice in the absence of a history suggestive of gall stones is common and is often associated with distension of the gall bladder, which can be palpated beneath the lower edge of the right lobe of the liver (Courvosier's law—see Fig. 14.3).

Special investigations

If infiltration of the medial wall of the second part of the duodenum has occurred this can be seen as irregularity on barium meal examination. As the head of the pancreas is expanded by the tumour the alteration in shape will also be detected on barium meal. A classic but rather unusual sign is the inverted '3' sign produced by bulging of the head of the pancreas around the ampulla of Vater.

Treatment

Treatment can be divided into two types:

1. *Curative treatment*

If the tumour is small and has not infiltrated the neck of the gland to the left of the portal vein, it is possible to remove the head of the pancreas, the neck and part of the body together with the duodenum and part of the stomach (Fig. 14.20) in a pancreaticoduodenectomy (Whipple's operation). Unfortunately, the long-term results from this operation are not good, the five-year survival being only of the order of 5%.

2. *Palliative*

So often this condition presents with obstructive jaundice and since this leads to rapid liver function deterioration and is associated with very severe itching, its relief is important. This may be secured by performing cholecystjejunostomy, a remarkably effective procedure producing good palliation (Fig. 14.6).

If no other palliation is possible, cytotoxic agents such as 5-Fluorouracil may be employed.

ISLET CELL TUMOURS

INSULINOMA

This is a tumour of the beta cells of the islet tissue which may be either benign of malignant. If considerably dedifferentiated the production of insulin is unlikely. Usually the tumour is benign and

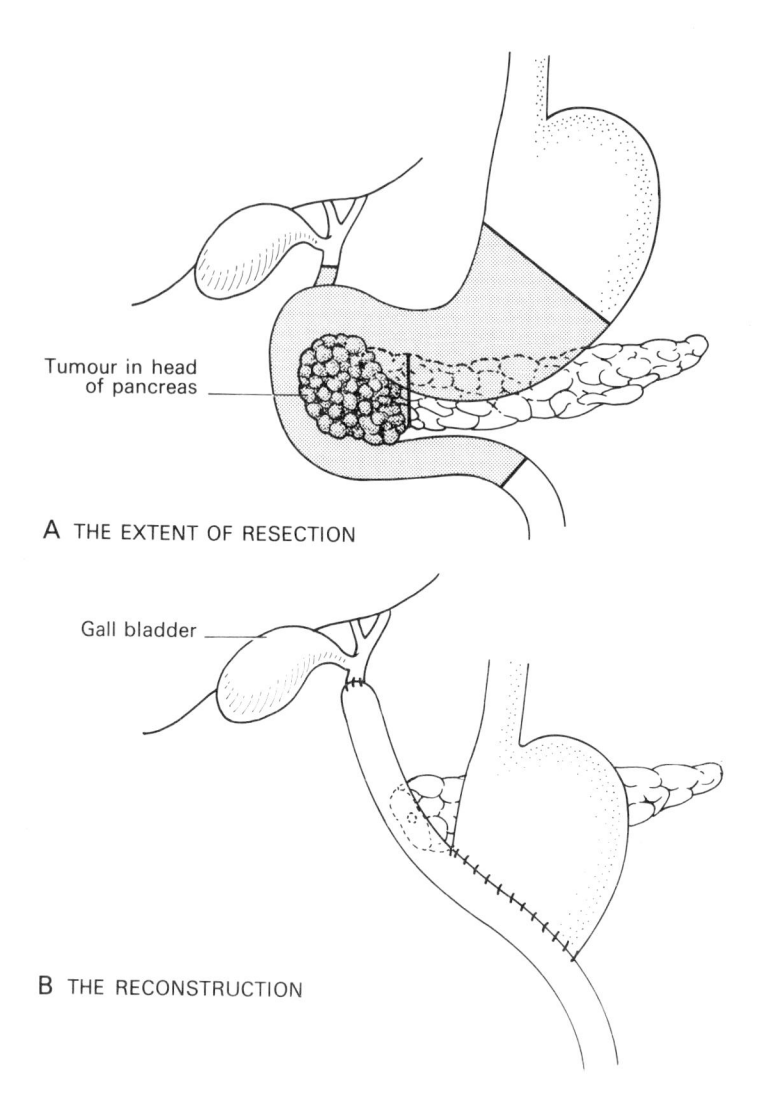

Fig. 14.20. Whipple's operation, pancreaticoduodenectomy.

- A THE EXTENT OF RESECTION
- B THE RECONSTRUCTION

inappropriate secretion of insulin does occur. Presentation consequently is by hyperinsulinism which, in extreme cases, produces profound coma but more commonly the unfortunate subject appears to undergo bouts of severe mental change, which includes antisocial manic behaviour, when in reality they are merely hypoglycaemic. In the past, before this syndrome was widely recognised, these unfortunate patients found their way into mental hospitals where commonly they died from long continued bouts of hypoglycaemia. Diagnosis is made on the basis of a prolonged sugar tolerance test which demonstrates hypoglycaemia precipitated by fasting.

Treatment

Treatment is excision of the tumour. Unfortunately this is not always easy as the tumours may be quite small and difficult to find and within the substance of the pancreas.

ZOLLINGER-ELLISON SYNDROME

This extremely rare syndrome was first described in 1955 and consists of:
1. Fulminating duodenal ulcer diathysis, the ulcerative process usually extending into the upper jejunum.
2. Considerable gastric hyper-secretion of acid.
3. A tumour of the islet cells of the pancreas, which has the extraordinary property of producing the hormone gastrin.

So far over 500 cases have been described and catalogued, from all over the world.

Two-thirds of these tumours are malignant and of these two-thirds have metastases by the time the patient presents for treatment. The tumours may be distributed anywhere in the pancreatic tissue and occasionally exist in an unusual situation, for example the hilum of the spleen, the duodenum or the stomach. The syndrome is more common in males than in females in the ratio of 3 : 2 and the peak age incidence is in the 3rd, 4th and 5th decades. Adenomas of other endocrine glands occur in one patient out of four, including the pituitary, adrenal, parathyroid and in a combination of these glands.

Special investigations

Diagnosis is confirmed either by estimation of the hormone gastrin in the blood, when truly enormously high levels are found, or by the demonstration of a fasting gastric acid secretion which is at least 60% of the secretion that results from the injection of a maximum dose of pentagastrin.

Treatment

The treatment of choice is total gastrectomy. If subtotal pancreatectomy is attempted there is considerable danger that a small unheeded tumour may be left behind and this could be quite sufficient to produce disastrous recurrent ulceration. Total pancreatectomy leaves the patient with the problem of diabetes of a type which is very difficult to control, together with a considerable digestive defect and the quality of life following total pancreatectomy is not as good as that following total gastrectomy. Even though two-thirds of the Zollinger-Ellison tumours are malignant they appear to be very slow-growing and even when metastases have been found at operation, patients have lived for many years.

CYSTS ASSOCIATED WITH THE PANCREAS

TRUE PANCREATIC CYSTS

Generally these are small and may be associated with cysts occurring in the kidney and the liver. They are due to obstruction to one or more of the ducts. No treatment is required and they do not give rise to symptoms.

PSEUDOCYSTS OF THE PANCREAS

In this condition the lesser sac of the peritoneal cavity becomes filled with fluid. The reason for this is that the opening into the lesser sac, the foramen of Winslow, becomes blocked because of an attack of pancreatitis. The inflammatory exudate which accumulates in the lesser sac from the anterior surface of the pancreas cannot find its way into the general peritoneal cavity and at the same time there must be a change in the permeability of the peritoneum lining the lesser sac, presumably due to the inflammatory processes.

Clinical features

The patient presents usually with central upper abdominal pain which may radiate through to the back. There may be a history of preceding pancreatitis and there may be a primary history of one of the precipitating causes of this, for example alcoholism. On examination a deep-seated mass is felt in the epigastrium, above the level of the umbilicus. It is usually difficult to define the borders of this mass accurately, impossible to get above it, and the mass may extend to diameters of 20 cm.

Special investigations

Plain X-ray of the abdomen will often reveal the edges of the cyst and there may be associated calcification within the pancreas. Barium meal demonstrates the stomach to be stretched over the front of the cyst and there may be distortion of the second part of the duodenum by the previously occurring pancreatitis (Fig. 14.21).

Treatment

Treatment is by making a wide anastomosis between the wall of the cyst and the posterior aspect of the stomach (Fig. 14.22). When this is done it might be supposed that the contents of the stomach leak

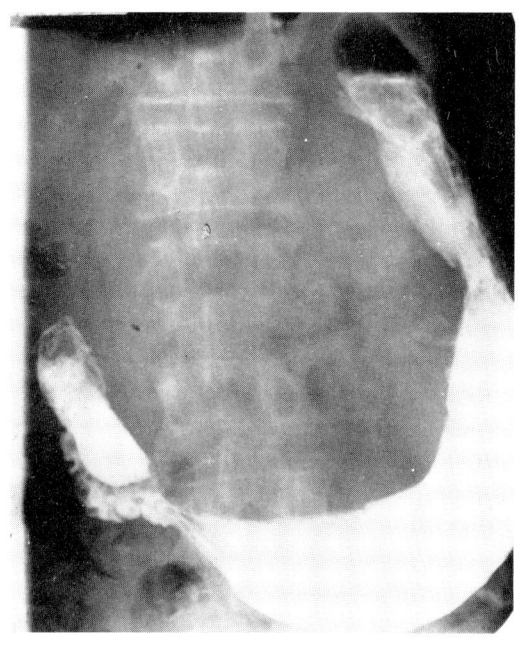

Fig. 14.21. Barium meal in a patient with a pseudocyst of the pancreas. Note the way that the barium within the stomach is stretched over the cyst.

into the cyst with disastrous results. This does not happen, however; fluid from the cyst drains into the stomach and if a barium meal is repeated after a few months in many cases it is found that there is no evidence either of the stoma or of the cyst, the latter having collapsed and become permanently closed.

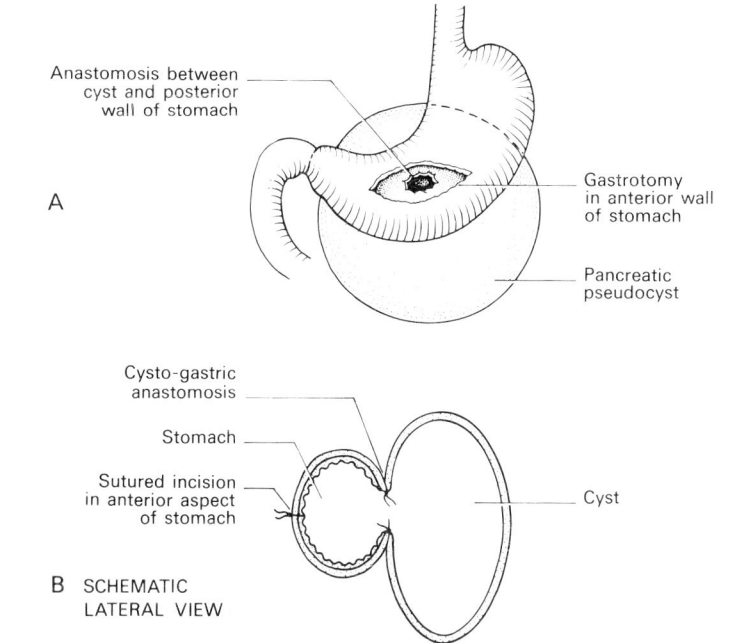

Fig. 14.22. Drainage of a pancreatic pseudocyst into the posterior aspect of the stomach.

Chapter 15. The urinary tract

The kidney and ureter

Anatomy

The kidneys lie retroperitoneally on the posterior abdominal wall. The right kidney is half an inch lower than the left, presumably because of its downward displacement by the bulk of the liver.

Each kidney lies against the diaphragm and the muscles of the posterior abdominal wall. Anteriorly the right kidney is related to the liver, duodenum (which may be accidentally injured in performing a right nephrectomy) and the hepatic flexure of the colon. In front of the left kidney lie the stomach, the pancreas, the spleen and the descending colon. On each side the adrenal sits as a cap on the kidney's upper pole (Fig. 15.1). The medial aspect of the kidney presents a deep vertical slit, the *hilum*, which transmits the renal

Fig. 15.1. The anterior relations of the kidneys.

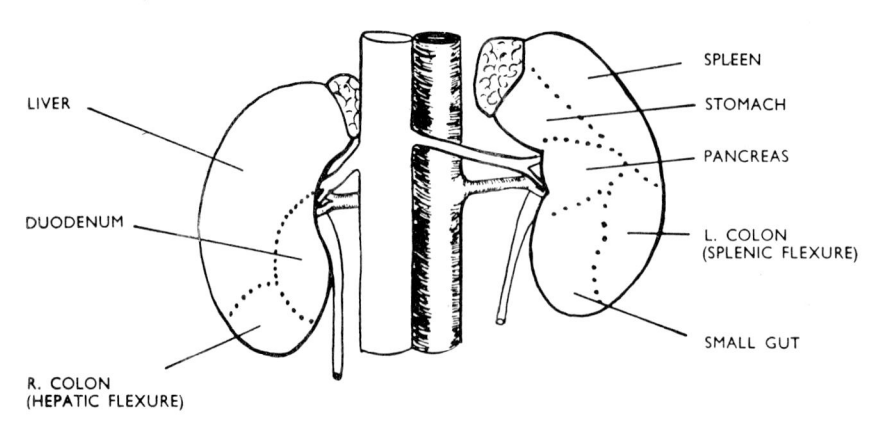

artery, renal vein and the pelvis of the ureter. Within the kidney, the pelvis of the ureter divides into two or three major *calyces*, each of which divides into a number of minor calyces and each of these, in turn, is indented by a papilla of renal tissue onto which the collecting tubules of the kidney discharge urine.

The renal artery is derived directly from the aorta and is a massive vessel; indeed about 1/5th of the total circulation is passing through the kidneys at any one time.

The ureter is 10 inches long and runs as a muscular tube from the renal pelvis to the bladder. It passes first down the posterior abdominal wall, then on the lateral wall of the pelvis in front of the internal iliac artery. It has a thick muscular wall which is seen in the operating theatre to undergo typical worm-like writhing movements and it is this that enables the surgeon to identify it during pelvic and retroperitoneal operations.

EMBRYOLOGY AND CONGENITAL ANOMALIES

The ureter develops from the *metanephric duct*, a bud which pushes out from the cloaca, the common tube which is later to split up into bladder and rectum. On top of this metanephric duct develops a cap of tissue called the *metanephros*. The duct will form the ureter, the renal pelvis and the calyces; the metanephros will give rise to the kidney tissue itself. The kidney originally develops in the pelvis of the embryo then migrates headwards to reach the posterior abdominal wall. As it migrates, it acquires successively a fresh blood supply from higher and higher along the aorta.

This complex developmental process explains the high frequency with which congenital anomalies of the kidney, ureter and renal blood supply are found. Among the more important of these are (Fig. 15.2):

1. *Pelvic kidney*—due to failure of migration of the developing kidney upwards into the abdomen.

2. *Horse-shoe kidney*—produced by fusion of the two metanephric masses across the midline.

3. *Double ureter and/or kidneys*—due to reduplication of the metanephric bud.

4. *Congenital absence*—in one in every 2400 births there is complete failure of the development of one kidney.

5. *Aberrent renal arteries*—it is not uncommon for there to be one or more additional arteries passing to the lower pole of the kidney; they represent persistence of aortic branches which pass to the kidney in its lower embryonic position.

6. *Polycystic disease* of the kidney results from failure of fusion of

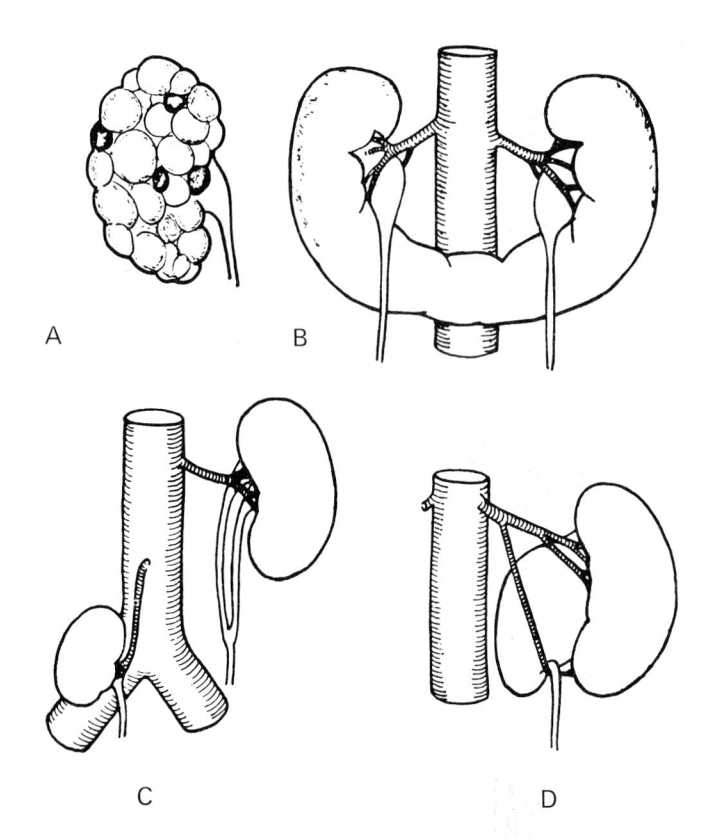

Fig. 15.2. Common renal abnormalities. A, polycystic kidney; B, horseshoe kidney; C, pelvic kidney and double ureter; D, aberrant renal arteries and hydronephrosis.

the metanephros with its ducts—the result is multiple cyst formation throughout the renal substance, nearly always affecting both kidneys. Eventually the patient may die of renal failure or of hypertension.

It is important to note that polycystic disease, double kidneys and ureters and congenitally misplaced kidneys are all associated with an increased likelihood of infection when compared with kidneys that are anatomically normal. A child with recurrent episodes of urinary infection thus requires investigation to see whether some congenital urological abnormality may be present.

Renal physiology

The kidney functions to maintain water and electrolyte balance and has an important part to play in the regulation of the pH (acid/base relationship) of the blood, as well as acting as the excretory organ for many waste products of the body's metabolism and of foreign toxic substances.

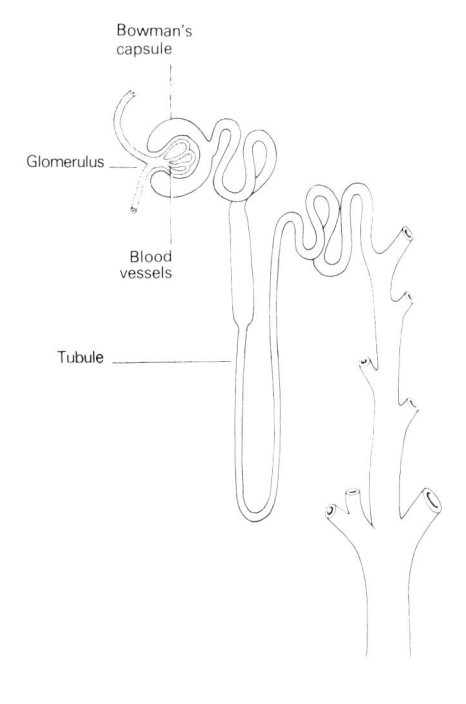

Fig. 15.3. Diagram of a nephron, comprising a Bowman's capsule and a tubule.

Each kidney is made up of approximately one million functioning units termed *nephrons* (Fig. 15.3) each comprising a glomerulus and a tubule. The *glomerulus* itself is made up of the expanded and thinned blind end of the renal tubule (termed Bowman's capsule) which is invaginated by a clump of capillaries.

The glomerulus acts as a simple filter through which the enormous amount of 180 litres of protein-free fluid is filtered from the bloodstream daily. This contains water, electrolytes and water-soluble substances such as glucose and urea. This filter is activated by the blood pressure—if the blood pressure falls then filtration slows or ceases.

In the *tubules* the greater part of this water is reabsorbed. Indeed since we produce approximately 1.5 litres of urine daily it means that 178 litres of glomerular filtrate is pumped back into the blood stream every 24 hours. The tubules select those substances which the body requires—all the glucose, for example, is completely reabsorbed in normal people—and lets pass those substances that are in excess and require elimination. In addition to this many toxic substances and poisonous chemicals, for example barbiturates, are cleared in this way.

Absorption is a property of the whole extent of the tubule, but the distal part is also capable of excreting substances into the urine, particularly hydrogen and potassium ions, and thus the distal duct plays an important part in maintaining the pH of the blood. It should be noticed that the tubules' power of absorption is limited so that, for example, if the blood glucose level is raised in diabetes mellitus not all the glucose can be absorbed by the tubules and this will then appear in the urine (glycosuria).

Water reabsorption is controlled by the anti-diuretic hormone of the posterior pituitary and sodium and chloride absorption is under the influence of aldosterone, one of the important hormones secreted by the adrenal cortex.

ANURIA

Having considered the normal physiology of the kidney we must now turn to the causes and treatment of failure of urine production of the kidney (*anuria*) or the only marginally less serious situation when the urine production falls to a level insufficient to maintain the body in health (*oliguria*).

The causes of this situation fall into three groups:

1. *Pre-renal*—here the kidneys themselves are initially healthy but if the blood pressure falls below the level necessary to maintain filtration through the glomeruli (usually below 80 mm of mercury), then renal function is impaired.

2. *Renal*—bilateral renal disease may be so severe that little or no urine can be produced. Examples are damage from certain poisons such as mercury, advanced chronic renal disease, transfusion reaction or tubular necrosis (see below).

3. *Post-renal*—complete bilateral obstruction of the renal drainage system, particularly by calculi or, fortunately rarely, by surgical injury.

ACUTE TUBULAR NECROSIS

The commonest cause of oliguria and anuria in modern surgical practice is acute tubular necrosis. This results from damage to the renal tubules as a result of ischaemia which may follow severe haemorrhage or result from the hypotension of severe toxaemia or burns. The damaged tubules become swollen, with blockage of their lumen, and suppression of urinary excretion takes place. Note that a patient who has a severe haemorrhage and becomes shocked may at first fail to produce urine because there is insufficient blood pressure to maintain filtration. However, if this state of affairs persists for several hours, there may then be the much more serious changes of tubular necrosis in the ischaemic kidneys and the anuria now becomes renal in origin.

Clinical features

There is always a good reason for the patient to become anuric—this may follow a serious accident, burns or heavy blood loss during operation which would suggest a pre-renal anuria which may proceed to acute tubular necrosis. The patient may be known to be suffering from severe chronic renal disease and the anuria is the end-stage of this condition. Anuria following hysterectomy indicates operative ligation of the ureters, or severe attacks of colicky pain, preceding the anuria suggests calculous obstruction.

The patient fails to pass urine but, unlike retention of urine, the bladder is empty on clinical examination. If necessary this diagnosis is clinched by passing a catheter under full sterile precautions, when only a few drops of urine are obtained. At first the patient appears reasonably well, but then, within a few days, he becomes drowsy and thirsty with a dry brown tongue, develops anorexia, hiccups and effortless vomiting, and then lapses into coma. The progression of the condition can be monitored by estimation of the blood urea since the kidneys are now unable to excrete this product of protein breakdown. It is not the urea itself which is particularly dangerous to the patient, but the retention of unexcreted electrolytes (particularly potassium, which, in high concentration, is toxic to the heart), the accumulation of non-excreted water which produces cerebral and pulmonary oedema, and the development of acidosis due to protein break-down.

Treatment

This will depend on the aetiology of the renal shutdown.

Pre-renal anuria requires replacement of blood volume, either by blood transfusion in haemorrhagic shock, plasma or plasma substitutes in severe burns, or saline in fluid depletion from vomiting or diarrhoea.

Post-renal anuria calls for surgical relief of the obstruction, for example, by catheterisation of the ureters blocked by stone (see page 337).

Tubular necrosis is the commonest variety of renal anuria. This is a reversible lesion and the aim of treatment is to keep the patient alive until the cells of the renal tubules recover. It is important not to overload the patient with water and electrolytes which cannot be excreted by the damaged kidneys, and to reduce protein metabolism as much as possible in order to limit the formation of protein breakdown products, such as urea and potassium. The following regime is therefore instituted:

Fluid balance

The daily allowance of water is cut down to a basic 1 litre in 24 hours; this replaces the water lost in sweat and the water vapour excreted in the breath. To this ration must be added any additional fluid loss which occurs in vomiting, diarrhoea, a bowel fistula, or any other causes.

It may be necessary to give sodium bicarbonate to treat acidosis, but unless there are special circumstances such as this, the patient should not receive any electrolytes during the period of anuria.

Calorie replacement

If the patient is starved, he will simply utilise tissue protein and add to the toxic breakdown products already accumulating in the tissues. To reduce this as much as possible, the patient should be given Dextrose in 40% solution in his daily water ration. Since a gram of sugar produces four calories, one litre of 40% solution provides 1600 calories daily. This may be given in some cases orally or by naso-gastric tube, but more often the concentrated solution can only be tolerated by a nauseated patient if administered as an intravenous drip. Since the concentrated sugar solution will produce thrombosis in peripheral veins, it must be given by means of a caval drip via a fine catheter threaded into the inferior or superior vena cava via either the long saphenous vein or an arm vein.

Dialysis

In some cases this treatment alone will suffice, particularly if the patient's general condition is good at the onset of the anuria and the period of tubular necrosis only lasts for a few days. However, if the patient's general condition deteriorates, the blood urea continues to rise and if the serum potassium reaches a dangerous level of about 7 m Eq/litre, it becomes necessary to maintain the patient by *haemodialysis* using the artificial kidney, which may be needed 2 or 3 times a week, or by *peritoneal dialysis*.

Haemodialysis. The principle of the artificial kidney is to pass the patient's blood through a coil of cellophane (a semi-permeable membrane), which is immersed in a bath of water to which electrolytes and sugar are added. Unwanted soluble substances in the patient's plasma (in particular, urea and potassium) pass from high concentration in the blood stream across the membrane into the bath fluid. (Fig. 15.4). During dialysis coagulation of the blood within the

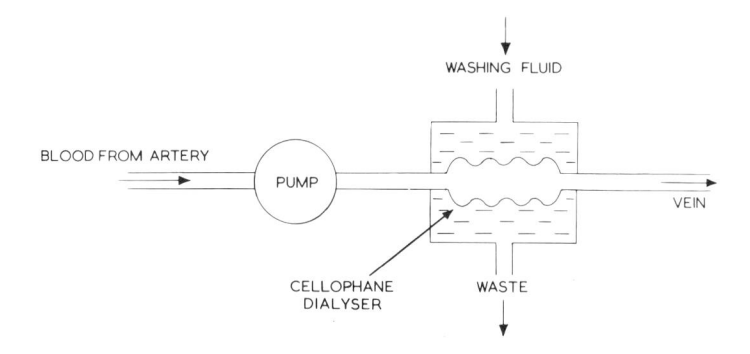

Fig. 15.4. Diagram of the circuit used in haemodialysis.

machine is prevented by heparinisation. Cannulae are placed in a suitable peripheral artery and vein and these can be used repeatedly by connecting the cannulae together, when not in use, by a plastic tube which maintains circulation and thus prevents clotting (the Scribner shunt Fig. 15.5). Another technique, recently introduced, is to anastomose a peripheral artery to its adjacent vein. Both vessels become distended in this artificial arteriovenous fistula and it is relatively easy to place large bore needles into these vessels under local anaesthesia whenever haemodialysis is required. This method is used when repeated dialyses are required in the treatment of chronic renal failure.

Peritoneal dialysis. The principle of this method is to use the peritoneal cavity as the semipermeable dialysing membrane. A plastic catheter is inserted into the peritoneal cavity and repeated lavage is carried out using an electrolyte-sugar solution similar to that employed in the bath of the artificial kidney (Fig. 15.6). The technique is relatively simple but strict precautions are required because of the risk of peritoneal infection.

Fig. 15.5. The Scribner shunt. This enables repeated dialyses to be performed, the arterio-venous shunt being re-connected after each session.

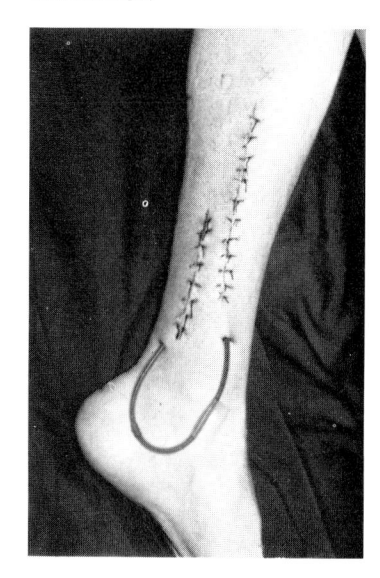

THE INVESTIGATION OF URINARY TRACT DISEASE

Thanks to modern laboratory and X-ray techniques, surgical conditions of the urinary tract can now be diagnosed with considerable precision. Like every other system in the body, the surgeon proceeds through three logical steps in making a diagnosis. First, a detailed history is taken, second a careful clinical examination is carried out and third, if the diagnosis is still in doubt or requires confirmation, special investigations are performed.

Three important points must be emphasized in diseases of the urinary system:
1. It is wise to think of the whole urinary tract as a unit rather than as a series of independent structures since disease of any one part

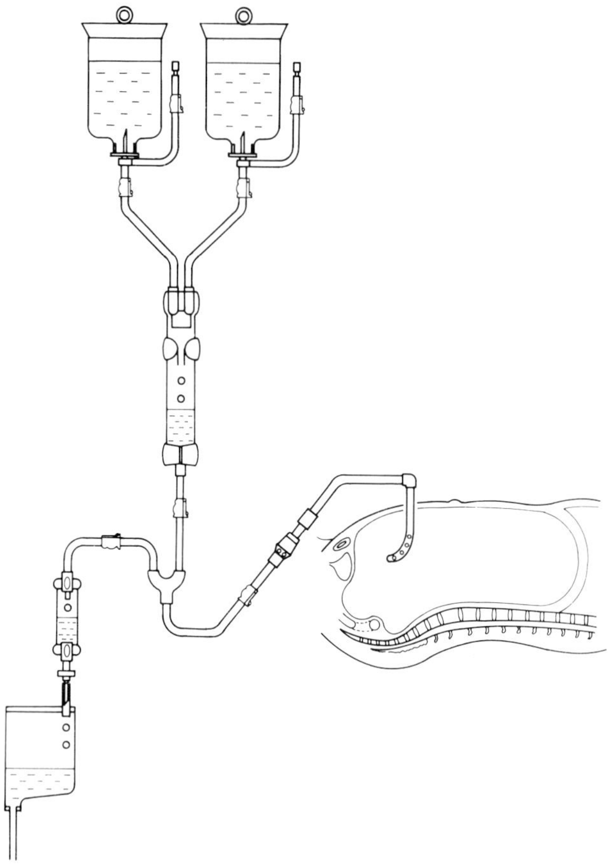

Fig. 15.6. The apparatus used in peritoneal dialysis. Repeated lavage is carried out and waste products passing from the blood stream across the peritoneum are removed in the effluent fluid.

may often have effects elsewhere. For example, a tumour of the bladder may present because it is producing haematuria (blood in the urine); however, it may grow over and obstruct the ureteric orifice, produce hydronephrosis of the occluded kidney and the patient presents to the doctor not with bladder symptoms but with pain in the loin from his obstructed kidney (Fig. 15.7). As another example, a patient with tuberculosis of the kidney may not have any symptoms referrable to the kidney itself, but may complain only of frequency of micturition and dysuria (pain on passing urine) from secondary tuberculous infection of the bladder.

2. As a corollary to this, many of the principal symptoms of urinary disease, for example blood or pus in the urine, pain or frequency of micturition or passage of stones in the urine, may come from any part of the urinary tract and it is wise to tick off the organs one by one from the kidney down to the urethra. As an example, haematuria

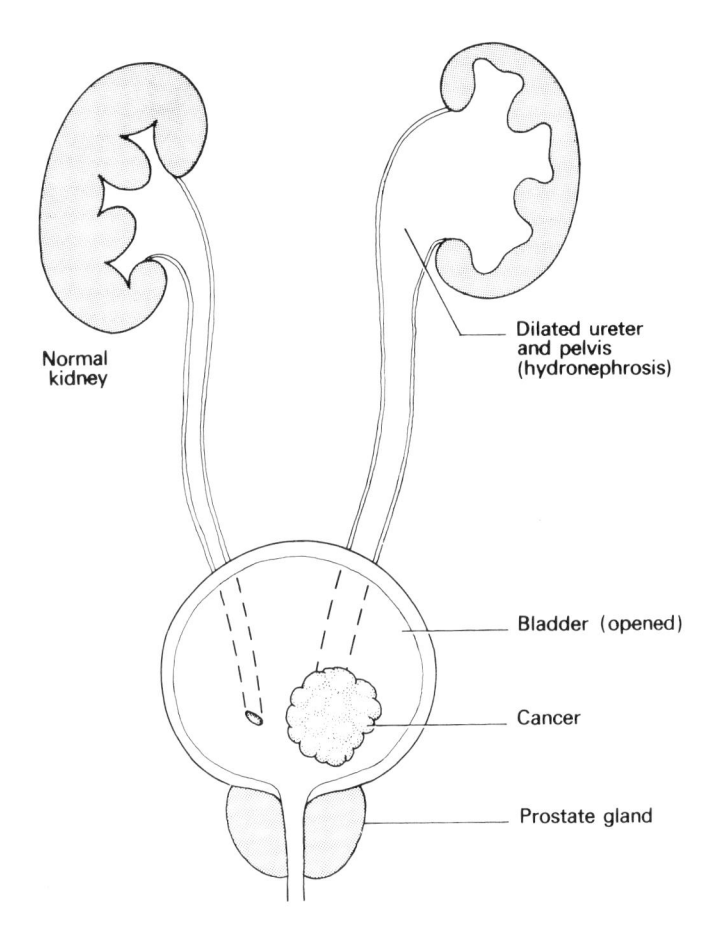

Fig. 15.7. Carcinoma of the bladder producing a hydronephrosis as a result of ureteric obstruction.

may arise from the kidney (trauma, stone, tumour, tuberculosis), the ureter (stone or tumour), the bladder (trauma, cystitis, benign and malignant tumours), the prostate ('prostatic varices', which are distended veins over an enlarged prostate) or from the urethra (trauma). This is illustrated in diagram form in Fig. 15.8.

3. Patients can lead a normal life with only one kidney provided that this is reasonably healthy. However, many examples of urinary tract disease have bilateral renal involvement. Here the patient may present with not so much urinary symptoms as with the features of renal failure (*uraemia*)—lethargy, mental impairment, headache, vomiting and diarrhoea. It is obvious that unless disturbance of the urinary tract is thought of, the patient may well find himself in a clinic dealing with gastro-intestinal, neurological or even psychiatric illness!

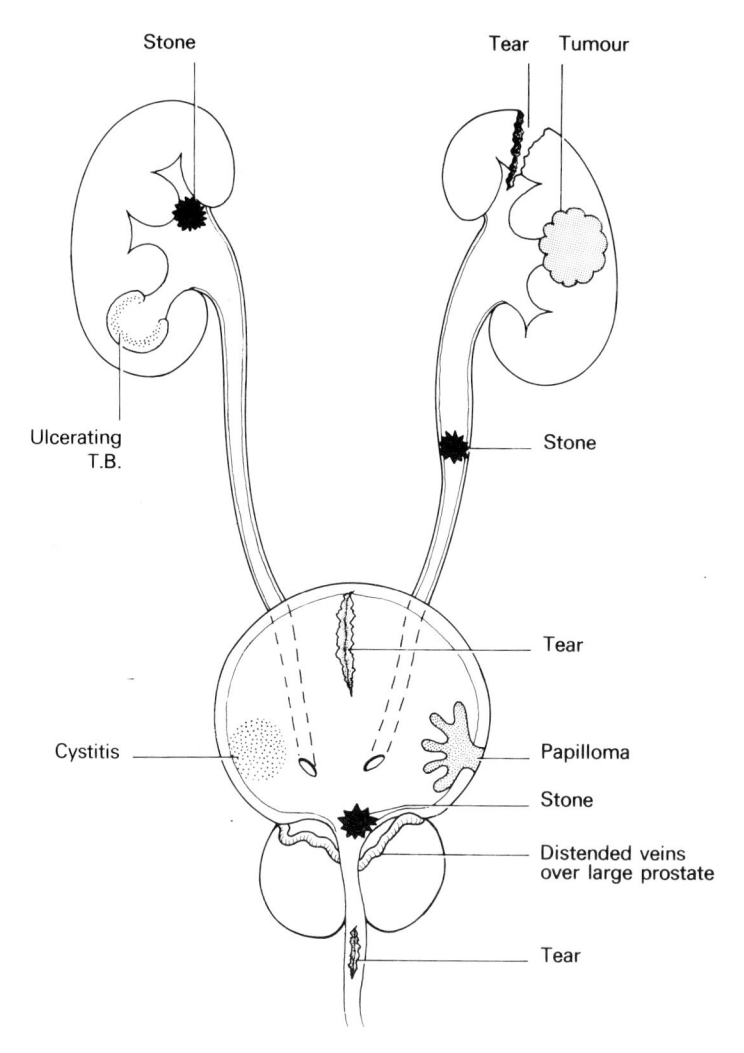

Fig. 15.8. Some important causes of bleeding in the urinary tract.

History

The majority of patients with surgical disease affecting the urinary tract present with one or more of the following symptoms:
1. Disturbance of micturition
2. Haematuria
3. Pain

Disturbance of micturition

Normal micturition (the act of urination) occurs three or four times during the day and depends to a large extent on the amount of fluid intake. It is rare for healthy people to have to pass urine at night (*nocturia*). Frequency, urgency to pass urine and *dysuria* (painful, difficult micturition) suggest urinary infection or prostatic obstruction, but note that patients with a perfectly healthy urinary tract but suffering from diabetes mellitus or diabetes insipidus may have very severe frequency.

Incontinence of urine may be due to damage to the bladder sphincter mechanism, enlargement of the prostate or 'overflow', when a chronically obstructed bladder trickles urine almost continuously. *Retention* of urine usually indicates obstruction of the bladder outlet. However, note that both urinary incontinence and retention may also be caused by diseases of the central nervous system, for example multiple sclerosis or spinal tumour, which interfere with the nervous pathways concerned with micturition.

Haematuria (blood in the urine)

Haematuria always calls for most careful investigation, and may be due to lesions anywhere along the urinary tract (see Fig. 15.8). Occasionally haematuria occurs in a patient with a perfectly normal urinary system but who has a bleeding tendency. The commonest cause of this is an overdose of one of the anticoagulants, for example heparin or dicoumarol.

Pain

A diseased kidney may give a dull aching pain in the loin which may cause the patient to complain of 'backache'. Obstruction of the pelvis of the kidney or of the ureter, especially by a calculus, results in typical ureteric colic, which is extremely severe, usually continuous, radiates along the course of the ureter into the scrotum or vulva and may make the victim roll about in agony. It is often accompanied by vomiting and sweating. Bladder pain is localised in the suprapubic region and is often accompanied by *dysuria* (pain on passing urine) or *strangury* (repeated painful attempts to micturate).

Examination

The general examination is important; renal failure may give rise to the typical uraemic picture of an anaemic, drowsy, dehydrated patient with a dry, brown tongue.

Local examination may reveal an enlarged kidney or renal tenderness, distension of the bladder or evidence of localised testicular disease. Rectal examination is extremely important because of the considerable information it gives about the status of the prostate gland.

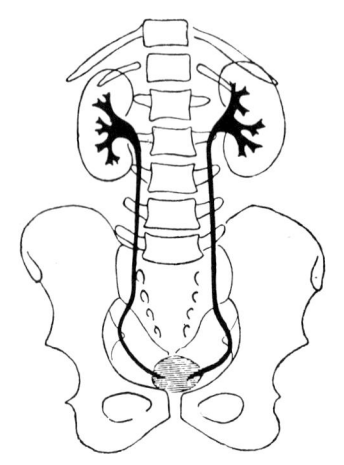

Fig. 15.9. Tracing from a normal intravenous pyelogram.

Fig. 15.10. Cystoscopes. The uppermost photograph shows the telescope which slides along the shaft of the cystoscope. The middle instrument is the examining cystoscope, the lowermost the operating cystoscope, through which a ureteric catheter or diathermy probe can be introduced into the bladder.

Laboratory and X-ray examinations

Urine. It goes without saying that the first investigation of urinary tract disease is a full ward test of the urine, followed, if necessary, by chemical and bacteriological studies for protein, blood, white cells and organisms. For the latter, a midstream specimen of urine is required.

The blood urea is a useful test of renal function. The normal value is below 40 mg %; a value of 60 or 70 mg % indicates definite impairment of renal function. In severe uraemia the level may rise to 300 or 400 mg %.

The intravenous pyelogram (IVP) depends on the excretion of a radio-opaque dye by the kidneys after intravenous injection. The pelvis of the kidneys, the ureters and the bladder are outlined. A further X-ray of the bladder is taken immediately following micturition to give a measure of the amount of residual urine in the bladder (Fig. 15.9).

Patients with poor renal function (indicated by a raised blood urea) fail to excrete an adequate amount of the dye so that under these circumstances the procedure is useless. Some patients are sensitive to iodine and since the dye contains this material an IVP is contraindicated.

Urethroscopy and cystoscopy. By means of these instruments the inside of the urethra and bladder can be directly inspected, together with the ureteric orifices (Fig. 15.10). Tumours and other lesions can be visualised and a biopsy taken for microscopic examination. If

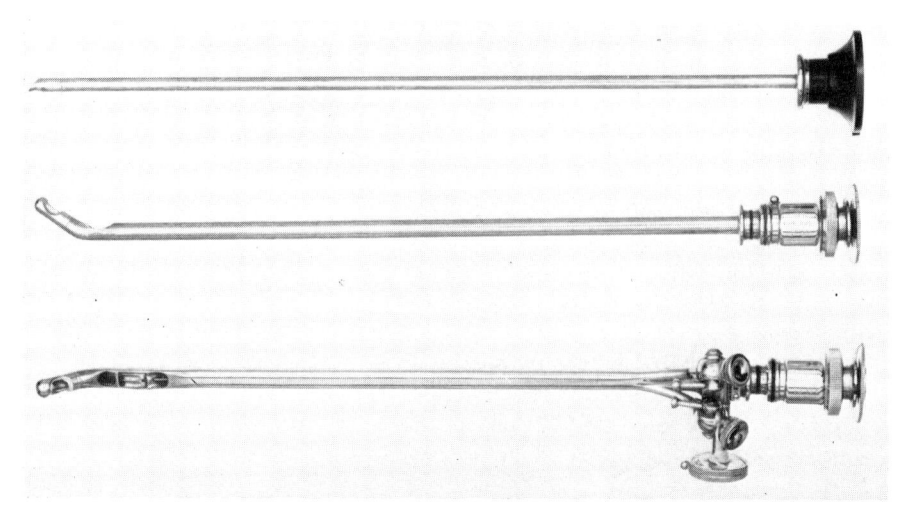

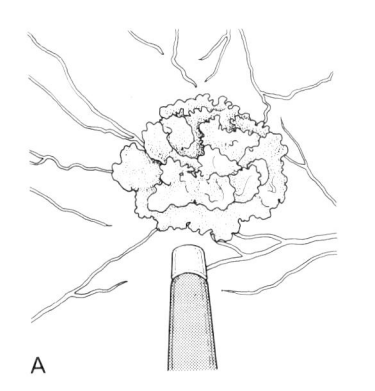

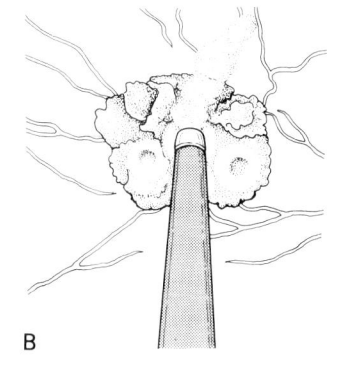

Fig. 15.11. Appearance of a bladder papilloma seen through a cystoscope (A). This can be treated by diathermy coagulation using a fine electrode threaded along the cystoscope (B).

necessary, diathermy coagulation can be performed. (Fig. 15.11). A fine ureteric catheter can be inserted into the ureter via an operating cystoscope so that a specimen of urine can be obtained from each kidney and by injecting radio-opaque dye through the catheter, the pelvis of the kidney can be outlined even if the organ is functioning so poorly that it cannot be demonstrated on an IVP (*retrograde pyelography*).

Micturating cystogram. The bladder can be outlined by injecting radio-opaque dye into its cavity via a fine catheter (cystography). X-rays taken during the act of micturition are useful in the demonstration of abnormal reflux of urine from the bladder into the ureters (vesico-ureteric reflux) which may be responsible for recurrent urinary tract infections. This technique can also be used to outline the outflow tract from the bladder.

Arteriography. In some cases an aortogram is necessary in the detailed investigation of a renal mass. It may be used, for example, to differentiate between a renal cyst and a carcinoma of the kidney. (Fig. 15.12).

KIDNEY TRAUMA

The kidney may be injured by a direct blow in the loin (for example, a kick at football) or occasionally by a penetrating wound. The degree of damage varies from a slight bruise to complete rupture of the organ or avulsion of the kidney from its pedicle (see Fig. 15.8).

Clinical features

Following the accident, there is local pain and tenderness in the flank and a tender mass may develop in the loin. The clue to the

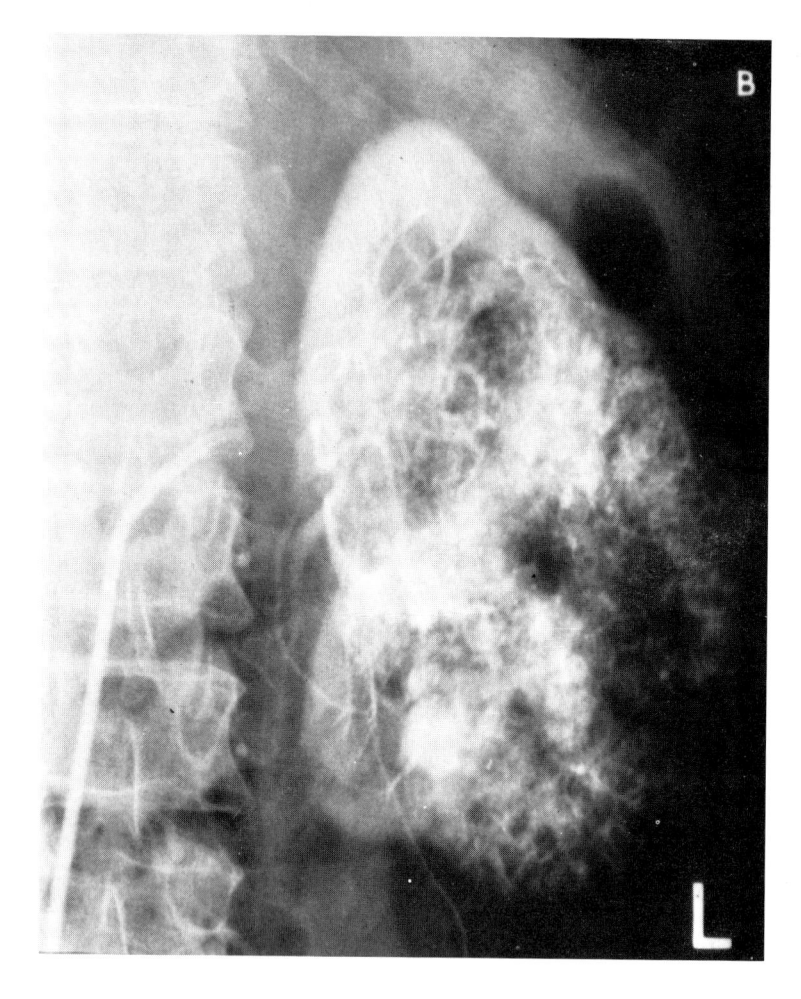

Fig. 15.12. An arteriogram in a case of renal carcinoma. Notice the extraordinarily rich blood supply of the tumour which occupies all but the uppermost part of the kidney. The catheter (which has been passed via the femoral artery, along the aorta and into the left renal artery), can be clearly seen.

renal damage is the presence of blood in the urine but it should be noted that occasionally the ureter is torn away from the kidney so that there may be severe internal bleeding without haematuria.

With modern high speed traffic accidents, it is not unusual for rupture of the kidney to be only a part of multiple injuries and it goes without saying that full examination must be carried out to determine whether there are accompanying fractures, chest injury, etc.

Treatment

Associated injuries will require appropriate treatment. Morphia is administered and shock treated if present by means of a blood transfusion. The patient is placed on a careful shock chart and each specimen of urine that is passed is saved so that it can be seen very readily whether the haematuria is increasing or getting less.

Fortunately, the great majority of renal injuries resolve with bed rest but nephrectomy, or partial nephrectomy, is required if signs of intra-abdominal bleeding continue. An emergency IVP is first taken to ensure that there is a functioning kidney on the other side!

HYDRONEPHROSIS

Hydronephrosis can be defined as an aseptic dilation of the renal pelvis and calyces. There may be an associated dilation of the ureter (hydro-ureter). One or both kidneys may be affected.

The causes of hydronephrosis fall into three large groups:
1. *Congenital.* This is found, as its name would imply, in children and young adults. Although no organic obstruction can be detected at the junction between the dilated pelvis of the kidney and the normal ureter, it is thought that some functional disturbances of peristalsis takes place across the smooth muscle fibres at this zone (Fig. 15.13).
2. *Obstructive.* Anything that produces a partial or intermittent obstruction of urinary outflow will produce hydronephrosis. This obstruction may be unilateral, (for example due to a stone in the ureter), or the block may involve the urethra, (for example a urethral stricture or prostatic hypertrophy) with resultant bilateral hydronephrosis.
3. *Associated with pregnancy.* Some degree of hydronephrosis occurs in pregnancy, the right kidney being rather more affected than the left. It is considered to be due in the main to relaxation of the ureteric muscle as a result of the high circulating level of progesterone. Pressure of the fetal head on the ureters may play some part by causing ureteric obstruction during the later part of the pregnancy.

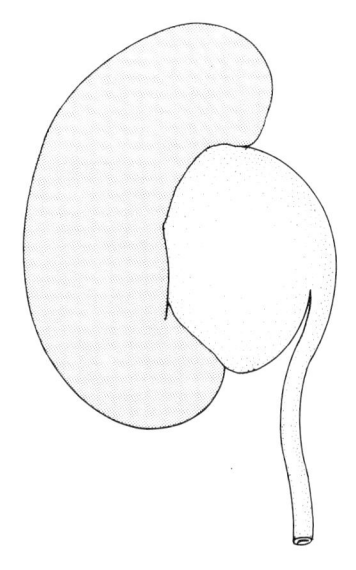

Fig. 15.13. Diagram of a typical hydronephrosis. Note the normal ureter and dilated pelvis.

Clinical features

Uncomplicated hydronephrosis may be symptomless, but more often the patient complains of a dull aching pain in the loin which is often mistaken for 'backache'. If both kidneys are severely affected, there may be the clinical picture of uraemia (see page 321). There may also be the symptoms produced by the underlying cause, for example the ureteric stone or the enlarged prostate.

The great dangers of hydronephrosis are its complications, which are as follows:
1. *Infection*—obviously the stagnant urine is very prone to infec-

tion and any carelessness in catheterizing such a patient may be disastrous. An infected hydroephrosis is termed a *pyonephrosis*.

2. *Stone formation*—phosphatic stones readily deposit in the infected stagnant urine of a pyonephrosis.

3. *Uraemia*—where there is extensive bilateral destruction of renal tissue. This destruction may be aggravated further by stone formation and infection.

4. *Hypertension*—secondary to renal ischaemia.

Special investigations

The urine is examined, but it should be noted that even if the hydronephrosis is infected, obstruction to the ureter may prevent pus from passing down into the bladder.

An intravenous pyelogram demonstrates the enlarged renal pelvis and the swollen, dilated, club-like calyces (Fig. 15.14). If renal func-

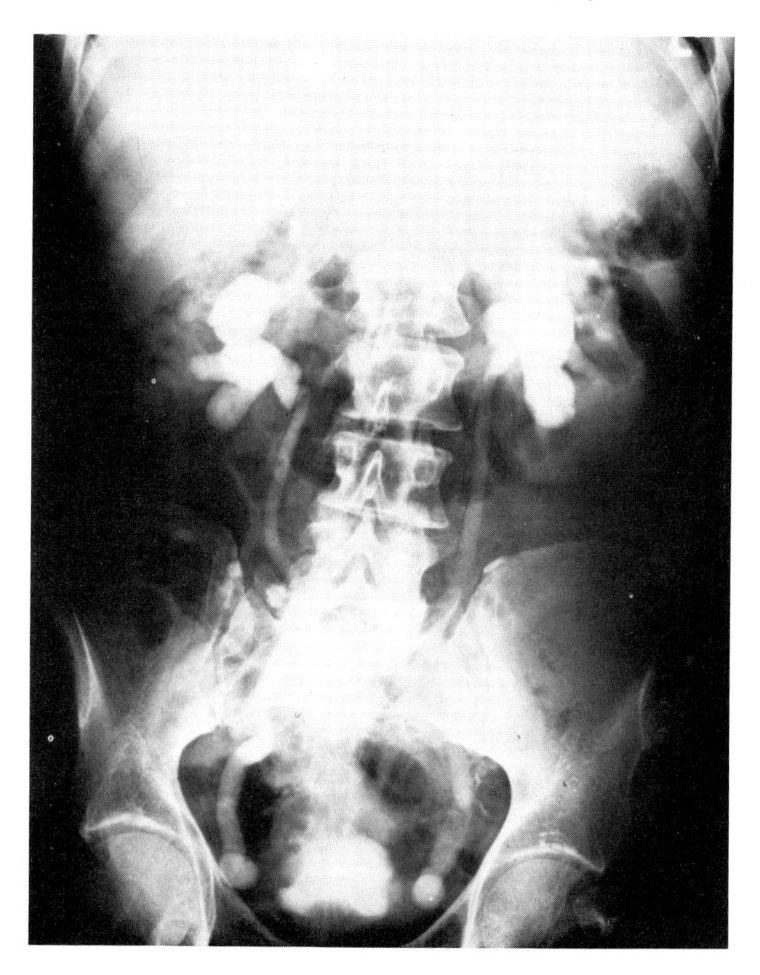

Fig. 15.14. Intravenous pyelogram of bilateral hydronephrosis due to prostatic obstruction.

tion is severely impaired, the kidney may not secrete dye and all that will be seen on X-ray is the outline of the distended kidney. In such a case a retrograde pyelogram may be required to show the exact anatomy of the hydronephrosis and to demonstrate any obstructive cause in the ureter. This is performed by passing a ureteric catheter up the ureter via an operating cystoscope.

Treatment

This is directed at removal of any underlying obstructive cause of the hydronephrosis. In the congenital group, a plastic operation at the pelvi-ureteric junction may save the kidney from progressive damage; the most popular operation is the Anderson-Hynes procedure (Fig. 15.15). A completely useless kidney, particularly if it is infected or almost replaced by a staghorn calculus, requires nephrectomy but obviously the surgeon must first satisfy himself that there is adequate function of the opposite kidney.

RENAL TUBERCULOSIS

With the general decline of tuberculosis in the Western world, involvement of the urogenital tract is also being seen with decreasing frequency.

Pathology (Fig. 15.16)

Tuberculosis of the urinary tract must obviously be secondary to a primary focus elsewhere, since the bacilli can only enter the body

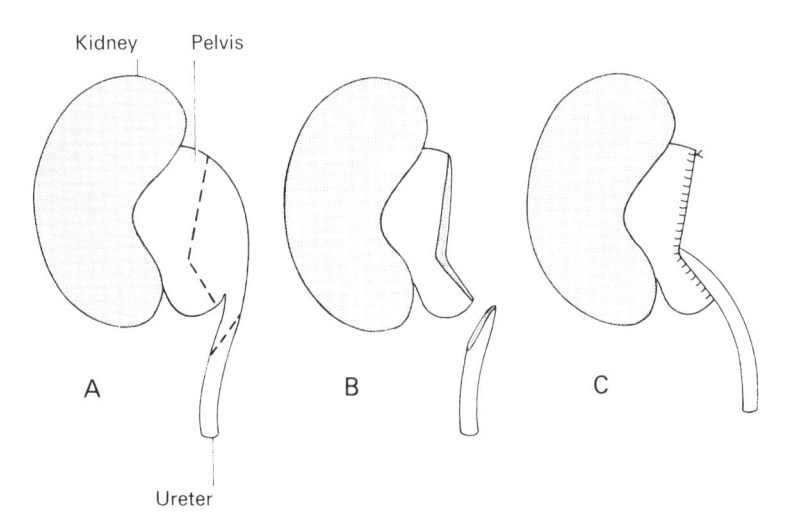

Fig. 15.15. The Anderson-Hynes pyeloplasty. A greater part of the dilated pelvis is excised together with the pelvi-ureteric obstruction. A plastic reconstruction of the pelvis is then performed.

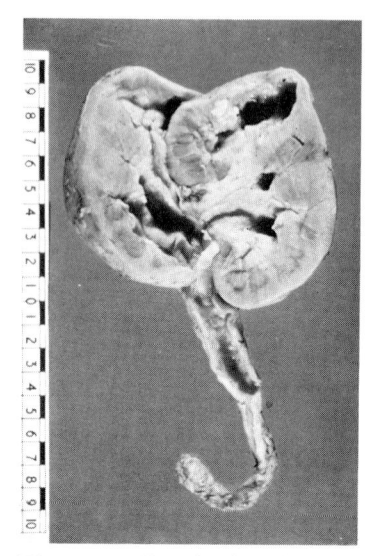

Fig. 15.16. Renal tuberculosis; an operative specimen. The pelvis is hydronephrotic and the renal substance is studded with tuberculous abscesses containing caseous material.

either via the lungs or the gut. About one quarter of the cases have pulmonary tuberculosis but in many patients the original focus may be quiescent at the time of active renal disease.

Bacteria reach the kidneys via the blood stream and early lesions are found near the junction of the cortex and medulla of the kidney. These enlarge, coalesce and eventually produce extensive destruction of the renal substance. The tuberculous abscess, full of cheesy (caseous) pus, then ruptures into the pelvis of the kidney. The infection spreads by infiltrating the ureter and frequently involves the bladder in a tuberculous cystitis. In the male, the epididymis and seminal vesicles may become implicated. Thickening of the ureter may produce obstruction which can lead to tuberculous pyonephrosis and the useless bag of pus may eventually become calcified. Untreated, the opposite kidney often becomes involved, but this probably represents a separate blood stream spread.

The introduction of modern antituberculous drugs has modified the classical pathological picture of this disease. In most patients nowadays the disease process is arrested and healing takes place with the production of fibrous tissue. In early cases this merely produces a small scar in the kidney but if treatment is only commenced when the disease is advanced, then this fibrous scar tissue may lead to stricture formation within the pelvi-ureteric system and this results in secondary hydronephrosis. Fibrosis of the infected bladder may produce gross contraction on healing ('the golf ball bladder').

Clinical features

The patient is usually a young adult, often between the ages of 20 and 40. Frequently there is a history of present or previous tuberculosis elsewhere. In the early stages the symptoms are mild and may indeed be entirely absent. Usually the patient first complains of frequency of micturition which results from the tuberculous cystitis. There may also be pain on micturition, and the patient may notice either pus or blood in the urine. In more advanced cases, the pain and frequency of micturition becomes intense because of extensive involvement of the bladder and its diminished capacity from fibrosis. The constitutional symptoms of tuberculosis—fever, night sweats, loss of weight and anaemia—may then become manifest.

Examination is usually negative but the affected kidney may be tender and is sometimes palpable. The epididymis may become hard and thickened if diseased, and rectal examination may show thickening of the involved prostate and seminal vesicles.

Special investigations

Urine. The examination of the urine is all-important in making a diagnosis of tuberculosis of the kidney. Routine ward testing often reveals the presence of protein, pus and blood; the last two are easily confirmed by examining a drop of urine under the microscope. The reaction is usually acid. Ordinary techniques of culturing the urine for bacteria give no growth because the tubercle bacilli are delicate organisms which do not grow on ordinary agar plates; (for this reason one is always very suspicious of a urine which is acid in reaction, contains pus cells and yet is apparently sterile on routine laboratory examination—tuberculosis *must* be excluded). Early morning (and therefore concentrated) mid-stream specimens of urine are to be examined on at least three occasions; the bacteriologist spins down some of the urine and stains it with Ziehl-Nielsen's stain which involves washing the stained slide in acid. Most bacteria give up the stain under this treatment but the tuberculous bacilli are 'acid-fast' and, if present in sufficient numbers, can be seen under the microscope. The next step is to carry out a special culture of the urine on Lowenstein Jensen's medium, which is specially enriched and on which the delicate tubercle bacilli thrive. Whereas most organisms grow within 24 hours or so, these bacilli must be cultured for up to 6 weeks before they can be seen in colonies on this medium. Finally the urine is injected into a guinea-pig which is sacrificed after 6 weeks and, in most cases, will be found to have foci of tuberculosis within its body.

IVP. An excretory pyelogram will demonstrate the destruction of kidney tissue—there may be irregularity of the calyces or cavitation. Hydronephrosis may be evident and in late cases there may be no function of the destroyed kidney. Frequently calcification occurs in the tuberculous caseating pus and this shows up as patchy white spots on the X-ray.

Cystoscopy may reveal a decreased capacity of the bladder the wall of which may be inflamed and may show white tubercles. The ureteric orifices may be seen to be held rigidly open by fibrosis ('golf hole ureters').

Treatment

Specific chemotherapy must not be commenced until diagnosis has been confirmed by the bacteriologist, since, once undertaken, treatment must be continuous and prolonged. In the first instance streptomycin 1 gm, I.N.A.H. 400 mg and P.A.S. 15 gm are prescribed daily. The urine is checked by culture each month and the treatment is continued until the urine has remained sterile for six months; this usually means about a year of intensive therapy. During this time sanatorium care is probably advisable so that the patient's general condition can be maintained and strict supervision of drug treatment carried out.

Surgery is only indicated in a minority of patients with advanced disease or where complications occur. A totally destroyed kidney, for example, may require nephrectomy. The damage produced by fibrosis may also indicate surgery. Thus late hydronephrosis with a totally destroyed kidney secondary to fibrosis of the ureter may require nephrectomy and a contracted bladder may require a plastic enlargement or transplantation of the ureters into an isolated segment of ileum draining as an ileostomy (see Fig. 15.25).

STONE IN THE URINARY TRACT

It is convenient to consider under one heading the topic of stone formation throughout the urinary system.

Aetiology

Predisposing factors can be grouped under three headings—inadequate drainage, excess of normal constituents in the urine, and the presence of abnormal constituents. It must be admitted, however, that many stones form without any apparent explanation so that obviously there are other factors of which, at present, we are quite ignorant.

1. Inadequate drainage

In any situation where urine stagnates, there calculi may deposit. This may be within a hydronephrosis, in a diverticulum of the bladder, or in the inadequately drained bladder which results from enlargement of the prostate or from a stricture of the urethra.

2. Excess of normal constituents

Kidney stones are especially likely to occur in tropical countries where dehydration results in an extremely concentrated urine. Patients with gout have an excess of uric acid in the serum which is excreted in the urine and which may be accompanied by uric acid stone formation. Hyperparathyroidism (see page 380) produces an increase in serum calcium and therefore urinary calcium; stone formation is the commonest manifestation of this condition.

3. *Presence of abnormal constituents*

Infection in the urine produces epithelial sloughs upon which stones may deposit, and this is particularly likely to occur in the presence of obstruction (e.g. pyonephrosis or chronic urinary retention). Any foreign body introduced into the urinary tract may form a nidus upon which calculi may form; thus stones may deposit on unabsorbable sutures inserted at operation or on a fragment of broken-off catheter tip. Patients have been known to introduce all sorts of strange objects into the bladder and most Hospital museums have stones with a centre made up of such things as hair pins. In the museum at Westminster Hospital we have a stone whose core is the rubber from a windscreen wiper. Another example of an abnormal constituent is cystinuria; in this condition the patient has an inborn defect in which the kidney tubules are unable to reabsorb the amino-acid cystine, which may then be deposited as cystine stones.

Patients who are immobilised on their backs for many months at a time, for example, long-stay orthopaedic cases or paraplegics, are particularly prone to develop calculi in the urinary tract. All three mechanisms that we have described may be at play; in the first place the urine stagnates in the kidney in the recumbent position and so we have the factor of inadequate drainage. Mobilisation of calcium takes place from the skeleton in these bed-bound patients and the excess is excreted in the kidneys. Finally, many of the paraplegics will have undergone repeated catheterisation, so that the third factor, purulent material in the urinary tract, may be present.

An important part of the nurse's duties in looking after paraplegic patients is prophylaxis against stone formation; this comprises regular moving of the patient, to promote urinary drainage, maintaining adequate fluid input, meticulous care of any catheter drainage system and regular testing of the urine for the presence of blood or pus.

Composition of urinary stones

The three common stones are phosphate, oxalate and urate (Fig. 15.17).

Phosphatic calculi are composed of a mixture of calcium, ammonium and magnesium phosphate ('triple phosphate stone'). These are hard, white, crumbly and rather like chalk. They are nearly always

Fig. 15.17. The three common varieties of urinary stone: left, a 'staghorn' phosphatic stone, middle, a smooth urate stone, right, a spiky oxalate stone.

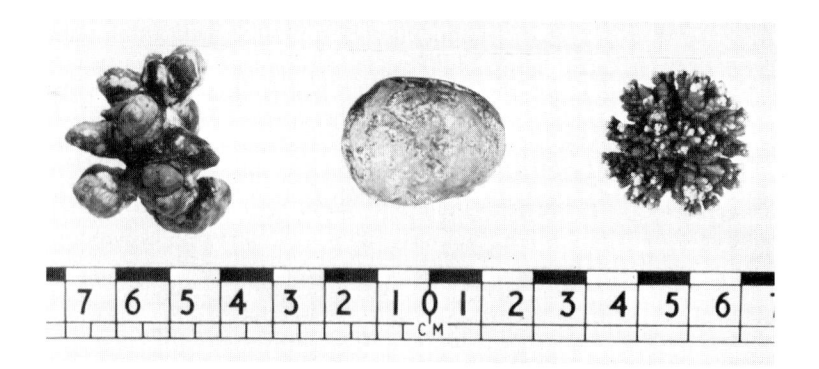

found in infected urine and produce a large 'staghorn' calculus which is found within a pyonephrosis.

Calcium oxalate calculi are hard with sharp spikes. These damage the urinary epithelium and the resultant bleeding usually colours the stone dark brown or black.

Uric acid and urate calculi are hard, brown and smooth. Pure uric acid stones are radio-translucent but, fortunately for diagnosis, most contain enough calcium to make them visible on X-rays.

Clinical features (Fig. 15.18).

Kidney. If the stone is embedded within the substance of the kidney, it may be symptom-free. If it is situated in the renal pelvis, the stone produces a dull loin pain. Impaction of the stone at the pelvi-ureteric junction, or its migration down the ureter, produces the dreadful agony of ureteric colic. The pain now radiates from the loin to the groin, is of great severity and is accompanied by restlessness, so that the patient is quite unable to lie still. There is often accompanying nausea, vomiting and sweating. Haematuria is frequently present and may be either obvious to the naked eye or may be detected under the microscope only; its presence is an extremely helpful means of clinching the clinical diagnosis.

Bladder. The typical triad of symptoms of bladder stone comprises *frequency* of micturition, severe *pain* (which is felt above the pubis, in the perineum or in the tip of the penis), and *haematuria*. Symptoms are particularly marked when the patient is in the upright position so that the stone lies over the bladder neck.

Urethra. The passage of a stone along the urethra may be accompanied by pain or may be hardly noticed. A large stone may impact and produce retention of urine, although this is surprisingly unusual.

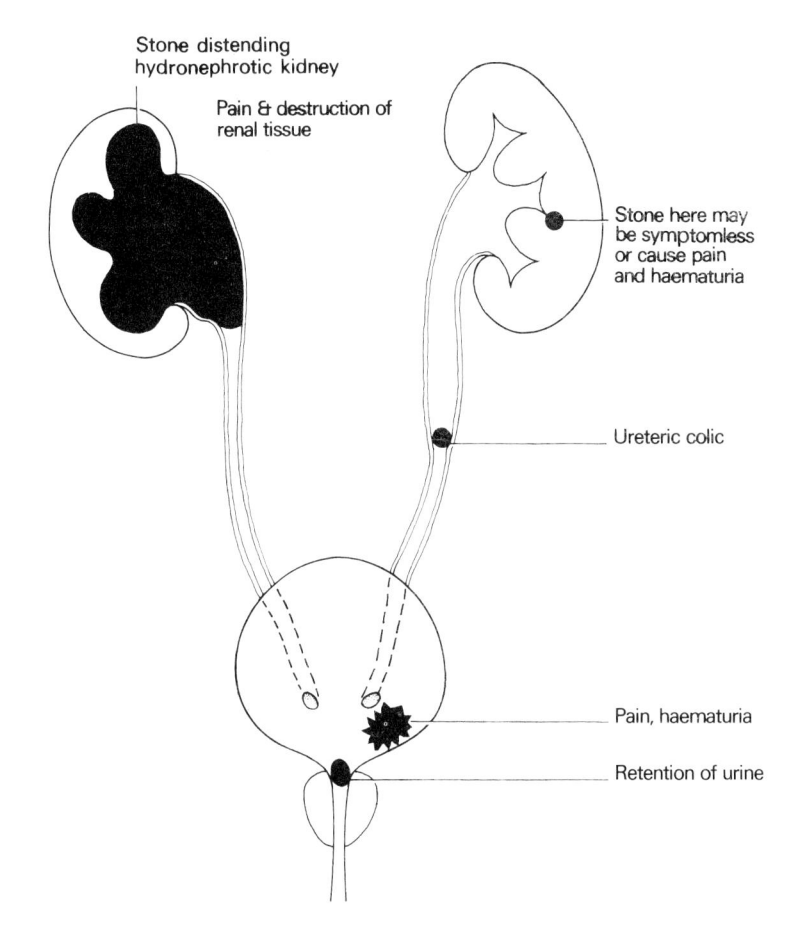

Fig. 15.18. Diagram of the effects of urinary calculi.

Special investigations

The following laboratory and X-ray investigations are carried out in patients with suspected stone:
1. *The urine* is tested for the presence of blood.
2. *A plain abdominal X-ray* will show the presence of a stone in 90% of cases (Fig. 15.19).
3. *An intravenous pyelogram* will demonstrate the exact anatomy of the urinary system, e.g. the presence of associated hydronephrosis, although a completely obstructed kidney may show no function whatsoever (see Fig. 15.19).
4. *Cystoscopy* is used to visualise bladder stones.

When a stone is present, it is important to try to determine its aetiology; the urine is therefore cultured for bacteria and examined microscopically and chemically for the presence of cystine crystals. A serum calcium estimation is carried out and a value above 11 mg%

Fig. 15.19. A plain X-ray of the abdomen reveals a large calculus in the right kidney (A). An intravenous pyelogram demonstrates the dilated pelvis of the right kidney and the normal function on the left side (B).

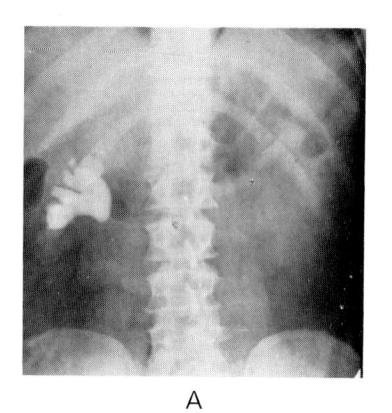

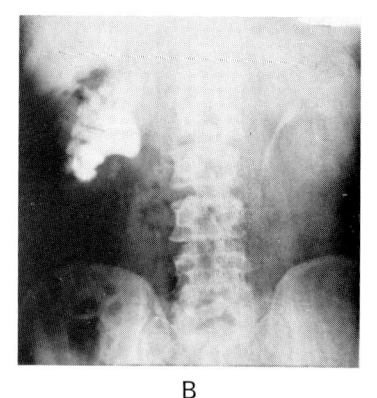

is very suspicious of the presence of a parathyroid tumour. A high serum uric acid may be found with urate stones.

Complications of urinary stone

1. *Hydronephrosis*—this results from an intermittent or incomplete obstruction of the ureter by a stone.
2. *Infection*—(pyelonephritis, pyonephrosis).
3. *Anuria*—due either to impaction of stones into the ureter on each side or blockage of the ureter in a remaining solitary kidney, the other kidney having either been previously removed or destroyed by disease. Very occasionally reflex anuria may result from a stone blocking one ureter with 'shut-down' of the normal opposite kidney.
4. *Retention of urine*—an unusual complication due to a stone becoming impacted in the urethra.

Treatment of stone in the urinary tract

Kidney

A small stone lodged in the kidney substance and not producing symptoms can be left alone although the patient must be kept under periodic X-ray survey. Large stones must be removed either by an incision through the substance of the kidney (*nephrolithotomy*) or, if at all possible, through the pelvis of the kidney (*pyelolithotomy*) since obviously this latter procedure can be effected with less damage to kidney tissue. If there is an associated hydronephrosis, removal of the stone alone is rarely sufficient and, indeed, may be followed in only a few months by recurrence of the calculus. It may be necessary to remove the lower pole of the kidney (*partial nephrectomy*) in order to ensure adequate drainage or to carry out a plastic operation on the pelvi-ureteric junction. Where the kidney is grossly and irreparably damaged, *nephrectomy* should be performed.

The ureter

Acute ureteric colic is treated by repeated injections of pethidine to relieve severe pain, together with a high fluid intake. The great majority of small stones within the ureter pass spontaneously. The smaller the calculus and lower down the ureter that the stone is situated, the more likely it is to pass, but stones up to the size and shape of a date stone, particularly if they are smooth, can be passed spontaneously.

If pain continues and x-rays show that the stone is not advancing, it may be possible to dilate the ureter via a ureteric catheter passed through a cystoscope, or it may be possible to fish out the stone by means of a number of ingenious snares and baskets which can be passed along catheters into the ureter under X-ray control in the operating theatre (Fig. 15.20). If these procedures fail then the stone must be removed surgically (*ureterolithotomy*).

Acute calculous anuria, due to blockage of both ureters by stone (or of the only remaining ureter where one kidney has already been destroyed by calculi, or removed surgically), is treated by catheterising the ureters. If the ureteric catheter cannot be passed beyond the obstruction, the impacted stone must be removed at operation. If the patient is severely uraemic his general condition must first be improved, either by haemodialysis or peritoneal dialysis.

Bladder

If the stone is small it may pass spontaneously, but if not it may be removed either by means of crushing with a *lithotrite* (Fig. 15.21)

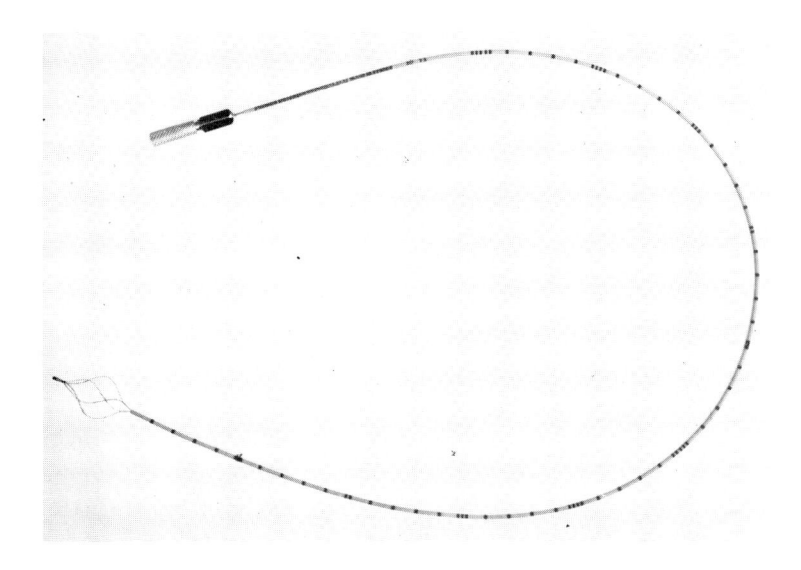

Fig. 15.20. A Dormia basket, which can be threaded through a cystoscope into the ureter for removal of a small ureteric calculus.

Fig. 15.21. A lithotrite used for crushing a bladder stone.

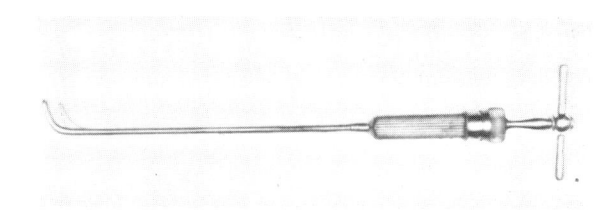

or more commonly by open cystotomy through a suprapubic incision. At this operation, any underlying cause, such as a large obstructing prostate, must be dealt with or the stone will simply recur.

In every case of stone in the urinary tract an attempt is made to determine any predisposing factor and to eliminate this; thus renal infection is dealt with and any obstructive lesion within the urinary tract may require surgical correction. A small percentage of recurrent and bilateral stones are found to be due to a parathyroid tumour (see page 380) removal of which will prevent further recurrences. In every case the patient should be instructed to drink liberal amounts of fluid of any sort, in order to encourage the production of a copious, dilute urine.

TUMOURS OF THE KIDNEY

Renal tumours are divided into those arising from the kidney itself and those derived from the renal pelvis. The latter grow from the transitional cell epithelium which lines the pelvis of the kidney as well as the ureter, the bladder and prostatic part of the urethra ('the uro-epithelium') so that tumours arising anywhere along this pathway are pathologically identical.

The two principal tumours of the kidney are the *nephroblastoma*, which usually occurs in children under four, and the *adenocarcinoma*, which usually occurs over the age of forty. Benign tumours and secondary tumours of the kidney are rare.

Tumours of the renal pelvis are the benign papilloma and malignant carcinoma.

NEPHROBLASTOMA

This is the commonest name for a cancer which is also termed Wilm's tumour, embryoma or adenomyosarcoma.

It it an extremely rapidly growing tumour which usually arises in children, although occasionally it affects adolescents. The tumour originates in the embryonic renal tissue and is made up of both epithelial and connective tissue elements. It is rapidly growing, soon invades surrounding tissues and the regional lymph nodes, and then spreads via the blood stream to the lungs and liver.

Clinical features

Rapid growth produces a large mass in the loin. Rather surprisingly, the renal pelvis is only involved late in the disease and therefore haematuria is relatively uncommon.

Treatment

If possible nephrectomy is performed and this is usually followed by radiotherapy. Occasionally a massive tumour may be shrunk down sufficiently by pre-operative irradiation to allow subsequent removal. In advanced cases cytotoxic agents may be employed.

ADENOCARCINOMA

This tumour is also termed the *Grawitz tumour*, after the German professor of pathology who first described it, or a *Hypernephroma*, an old term which dates back to the days when it was thought to arise from suprarenal tissue above the kidney.

Pathology

This tumour is the commonest of all renal growths. Men are more often affected than women and the patients are usually 40 years of age or over. The tumour appears as a large, vascular golden-yellow mass and is usually situated in one or other pole of the kidney (Fig. 15.22).

The tumour spreads directly through the renal substance and then invades the fatty capsule around the kidney. It disseminates by

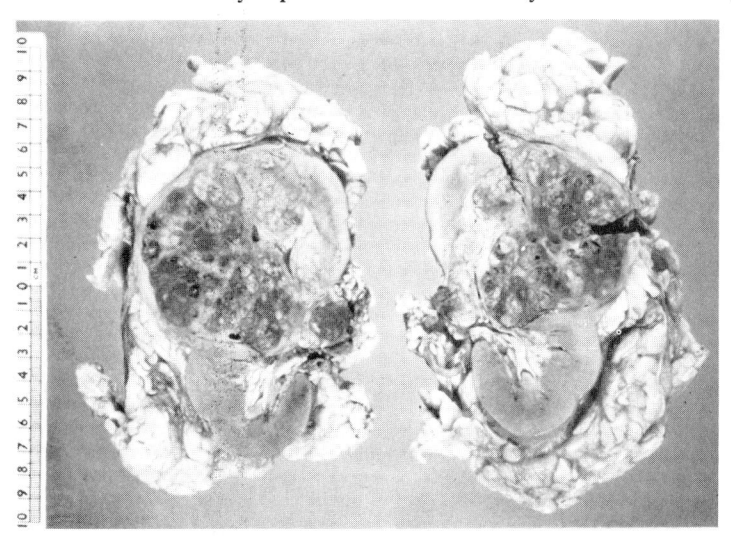

Fig. 15.22. A renal carcinoma (hypernephroma). The kidney has been bisected to show the massive tumour which occupies the upper half of the organ.

the lymphatics to the lymph nodes adjacent to the aorta and also tends to grow along the renal vein into the inferior vena cava; it then spreads by the blood stream to the lung, bones, brain and elsewhere.

Clinical features

About 40% of the patients present with haematuria; another 40% notice a mass in the abdomen or aching pain in the loin. The remaining 20% of patients manifest either with secondary deposits, for example a pathological fracture (Fig. 15.23), or else with the general features of malignant disease—anaemia, loss of weight and anorexia.

Investigations

The urine nearly always contains blood, which may be detected macroscopically or require microscopic examination. *The intra-*

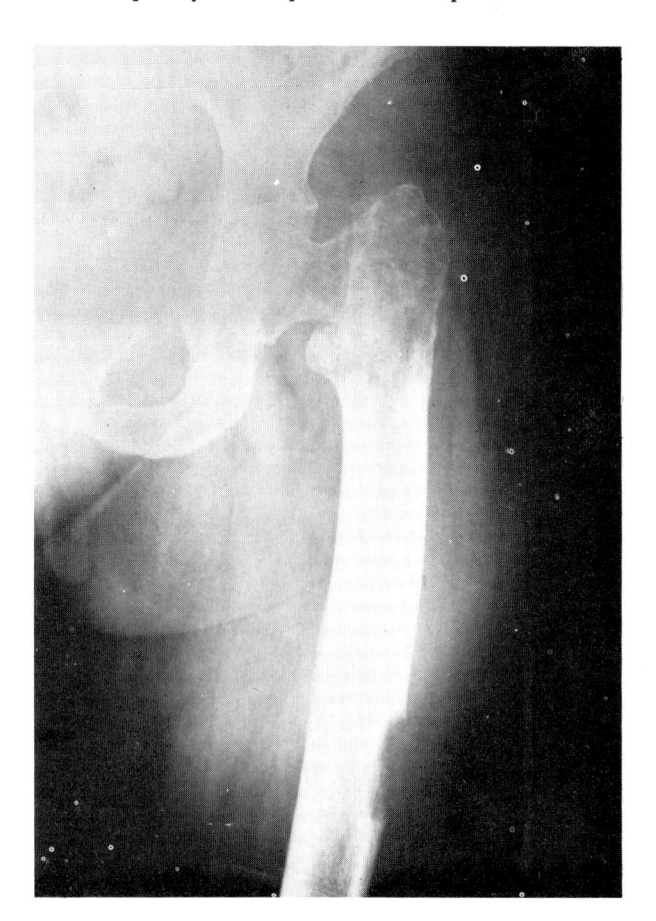

Fig. 15.23. A pathological fracture through a secondary deposit in the femoral neck. Notice a further deposit in the shaft of the femur. The patient had a renal carcinoma.

venous pyelogram shows distortion of the kidney by the tumour (Fig. 15.24). *Aortography* may be useful in doubtful cases. It demonstrates a typical tumour circulation and differentiates the avascular filling defect of a renal cyst (see Fig. 15.12).

A chest X-ray should always be performed for possible lung secondary deposits, which, if present, have a typical cannon-ball appearance.

Treatment

Nephrectomy is carried out provided there is no evidence of distant spread of the tumour.

TUMOURS OF THE RENAL PELVIS

Tumours arising from the transitional cell epithelium of the renal pelvis and ureter vary in malignancy from benign papillomas to invasive carcinomas.

Patients present either with haematuria or with hydronephrosis due to ureteric obstruction.

Treatment comprises nephrectomy combined with excision of the ureter, if this is involved.

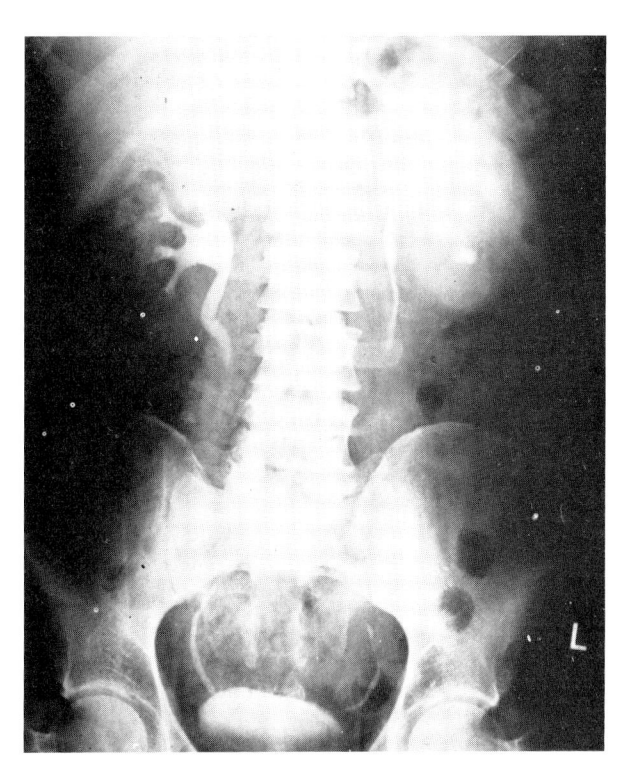

Fig. 15.24. An intravenous pyelogram showing a left-sided renal carcinoma. The kidney is enlarged and there is gross distortion of the calyces.

The bladder

Anatomy

The urinary bladder of a normal subject is uncomfortably distended by half a pint (250 ml) of fluid. When fully distended, the adult bladder projects from the pelvic cavity into the abdomen, stripping the peritoneum upwards from the anterior abdominal wall. The surgeon utilises this fact in carrying out an extra-peritoneal incision into the bladder. The bladder lining is made up of transitional epithelium which, unlike any other epithelium, is completely resistant to continuous soaking with urine. The muscle coat is formed by a crisscross arrangement of involuntary muscle fibres which condense around the orifice of the bladder to form the *internal urethral sphincter*. The ureters enter the bladder posteriorly and the triangular area bounded by the ureteric orifices and the junction with the urethra is termed the *trigone*. In this area the mucosa is adherent to the underlying muscle, whereas elsewhere it is only loosely attached and is thrown into folds when the bladder is empty.

CONGENITAL ABNORMALITIES

Fortunately these are uncommon. The bladder may fail to develop normally so that the ureters and the trigone open directly on to the anterior abdominal wall, a condition termed *ectopia vesicae*. There is frequently an associated maldevelopment of the pubic bones, with failure of the pubes to meet at the symphysis. The child is, of course, completely incontinent of urine and may eventually die of ascending urinary infection. Malignant change may take place in the exposed bladder mucosa.

Treatment

The most satisfactory procedure is to implant the ureters, either into the colon or into an ileal loop with an ileostomy (uretero-ileostomy), combined with excision of the bladder mucosa (Fig. 15.25). Other surgeons attempt to reconstruct the bladder but in many cases this proves unsuccessful.

RUPTURE OF THE BLADDER

The bladder may be ruptured either into the peritoneal cavity or into the extra-peritoneal tissues. *Rupture into the peritoneum* may follow

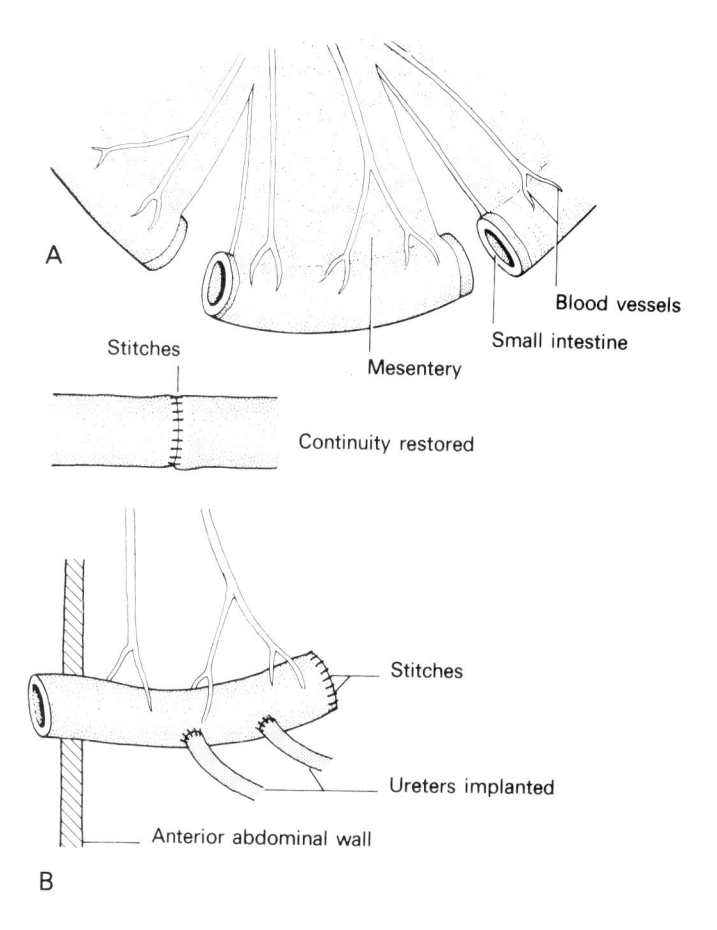

Fig. 15.25. Ureteric transplantation into an ileal loop.

a penetrating wound (for example a bullet) or a crush injury to the pelvis when the bladder is distended. Occasionally the bladder may be perforated by a cystoscope or by a rigid catheter and rarely the over-distended bladder in acute retention may rupture spontaneously. *Extra-peritoneal rupture* is more common; the bladder may be penetrated by a fragment of bone in fracture of the pelvis, or is sometimes wounded during a hernia operation or in a vaginal repair of a cystocele.

Clinical features

If the bladder ruptures into the peritoneal cavity there results the typical picture of a peritonitis, with severe generalised pain and rigidity of the abdominal wall. Extra-peritoneal rupture is associated with extravasation of a mixture of blood and urine into the pelvic tissues which produces a painful swelling rising out of the pelvis.

Treatment

An intra-peritoneal rupture is sutured and the bladder drained by means of a catheter. An extra-peritoneal rupture may be sutured, but if it is inaccessible at the base of the bladder then a suprapubic catheter is inserted to keep the bladder empty and to allow healing to take place.

CYSTITIS

Cystitis is a term applied to inflammation of the bladder. This may be either acute and chronic, affects any age, and may occur in both sexes, but it is extremely common in young women.

Aetiology

There must always be a cause for cystitis, but it must be confessed at once that in many patients, especially women, this cannot be found! Possible sources are:
1. The bladder itself—the presence of a stone, foreign body or ulcerating tumour.
2. Ascending from the urethra—this is by far the commonest cause in women. The short urethra may be traumatised during intercourse ('honeymoon cystitis') and may admit organisms from adjacent vaginal infection. The passage of a catheter without full aseptic precautions may infect the bladder and this is particularly dangerous if there is any obstruction to bladder drainage as the result of prostatic obstruction, urethral stricture, etc.
3. Descending infection—may occur from the kidney and this is particularly so in tuberculous cystitis secondary to renal tuberculosis. (Note also that the opposite may occur, that is to say, that pyelitis may result from an ascending infection of the kidney from the infected bladder).

Clinical features

Acute cystitis is accompanied by frequency and pain on micturition. There may be haematuria and there may be obvious pus in the urine. The patient is often febrile and the bladder may be tender on suprapubic pressure.

Special investigations

It is essential that a mid-stream specimen of urine be sent to the laboratory at once for bacteriological examination. It is extremely bad practice to start any treatment until this simple step has been taken since if antibiotics are commenced it may then be quite impossible to determine the precise bacteriological diagnosis.

Treatment

This comprises specific antibiotic therapy determined by the bacteriological reports. Always keep tuberculosis in mind and in any suspicious case, specific tests for this are carried out (see page 331).

Once the acute infection is under control it is then necessary to try to determine whether there is an underlying cause—this will include carrying out an intravenous pyelogram and a cystoscopic examination of the bladder.

BLADDER TUMOURS

Bladder tumours may be benign or malignant. The former are papillomas, the latter, carcinomas.

Secondary invasion may sometimes take place from adjacent cancers of the rectum, ovary, uterus or prostate.

The benign papilloma forms a pedunculated growth which resembles sea-weed floating in the urine. A carcinoma, in contrast, is flat, solid, infiltrates the bladder wall and then ulcerates (Fig. 15.26). The malignant tumour may obstruct one or both ureters,

Fig. 15.26. A benign bladder papilloma (A) contrasted with a carcinoma (B).

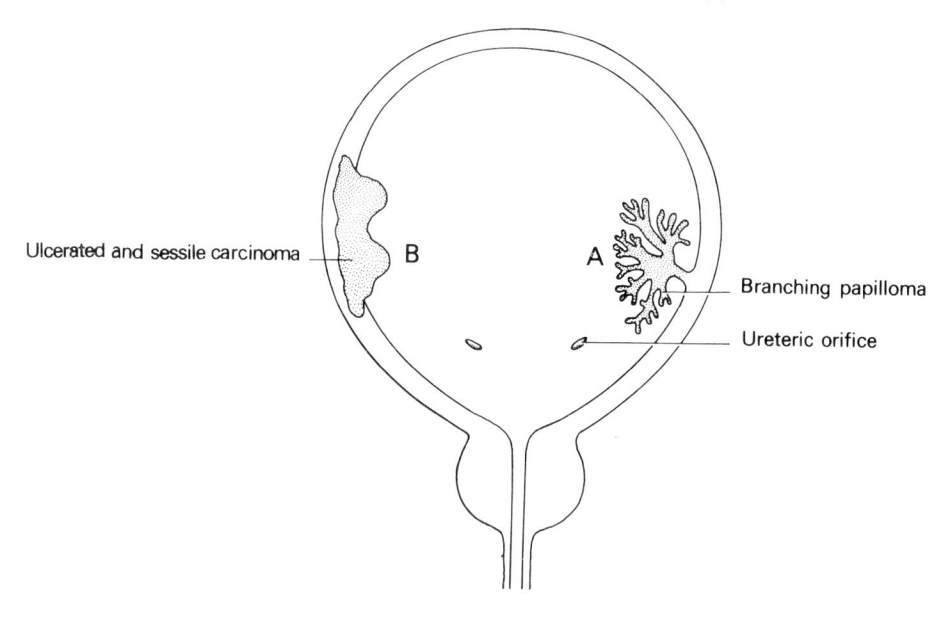

producing hydronephrosis (see Fig. 15.7) or may obstruct the urethra with retention of urine.

Clinical features

Bladder tumours nearly always present with painless haematuria, although a malignant tumour which ulcerates and invades may also produce frequency, urgency and pain on micturition. Occasionally the patient may present with hydronephrosis due to ureteric obstruction, or with retention of urine due to the growth having involved the urethra.

Special investigations

Urine examinations usually reveals blood, either to the naked eye or under the microscope. The skilled pathologist may be able to detect malignant cells in the urinary deposit.

An intravenous pyelogram may demonstrate a filling defect in the bladder and perhaps also ureteric obstruction or hydronephrosis.

Cystoscopy is the most valuable investigation since the tumour can be visualised and a biopsy obtained for microscopic examination.

Treatment

Most benign papillomas can be controlled by diathermy carried out through an operating cystoscope (Fig. 15.11). Since the lesion may recur, or others may appear the patient should be supervised by regular cystoscopic examinations.

The management of bladder carcinoma is difficult and the results are often poor. Occasionally a localised tumour can be excised by partial cystectomy. More extensive tumours are treated by high voltage X-ray therapy. If the growth does not respond, or if it recurs, then total cystectomy may be required with transplantation of the ureters, either into the colon or into an isolated loop of ileum, the urine then draining through an ileostomy stoma into a bag.

The male urethra

CONGENITAL ABNORMALITIES

The urethra may be mal-positioned during its development so that it may open anywhere along the lower aspect of the penis or, much more rarely, along its dorsal aspect. These abnormalities are termed *hypospadias* (Fig. 15.27) and *epispadias* respectively. The latter is usually associated with ectopia vesicae. These conditions require plastic surgical repair.

The other important congenital anomaly is the presence of urethral valves which can obstruct the flow of urine and result in chronic retention and uraemia in infants.

RUPTURE OF THE URETHRA

This most unpleasant injury can be classified into rupture of the bulb of the urethra, and rupture of the urethra within the pelvis in its membranous part (Fig. 15.28).

The bulbous urethra may be damaged by a direct blow, for example, falling off a tree astride a fence. It may also be torn by the surgeon during forcible dilatation or cystoscopy. There is severe pain in the perineum and bright red blood will be seen to drip from the external meatus. There will be marked bruising in the region of the injury.

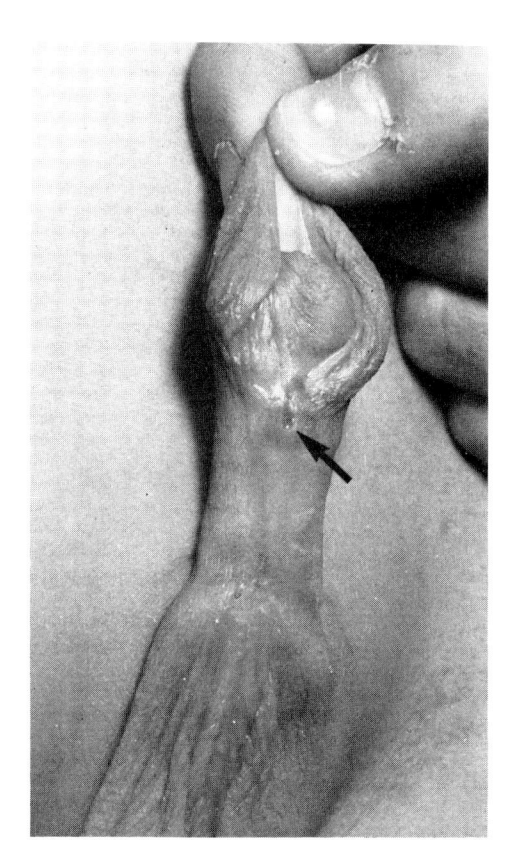

Fig. 15.27. Hypospadias. The arrow points to the urethra, which opens along the inferior aspect of the shaft of the penis.

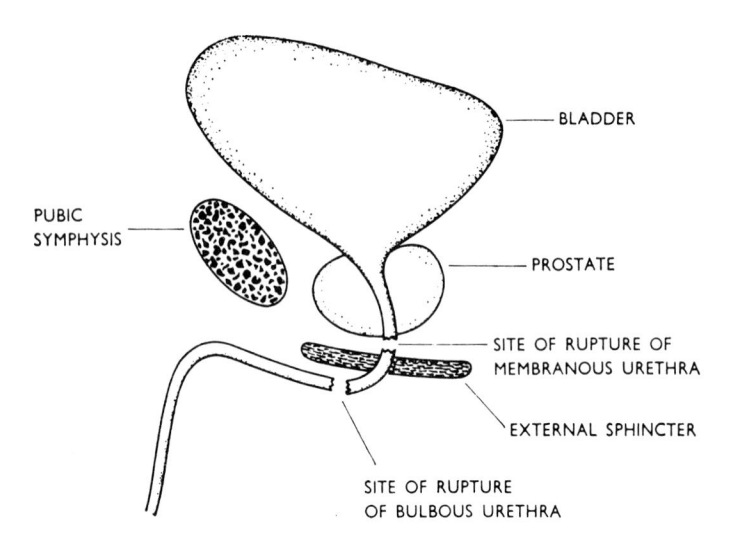

Fig. 15.28. The two common sites of urethral rupture.

The membranous urethra may be injured in fracture of the pelvis, the tear occurring at the junction with the prostatic urethra. As with extra-peritoneal rupture of the bladder (page 342), blood and urine leak out into the extraperitoneal space and produce a swelling which extends above the urethra.

Treatment

Rupture of the *bulbous urethra* may be partial or complete. If a catheter can be passed easily into the bladder, then obviously there has only been incomplete tearing of the urethra. Catheter drainage allows the damaged wall to heal. However, with complete laceration, suture of the torn urethra must be carried out via a perineal approach. Rupture of the *membranous urethra* requires abdominal exploration. The surgeon's first duty is to see whether the cause is an extra-peritoneal rupture of the bladder or a tear of the pelvic urethra; in the former situation, the bladder is completely empty (the urine having escaped through its torn wall) whereas in the latter it contains urine. The torn urethra cannot be sutured directly, so it is necessary to maintain the ruptured ends of the urethra approximated by means of a Foley balloon catheter to which a half-pound weight is attached (Fig. 15.29). At the same time a suprapubic catheter is inserted in the bladder to ensure adequate drainage.

Injuries to the urethra are nearly always followed by stricture formation due to scarring. Subsequent regular dilatations by urethral bougies are necessary.

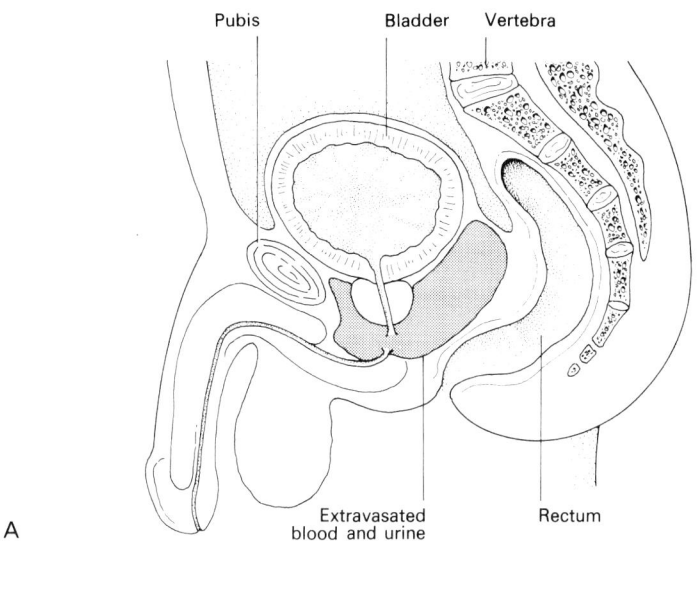

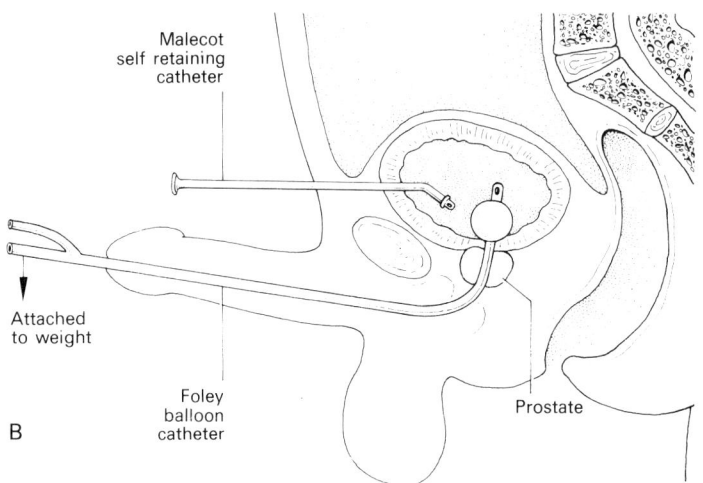

Fig. 15.29. Splintage of a ruptured membranous urethra by means of traction on a Foley balloon catheter.

URETHRAL STRICTURE

Urethral stricture used to be extremely common in this country as a result of gonorrhoea which, untreated, results in chronic infection and fibrosis of the urethra. Since the introduction of antibiotic treatment this has become much less common, but it is still seen quite frequently in Africa, the West Indies and other emerging areas.

A commoner cause of stricture today is post-traumatic. This may result from rupture of the urethra, injury as a result of the use of an indwelling catheter for a prolonged period, or scarring following damage at the time of prostatectomy or the forcible passage of an instrument along the urethra.

Clinical features

A patient with a urethral stricture complains of difficulty in passing urine with a poor stream. He has to strain to empty his bladder and may develop retention of urine.

Treatment

Most patients are subjected to regular dilatations of the urethra; some require this as often as every week, whereas others require dilatation every few months or even yearly. A variety of instruments may be used (Fig. 15.30). These include:

1. *Lister's metal bougies.* These can be sterilised by boiling or autoclaving and the numbers on the handle refer to the circumference of the narrowest and widest part of the instrument measured in millimetres.
2. *Olivary-headed plastic bougies.* These were formerly made of gum elastic but are now made of plastic material.
3. *Filiform bougies.* They are very useful in difficult strictures since a number of these can be introduced into the urethra and, by mani-

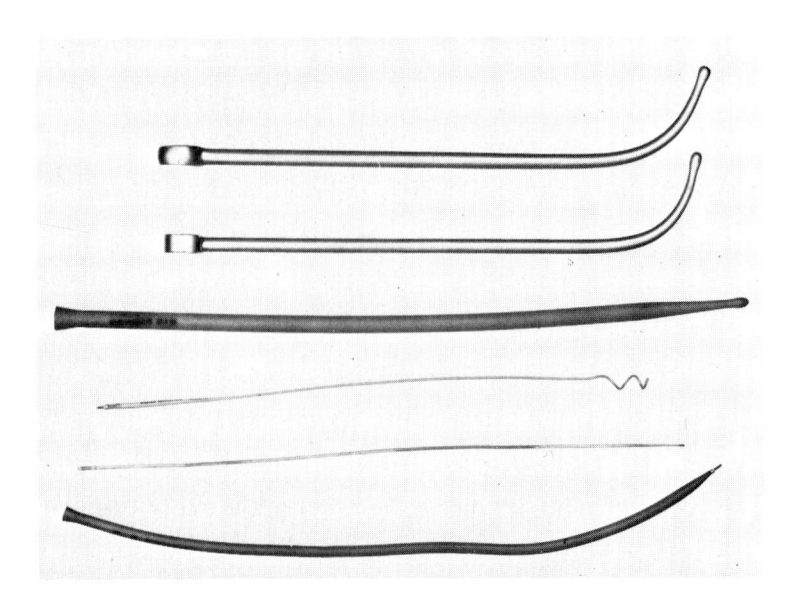

Fig. 15.30. Instruments used in urethral dilatation. From above down: Lister's metal bougies, olivary headed plastic bougie, and filiform bougies with dilator which screws in to the proximal end.

pulation, one can eventually be persuaded to pass through the stricture. Each of these fine bougies is provided with a screw end to which larger bougies can be attached and threaded through the stricture by 'rail-roading' along the passage determined by the filiform bougie.

In some cases it is possible to carry out a plastic repair of the urethral stricture.

The management of retention in cases of urethral stricture is dealt with on page 358.

The prostate

The prostate is a fibro-muscular and glandular organ which surrounds the urethra as this emerges from the bladder (Fig. 15.31). It is $1\frac{1}{4}$ inches long and is the size and shape of a chestnut.

There are only two common conditions which affect the prostate but these are both immensely important—benign enlargement and carcinoma.

BENIGN PROSTATIC ENLARGEMENT

Some degree of enlargement of the prostate is extremely common from the age of 45 onwards, but this enlargement often produces either no symptoms or only minor ones. The reason for this enlargement is not known, but the prostate, like the breast and thyroid, is an organ which has periods of activity and involution throughout

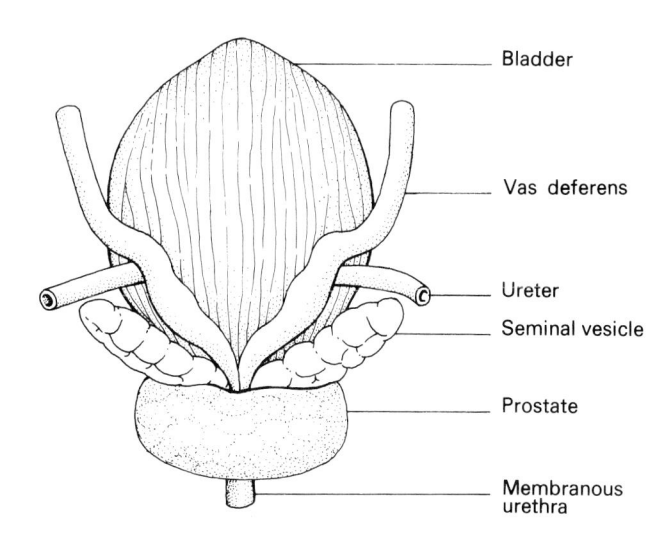

Fig. 15.31. The prostate and adjacent structures, posterior view.

life—the condition of benign enlargement is therefore somewhat similar to the development of a nodular goitre or chronic mastitis.

At the prostate enlarges, the urethra may become obstructed. This obstruction may result in secondary hypertrophy of the muscle wall of the bladder. The obstructed bladder may become infected (especially after catheterisation) and bladder stones may form in the infected pool of stagnant urine. Back pressure on the ureters and kidneys may cause a progressive hydronephrosis and eventually renal failure (see Fig. 15.14).

Clinical features

The symptoms produced by an enlarged prostate may be divided into three broad groups:

1. *Disturbance of micturition*—the patient experiences increasing frequency and often has to get up from his bed several times at night to pass urine (nocturia). The stream becomes poor and hesitant and the whole act of passing urine may be converted into a long, slow, tedious dribble. Occasionally the congested veins over the enlarged prostate bleed, with resultant haematuria.

2. *Retention of urine*—this may be *acute* with sudden onset of severe pain, or *chronic*, in which the bladder gradually becomes distended and the patient develops dribbling overflow incontinence, with little or no pain. One Irish patient with this complaint told us that he was 'passing his urine wonderfully often'—a brilliant description of this situation.

3. *Uraemia*—progressive obstruction to the bladder outflow may result in renal failure so that the patient complains of headache, drowsiness, anorexia, nausea and mental deterioration.

Examination of the abdomen will reveal whether or not the bladder is distended. The prostate is assessed by rectal examination; the benignly enlarged gland can be felt as a rubbery swelling.

The patient is carefully examined for evidence of uraemia, characterised by a dried furred tongue, anaemia and mental confusion.

Special investigations

Patients with symptoms of prostatic enlargement should have the following studies performed:

The haemoglobin is estimated, since uraemia is often associated with anaemia.

The blood urea is measured—it should be under 40 mg% if renal function is normal.

The serum acid phosphatase is determined. This is useful in making a differential diagnosis from carcinoma of the prostate since in the latter situation it is raised above 3 units in 50% of cases.

A mid stream specimen of urine is sent to the laboratory for full examination and culture. Most patients with prostatic disease have a sterile urine unless infected by catheterisation.

An intravenous pyelogram gives useful evidence of kidney function, the amount of prostatic enlargement (which can be seen as a globular filling defect in the base of the bladder) and the amount of residual urine, which is studied by taking a further X-ray after micturition (Fig. 15.32).

Treatment

This depends on whether the patient is an elective case, due to troublesome prostatic symptoms, or whether he presents as an urgent problem of retention of urine. (This is dealt with on page 358).

There are three routes of surgical approach to the prostate (Fig. 15.33).

These are:
1. Retro-pubic.
2. Transvesical.
3. Endoscopic (Transurethral).

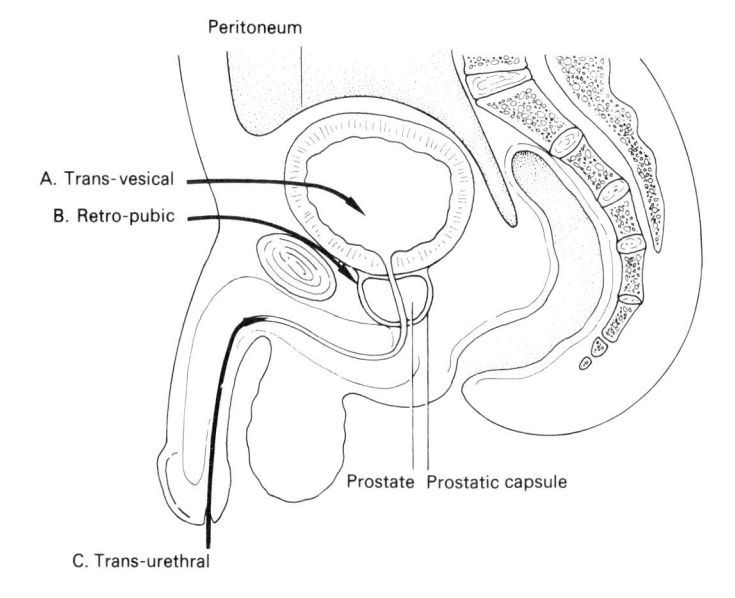

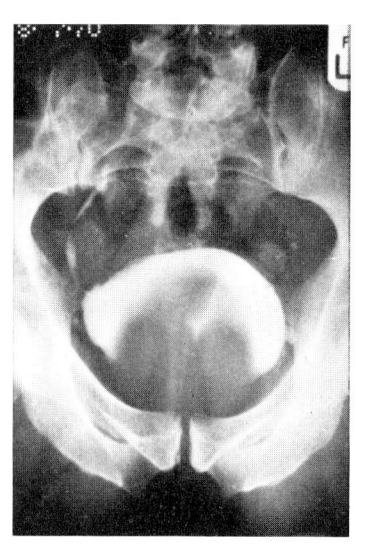

Fig. 15.32. A very large prostate demonstrated on intravenous pyelography. The patient has just passed urine but there is still a considerable residuum in the bladder.

Fig. 15.33. The three approaches to the prostate.

1. The *retropubic prostatectomy* was devised by Terence Millin, after whom it is named. The capsule of the prostate is exposed by dissecting through the fatty tissue behind the pubis. The capsule is then incised, the enlarged prostate enucleated, a wedge removed from the posterior margin of the bladder neck to avoid stricture formation, and the prostatic capsule then sutured after the passage of a Foley self-retaining catheter. Since the inside of the bladder cannot be fully explored at this operation, the surgeon commences the procedure by carrying out a cystoscopy to make sure that he is not overlooking any calculi or a small tumour in the bladder, and to ensure that there is no stricture along the urethra.

2. The *transvesical operation* involves the enucleation of the prostate via an incision in the bladder. In the original operation no attempt at haemostasis was made, but a large tube was placed in the bladder to enable clots to escape freely. This operation had the advantage of speed and safety, but involved a long convalescence while the suprapubic fistula healed. Named after Sir Peter Freyer, it is now seldom performed. It was modified by Harris and by Wilson Hey, who introduced careful haemostasis followed by suture of the bladder, either with a urethral catheter alone, or with the addition of a small suprapubic catheter drainage.

3. *Endoscopic prostatectomy* is carried out with an operating cystoscope—either a diathermy loop (McCarthy) or else with a cutting punch (Thompson). The surgeon pares away slices of the prostate surrounding the urethra; this is particularly suitable for small fibrous prostates and for carcinoma of the prostate (see below). Following operation, a Foley catheter is left in place until bleeding ceases.

Post-operative care and complications

Prostatectomy is a common operation and a particularly challenging one to the nursing staff of a surgical ward. The patients are often elderly, frequently with pre-existing pulmonary or cardiac disease, who are then submitted to a major, unpleasant and uncomfortable procedure. As well as being on the alert for all the usual post-operative complications there are a number of specific problems:

Fluid balance. A careful fluid chart is vital and is complicated by the fact that we must take into consideration the fluid that is being used in the bladder irrigation; this must, of course, be deducted from the amount in the urine drainage bottle to give the actual urinary output. The patient needs a high fluid intake to ensure diuresis and lavage to the bladder—yet he may be loath to drink. He may be tempted by being given his favourite drink and tea is usually welcomed by the average elderly Englishman. Intravenous supplement is required in most patients for the first day or two.

Prevention of infection. The raw prostatic bed plus the presence of an indwelling catheter makes infection a particular risk. Most surgeons cover the operation with a broad spectrum antibiotic, for example ampicillin or one of the sulphonamides, of which, sulphamethizole (Urolucosil) 0.5 gm 6 hourly or sulphatriad 1 gm 3 times daily are especially useful. The drug may need changing according to the sensitivity of any organisms grown in the urine. Particularly important is that a 'closed' system of bladder drainage is employed, the catheter emptying either into a sterile bottle below the level of an antiseptic solution or into a disposable bag (Fig. 15.34). If the system is disconnected for a bladder wash-out or any other purpose, this must be done under the strictest aseptic precautions.

Clot retention. It is everybody's duty to ensure that a continuous drip of urine takes place from the catheter post-operatively. If this stops it is due to one of the two causes. Either the catheter has been dragged down by the weight of the tubing into the urethra, or its lumen has been blocked by blood clot. The first is easily remedied by cleansing the catheter and replacing it in its proper position—but it should never be allowed to occur by ensuring that the catheter is soundly fastened by adhesive strapping to the thigh so that it lies

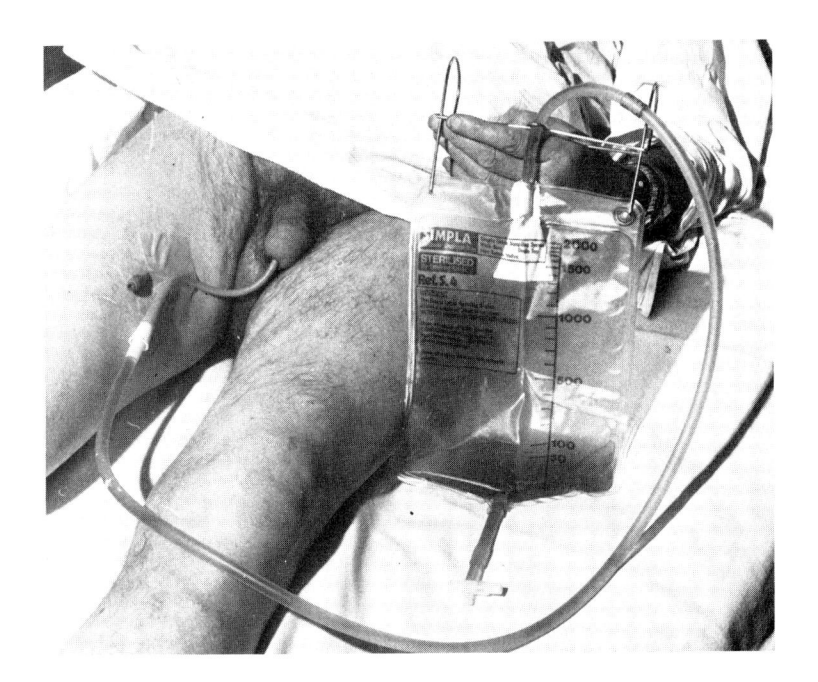

Fig. 15.34. Closed catheter drainage of the bladder. The Foley balloon catheter is strapped to the patient's thigh to prevent the weight of the tubing dragging on the bladder base.

at the correct level within the bladder. Clot retention is a much more serious state of affairs. Left untreated, the bladder rapidly fills with clot and the patient not only becomes severely distressed and in pain but also may become shocked from loss of blood. If diagnosed at once the situation can be remedied by washing out the catheter under full aseptic precautions. If this is unsuccessful, the patient must be taken back to the operating theatre and an attempt made to evacuate the clot using a wide bore metal catheter and a Bigelow evacuator (Fig. 15.35). If this fails the wound must be re-opened, the clot is cleared and a suprapubic tube inserted. Blood loss is replaced by transfusion.

CARCINOMA OF THE PROSTATE

Pathology

Cancer of the prostate is the fourth commonest cause of death from malignant disease in males in this country. It is rare below the age of 50 but becomes particularly common in the elderly.

The tumour is an adenocarcinoma, which arises from the glandular tissue of the prostate. Having spread through the prostate itself the tumour then invades adjacent organs—the bladder, urethra and, rarely, the rectum. It spreads into the lymph nodes along the iliac vessels and also by the blood stream, with a particular tendency to metastasize to the bones of the pelvis, spine, and skull. Deposits may also be found in the liver and lung.

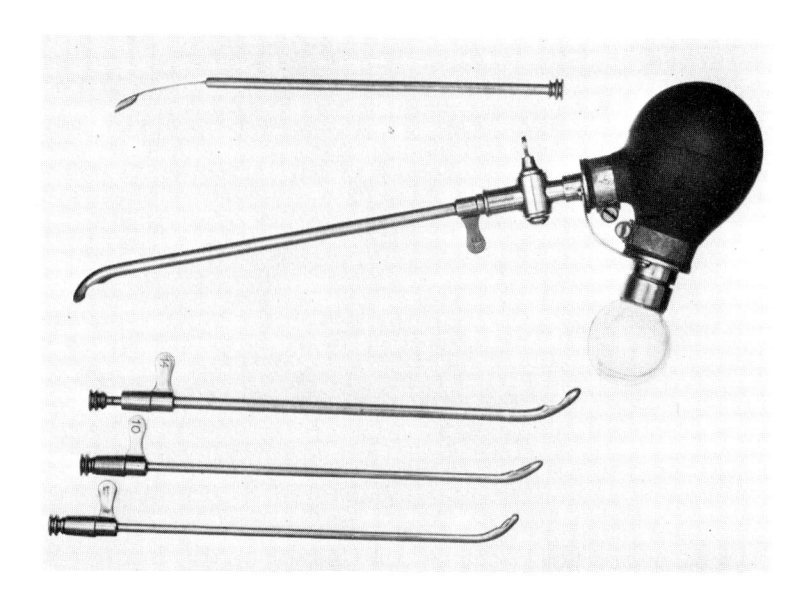

Fig. 15.35. Bigelow's evacuator with metal catheters.

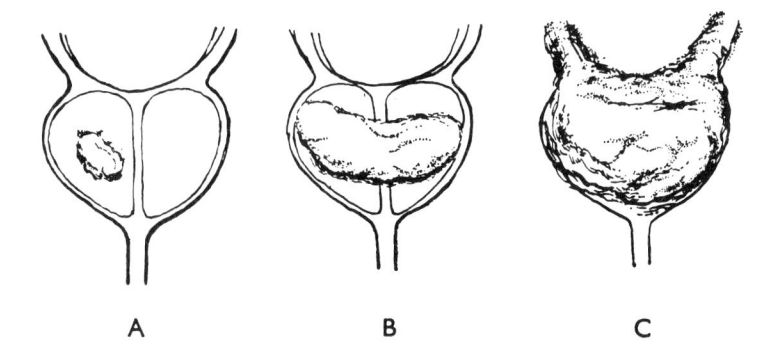

Fig. 15.36. The clinical stages of prostatic carcinoma, A, a hard nodule in the prostate; B, a mass obliterating the median sulcus; C, infiltration outside the prostatic capsule.

Clinical features

The symptoms of carcinoma of the prostate are usually identical to those of benign enlargement, but, in addition, the patient may present with symptoms due to secondary deposits, particularly pain in the back due to vertebral or pelvic involvement.

The diagnosis can usually be at least suspected by the surgeon when he examines the prostate per rectum. Instead of feeling the usual elastic gland, he notes that the malignant prostate is hard, irregular, and may infiltrate adjacent tissues. (Fig. 15.36).

Special investigations

The same investigations are performed as described under benign enlargement. The particularly useful finding in differentiating the malignant gland is the high serum acid phosphatase (above 3 units) which is present in about 50% of cancer cases. Some 25% have X-ray evidence of bony secondary deposits which, unlike most other secondaries, are usually osteosclerotic, that is to say, that they are more dense than normal bone (Fig. 15.37).

Fig. 15.37. A sclerotic deposit from a carcinoma of the prostate in the fourth lumbar vertebra.

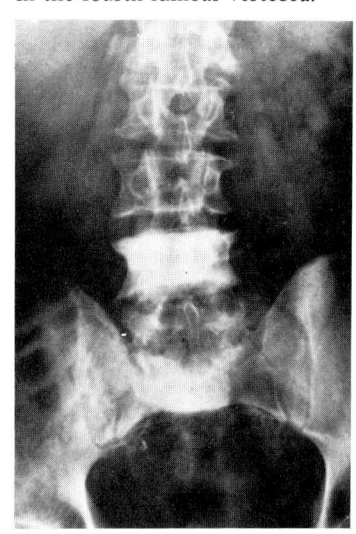

Treatment

Occasionally an apparently benign prostate is removed and found to contain a small focus of carcinoma. Under such circumstances, no further treatment is usually required. More often, carcinoma of the prostate is only discovered at a stage when it has already spread beyond its capsule and may well have involved other organs, particularly the pelvic cellular tissues, the base of the bladder, and perhaps also spread to the bones. Many of these patients respond to treatment with stilboestrol or to bilateral orchidectomy. The former treatment is usually preferred but orchidectomy is advised if the patient is unable to tolerate the stilboestrol or other oestrogens.

The side effects of these hormones include fluid retention, nausea and vomiting, gynaecomastia (enlargement of the breasts) and testicular atrophy.

Carcinoma of the prostate may produce urinary obstruction and this may be relieved by stilboestrol. If not, an endoscopic prostatectomy is indicated. (See page 354).

URINARY RETENTION

A common surgical emergency is retention of urine. This may be *acute*, which is a painful condition (except when due to diseases of the central nervous system) or *chronic*, when the patient develops progressive obstruction which leads to dribbling overflow incontinence and which is painless.

It is first necessary to determine the cause of the retention and this may be either due to some *general* cause, (with no organic obstruction to urinary flow), or to a *local* cause.

The commonest general cause is undoubtedly post-operative retention of urine. Indeed, this is the commonest of all causes of retention. It is well known to any experienced nurse how frequent it is for a patient following any surgical procedure (but especially an abdominal, pelvic or perineal operation) to be unable to pass urine in the post-operative period. This is due to a combination of the pain produced by straining, the difficulty in passing urine in the lying position, and perhaps also, in elderly patients, to some degree of prostatic obstruction aggravated by this situation.

Any disease or injury of the spinal cord may interrupt the reflex pathway of micturition, so retention of urine is commonly seen in patients with disseminated sclerosis, transverse myelitis or a spinal tumour, and is invariable in patients with paraplegia due to fracture of the spine.

Local causes are due to some obstruction of the urethra. Obstruction of any tube in the body must be classified into causes in the lumen of the tube, causes in its wall and causes pressing on the wall from outside. The urethra is no exception and so we have:
1. *Causes in the lumen*—calculus or blood clot (clot retention)
2. *In the wall*—urethral stricture.
3. *Outside the wall*—prostatic enlargement (benign or malignant), faecal impaction, pelvic tumour or pregnant uterus.

The diagnosis of the cause of retention is made on the history, examination and special investigations.

The history may reveal the typical progressive symptoms of prostatism, a story of urethral infection suggesting stricture, or associated leg weakness and numbness, indicating some neurological lesion.

Examination includes a rectal examination to determine the size and nature of the prostate, palpation of the urethra for stone or stricture, inspection of the urethral orifice to detect meatal stenosis or phimosis, and careful examination of the central nervous system.

Special investigations include estimation of the serum acid phosphatase which, if raised above 3 units, suggests carcinoma of the prostate, and X-ray of the pelvis, which may reveal a calculus at the bladder base or bony secondaries from metastatic carcinoma of the prostate.

In addition to establishing the diagnosis, the surgeon needs to know two other things about a patient with urinary retention before deciding on definitive treatment. These are:

1. *The general condition of the patient*—the average patient with retention of urine admitted to hospital is an elderly gentleman. Before proceeding to major surgery, his general condition must obviously be carefully investigated.
2. *The renal function*—the patient with retention of urine may potentially have damaged his kidneys by back pressure. This is assessed by the general condition of the patient and by estimation of the blood urea. Elevation above 40 mg% suggests renal impairment.

Management of urinary retention

Treatment naturally depends on the cause of the retention.

Post-operative retention

This can usually be overcome by giving the patient an injection of morphia and sitting him with his legs over the side of the bed. If this does not succeed, catheterisation may be required. The catheter can either be removed as soon as the bladder has been emptied, or, if the patient is particularly ill, can be left in place until the following day. Carbachol should not be used; it causes intense pain and there is risk of rupture of the bladder if any obstruction is present. Sometimes in a patient with an enlarged prostate retention of urine is precipitated by some other surgical procedure and can only be relieved by eventually proceeding to prostatectomy.

Patients with diseases of the central nervous system complicated by retention of urine are managed by means of indwelling self-retaining catheter.

The three common causes for an emergency surgical admission of a man with acute urinary retention are urethral stricture, benign prostatic hypertrophy, and malignant disease of the prostate.

Urethral stricture

A catheter cannot be passed through the narrowed urethra, which must be gently dilated with bougies under local or general anaesthetic. Following this, it is then possible to catheterise the patient and relieve the retention. Subsequently the patient must continue with regular urethral dilatations. Rarely the stricture is impassable and the patient then requires a temporary subrapubic cystotomy with insertion of a self-retaining catheter in the bladder. Once the oedema has been allowed to subside, it is then often possible to dilate the urethra after about a week to allow the suprapubic fistula to close.

Benign prostatic enlargement

The patient is catheterised under full aseptic precautions and prostatectomy can be carried out as soon as convenient if the renal function and general condition of the patient are satisfactory. If renal damage or the patient's poor general condition preclude operation, catheter drainage is continued until these can be improved. If the patient is in such poor health that operation will obviously never be possible, for example, a bed ridden cardiac cripple, then he is best managed by a permanent urethral drainage, the catheter being changed weekly and urinary antiseptics being used should urinary infections occur. The modern plastic self-retaining catheter is far kinder to the patient than a leaking and odorous permanent suprapubic cystotomy tube.

Catheters and catheterisation

There are a large variety of urinary catheters, each subserving a useful function (Fig. 15.38).

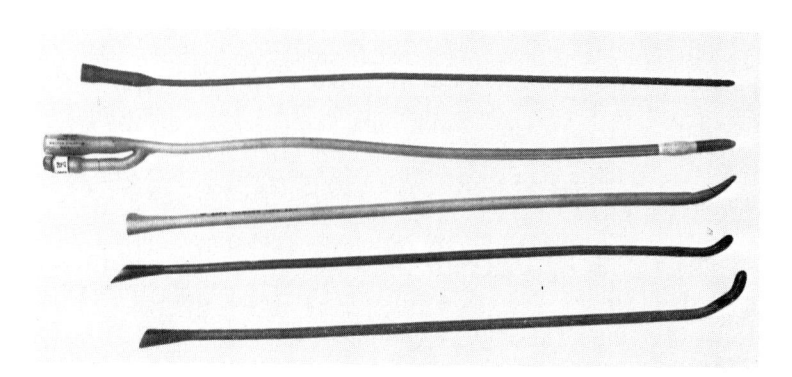

Fig. 15.38. Urinary catheters. From above down: rubber, Foley balloon, Tiemann, coudé and bi-coudé gum elastic.

Jaques' plastic catheter is convenient for a single catheterisation, especially in the female, when it is not intended to leave a catheter in place. It can, if necessary, easily be sterilized by boiling, but it is usually available already sterilized and disposable.

Foley's balloon catheter is made of latex-rubber or polythene with a thin balloon which can be distended with sterile water injected through a side tube. A modification has a second side tube which can be used for bladder irrigation. This catheter is the most commonly used of the self-retaining catheters and, these days, is usually disposable and already sterilized by gamma irradiation.

Tiemann's catheter is made of hard rubber with a curved solid tip. This is used in male catheterisation when there is difficulty due to prostatic enlargement.

Gum-elastic catheters are semi-rigid catheters used in difficult cases of prostatic obstruction. They may have an olivary tip, a single bend (coudé) or a double bend of the tip (bi-coudé). The original gum-elastic material could not be boiled and had to be sterilised in formalin vapour. These catheters are now archaic and have been replaced by semi-rigid plastic material which can be boiled in the usual way.

Gibbon's catheter is a fine plastic catheter provided with plastic wings to attach the catheter to the penis. The long end of the catheter can be attached directly to a drainage bottle. This catheter is particularly useful in long-term catheterisation of paraplegic patients.

Whatever the catheter used, the strictest aseptic precautions must be employed. The operator wears a mask and sterile gloves. The urethral meatus is thoroughly cleansed with an antiseptic such as Hibitane or Cetrimide, sterile towels are employed and the catheter passed, if possible, by a no-touch technique using a sterile pair of forceps. If drainage is to be continued the catheter is immediately connected to a sterile drainage system (see Fig. 15.34).

The testis

Anatomy

Each testis is contained by a white fibrous capsule, the *tunica albuginea*, and each is invaginated anteriorly into a double serous covering termed the *tunica vaginalis*, just as the intestine is invaginated anteriorly into the peritoneum. Along the posterior border of the testis lies the *epididymis*, which is divided into an expanded head, a body and a tail (Fig. 15.39A).

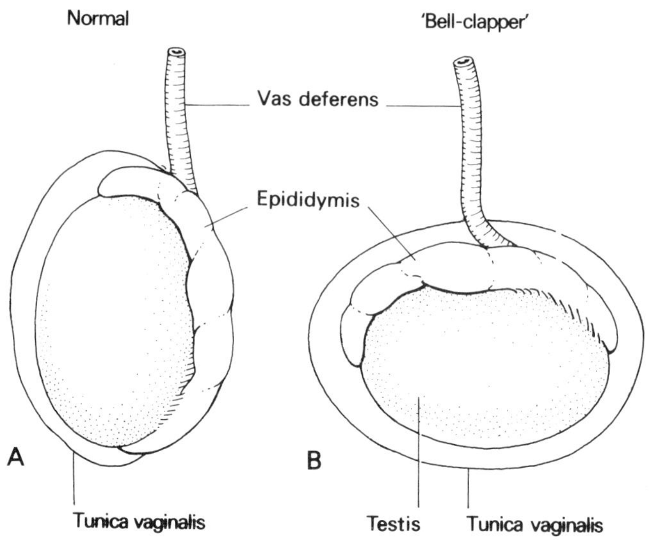

Fig. 15.39. A, The anatomy of the normal testis; B, The 'bell-clapper' deformity in which the testis hangs within the tunica vaginalis.

The testis is supplied by the testicular artery, which arises from the aorta at the level of the renal vessels. Its venous drainage is via the *pampiniform plexus* which joins to form the testicular vein. On the right this drains into the inferior vena cava, on the left into the renal vein. The lymphatic drainage of the testis obeys the usual rule; it accompanies the venous drainage and thus passes to the para-aortic lymph nodes at the level of the renal vessels.

The testis is made up of coiled seminiferous tubules, each about two feet in length. These tubules drain posteriorly into about a dozen fine efferent ducts which pass into the head of the epididymis. The epididymis itself is made up of a considerably convoluted tube which drains into the vas deferens.

Development of the testis

This is important and the key to several features of clinical interest.

The testis arises from the posterior wall of the abdomen in the fetus and links up with a tube termed the mesonephric duct which is to form the epididymis and vas. From the third to ninth month of foetal life the testis migrates down the posterior wall of the abdomen and then along the inguinal canal until it reaches the scrotum, just before birth. A prolongation of peritoneum called the *processus vaginalis* projects into the fetal scrotum; the testis slides behind this and is thus covered on its front and sides by peritoneum. The processus becomes obliterated at about the time of birth, leaving the testis covered by the tunica vaginalis.

ABNORMALITIES OF TESTICULAR DESCENT

Three important abnormalities of the testis must be differentiated from each other:
1. Retractile testis.
2. Ectopic testis.
3. Maldescended testis.

The retractile testis is a normal organ which is drawn up into the groin by excess activity of the cremaster muscle which surrounds the spermatic cord.

An ectopic testis means one which is lying in an abnormal site, (just as an ectopic pregnancy is one taking place in an abnormal site in the fallopian tube rather than in the uterus). A common anomaly is for the testis to emerge through the external ring and then, instead of descending into the scrotum, to come to lie in the superficial tissues of the groin. Other less common situations are in the perineum or at the root of the penis.

A maldescended testis lies in the normal course of descent anywhere from the abdominal cavity to the inguinal canal. The vast majority represent some local defect in development. Unilateral undescended testes are four times as common as bilateral.

Most, if not all, testes which *are* going to descend do so within the first few months of life.

Diagnosis

A retractile testis is a common condition and often the parents think that one or both testes have failed to descend. However, careful manipulation enables the infant's testis to be coaxed into the scrotum.

If the testis is easily palpable in the groin, then it is lying in an ectopic position and not in the inguinal canal where it is usually impalpable, or, at the most, in a thin boy, detected as a vague tender bulge.

Treatment

The child with retractile testes is perfectly normal, and all that is required is reassurance of the parents.

The ectopic or maldescended testis must be placed in the scrotum before the child reaches puberty if it is to function as a sperm-producing organ. The operation is therefore carried out when the child is about six or seven years of age and comprises mobilisation of the testis, removal of the co-existing inguinal hernia sac (the persistent processus vaginalis) and fixation of the testis within the scrotum without tension.

Left untreated the undescended testis will not produce sperm so that sterility will result in bilateral cases. In addition there is an increased risk of trauma, torsion and malignant disease in the maldescended testis.

TORSION OF THE TESTIS

Usually this is a torsion of the spermatic cord in a congenitally abnormal testis which is often hanging like a bell-clapper within a completely investing tunica vaginalis (Fig. 15.39B). It is probably impossible for a torsion to occur in a completely normal testis. Left untreated for more than a few hours, irreversible gangrenous change occurs in the organ.

Clinical features

Torsion usually occurs in children and adolescents. There is an acute onset of pain and the affected testis becomes swollen and extremely tender. The main difficulty is differential diagnosis from acute epididymitis. In the latter condition there is usually a pyrexia, a history of urinary tract infection, with pus cells and organisms in the urine, and the white cell count is raised. A useful factor in differential diagnosis is the age of the patient, since torsion of the testis is unusual after 20, whereas epididymitis is rare before that age.

Treatment

It may be possible in a very early case to untwist the torsion manually. If not, it is best to explore the testis if there is any doubt about the diagnosis, since every hour increases the likelihood of irreversible damage. If still viable, the testis is untwisted and sutured to the tunica vaginalis to prevent recurrence; if gangrenous, it is removed. In every case fixation of the other testis should be performed at the same time, since any congenital anomaly is likely to be bilateral and torsion of the opposite testis may therefore occur.

CYSTS WITHIN THE SCROTUM

There are two very common cysts associated with the testis. The first is a *hydrocele*, which is a collection of clear yellow fluid in the tunica vaginalis. This is usually without any obvious underlying cause, but it may be secondary to some inflammatory or malignant disease of the testis. The other condition is *cyst of the epididymis* which arises above and behind the testis and may contain either clear or milky fluid (Fig. 15.40).

Both types of cyst usually require surgical removal and it is important in hydrocele that the underlying testis should be carefully inspected to exclude any underlying testicular disease.

INFECTION OF THE TESTIS

Infection of the testis itself is unusual but may complicate mumps (*mumps orchitis*). A *gumma* of the testis due to late syphilis was once common, but is now extremely rare. Much more commonly the epididymis is affected as an ascending infection from the urinary tract, either due to gonorrhoea or to a coliform infection of the urine. Usually *acute epididymitis* resolves with antibiotic treatment. *Chronic epididymitis* may be due to tuberculosis, which is now becoming relatively uncommon, but is more likely to be due to a chronic phase of acute epididymitis which has not completely resolved following antibiotic treatment.

TUMOURS OF THE TESTIS

There are two main forms of malignant tumour of the testis—the seminoma and the teratoma.

The seminoma arises from the cells of the seminiferous tubules,

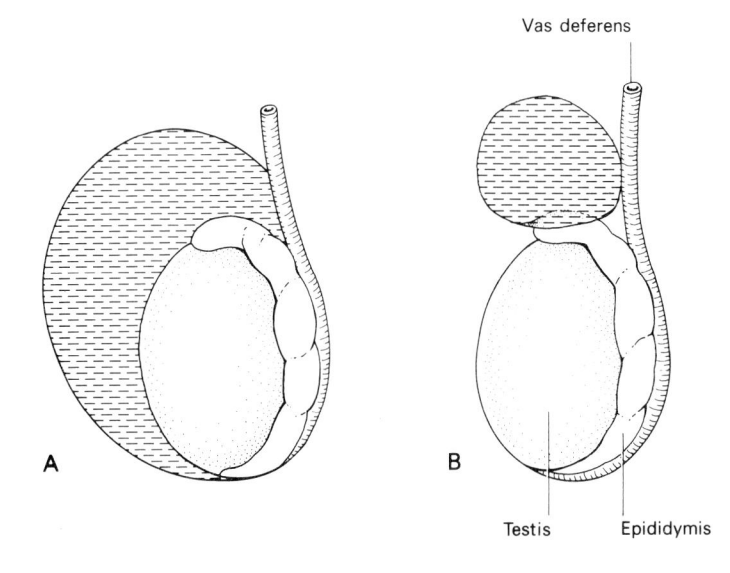

Fig. 15.40. A, Hydrocele. B, Cyst of epididymis.

usually in men between 20 and 40 years of age. The tumour is solid and white in appearance. About 10% arise in undescended testes.

The teratoma occurs in younger men, the peak incidence being 20 to 30 years. It is thought to arise from primitive germinal cells and has a markedly cystic appearance. Under the microscope the cells are very variable and the tumour may contain cartilage, bone, muscle, fat and other tissues.

Local spread of the tumour gradually destroys the testis. Lymphatic spread is to the para-aortic nodes on the posterior abdominal wall and in advanced cases there may be enlargement of the supraclavicular nodes on the left side of the neck due to thoracic duct invasion. Blood borne spread occurs to the lungs and liver.

The tumour usually presents as a lump in the testis which may rapidly enlarge in size and may be mistaken for an inflammatory condition. Some patients present with metastases—for example, a mass in the abdomen due to abdominal lymph nodes.

Treatment

This comprises orchidectomy, with radiotherapy to the paraaortic lymph nodes.

Penis

NON-RETRACTILE PREPUCE

It is extremely common for male infants in this country to be brought to the doctor or nurse because the parents notice that the prepuce cannot be retracted. In fact, the foreskin is non-retractile in 95% of infants at birth; 50% retract in the first year and the vast majority can be retracted by the third or fourth year as congenital adhesions between the glans and the prepuce break down (Fig. 15.41). Inability to retract the prepuce in the infant is no indication in itself for circumcision; indeed in the 'nappy' stage, the prepuce protects the delicate glans and the urethral orifice from the excoriation of ammoniacal dermatitis, which is liable to occur if the child's diapers are not frequently changed and are allowed to remain wet. Forcible attempts to retract the foreskin simply injure the tissues and the resultant scarring may lead to a true phimosis.

Circumcision is an operation which dates back some 15,000 years and which is steeped in religious, mystical, medical, social, hygienic

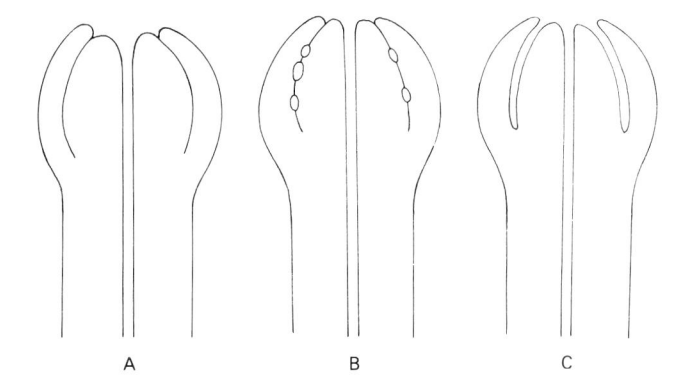

Fig. 15.41. The prepuce in the newborn baby is adherent to the glans penis (A). The adhesions gradually break down (B) until by the age of 3 or 4 the great majority of children have a prepuce which can be easily retracted (C).

and sexual traditions, misconceptions, myths and customs. Our practice is to carry out circumcision if requested by the parents on religious grounds, in the occasional case where the prepuce cannot be retracted in a child over the age of 4, or when an organic phimosis is present.

PHIMOSIS

This is a condition of gross narrowing of the orifice of the prepuce. (Fig. 15.42). It occurs rarely as a congenital lesion but may follow the scarring produced by attempts at forcible retraction of the prepuce (see above), or may result from chronic inflammation of the prepuce (*balanitis*).

In extreme cases it may produce obstruction to the urinary stream. *Treatment* is by circumcision.

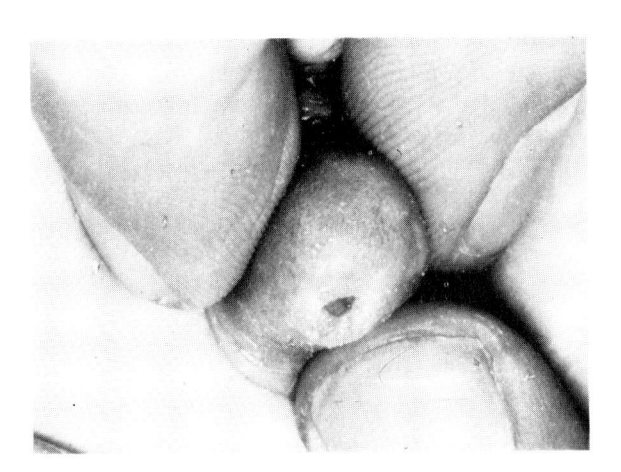

Fig. 15.42. Gross phimosis in a baby. This has resulted from attempted forcible stretching of the prepuce.

PARAPHIMOSIS

A condition in which the foreskin becomes retracted around the glans, interferes with venous return and results in swelling of the glans and extreme pain. There is an important practical nursing point here; always ensure that the patient's prepuce is pulled forward again after the insertion of an indwelling catheter—if not, a paraphimosis may well follow.

Treatment

Once the lesion has become established it is often too tender to manipulate without an anaesthetic. However, when this is administered the prepuce can usually be pulled forward into position; if not, a dorsal slit of the prepuce may be necessary.

CARCINOMA OF THE PENIS

This tumour usually affects elderly subjects (Fig. 15.43) and is practically never seen in circumcised men. Its most frequent site is in the groove between the glans and the prepuce. The tumour gradually erodes the penis and spreads to the lymph nodes in the groins. Indeed it is haemorrhage from fungation of these nodes that is likely to be the cause of death in cancer of the penis. Surprisingly enough the tumour never seems to occlude the urethra sufficiently to produce retention of urine.

Treatment

The diagnosis must always be confirmed by microscopic examination of a biopsy specimen.

Radiotherapy may be used in early cases but amputation must be carried out when the urethra is involved. If the groin lymph nodes are involved, block dissection is performed. Inoperably fixed nodes are treated by palliative irradiation.

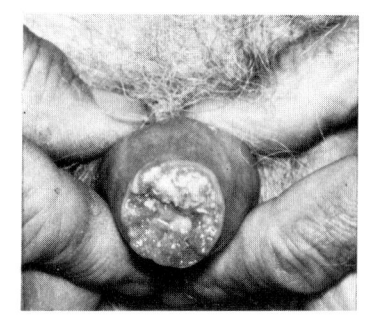

Fig. 15.43. An extensive carcinoma of the penis.

Chapter 16. The endocrine glands

The thyroid

Anatomy

The thyroid gland is made up of the isthmus, which overlies the second, third and fourth rings of the trachea, and the lateral lobes, each of which extends from the side of the thyroid cartilage down to the sixth tracheal ring (Fig. 16.1). On its deep aspect lie the larynx and the trachea, with the pharynx and oesophagus behind and the common carotid and internal jugular vein on either side. In the groove between the trachea and oesophagus lies the recurrent laryngeal nerve, which runs up into the larynx to supply its intrinsic muscles. The parathyroid glands are each about the size of a split pea and lie on, or buried in, the posterior aspects of each lateral lobe. They are usually four in number, a superior and inferior on either side.

Development

The thyroid develops from a bud which pushes downwards from the floor of the tongue. This outgrowth then descends to its adult posi-

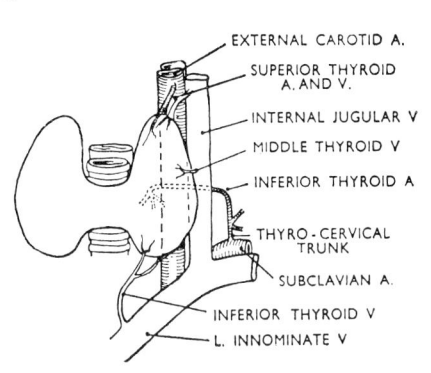

Fig. 16.1. The thyroid gland to show its immediate relationships and its blood vessels.

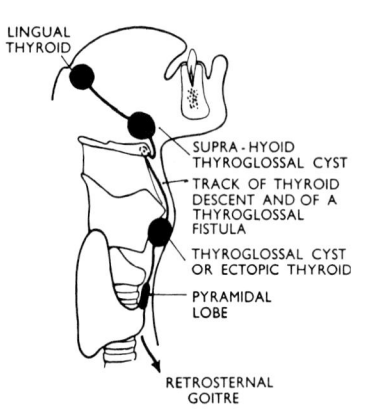

Fig. 16.2. The descent of the thyroid, showing possible sites of ectopic thyroid tissue or thyroglossal fistula. The arrow shows the further descent of the thyroid which may take place into the retrosternal position.

tion in the neck. Normally it loses all connection with its origin which is commemorated, however, by the little pit termed the *foramen caecum*, which lies at the junction of the middle and posterior thirds of the tongue.

Congenital anomalies

The embryological line of descent of the thyroid from the base of the tongue to its normal position in the neck may be the site of fistula or cyst formation (Fig. 16.2). A *thyroglossal fistula* appears as an orifice in the midline of the neck which discharges watery fluid. A *thyroglossal cyst* forms a round cystic swelling in the midline of the neck which typically moves upwards when the patient protrudes the tongue, because of its attachment to the track of the thyroid descent.

Rarely the thyroid fails to descend properly into the neck and such a patient may present with a lump at the foramen caecum on the dorsum of the tongue, and which represents the whole of the thyroid tissue (*lingual thyroid*). On some occasions the thyroid descends beyond its normal station into the superior mediastinum so that the whole of the thyroid is situated within the chest (*retrosternal thyroid*).

THYROID PHYSIOLOGY

The function of the thyroid gland is to manufacture, store and secrete two iodine-containing hormones, *thyroxine*, amounting to about 80% of the hormone secretion, and *triiodothyronine*. These hormones are stored in the colloid contained within the follicles of the thyroid gland. The thyroid hormones are linked to protein in this colloid (*thyroglobulin*). The hormones are liberated into the bloodstream mostly bound to protein, although small amounts of both hormones are in their free active form. The rate of manufacture of the thyroid hormones and of their secretion into the blood is regulated by the thyroid stimulating hormone (TSH) secreted by the anterior lobe of the pituitary.

The thyroid hormones increase the metabolic activities of all the tissues of the body.

Hyper- and hypo-thyroidism

When the thyroid activity is normal the patient is said to be in a *euthyroid* state. If the thyroid is secreting an excess of thyroid hormones, the patient is said to be suffering from *hyperthyroidism* (or *thyrotoxicosis*), whereas if a subnormal secretion of thyroid hormone is taking place the condition is termed *hypothyroidism* or *myxoedema*.

Patients with hyperthyroidism show some or all of the following clinical features:

1. Central nervous system—the patient is irritable, nervous and demonstrates tremor of the outstretched fingers.
2. The skin—is moist and hot, the patient prefers winter to summer because she is so hot and sweaty in the warm weather.
3. The thyroid—this is usually enlarged but not invariably so. It may be highly vascular, which can be demonstrated by feeling the thrill of blood rushing through the thyroid when this is gently palpated.
4. The cardiovascular system—a rapid pulse is almost invariable and typically the sleeping pulse is also raised. There may be auricular fibrillation and, indeed, the patient may present with heart failure.
5. Alimentary system—the patient's appetite is increased and yet weight is lost. Diarrhoea is an occasional feature.

Many patients with thyrotoxicosis demonstrate exophthalmos. This is due to oedema and an actual increase in the mass of fat within the orbit and in the extrinsic muscles of the eye. Its cause remains unknown but the appearance is very typical (Fig. 16.3).

Hypothyroidism produces almost the complete opposite in the way of physical signs. Congenital hypothyroidism or *cretinism* is a condition in which the child is born with little or no functioning thyroid. He is stunted and mentally defective, with puffy lips, a large tongue and a swollen abdomen.

In the adult, hypothyroidism or myxoedema usually affects women and most often occurs in the middle aged or elderly. This patients have a slow deep voice, are overweight and apathetic with a dry coarse skin and thin hair (Fig. 16.4). They usually feel cold even in hot weather, have a slow pulse and are constipated.

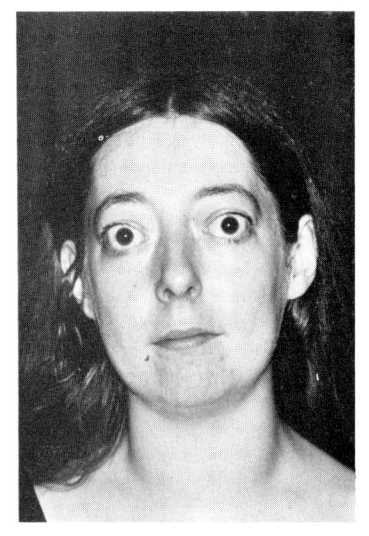

Fig. 16.3. Marked exophthalmos in a girl with severe thyrotoxicosis.

Fig. 16.4. Myxoedema. The patient is apathetic, the skin is thickened and coarse, and there has been loss of hair. This patient responded dramatically to treatment with thyroxine.

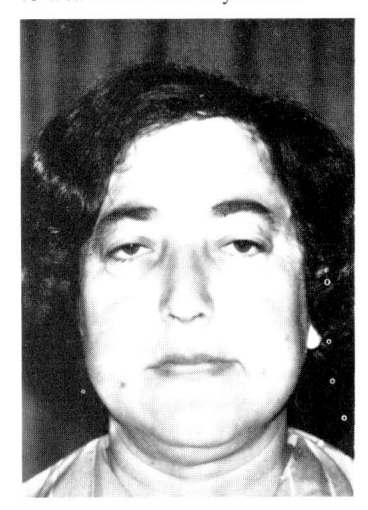

Tests of thyroid function

The sleeping pulse rate. This is a simple and reliable test. A great difficulty in the clinical diagnosis of hyperthyroidism is its differentiation from an acute anxiety state. However, such patients when sleeping will have a normal pulse rate while patients with hyperthyroidism continue to have a rapid pulse even when asleep.

Laboratory tests of thyroid function fall into two main groups. The first measures the amount of iodine taken up by the thyroid gland, since this is usually increased in hyperthyroidism and depressed in myxoedema. A small dose of radioactive iodine is injected intravenously and its uptake into the thyroid measured by means of a Gamma ray detector; the count is proportional to the activity of the thyroid. The second group of tests measures the amount of thyroid

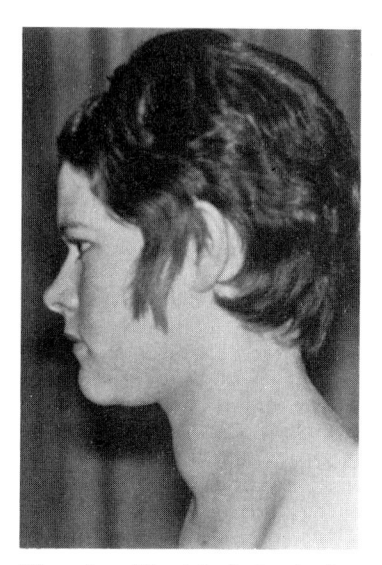

Fig. 16.5. 'Physiological goitre'; This young girl's thyroid became diffusely enlarged at puberty.

Fig. 16.6. A large nodular but non-toxic thyroid.

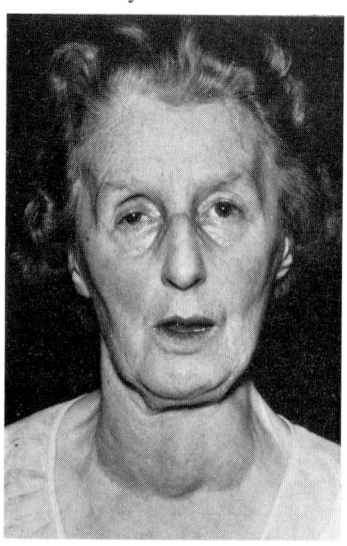

hormones circulating in the blood stream in the protein-bound form. This is normally raised in thyrotoxicosis and depressed in myxoedema, although false high values may be obtained in patients who have taken medicines such as cough mixture which contain iodine. A direct estimation can also be made of the serum level of thyroxine (the T4 level) and this is the most accurate of the laboratory tests in current use.

TYPES OF THYROID ENLARGEMENT

The clinical examination of a patient with enlargement of the thyroid gland falls into two phases. In the first place the physical characteristics of the gland must be determined to see whether it is smoothly enlarged, nodular, or infiltrating and invading adjacent tissues. Second, we must determine the endocrine state in order to see whether the patient is hyper-, hypo- or eu-thyroid.

A synthesis of these two phases gives a simple clinical classification of the vast majority of thyroid swellings.

(Note that 'goitre' is an old world that simply means 'any sort of thyroid enlargement').

The common conditions are:

1. A smooth, non-toxic enlargement of the thyroid gland; this is the *'physiological'* goitre. It is particularly found in mountainous areas in which the water and diet are low in iodine; examples are in Switzerland, the Himalayas, Ethiopia and, in England, Derbyshire (hence the term 'Derbyshire neck'). Lack of iodine results in a raised secretion of the thyroid-stimulating hormone of the pituitary with consequent thyroid enlargement. A similar situation may occur when there is increased requirement of thyroid hormone, which accounts for the enlargement of the gland which may occur during puberty or pregnancy (Fig. 16.5).

2. A nodular, non-toxic gland; this is the commonest thyroid abnormality found in this country, there being either a solitary or multiple nodules present (Fig. 16.6).

3. A smooth, toxic goitre. This is termed *primary thyrotoxicosis* or Graves' disease.

4. A nodular enlargement of the thyroid in the presence of toxicity; this is termed *secondary thyrotoxicosis* and is due to a previous nodular non-toxic gland becoming toxic.

5. Smooth enlargement of the thyroid with myxoedema, usually in a middle-aged female, is the condition known as *Hashimoto's disease*.

6. An invasive enlargement of the thyroid is probably due to *malignant disease* (Fig. 16.7). Note that carcinoma of the thyroid is relatively unusual but must be suspected in any solitary nodule in the thyroid gland.

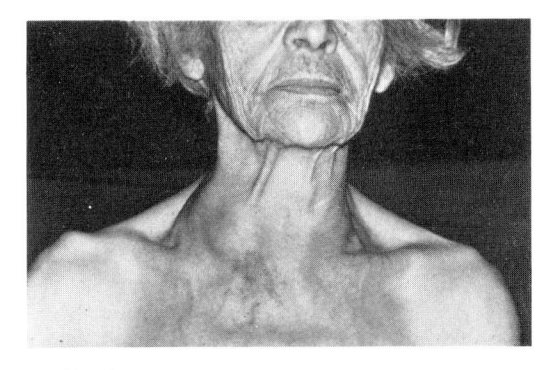

Fig. 16.7. An extensive carcinoma of the thyroid gland which is invading surrounding structures.

Outline of treatment of goitre

NON-TOXIC ENLARGEMENT

In endemic areas of goitre, the incidence of this condition has been greatly reduced by adding traces of potassium iodide to the table salt. In early stages of smooth enlargement, the condition may be reversible by administering thyroxine. However, if the physiological enlargement has failed to regress on this treatment and is producing symptoms of pressure on the trachea (Fig. 16.8) then partial thyroidectomy is necessary.

The single nodule in the thyroid or the non-toxic nodular enlargement will not improve on iodine or thyroxine treatment. In elderly patients with a long-standing goitre without symptoms it is probably best to leave well alone, but in nearly all other circumstances operative treatment is advisable for the following reasons:

1. Cosmetic appearance—often the patient is concerned about the appearance of her swollen neck.
2. There may be compression of the trachea and there is the risk of haemorrhage into a thyroid cyst which may produce acute airway compression.
3. Just as every solitary lump in a woman's breast is best removed, it is similarly wise to advise excision of any solitary thyroid nodule, since a small proportion of these prove to be carcinomatous.
4. There is a small risk that any nodular enlargement of the thyroid may undergo either malignant change or become toxic ('secondary thyrotoxicosis').

TOXIC GOITRE

The available methods of treatment in thyrotoxicosis are:
1. Medical treatment—antithyroid drugs.
2. Thyroidectomy after the patient has been rendered euthyroid by drug treatment.
3. Radio-active iodine.

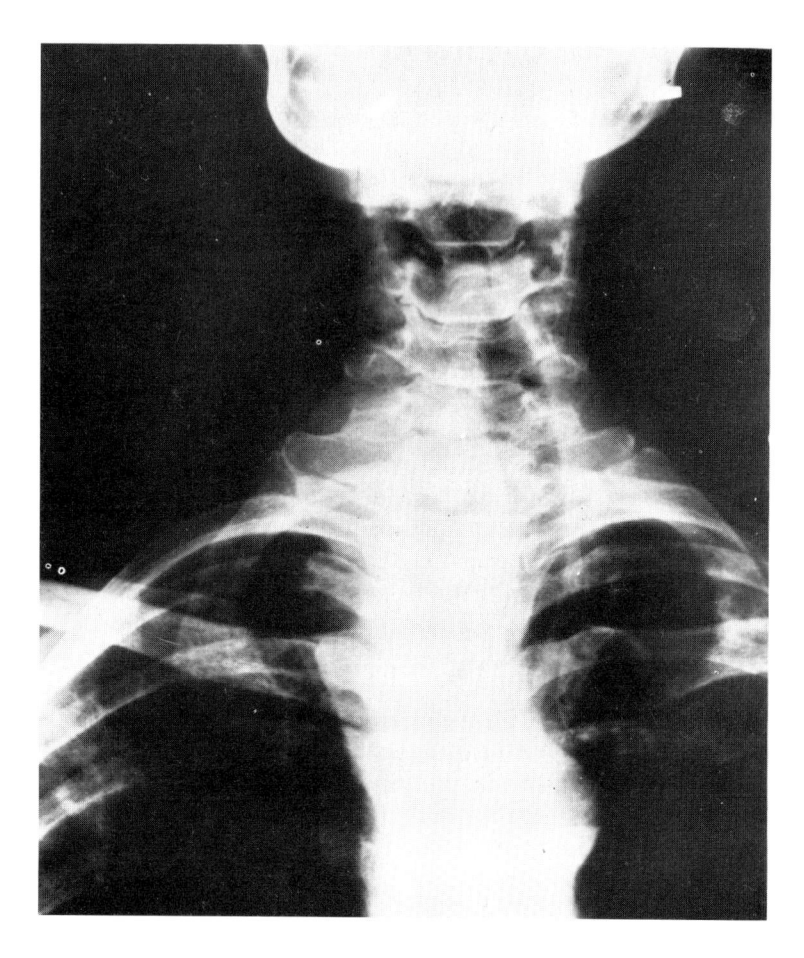

Fig. 16.8. X-ray of the thoracic inlet. The air-filled shadow of the trachea is displaced well over to the left by a nodular goitre mainly involving the right lobe.

Medical treatment

This usually comprises carbimazole (proprietary name Neomercazole) which is given in a dosage of 10 mg three times daily, combined with sedation and bed rest in the acute phase of thyrotoxicosis. There is rapid regression of symptoms and the patient begins to feel better within about two weeks. Unfortunately, there is a high relapse rate after ending treatment, even if this is prolonged for two or more years. Medical treatment alone is usually confined to the management of primary thyrotoxicosis in children and adolescents.

Toxic effects include skin rash, fever and agranulocytosis in which the polymorph white cell count in the blood drops almost to zero. The first symptom of this is a sore throat in which the normal commensal bacteria in the mouth begin to invade the tonsil region. Patients on carbimazole must be warned to discontinue treatment immediately if this occurs and to report to Hospital. Antibiotic therapy is commenced, fresh blood transfusions are given if necessary and the patient is barrier nursed until the bone marrow recovers.

Drugs and surgery combined

The majority of adult patients in this country are treated by preliminary carbimazole until euthyroid and then given iodine (potassium iodide 60 mg three times daily for about ten days) to reduce the vascularity of the gland, following which they are submitted to subtotal thyroidectomy; a small amount of thyroid tissue, about enough to fill a teaspoon, is left on either side.

Radio-active iodine

From the patient's point of view this treatment is miraculous! All she has to do is to swallow a glass of water containing the tasteless radio-iodine. There is no need to take tablets continuously, nor are there the risks of operation. It usually takes two or three months before the patient is rendered euthyroid and if seriously toxic it may be necessary to give carbimazole during this period.

There is a theoretical risk of carcinogenic change in the irradiated gland (although no case has yet been reported) and, because of this, it is current practice not to use radio-iodine in patients under the age of forty-five. It is not employed in young women who may become pregnant during treatment, since there is a danger of affecting the thyroid of the fetus.

The greatest disadvantage of this treatment is the production of hypothyroidism which increases in incidence with the passage of time and rises to nearly 13% after 10 years. When this occurs, thyroxine is used as replacement therapy.

Complications of thyroidectomy

Partial thyroidectomy is a common operation and the majority of cases make an uneventful recovery. However, there are a large number of possible post-operative complications which may occur, so that nurses on a surgical ward must always be on their toes when they are looking after thyroidectomy cases.

It is convenient to group these complications into three categories:
1. *The complications of any operation*
    Especially:
        Haemorrhage

Wound infection
Post-operative pulmonary collapse and chest infection
2. *Hormonal disturbance*
(of the thyroid itself and the adjacent parathyroid glands).
Thyroid crisis.
Myxoedema (due to extensive removal of thyroid tissue). Late recurrence of toxicity (inadequate operation in the toxic gland).
Tetany (due to damage or bruising of the parathyroid glands).
3. *Damage to related anatomical structures*
Recurrent laryngeal nerve injury with vocal cord paralysis.
Injury to the trachea.
Pneumothorax due to injury of the dome of the pleura.
Some of these complications require further consideration here.

Haemorrhage

Haemorrhage immediately after thyroidectomy is a dangerous condition, since bleeding into the tissues of the neck may compress the trachea. The situation must be dealt with at once by removing the skin and subcutaneous sutures, in the ward if necessary, in order to decompress the neck. The patient can then be transferred to the theatre, any bleeding points secured and the wound re-sutured. Blood loss may require transfusion replacement.

Thyroid crisis

An acute exacerbation of thyrotoxicosis may occur immediately after operation but this complication is now extremely rare because of careful pre-operative preparation. It is thought to be due to massive release of thyroxine from the hyperactive gland during surgery.

Treatment comprises heavy sedation, intravenous iodine and cooling the patient by means of ice packs.

Hypoparathyroidism

Accidental removal of the parathyroids or their bruising during operation will be followed by the development of tetany a few days post-operatively, with typical tetanic spasms affecting hands and legs. This may be precipitated by inflating a blood pressure cuff around the arm (Trousseau's sign). The serum calcium falls from its normal 10 mg to below 6 mg%.

In addition to frank tetany, (occurring in about 1% of cases), milder degrees of hypoparathyroidism may occur, and present months or even years later with mental depression, skin rashes or bilateral cataracts.

Treatment. Tetany is treated by giving 10 ml of 20% calcium gluconate intravenously. This is followed by calcium lactate 15 gm daily by mouth.

Recurrent laryngeal nerve injury

The recurrent laryngeal nerve lies in the groove between the oesophagus and the trachea, in close relationship to the inferior thyroid artery as this vessel passes forward into the posterior aspect of the thyroid gland (Fig. 16.9). Here the nerve is at risk of damage during thyroidectomy.

If only one nerve is damaged the patient develops slight hoarseness, which may gradually fade because the opposite vocal cord compensates by passing across the midline during speech. However, if both recurrent laryngeal nerves are injured, there is almost complete loss of voice and also serious narrowing of the airway, so that a permanent tracheostomy may be required. It is estimated that the nerve is injured in about 2% of thyroidectomies. Following operation, it should be routine practice to examine the vocal cords by means of a laryngoscope. Full movements of the cords during phonation means that the nerves are intact; damage to the nerve is shown by paralysis of the cord on the affected side.

CARCINOMA OF THE THYROID

Cancer of the thyroid is fortunately an unusual condition and accounts for about 400 deaths yearly in England and Wales. It is roughly three times more common in women than in men, may arise in a pre-existing goitre, and may follow irradiation of the neck in childhood.

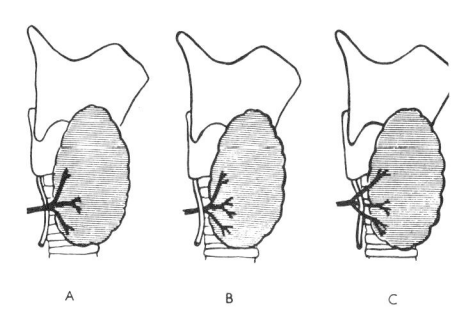

Fig. 16.9. The close relationship of the recurrent laryngeal nerve to the thyroid gland and the inferior artery. (A) The nerve is usually deep to the artery but (B) may be superficial to it or (C) passed through its branches.

Thyroid cancers fall into two main groups:

1. *Well-differentiated tumours* which, under the microscope, may have either a *papillary* or *follicular* appearance. The first is arranged in a frond-like pattern, the second resembles normal thyroid tissue. Quite often both types occur in the same tumour.

2. *Anaplastic carcinoma*, which is undifferentiated and is made up of masses of rapidly growing cancer cells.

Such important differences occur between these two groups that they might almost be considered as separate diseases.

The well-differentiated tumours occur in young adults, adolescents or even children. They are slow-growing, although they may spread to the regional lymph nodes and, as a late affair, by the blood stream to the bones, lungs etc. The anaplastic carcinomas, in contrast, occur in the elderly (see Fig. 16.7). Rapid local spread takes place, with compression and invasion of the trachea and involvement of the recurrent laryngeal nerve, resulting in hoarseness. There is an early lymphatic spread to the nodes in the neck and dissemination via the blood stream to the lungs, skeleton and the brain.

Treatment

The well-differentiated carcinoma presents as a localised mass in the thyroid and is treated by total removal of the affected lobe of the gland. If adjacent lymph nodes are involved these too are excised.

Many well-differentiated tumours take up radio-active iodine and it is possible to treat recurrences or metastases by this means.

The thyroid cells are under the control of the anterior pituitary and this applies also to the well-differentiated cells in thyroid cancer. It has been shown that giving thyroid will suppress the thyrotrophic hormone of the pituitary, and there have been remarkable examples of regression of thyroid cancer when large doses of thyroxine are given.

The anaplastic carcinomas may be treated by radical thyroidectomy but usually these patients present with an already inoperable mass in the neck. Palliative radiotherapy may give temporary relief and tracheostomy may be required for obstruction of the airway.

Prognosis

This is very different in the two groups of cases; the well-differentiated tumours may be associated with long survival, even in the presence of lymph node deposits, whereas patients with anaplastic tumours generally have a very poor outlook.

HASHIMOTO'S DISEASE

This is an uncommon disease which has, however, received considerable attention because it was demonstrated some years ago that in this condition the patient produces antibodies to her own thyroid tissue. This was the first of the group of conditions termed 'the autoimmune diseases'.

The patient is usually a middle aged female with an enlarged thyroid gland and evidence of hypothyroidism. Under the microscope the thyroid is diffusely infiltrated with lymphocytes and fibrous tissue. About 90% of these patients can be shown to have antibodies in their blood which react against thyroglobulin.

Biopsy may be necessary to confirm the diagnosis. The condition is treated by thyroxine, the maintenance dose of which varies between 0.1 and 0.3 mg daily.

The parathyroid glands

Anatomy

The parathyroid glands are four in number, each about the size of a split pea, which usually lie in two pairs behind the lateral lobes of the thyroid gland. The inferior parathyroids may lie occasionally almost anywhere in the neck or even descend into the superior mediastinum (Fig. 16.10).

Physiology

The function of the parathyroids is to secrete *parathormone*, which maintains the normal plasma calcium level. If the calcium in the

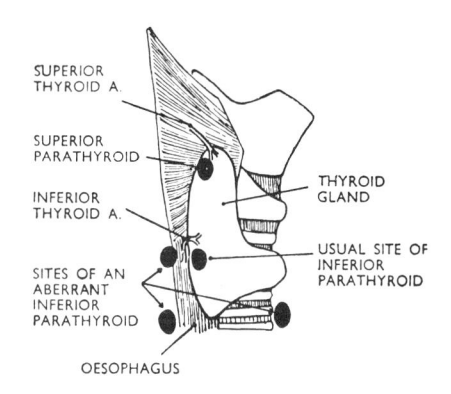

Fig. 16.10. The normal and abnormal sites of the parathyroid glands.

blood falls, the parathyroid glands are stimulated to secrete more hormone and vice-versa. The exact mechanisms of the action of this hormone are not known. The most popular theory is that parathormone mobilises calcium from bones but it may also act by producing excessive excretion of phosphate from the kidney.

Tetany

Lack of parathormone produces a low serum calcium; this results in hyper-irritability of the skeletal muscles with spasms, the syndrome being termed *tetany*. This is liable to occur if the serum calcium falls below the normal level of 10 mg% to the region of 6 mg%. The muscle spasms may affect any part of the body, but typically the hands and feet are involved. The wrist becomes flexed and the fingers are drawn together, rather fancifully like the hand of an obstetrician ('main d'accoucheur'). This spasm may be induced by inflating a blood pressure cuff around the arm (*Trousseau's sign*).

Parathyroid tumours

Parathyroid tumours are mostly benign adenomas; carcinoma may occur but it is fortunately rare. The importance of these tumours is that they produce an excessive secretion of parathormone. Occasionally this results from hyperplasia of the parathyroid glands.

The symptoms of excess parathormone secretion may fall under one or more of the following headings:

1. *Renal effects*. The commonest presentation of hyperparathyroidism is renal stone formation due to the excessive excretion of calcium in the urine.
2. *Bone changes*. There may be decalcification of bones with cyst formation and even spontaneous fractures. This condition is known as osteitis fibrosa cystica, which, as the name implies, means fibrosis and cyst formation in bone. It is also termed Von Recklinghausen's disease of bone.
3. *Features due to the high serum calcium*. These include lassitude, weakness, anorexia, loss of weight, and excessive thirst.
4. *Peptic ulceration*. Indigestion or duodenal ulceration is sometimes associated with a high serum calcium.

We can sum up the main effects as 'stones, bones, abdominal groans'.

The diagnosis is confirmed by estimation of the serum calcium, which is raised to 11 mg% or above. Other causes of a raised serum calcium include widespread malignant disease, sarcoid and excessive administration of Vitamin D. In these conditions the serum calcium falls to normal if a 10-day course of hydrocortisone is given (the cortisone suppression test).

Treatment. The parathyroid adenoma requires surgical removal. This can be rather difficult to find as the tumour may be small and may be lying in an ectopic position.

Hypoparathyroidism

This is usually secondary to surgery in the neck, especially thyroidectomy, and is considered on page 376.

The adrenal glands

Anatomy

The adrenal, or suprarenal, glands cap the upper poles of the kidneys and lie against the diaphragm. The left is related anteriorly to the stomach, whereas the right lies behind the right lobe of the liver and tucks itself on its inner side behind the inferior vena cava.

The adrenal gland is a good example of where two organs with entirely separate functions are fused into one anatomical structure. Other examples are the anterior and posterior lobes of the pituitary, and the insulin-secreting islet cells embedded in the enzyme-secreting glandular tissue of the pancreas. If the adrenal gland is cut across it will be seen to comprise a golden yellow *cortex* and a dark red central *medulla*. The latter is derived from the neural crest of the embryo, which also gives rise to the sympathetic ganglia. The cortex is derived from mesoderm. These two parts of the gland have entirely separate origins, functions and diseases and it is therefore also necessary to consider them quite separately.

THE ADRENAL MEDULLA

Physiology

The medulla of the adrenal gland is made up of large cells which stain yellow with chromic acid; for this reason they are termed *chromaffin cells*. Stimulation of the sympathetic nerves causes these cells to secrete adrenaline and noradrenaline into the blood stream. *Adrenaline* increases the heart rate and the cardiac output and, because of this, raises the blood pressure. Another effect is to mobilise sugar from the liver and thus to increase the blood glucose level.

Noradrenaline particularly acts by producing constriction of peripheral blood vessels.

Tumours of the adrenal medulla

From the surgical point of view the adrenal medulla is of importance because a number of rather unusual tumours may arise within it. These are:
1. Ganglioneuroma
2. Neuroblastoma
3. Phaeochromocytoma
4. Secondaries (a site for deposits from carcinoma of the breast and bronchus).

Ganglioneuroma

A benign tumour which may arise from cells in the sympathetic ganglia or, in 15% of cases, in the cells of the adrenal medulla.

Neuroblastoma

A highly malignant tumour of sympathetic ganglion cells which occurs in young children. There is early dissemination to lymph nodes, the skeleton and the liver.

PHAEOCHROMOCYTOMA

Although this tumour is rather rare it is of considerable importance because it represents a cause of severe hypertension which can be cured surgically. It is a physiologically active tumour of chromaffin cells which secretes noradrenaline and adrenaline. Ninety per cent occur within the adrenal glands themselves but 10% arise elsewhere in the sympathetic chain and it is useful to note that 10% are malignant and 10% are multiple. For this reason it has been given the nick-name of 'the ten per cent tumour'.

Any age may be affected, but the tumour is particularly found in young adults.

Clinical features

These are produced by the excess of circulating adrenaline and noradrenaline. The most important feature is the hypertension, which may be paroxysmal or sustained. This may be accompanied by palpitations, headache, blurred vision, fits and papilloedema. The intense constriction of peripheral blood vessels may produce episodes of pallor and there may be attacks of profuse sweating.

The excess secretion of adrenaline may produce hyperglycaemia with glycosuria; indeed about 10% of these patients have diabetes.

Special investigations

It is possible to measure the level of adrenaline or noradrenaline excreted in the urine. Most laboratories measure the major metabolite of these chemicals in the urine which is vanillyl mandelic acid (abbreviated to VMA).

The high blood pressure produced by phaeochromocytoma is brought down to normal by giving phentolamine, which is a noradrenaline antagonist.

If we are pretty certain that a tumour is present, attempts are then made to localise it to one or other adrenal, or to other parts of the sympathetic chain, by carrying out an aortogram or by outlining the retroperitoneal tissues for X-ray examination by insufflation with carbon dioxide.

Treatment

Having localised the tumour, surgical excision is carried out. This must be done with considerable care since manipulation of the tumour during the operation releases adrenaline and noradrenaline into the blood stream. The gross hypertension which may result is countered by intravenous phentolamine. Immediately after removal of the tumour the blood pressure may fall to very low levels and it may be necessary to counter this by blood transfusion and by a noradrenaline drip, which may have to be continued for a day or two after the operation (Fig. 16.11).

THE ADRENAL CORTEX

Physiology

The adrenal cortex is essential to life because of the important hormones which it secretes. Unless these are replaced, the adrenalectomised patient will certainly die. These hormones are varieties of chemicals called steroids and it is interesting that this chemical structure is also the basis of cholesterol, bile salts and the sex hormones.

The steroids secreted by the adrenal cortex overlap in their action, but they can be divided into three main groups:
1. *The glucocorticoids*—these regulate carbohydrate metabolism, protein break-down and the mobilisation of fat from tissue stores. Most important of these are cortisone and hydrocortisone.
2. *Sex hormones*—of both the male (androgenic) and female (oestrogenic) varieties.

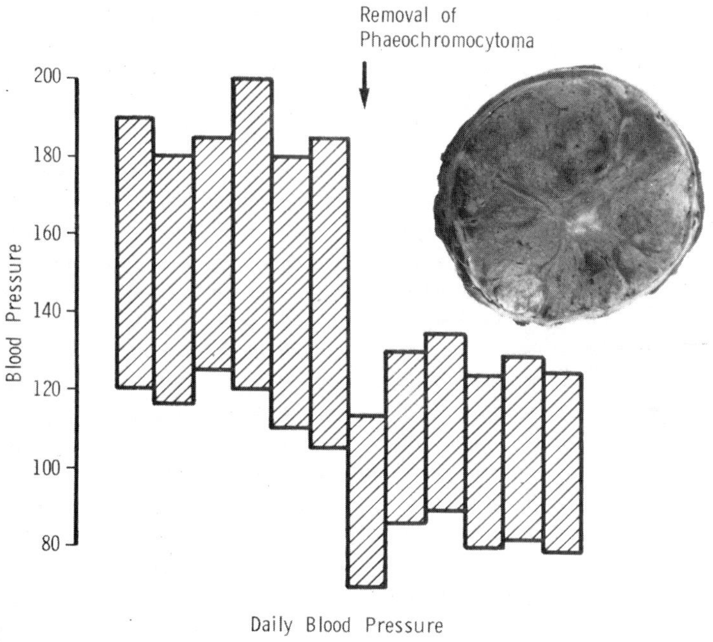

Fig. 16.11. Daily blood pressure readings before and after excision of a phaeochromocytoma. Note the dramatic fall in pressure after surgery. The inset shows the cut surface of the tumour.

3. *Mineral corticoids*—these regulate salt and water metabolism. The most important of these is aldosterone which acts to retain sodium and water and to regulate potassium excretion by the kidney.

It should be noted that representatives of these groups may overlap in their action. Thus although cortisone is an important member of the glucocorticoid group, it also affects salt and water metabolism and has androgenic effects (acne and excessive hair growth) if given in large amounts.

The secretion of hormones by the adrenal cortex is under the control of the anterior lobe of the pituitary, which produces adrenocorticotropic hormone (ACTH), a specific stimulant to the adrenal cortex. If excess cortisone is produced, there is what is termed a 'feed back' mechanism which inhibits the output of ACTH in an attempt to reduce cortisone secretion.

Hyperadrenocorticism

Overaction of the adrenal cortex, with excessive secretion of its hormones, may be due to a number of causes: hyperplasia of the gland, a functioning tumour of the cortex (either a benign adenoma or a malignant carcinoma) or occasionally the condition may be secondary to a pituitary tumour producing an excess of ACTH.

The clinical pictures produced by hyperfunction of the adrenal

cortex can be attributed to excess of each of its three groups of hormones:
1. Cushing's syndrome—glucocorticoid excess.
2. The adrenogenital syndrome, or virilism—due to excess androgen production.
3. Conn's syndrome or primary aldosteronism—oversecretion of aldosterone, the important mineral corticoid.

CUSHING'S SYNDROME

This syndrome was first described by Harvey Cushing of Boston, one of the pioneers of neurosurgery. It results from an over secretion of adrenal corticosteroids and is also reproduced exactly by patients who are receiving large doses of cortisone (Fig. 16.12). The majority of cases are due to hyperplasia of the adrenal cortex, but some are due to benign or malignant tumours and rarely to a tumour of the anterior lobe of the pituitary.

Clinical features

The syndrome usually affects young adults, females much more often than males. The appearance is quite typical. The patient is obese, but the fat is distributed centrally, mostly over the trunk, face and neck, giving the typical 'moon face'; the arms and legs are, in contrast, relatively thin. The skin of the face is red, acne is common and there is often an increased growth of hair on the face so that the unfortunate woman may have to shave each day. Ugly red striae appear on the abdomen, exactly like the 'stretch marks' which follow pregnancy. The periods cease, the blood pressure is increased, the bones become thinned (osteoporosis) and diabetes is common.

Special investigations

The raised level of steroid production can be measured by estimating the excretion of ketosteroids in the urine. X-rays of the abdomen after injection of carbon dioxide into the retroperitoneal space may enable the radiologist to localise the adrenal tumour. The adrenals can also be outlined by aortography. An X-ray of the skull may sometimes reveal an enlarged pituitary fossa, which suggests the presence of a pituitary tumour.

Treatment

Bilateral adrenalectomy is performed for bilateral hyperplasia and the patient is then maintained on cortisone. In cases of adrenal tumour, the affected gland is removed (Fig. 16.13).

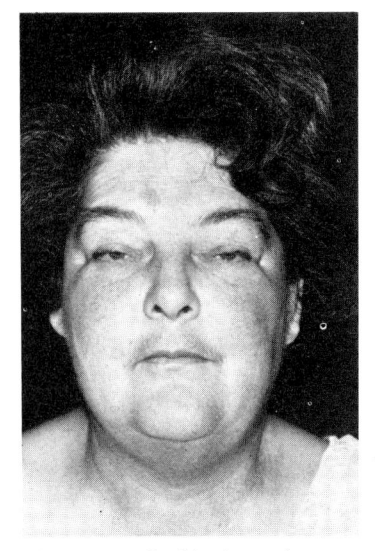

Fig. 16.12. Cushing's syndrome. Note the 'Moon-face'.

Fig. 16.13. A large adenoma of the adrenal cortex.

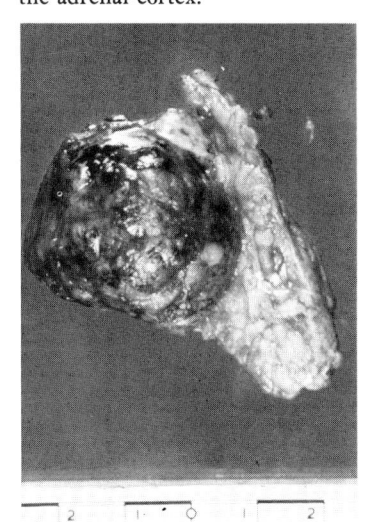

The rare examples which are due to pituitary tumour may respond to hypophysectomy.

THE ADRENOGENITAL SYNDROME

This syndrome results from an over secretion of androgens by the adrenal cortex and can be divided into a congenital and an acquired type:

1. *The congenital form* appears to be due to a failure of the adrenal cortex to synthesise hydrocortisone. The pituitary therefore produces an excess of ACTH which results in hyperplasia of the adrenal cortex and hypersecretion of cortical androgens.

2. *The acquired variety* in children is always due to a tumour of the adrenal cortex, usually malignant. In young adults it may be due either to a tumour or to hyperplasia of the gland in examples of Cushing's syndrome where androgen production is excessive.

Clinical features

These fall conveniently into three groups, depending on the age of onset.

1. *Congenital.* In this variety, the new born female has an enlarged clitoris and is often mistaken for a male (female pseudo-hermaphrodite). The child initially grows rapidly, but the epiphyses fuse early, so that eventually the youngster is stunted. There may be episodes of acute adrenal insufficiency especially precipitated by stress or infection.

2. *Childhood.* In the female there is virilisation and in the male child precocious sexual development (the 'infant Hercules'). The changes have been summed up as 'little girls become little boys and little boys become little men'.

3. *Adults.* In the male feminisation is seen, but this is extremely rare. The condition is commoner in females, who show the features of Cushing's syndrome together with amenorrhoea, excessive hair growth and atrophy of the breasts.

The diagnosis is confirmed in the laboratory by determining the excretion of 17-ketosteroid in the urine, which is greatly raised in this condition.

Treatment

In infancy treatment comprises the administration of cortisone. This suppresses the excess ACTH secretion which, in turn cuts down the excessive excretion of androgens. In the acquired variety the adrenals are explored; if a tumour is present this is removed or if both glands show hyperplasia, bilateral adrenalectomy is performed with subsequent cortisone maintenance.

CONN'S SYNDROME

This is a rare disease produced by an aldosterone-secreting adenoma of the adrenal cortex. There is sodium retention and a fall in serum potassium, which results in muscular weakness. There is associated hypertension and it is the association of a raised blood pressure with a low potassium that gives rise to suspicion of this condition. The tumour is small, benign, and its removal cures the condition.

ADDISON'S DISEASE

This is a disease, first described by Thomas Addison of Guy's Hospital in 1849, of chronic insufficiency of the adrenal cortex. It may result from atrophy of the gland or its destruction by tuberculosis or malignant disease.

Clinical features

The sexes are equally affected. There is gross muscle weakness, low blood pressure and pigmentation of the skin from melanin deposition, which also occurs within the mouth.

Special investigations

Deficiency of the cortical hormones is reflected by a decreased sodium and chloride, together with potassium elevation in the plasma. The urinary excretion of steroids is also grossly diminished. Note that a similar picture (although without the pigmentation) is seen in patients following bilateral adrenalectomy who are not receiving sufficient steroid cover.

Treatment

This comprises the adequate replacement of cortisone.

Adrenalectomy for breast cancer

This is considered in Chapter 17.

The pituitary gland

See Chapter 10.

Chapter 17. The breast

Anatomy

The female breast overlies the 2nd to the 6th rib and rests on the pectoralis major and the serratus anterior muscles. It is made up of 15–20 lobules of glandular tissue which are embedded in fat. Each lobule drains on to the nipple by a separate duct. The nipple itself is surrounded by the pigmented areola which is lubricated by the glands of Montgomery. These are modified sebaceous glands and may occasionally become obstructed and distended into a sebaceous cyst.

The male breast is rudimentary and is made up of small ducts without gland tissue, but supported by fibrous tissue and fat. Although an insignificant structure it is still prone to all the major diseases that affect the female organ.

The breast has a rich blood supply derived from branches of the axillary, the internal mammary and the intercostal arteries with venous drainage to the corresponding veins.

The lymphatic drainage of the breast is of considerable importance in the spread of breast tumours and, as with any other organ, follows the same pathway as its blood supply. The lymphatics, therefore, travel along the tributaries of the axillary vessels to the axillary lymph nodes, and also along tributaries of the internal mammary vessels in each intercostal space to the lymph nodes which run along the internal mammary chain and which also receive lymphatics penetrating along the perforating branches of the intercostal vessels (Fig. 17.1). If these normal lymphatic pathways are interrupted by malignant deposits, lymphatic spread may occur further afield to the opposite breast, the opposite axilla, the lymph nodes in the groin and the nodes in the neck.

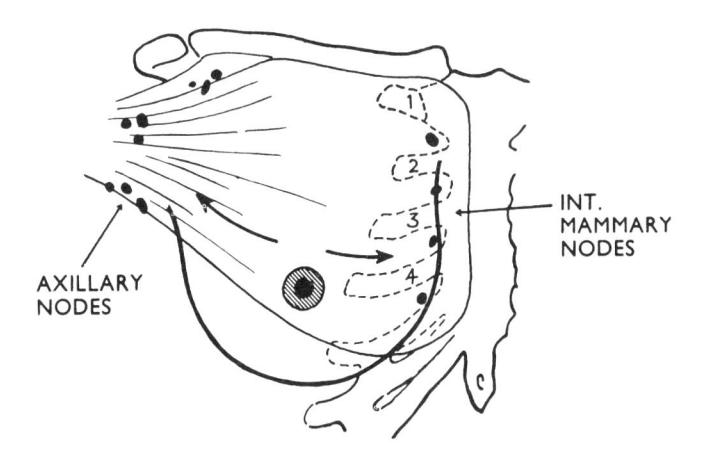

Fig. 17.1. Diagram of the principle pathways of lymph drainage of the breast. These follow the venous drainage of the breast to the axilla and to the internal mammary chain.

Development of the breast

The breast develops as an ingrowth of the skin of the chest wall which forms a series of branching ducts. Shortly before birth this site of invagination everts to form the nipple. At puberty, glandular tissue sprouts from the ducts and considerable fatty infiltration of the breast tissue takes place. With pregnancy there is a tremendous development of the duct system which, during lactation, secretes the fatty droplets of milk. At the menopause the gland tissue undergoes atrophy.

Developmental abnormalities of the breast are quite common. The nipple may remain inverted and create difficulties during attempts to breast feed. Supernumerary nipples or even additional breasts may occur and act as a reminder of the line of mammary glands found in more primitive mammals. In other cases the breast on one or both sides may fail to develop (*amazia*).

ACUTE INFLAMMATION OF THE BREAST

The commonest inflammation of the breast is due to the staphylococcus aureus which invades the breast tissue either through a crack in the skin of the nipple, or along one of the lactiferous ducts. It is especially likely to occur during lactation, when the breast is engorged with milk and the nipple is being traumatised by the baby's mouth. Under these circumstances inflammation is especially likely to take place in the first month of lactation and in the first pregnancy.

The infection commences as a cellulitis (see page 10), a spreading infection of the subcutaneous tissues. The patient is febrile and the affected segment of the breast is red, hot, swollen and tender. Within a few days, the infection localises into an abscess.

Treatment

Breast feeding is discontinued and the breast emptied of milk either by expression or by means of a breast pump. If seen within 24 hours of the onset of the symptoms, the infection is likely still to be in its spreading cellulitic phase and, at this stage, antibiotic treatment may abort the infection before abscess formation takes place. Since the majority of infections are acquired in hospital, the staphylococci are almost certain to be penicillin resistant and therefore it is necessary to use erythromycin or methicillin (celbenin). However, if infection is already established for several days, it can be assumed that tissue breakdown is already occurring with abscess formation. Antibiotic treatment at this stage will simply produce a chronic abscess walled off by dense fibrous tissue, a condition which has received the nicknames of 'antibioticoma' or 'penicillinoma'. In these circumstances it is surgical drainage that is necessary, not antibiotics. A small incision is made into the centre of the abscess, the finger used to break down any loculi and a soft drain inserted. The drain is subsequently shortened each day until the abscess cavity has healed from below upwards.

CHRONIC MASTITIS

This is the commonest by far of all conditions affecting the breast. In spite of its name, it is not an inflammatory condition at all. Many more scientific terms have been given to it, of which the best is fibroadenosis, but most people use the older and less accurate term.

Pathology

Any organ in the body which undergoes cyclical changes of proliferation and regression is prone to abnormalities of this process; these organs are the thyroid, prostate, ovary and breast. Since these cyclical changes only occur in the breast during the woman's menstrual life, the disturbances of chronic mastitis are seen between the age of about 30 and the menopause. The breast tissue is yellowy white, of rubbery, nodular consistency and may contain cysts. Under the microscope there is an increase of the connective tissue between the glandular elements, hyperplasia of the glandular tissue, formation of cysts, which vary from microscopic size to several inches in diameter, and infiltration by lymphocytes. It is, in fact, this infiltration of white cells which cause the early pathologists to label the condition 'chronic mastitis' in the mistaken belief that it was some sort of chronic inflammatory condition.

Clinical features

The patient usually complains of aching in one or both breasts, especially before the periods. A lump may be noticed in the breast or the patient may sometimes complain of discharge from the nipple, which may be blood stained, yellow or green. Examination may show a generalised lumpiness and granularity of both breasts or a mass confined to one sector of the breast which, for some unknown reason, is especially likely to be the upper, outer quadrant (Fig. 17.2). Less commonly there may be one or more cystic masses in the breast which may be of considerable size. Quite often the lymph nodes in the axillae are enlarged and rubbery.

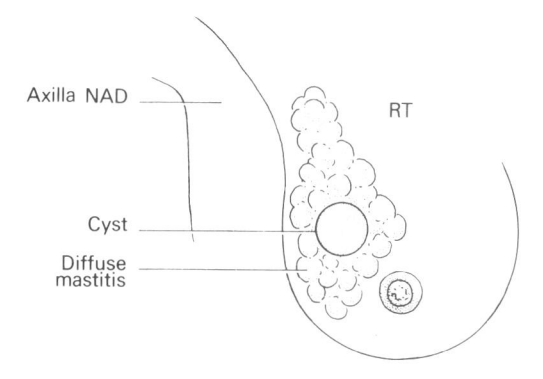

Fig. 17.2. Diagram of the typical findings in a patient with diffuse chronic mastitis and an associated cyst.

Management

Chronic mastitis is a harmless condition and there is no evidence that it predisposes to cancer of the breast. If the patient presents with diffuse granularity or nodularity in the breast and with no localised mass, nothing more is required than reassurance. However, if a discrete lump is discovered in the breast, then it is vitally important to make sure that this is not a cancer. The lump is removed and submitted to microscopic examination; if benign, no further treatment is needed, but if a tumour is found then appropriate surgery is carried out (see below).

If the surgeon thinks that the lump is a cyst, it is a common practice to perform aspiration under local anaesthesia (Fig. 17.3). If the fluid obtained is not blood stained (it is usually yellow, brown or green in colour) and if the lump disappears completely, we can be quite sure that the cyst is perfectly benign. If no fluid is obtained then, of course, excision of the lump must be carried out.

It is a wise saying that 'no lady should have a lump in the breast' and the diagnosis of any discrete lump in the breast must always be elucidated.

Fig. 17.3. Aspiration of a large cyst of the left breast. The mass disappeared completely and it did not recur.

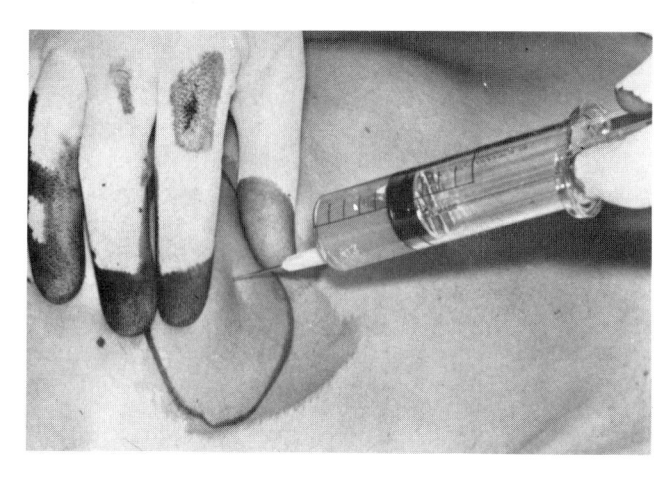

BENIGN TUMOURS OF THE BREAST

There are two common benign breast tumours, the duct papilloma, and the fibroadenoma.

Duct papilloma

This arises from the epithelium lining one of the main breast ducts. The usual complaint is of bleeding from the nipple and the surgeon examining the patient may find a small lump adjacent to the nipple, pressure on which produces a bloody discharge. In other cases he may be unable to feel the lump but pressure on one spot causes a discharge of blood.

Treatment comprises excision of the lump or of the affected segment from which the blood can be expressed. Of course it is important to submit the tissue to microscopic examination because in some cases the same signs and symptoms can be produced by an intraduct carcinoma.

Fibroadenoma

This is a benign encapsulated tumour made up of fibrous tissue which surrounds proliferating epithelial ducts (Fig. 17.4). It commonly occurs in young women, often in their teens, and presents as a highly mobile firm lump in the breast, so mobile, in fact, that it receives the nickname of a 'breast mouse'. Sometimes in middle aged or elderly women a very large lobular fibroadenoma occurs which may even ulcerate through the overlying skin by pressure necrosis and mimic an advanced malignant tumour (Brodie's disease of the breast). Occasionally, sarcomatous change may occur.

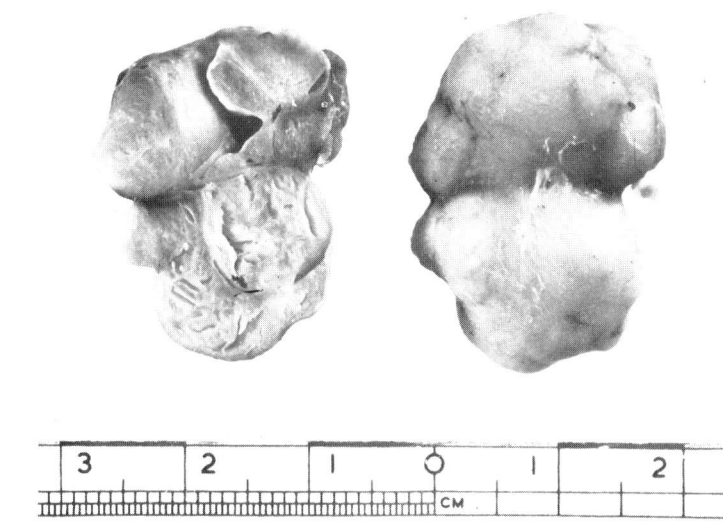

Fig. 17.4. Fibroadenoma of the breast. This is easily enucleated from the adjacent breast tissue.

Treatment. Remembering our aphorism that 'no lady has a lump in the breast', all fibroadenomas should be removed and submitted to examination under the microscope to confirm the diagnosis and to ensure that a small carcinoma has not been misdiagnosed as a benign lesion.

CARCINOMA OF THE BREAST

Cancer of the breast is an immensely important subject. It is the commonest cause of death from malignant disease in women in the United Kingdom and accounts for approximately 10,000 deaths per year in England and Wales (Fig. 17.5). In the population as a whole, it is only exceeded in frequency by carcinoma of the lung, the large intestine and the stomach. About 1% of cases occur in males. Any age may be affected but the condition is rare below 30, and the

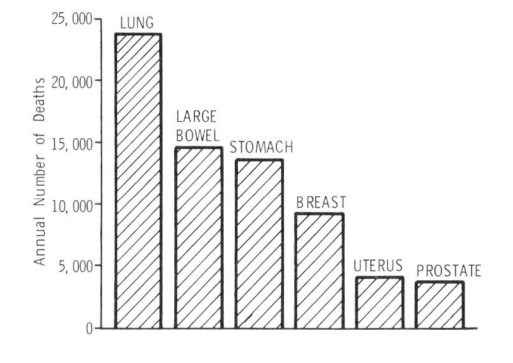

Fig. 17.5. Histogram of the common causes of death from cancer in England and Wales. Note that cancer of the breast is the fourth commonest for the sexes combined and the commonest cause of cancer deaths in women.

majority of patients present between the ages of 40 and 70. There is no definite evidence of any predisposing factors, although it is more commonly found in childless women. Any part of the breast may be involved, although the tumour is particularly likely to be found in the upper outer quadrant.

Pathology and Spread

Carcinoma of the breast usually arises from the glandular epithelium, although occasionally it arises in one of the milk ducts to form an intra-duct carcinoma. An unusual variety is termed *Paget's disease of the nipple* which is believed to be an intra-duct carcinoma of the breast which invades and ulcerates the nipple by extending along the main ducts from the primary tumour to become implanted in the epidermis (Fig. 17.6).

Tumour spread may occur as follows:

1. *By direct extension* first expanding through the breast substance, then involving the overlying skin, which is first dimpled over it, and may then become ulcerated (Fig. 17.7). The fibrous reaction around the tumour may produce retraction and elevation of the nipple (Fig. 17.8). Eventually, deep extension involves pectoralis major and even the chest wall itself.

2. *Lymphatic spread.* The main lymph channels pass directly to the axillary and internal mammary lymph nodes. The former may be palpated in the armpit but the latter cannot be detected clinically. Later spread occurs to the lymph nodes above the clavicle, to the groin and to the opposite axillary nodes. Obstruction of the dermal lymphatics of the skin of the breast leads to cutaneous oedema which is pitted by the orifices of the sweat ducts. This gives the appearance of orange peel ('peau d'orange') (Fig. 17.9). This lymphatic invasion

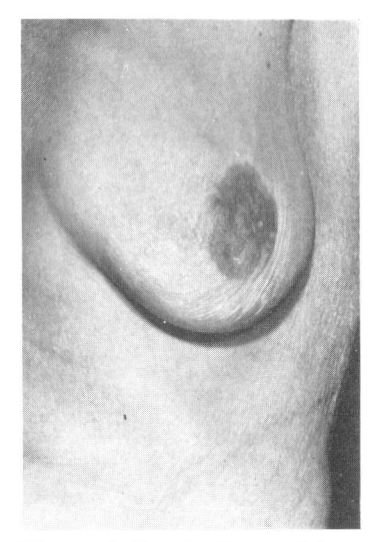

Fig. 17.6. Paget's disease of the nipple. The nipple is reddened and ulcerated.

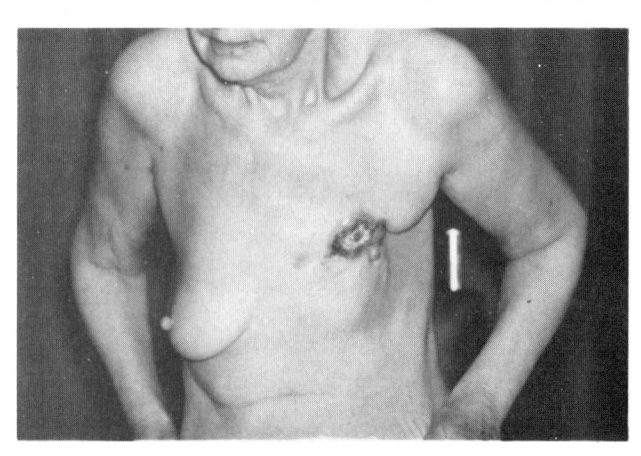

Fig. 17.7. Carcinoma of the breast which has involved and ulcerated the overlying skin.

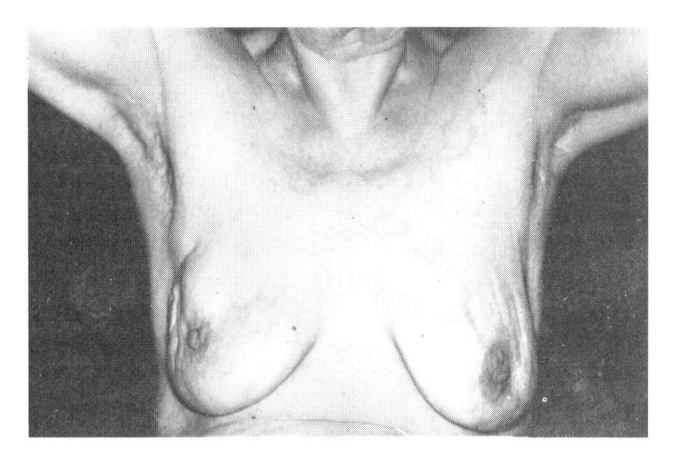

Fig. 17.8. Carcinoma of the right breast. Note the elevation and retraction of the nipple. The skin is tethered to the underlying tumour mass.

produces daughter skin nodules and eventually the whole chest wall may become a firm mass of tumour tissue rather like a suit of armour ('cancer en cuirasse') (Fig. 17.10).

3. *Blood spread.* The tumour may invade the small blood vessels of the breast, allowing tumour cells to disseminate widely by the blood stream. These deposits are especially prone to grow in the lungs, liver (see Fig. 5.5) and bones. The skull, vertebral column, pelvis, ribs, upper end of the femur and upper end of the humerus are especially likely to be involved. There is no mystery about this; these bones are the sites where red bone marrow persist in the adult, so that they have a particularly good blood supply and thus favour tumour growth. The brain, the ovaries and the adrenal glands are also frequent sites of tumour deposits.

4. *Trans-coelomic.* In advanced disease, tumour seeding may occur over the pleural and peritoneal surfaces, accompanied by the development of a pleural effusion (see Fig. 5.6) and ascites respectively.

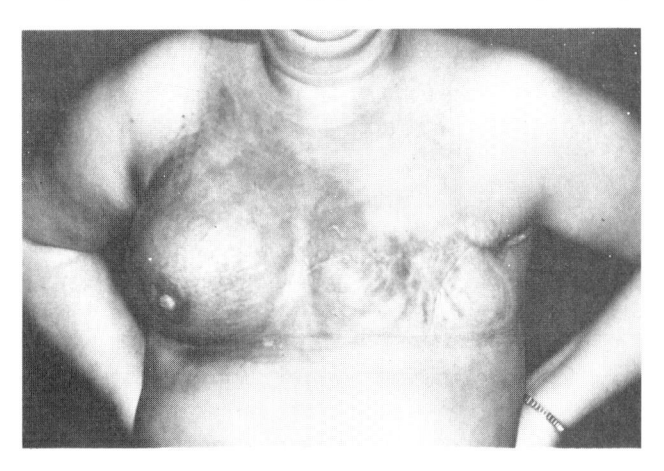

Fig. 17.9. 'Peau d'orange' due to lymphatic obstruction in an extensive carcinoma of the breast.

Fig. 17.10. 'Cancer en cuirasse'. This patient has already had a mastectomy for a carcinoma of the left breast. She now has an extensive tumour of the right breast involving the skin of the chest wall.

Clinical features

The commonest mode of presentation is for the patient to notice a painless lump in her breast or to have this detected during the course of a routine medical examination. Occasionally a pricking discomfort is noticed in the lump or the patient discovers recent indrawing of the nipple or a blood-stained discharge therefrom. A small proportion of patients present with symptoms produced by secondary deposits. A woman may discover a clump of enlarged nodes in the axilla, for example, or may complain of back-ache from spinal deposits, a pathological fracture, or breathlessness from involvement of the lung and pleura.

On examination, the surgeon may detect nothing more than a localised small lump in the breast and, without removal for microcopic examination, he may be unable to determine whether the lump is benign (a cyst, area of chronic mastitis or a fibroadenoma) or malignant. Signs which suggest malignant disease are retraction of the nipple, fixation of the skin to the underlying tumour, enlarged nodes in the axilla, or evidence of deposits elsewhere, for example enlargement of the liver, pleural effusion or ascites.

Note that only recent nipple retraction is significant, because the nipple may have been indrawn since birth or following a previous breast infection. If the retraction is recent it is significant; if of long standing, it can be discounted.

Special investigations

The chest is X-rayed and a radiographic skeletal survey is taken of the bones likely to be the sites of secondary deposits—skull, spine, pelvis, upper end of the femur and upper end of the humerus (the ribs, of course, will be visualised on the chest X-ray). Recently it has been shown that scanning of the bones following the injection of radio-active fluorine is an even more accurate way of detecting bony deposits than conventional X-rays but this technique can only be carried out in a number of special centres.

Clinical staging

Having carefully examined the patient, the surgeon can then place the tumour into one of the following stages:

Stage   I—the lump is confined to the breast
Stage   II—in addition the axillary lymph nodes are enlarged
Stage III—the tumour is invading the skin and/or the underlying muscles; the axillary nodes may also be fixed to surrounding tissues
Stage IV—distant metastases are present

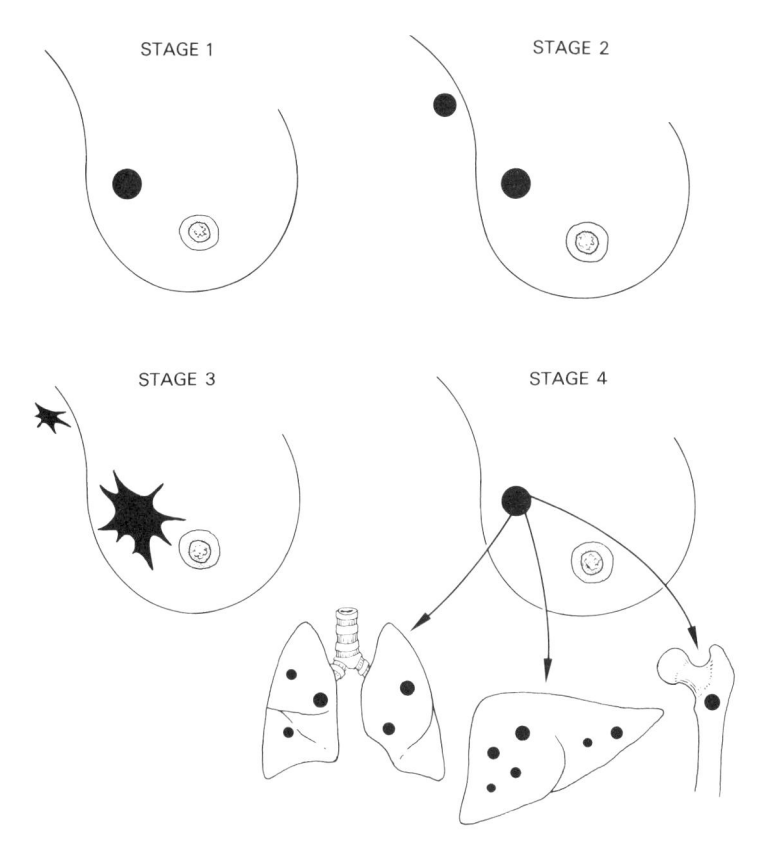

Fig. 17.11. The clinical staging of breast cancer.

This classification (Fig. 17.11), although useful, is fairly rough and ready. For example, although lymph nodes may not be palpable in the axilla, microscopic examination may subsequently reveal that they contain tumour deposits. Conversely, axillary nodes which are palpable may prove free from tumour. Although the tumour may appear clinically to be in Stage I, subsequent investigations by X-rays may reveal undetected bony deposits so that, in fact, we are dealing with a Stage IV case.

Treatment

This must be divided into 'curative' and 'palliative'.

When the disease is apparently confined to the breast tissue alone, or has only involved the axillary lymph nodes with no evidence of further spread, the surgeon hopes to be able to eradicate the disease and achieve a 'cure', (such patients fall into Stages I and II of the classification given above). Unfortunately, a proportion of these cases will already have microscopic metastases elsewhere in the body at the time that surgery is undertaken, and, inevitably, recurrence will eventually take place.

There is an enormous variation in the treatment of these early cases of breast cancer in different centres throughout the world. Some surgeons advise wide local removal of the tumour ('*lumpectomy*'). Others carry out a *simple mastectomy* in which the whole of the breast tissue is excised. In other centres, this procedure is combined with removal of the axillary lymph nodes, an operation which is termed '*extended simple mastectomy*'. In the long established operation of *radical mastectomy* the surgeon removes not only the breast and the axillary lymph nodes, together with wide sweep of overlying skin, but also the underlying muscles (the pectoralis major and pectoralis minor). In one or two hospitals the so called '*super-radical*' mastectomy is carried out, in which the internal mammary chain of lymph nodes is removed by resecting the anterior aspects of the ribs. Finally, some surgeons go so far as to advise, in addition, removal of the *opposite* breast at the time of the initial mastectomy. There is no uniformity of opinion as to which of these operations gives the best results, or indeed whether they should be combined with either pre- or post-operative radiotherapy. Fortunately, careful clinical trials comparing the various methods are now being carried out and within the next few years we should be able to state, quite clearly, which technique gives the most satisfactory results, both with regard to survival of the patient and, of great importance, the least disturbance of function. Obviously the more radical the treatment the more chance the patient may have of developing stiffness of the shoulder from scar formation and oedema of the arm from lymphatic interruption. Perhaps here we should state our own present practice, which is, in most instances, to carry out an extended simple mastectomy without post-operative radiotherapy.

Stage III cases

Once the tumour is invading surrounding structures, surgical clearance becomes impossible. Local radiotherapy often produces palliative regression although a 'toilet' operation may then be advisable to remove residual diseased tissue.

Stage IV, and recurrences after previous mastectomy

A solitary distant deposit, for example in one bone, or local recurrence in the scar following mastectomy can be controlled by radiotherapy treatment. Where dissemination is widespread, sex hormones or 'hormone surgery' are used. It is known that a proportion of breast tumours appear to be dependent for growth upon the hormone environment. Unfortunately it is at present impossible to determine whether a particular patient will or will not respond to therapy without trying it. Taking patients as a whole, it is found that about one third show objective response to such treatment (the tumour mass actually becoming smaller or disappearing), a third feel better or lose their pain, although we cannot measure shrinkage of the tumour (subjective response) and a third show absolutely no response at all to this therapy.

The possible methods of hormone treatment which are available include:

1. *Androgens*, which are usually employed in pre-menopausal patients (Durabolin 50 mg intramuscularly weekly).
2. *Stilboestrol* in post-menopausal patients (5 mg three times daily).
3. *Oophorectomy* (removal of the ovaries) particularly in pre-menopausal and early post-menopausal patients.
4. *Bilateral adrenalectomy* which is usually combined with bilateral oophorectomy, if this has not already been performed.
5. *Hypophysectomy* (removal of the pituitary gland) which may be performed either by a cranial operation, an approach through the nasal route, or by implanting radio-active material through a cannula under x-ray control.

In patients who fail to respond to hormone therapy, or who relapse after initial response, some temporary relief may be obtained by means of cytotoxic drugs (see Chapter 5).

THE CARE OF THE MASTECTOMY PATIENT

Women fear mastectomy probably more than any other commonly performed operation and it is the duty of the nursing as well as the medical staff to do as much as possible to allay the patient's anxiety and to make her stay in hospital as comfortable as possible. The words 'amputation of the breast' are cruel and should never be used. It should be explained to the patient that if the surgeon decides that the breast needs removal, this entails only removal of the breast substance and that the patient will wake up post-operatively with a linear scar across the chest wall. Some women are under the misconception that mastectomy must obviously leave a gaping hole where the breast has been removed and do not realize that they are to be left with quite a neat scar. It is worth pointing out to the patient that the mastectomy wound is easily disguised by the clothes and that the modern prosthesis worn within the brassiere enables the patient to wear evening dress, bathing costume etc. without anybody knowing that a mastectomy has been carried out.

At one time, the post-operative care of the mastectomy patient was bedevilled by the collection of blood or serum under the large skin flaps. Fortunately, this has now been overcome by the use of suction drainage by means of a low-pressure pump (Fig. 17.12). Suction should be continued until no further haemo-serous aspirate is obtained, usually about 3 days following operation. As a result of this, primary healing can be anticipated in the majority of cases. From time to time, (and this particularly applies to mastectomy for cancer in the male), the surgeon finds that there is inadequate skin for closure and in such cases a split skin graft from the thigh is required from the time of operation. The surgeon can usually anticipate this need, in which case the patient is warned before operation and the thigh prepared as a donor site by preliminary shaving and skin disinfection.

It was once the custom to torture the patient immediately postoperatively by insisting on violent exercise to the shoulder on the side of the mastectomy. This was due to the mistaken view that a few days of rest would result in stiffness of the shoulder. Of course, quite the reverse is true. It is a general principle throughout surgery that *damaged tissues should be placed at rest until healing has taken place*. Once this has been effected, then active movement will rapidly restore full function. Following mastectomy, the patient should be encouraged to use the elbow, wrist, and hand on the affected side but to keep the shoulder still, either by resting the arm on the pillow or (as in our practice) by supporting the arm in a

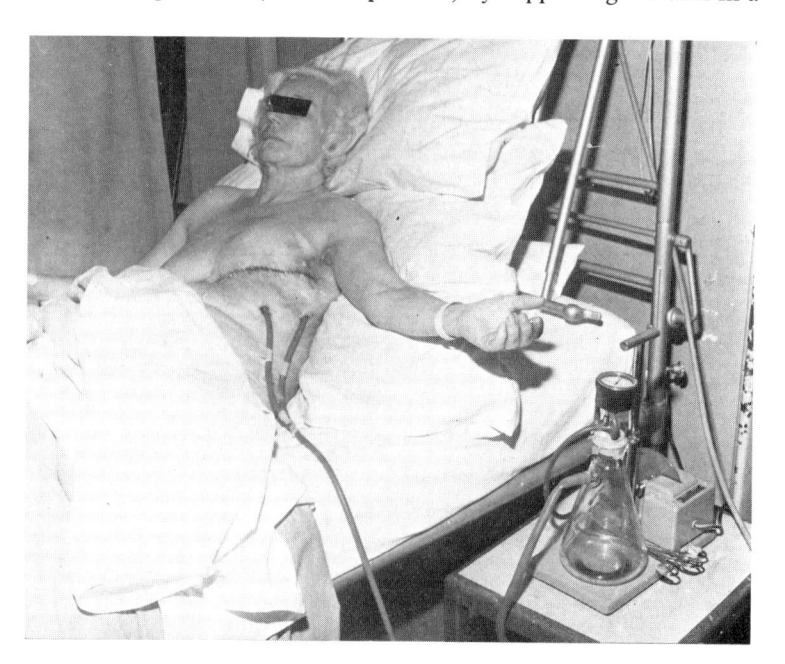

Fig. 17.12. Suction drainage following mastectomy; a Robert's pump is being used.

collar and cuff sling for a few days. Gentle movement is allowed after a week and, once the wound has healed, full movement of the shoulder is rapidly restored. With extended simple mastectomy, it is extremely rare for a patient to have any significant shoulder stiffness or oedema of the arm in the post-operative period. There is no hurry to remove the sutures. Following the mastectomy, the wound is sutured under a good deal of tension and early removal of the stitches may be followed by unpleasant gaping of the wound. It is our practice, therefore, to leave the sutures in place for 3 weeks.

SCREENING FOR BREAST CANCER

There are a number of ways of screening the adult female population in an attempt to diagnose breast cancer at an early stage. These include teaching women to examine themselves at regular intervals, regular medical examinations at 'Well Women Clinics' at the time of cervical smear examinations, thermography and mammography.

The majority of lumps are indeed diagnosed by the patients themselves, and self-examination once monthly is a reasonable suggestion to make to one's patients. Examination by a doctor will detect tumours at any early stage but is naturally time-consuming, expensive and would need to be repeated at least at yearly intervals. Many women, in addition, fail to attend such screening programmes. Thermography depends on the fact that breast cancer emits slightly more heat than normal breast tissue, and this can be picked up on a sensitive recording device. However, similar changes may be given by a variety of benign breast lesions, and in practice, this has proved of little value. Mammography produces a soft tissue X-ray of the breast and minute cancers of the breast can be detected as a small area of density which often shows specks of calcification. Once again, there are the disadvantages of time, expense, and failure of patients to attend for screening or who subsequently default from further appointments. At present an extensive trial in New York is taking place which should provide important data as to whether or not prognosis could be improved by such elaborate screening programmes. If it is shown to be so, then obviously further efforts must be made to introduce such screening programmes into this country regardless of their cost in time and money.

Chapter 18. The skin and its adnexae

Fig. 18.1. The structure of the skin. Note the clearly defined epidermis and the dermis and the adnexae to the skin—the hair follicle, sebaceous gland and sweat gland.

Structure and function

The skin is the largest organ of the body and extends over an area of about 1.5 sq. metres. It continues with the mucous membranes of the body's orifices (nose, mouth, anus, urethra and vagina) and is modified to form the conjunctiva and the ear drum. It is made up of two components, the epidermis and the dermis (Fig. 18.1).

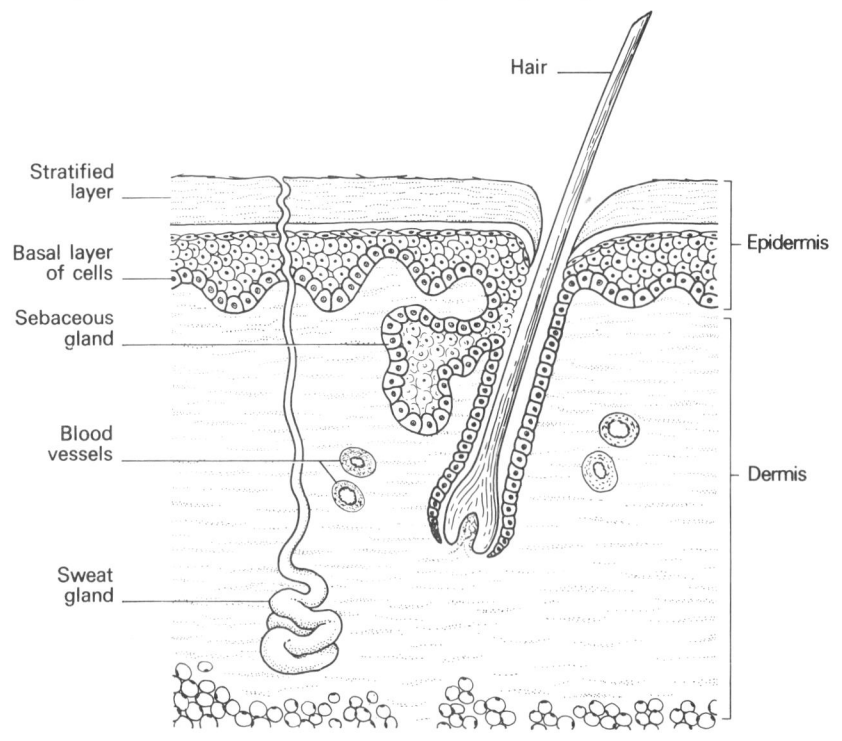

The epidermis is avascular and is formed by a stratified squamous epithelium. This is derived from a single layer of cells termed the basal layer or germinal layer. This continually proliferates cells which become flattened as they pass to the surface, and eventually die, so that the surface layer itself, the *stratum corneum* or horny layer, is made up of dry, flat, dead cells without obvious nuclei. These are continuously flaking away and are being replaced by further cells from below. The stratum corneum is especially thick over the palms of the hands and the soles of the feet, but becomes thickened at any place where the skin is subjected to prolonged and heavy friction.

The dermis is made up of fibro-fatty tissue containing the *sweat glands*, formed by coiled tubes which pass by thin ducts through the dermis to open onto the surface of the epidermis, the *hair roots or follicles*, which are, in fact, downward prolongations of the epidermis, and the *sebaceous glands* which discharge their fatty secretion, sebum, into the hair follicles from which they develop as outgrowths.

Sweat glands are universally distributed over the body, especially over the hands, feet and face. Hair follicles (and therefore their accompanying sebaceous glands) are absent over the palm of the hand and sole of the foot.

The skin has truly remarkable properties and functions, and is far more than being merely the outer wrapping of the body. It is extremely tough and waterproof and, as we have already noted, is able to thicken in areas exposed to excessive stress. By variations in blood flow through the skin and the amount of sweat production, the skin acts as an organ of body temperature regulation. Because of the rich supply of nerve endings in the dermis, it functions as an extensive sensory organ for perception of heat, cold, touch, and pain. Vitamin D is synthesized in the skin by the action of the ultra violet rays of the sun. Finally, by producing melanin pigment as required, the skin can protect itself from excessive exposure to the sun by becoming pigmented—surely it is one of the most versatile of all the organs of the body!

Skin bacteriology

The skin is constantly being contaminated with bacteria and this is especially so among doctors and nurses in hospital where contact with infected wounds, ulcers and other septic foci is almost inevitable. However, the skin has quite remarkable powers of disinfecting itself, so that within an hour of soiling the healthy skin has got rid of the contaminants and is left with only two types of resident bacteria, the *staphylococcus albus* and *diphtheroids*, both of which are rarely pathogenic and may actually themselves produce antibiotics which destroy invading organisms. The other mechanisms of skin auto-disinfection are desiccation (most bacteria require a moist environment in order to grow) and also the antibacterial effect of fatty acids derived from skin lipids.

Cleansing of the surgeon's and nurse's hands and of the patient's skin in the area of the operation is designed not to remove the harmless skin commensals but to clear away possible contaminants. This can be carried out effectively either by a vigorous scrub with soap and water or by the application of 0.5% chlorhexidine or iodine in 70% alcohol solution.

Skin infections—boils, carbuncles, cellulitis—see Chapter I.

SEBACEOUS CYST

A sebaceous cyst is a retention cyst produced by obstruction of an orifice of a sebaceous gland. The cyst can occur, therefore, on any part of the skin except those areas devoid of sebaceous glands—the palms of the hands and the soles of the feet. They are particularly common on the scalp, (which was the site of the most famous sebaceous cyst of all, that of King George IV, removed by Sir Astley Cooper of Guy's Hospital in 1821), the face, the lobule of the ear and the scrotum. It is an easy diagnosis to make (Fig. 18.2); a

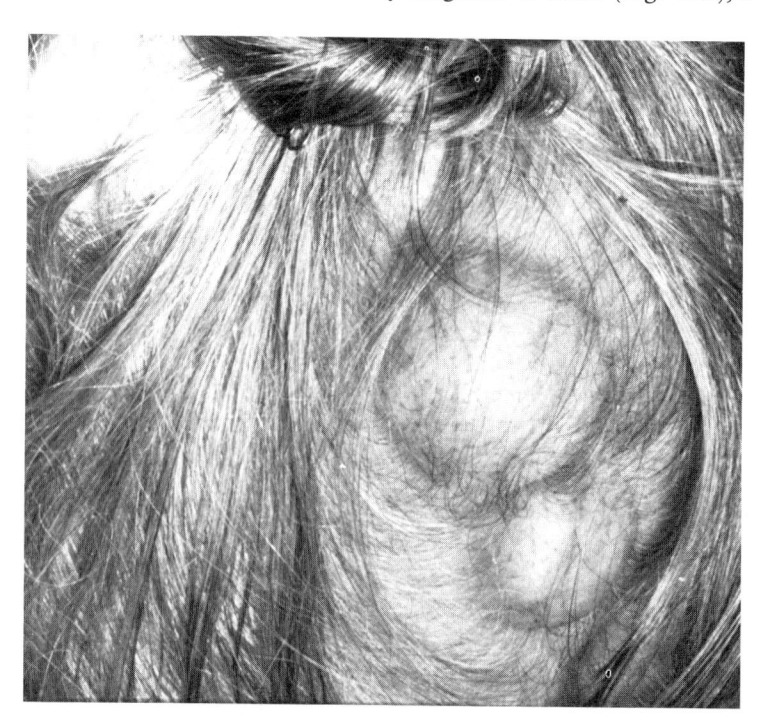

Fig. 18.2. Sebaceous cysts of the scalp.

soft elastic swelling, which is adherent to the skin and which may show the typical punctum of the obstructed duct at the apex of the cyst. Sometimes sebaceous material can be seen oozing from it. The lump may be quite tiny but occasionally reaches 5 cm or more in diameter before the patient seeks medical advice. The cyst contains cheesy, whitish-yellow material with an unpleasant smell and this is the inspissated secretion of the sebaceous gland.

Complications

Left untreated, the cyst is very likely to become infected and may ulcerate. The ulcerated surface may even resemble a fungating carcinoma and yet is, of course, still perfectly benign. For this reason it receives the name 'Cock's peculiar tumour', named after Edward Cock, a surgeon at Guy's Hospital in the 19th Century. It should be noted that malignant change does very rarely occur in a sebaceous cyst to form a sebaceous carcinoma.

Treatment

Sebaceous cysts should always be removed in order to prevent complications. When small, this can be done easily under a local anaesthetic. If infection has taken place, incision and drainage is required, followed subsequently by excision of the capsule wall.

A number of other common cysts occur in the skin and subcutaneous tissues. These include:

IMPLANTATION DERMOID (Fig. 18.3)

Occasionally a puncture injury may implant a fragment of epithelium into the subcutaneous tissues; growth and degeneration of these cells results in a cystic swelling. Because of its origin, the typical implantation dermoid is found on the index finger of a needle-woman!

Fig. 18.3. An implantation dermoid of the index finger which followed a puncture injury.

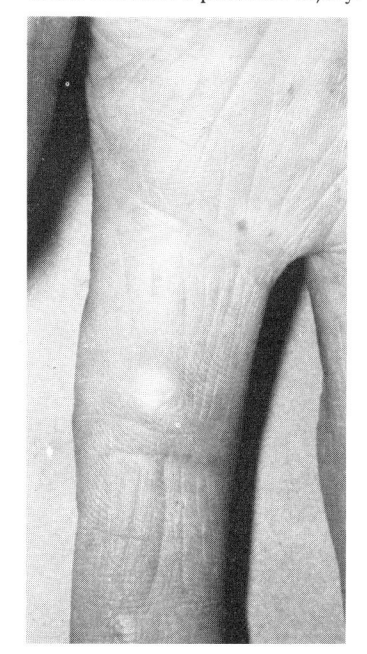

EXTERNAL ANGULAR DERMOID

Epithelial cells may become buried along the lines of fusion of the skin in embryonic life. The commonest place for this to happen is at the outer border of the eyebrow where the processes going to form the forehead and the face fuse together. It is very easy to diagnose this typical little cyst which begins to form in early childhood.

Fig. 18.4. A ganglion of the wrist.

GANGLION (Fig. 18.4)

Ganglia are among the commonest of all superficial cysts. They arise from a joint capsule or a tendon sheath and occur especially around the wrist joint, the dorsum of the foot, the anterior aspect of the fingers or along the peroneal tendons on the lateral side of the ankle. The cyst is thin walled and contains a sticky mucoid colourless fluid which exactly resembles Wharton's jelly in the umbilical cord.

Treatment

If the cyst is troubling the patient it should be excised under a general anaesthetic, using a tourniquet to produce a bloodless field. In the old days treatment comprised rupturing the cyst with a blow from the family Bible, but unfortunately recurrence invariably followed this traumatic experience.

PILONIDAL SINUS

The definition of a sinus is a blind track lined with granulation tissue which opens on to a surface; one of the best examples of this is a pilonidal sinus (Fig. 18.5).

The majority occur immediately above the anus in the cleft between the buttocks. The name is derived from the hair which is contained within the sinus, the word meaning 'nest of hair'. Pilonidal sinuses are also found in the clefts between the fingers in barbers (Fig 18.6) and, rarely, in the umbilicus, the perineum, between the toes and in the folds of skin on amputation stumps.

The origin of the pilonidal sinus has been the matter of some controversy but it is now agreed that the sinus forms from implantation of hair into the skin—this fits in with sinuses which develop on the hands of barbers and on the feet of men working in abattoirs,

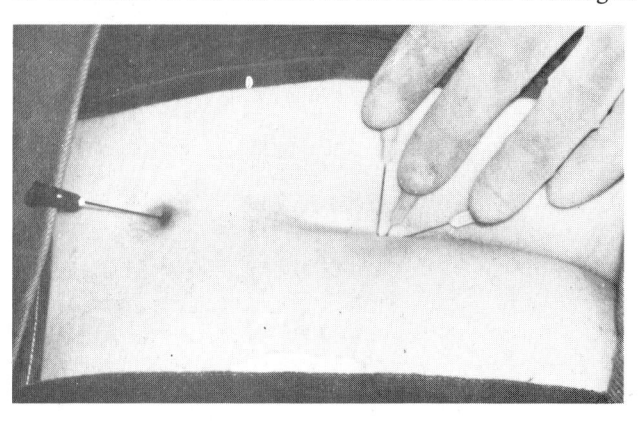

Fig. 18.5. Multiple pilonidal sinuses. The three small needles have been placed in the orifices of the three hair-containing sinuses. From these, a long track extends headwards and opens as a discharging abscess, which is marked by the larger needle.

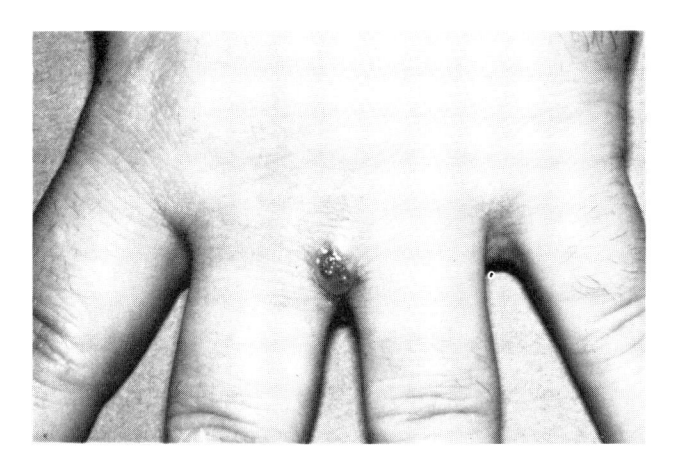

Fig. 18.6. A hair-containing pilonidal sinus between the fingers. The patient was a barber.

where the hair comes from the client and from the animals respectively. Once the hair has become implanted it sets up a foreign body reaction which produces a chronic infected sinus. The pilonidal sinus is symptomless until it becomes infected, following which recurrent abscesses occur; these either require drainage or discharge spontaneously.

Treatment

If there is an acute abscess present, this must be drained. In the quiescent phase the track is excised or laid open and allowed to heal by granulation. This may take a considerable time and it is the nurse's duty to ensure that the wound heals soundly from its depth upwards to the surface. If the epithelium is allowed to bridge over the defect, a persistent cavity will form and healing will be delayed. Further recurrence is prevented by keeping the surrounding skin free from hair by frequent cleaning and by rubbing with fine sand paper.

THE NAILS

The nails are the site of a number of common surgical conditions.

PARONYCHIA

A paronychia is an infection of the nail fold, usually of the finger but also quite commonly of the great toe as a complication of ingrowing toe-nail (see below). It is the commonest infection of the hand and makes up about one third of all such infections. The infecting organism is nearly always the staphylococcus aureus, which most commonly invades through a tear in the nail fold ('hang-nail'). The nail fold becomes red, swollen and tender and pus may become visible.

Treatment

If seen at an early stage before pus formation has occurred the infection may subside with antibiotic treatment combined with immobilisation of the finger in a splint and a sling to the arm. If pus is present, however, surgical drainage is required through a small incision which may need, in addition, removal of the base of the nail if the pus is tracking beneath it.

Chronic paronychia may be seen in women who have their hands constantly soaked in water but may also occur as the result of fungus infection of the nail and also in patients with poor peripheral circulation, for example, Raynaud's phenomenon. The affected finger must be kept dry. If fungal infection is present, this is treated with oral griseofulvin.

INGROWING TOE NAIL

This condition is nearly always confined to the great toe. It results from a combination of tight shoes and the habit of cutting the nail downwards into the nail fold so that the sharp cutting edge of the nail grows into the side of the nail bed with resultant ulceration and infection.

Treatment

If seen before infection has occurred, the patient is advised to cut the nail transversely rather than downwards into the nail fold and a wisp of cotton wool is tucked daily into the side of the nail bed. These simple steps, combined with the wearing of sensible, wide shoes, enable the nail to grow up out of the fold.

If acute paronychia is present, the nail will require avulsion in order to allow drainage of pus to take place. If the nail continues to give trouble, it should be obliterated by excision of the nail base (Zadek's operation) which prevents regrowth of the nail (Fig. 18.7).

ONYCHOGRYPHOSIS

Any of the toe nails may be affected by this 'ram's horn' deformity of the nail, but the hallux is the commonest site. It usually occurs in the elderly and may follow trauma to the nail bed.

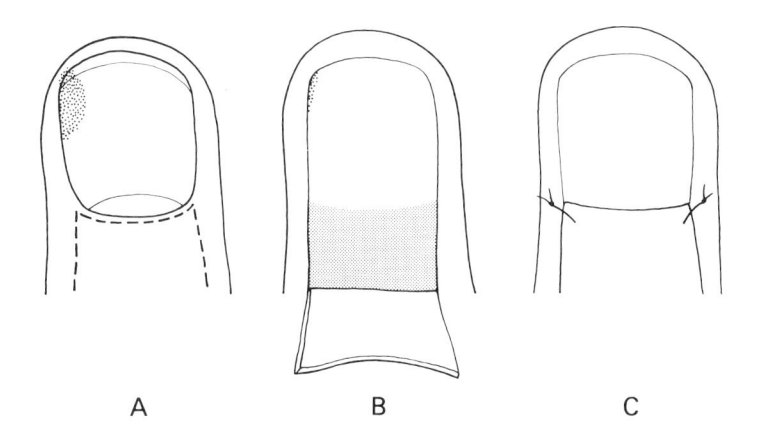

Fig. 18.7. Zadek's operation. A, the skin incisions to expose the nail base; B, the skin flap is reflected, the nail has been avulsed and the nail base (cross-hatched) from which the nail develops has been completely excised; C, the skin flap is now stitched back over the excised nail base.

Treatment

Mild examples can be kept under control by trimming the nail with bone cutting forceps. If the nail is simply avulsed recurrence invariably occurs and the only adequate surgical treatment is removal of the nail and excision of its base to prevent further growth (Zadek's operation).

LESIONS OF THE NAIL BED

There are a number of relatively common conditions which affect the nail bed. These are:

Haematoma

A crush injury to the terminal phalanx may result in a tense painful haematoma under the nail. This may be accompanied by fracture of the underlying bone. The clot should be evacuated by drilling through the insensitive nail either with a dental drill or a red hot wire. Surprisingly enough a small haematoma may develop without the patient remembering any injury and this may closely mimic a subungual melanoma.

Subungual exostosis

This is a bony lump lying under the nail, usually of the great toe, especially in young adults. The exostosis may ulcerate through the overlying nail to produce an infected granulating mass. An X-ray reveals the exostosis and treatment comprises removal of the nail and the underlying bone nodule.

Melanoma

The nail bed is a common site for malignant melanoma (see page 413).

Glomus tumour

The nail bed of the fingers and toes are common sites of this extremely painful lesion, which is a benign tumour arising from a subcutaneous glomus body. These are tiny arteriovenous communications in the skin which are concerned with temperature regulation. The tumour comprises a plexus of blood vessels and nerves which, although tiny, is exquisitely painful on pressure. It is benign and the treatment is surgical excision.

TUMOURS OF THE SKIN AND SUBCUTANEOUS TISSUES

A wide variety of tumours are found in the skin and subcutaneous tissues. The explanation for this is the presence of numerous structures—not only the skin itself but also nerves, fat, blood vessels, sweat glands, etc. from any of which growths may arise.

BENIGN TUMOURS

Papilloma is a common benign tumour, situated on a stalk and often pigmented with melanin. Rarely it may undergo change into a squamous cell carcinoma (see below).

Senile Keratosis. This is a small, hard, scaly tumour which occurs particularly on the face and hands of the elderly; again, this may rarely undergo malignant change.

Seborrhoeic Keratosis is common in the elderly and occurs as a yellowish or brown raised lesion on the face, arms, or trunk. It is often multiple. Because of its pigmentation it is a differential diagnosis from a melanoma.

Verruca Vulgaris. This is the common wart and results from a virus infection of the skin. It is found on the fingers, hands and especially on the sole of the foot (plantar warts). Often it disappears spontaneously but if troublesome a wart may be removed by repeated applications of silver nitrate or may be curetted away under local or general anaesthetic.

SQUAMOUS CELL CARCINOMA

This is a malignant tumour of the skin epithelium (epithelioma) and is particularly likely to appear in the elderly male, especially in skin areas exposed to the sunshine, for example the face and the

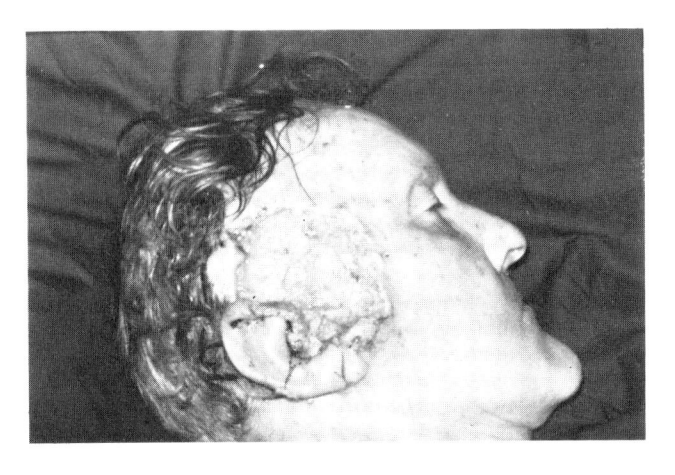

Fig. 18.8. An enormous squamous carcinoma of the temporal region. It has invaded the facial nerve and produced a facial paralysis.

backs of the hands (Fig. 18.8). It is common in white men who live in sunny, tropical areas. Not only sun, but anything that chronically irritates the skin may predispose to this malignant change so that squamous cell carcinoma may arise in a chronic varicose ulcer, an unhealed burn or the sinus discharging over an area of chronic osteomyelitis. Such malignant change in a chronic ulcer is termed a *Marjolin's ulcer*. Exposure to irradiation or to pitch, tar or soot also predispose skin to malignant change.

The tumour presents as a typical malignant ulcer with raised everted edges and a central scab. Spread occurs by local infiltration and then by lymphatic drainage to the regional lymph nodes, but blood spread is seen only in very late cases.

Treatment

This comprises either wide excision or radiotherapy and depends rather on the site of the lesion. Involvement of the regional lymph nodes is an indication for their surgical excision.

BASAL CELL CARCINOMA (Rodent ulcer)

This is an extremely common tumour which occurs particularly in elderly males. The vast majority occur on the face above a line which joins the angle of the mouth to the external auditory meatus. Occasionally multiple tumours may be found. Predisposing factors are exposure to sunlight or irradiation and, just like the squamous cell carcinoma, the tumour is particularly common in white-skinned subjects in sunny tropical regions.

The tumour has a typical appearance of pearly nodules over which fine blood vessels are seen (Fig. 18.9). Its edges are raised and rolled. As the nodule enlarges slowly its centre ulcerates and becomes

Fig. 18.9. A typical basal cell carcinoma (rodent ulcer) of the outer canthus.

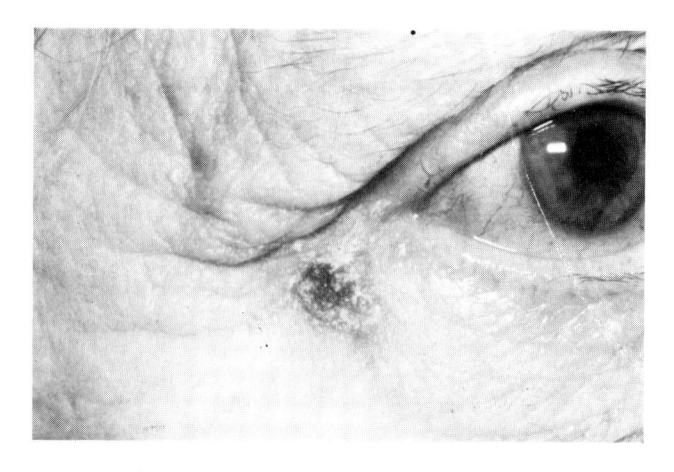

covered with a scab. The tumour arises from the basal layer of the epidermis and spreads by slow but steady infiltration. It destroys surrounding tissues and eventually erodes adjacent bone and other structures, eating away the tissues just like the rat after which it is named. It is interesting that spread by the lymphatics and blood occurs only with the greatest rarity.

Treatment

The tumour is very radiosensitive and can be treated with superficial x-ray therapy. Surgical excision can be carried out in those areas where gross deformity will not result.

MELANOMA

Melanin pigment in the skin is secreted by cells termed *melanocytes* which are situated in the basal layer of the epidermis. Pigmentation of the skin is produced by the melanocyte injecting melanin into adjacent basal cells of the epidermis via sharp needle-like processes. This injection or pigment is termed *cytocrinia*. Far more cytocrinia occurs, obviously, in black than in white skin and this phenomenon is also responsible for sunburn, and the formation of freckles. In the slightly raised pigment patches seen on the skin of elderly people (lentigo) the melanocytes are larger, increased in numbers and produce excess of melanin.

Normally the melanocytes occur as isolated cells. A *benign melanoma* or *naevus* or *mole* consists of a clump of melanocytes. Nearly every white skinned person possesses one or more of these, and some have hundreds, although they may not become apparent until after puberty. Moles which are situated entirely within the dermis (the *intradermal naevus*) remain benign, but a small percentage of the

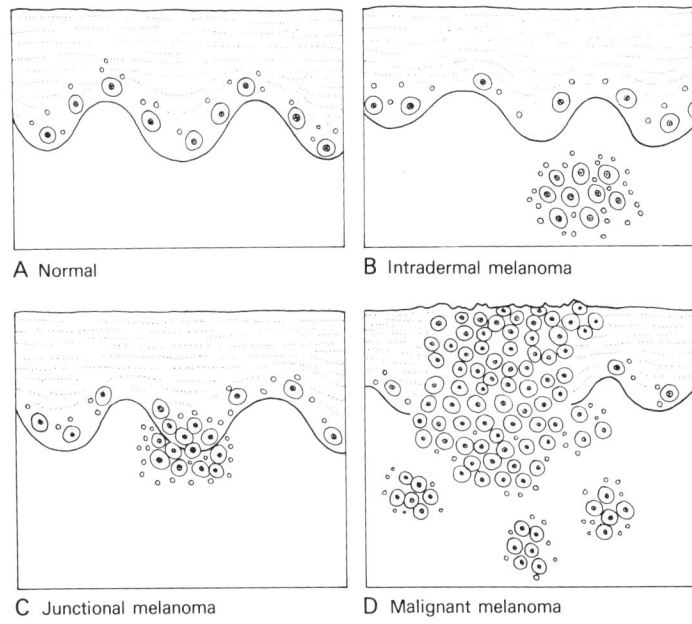

Fig. 18.10. (A) The normal skin contains melanocytes and melanin pigment. The pigment increases in sunburn and freckles. (B) A benign intradermal naevus; the melanocytes are clumped together in the dermis to form a localised benign tumour. (C) A junctional naevus with melanocytes clumping together in the basal layer of the epidermis. These are usually benign but may occasionally give rise (D) to an invasive malignant melanoma.

junctional naevi, so called because they occur in the basal layer of the epidermis at its junction with the dermis, may undergo malignant change.

These different pigment spots are shown in diagram form in Fig. 18.10.

Intradermal Naevus (Fig. 18.11)

This is the commonest variety of mole, may be light or dark in colour and is either flat or warty. A mole with hair growing out of it is nearly always intradermal. They may be found everywhere in the skin except the palms of the hand, the sole of the feet and the skin of the scrotum. They never become malignant.

Fig. 18.11. A benign intradermal naevus of the arm.

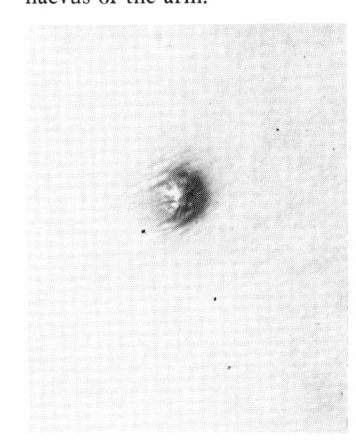

Junctional Naevus

This pigment spot may be any shade from light brown to almost black. It is usually flat, smooth and hairless and may occur anywhere in the body, including the palm, the sole and the genitalia. Only a small percentage of junctional naevi undergo malignant change but it is from this group that the majority of malignant melanomas arise.

Malignant Melanoma (Fig. 18.12)

Although malignant melanoma has a well-deserved dangerous reputation, it is fortunately a rare tumour. The majority occur in the skin but may be found also on the mucous membrane of the nose,

Fig. 18.12. Malignant melanoma of the foot. The tumour is growing rapidly and has eroded through the skin.

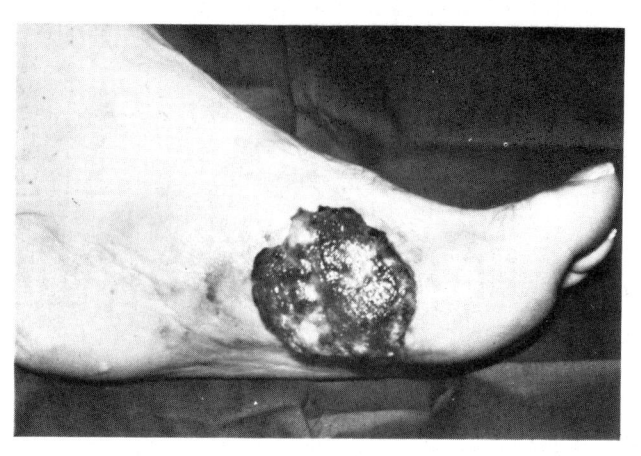

within the mouth, the anal canal and the intestine. Another important group arises from the pigment cells within the eye. Any part of the skin may be affected but especially the lower limb, the sole of the foot, the nailbeds and the head and neck.

The majority probably arise in pre-existent junctional naevi. The signs which suggest malignant change are: increase in size, increase in pigmentation, bleeding or ulceration of a pigment spot, spread of pigment from the edge of the tumour into the surrounding skin, formation of daughter nodules around the tumour and itching or pain within the naevus.

Spread. As well as local growth and ulceration, malignant melanomas permeate the lymphatics and produce cutaneous nodules by progressive spread. The regional lymph nodes then become enlarged and there is finally widespread dissemination by the bloodstream.

Treatment of pigmented lesions

Since every white skinned person has at least one, and usually dozens, of pigment spots, and since malignant melanomas are rare, there is obviously no need to be concerned about every single pigmented lesion. However, any pigmented tumour on the hand, the sole or the genitalia or any which are subjected to trauma (for example, a spot on face which is repeatedly injured while shaving) should be excised: these are the commonest amongst the naevi to undergo malignant change. Of course, if the pigment spot is giving cosmetic anxiety or if the patient is acutely unhappy about its presence (and this is a particularly common phenomenon among nurses) it should be removed and sent for careful microscopic examination.

If the pigmented lesion shows any of the features listed above which suggest that malignant change might have taken place, the tumor is excised and sent for urgent histological examination. If the diagnosis is confirmed, a wide local excision of the area is performed and the defect covered with a split skin graft. Many surgeons believe that some prophylactic treatment should be given to the regional lymph nodes, either by carrying out a block dissection or by injecting radioactive material into the lymphatic drainage from the area. Once gross enlargement of the regional lymph nodes has occurred, such intralymphatic therapy is no longer effective and surgical excision is necessary.

Prognosis

In cases which are diagnosed at an early stage before lymph node involvement has occurred, about 75% survive for 5 years or more. Once the regional nodes are involved, the 5-year survival drops to 20% and once more distant metastases have occurred prognosis is usually very poor.

SUBCUTANEOUS TUMOURS

Benign subcutaneous tumours may arise from blood vessels (haemangioma), lymph vessels (lymphangioma) and the sheaths of peripheral nerves (neurofibroma). Occasionally malignant tumours arise from these tissues (haemangiosarcoma, lymphangiosarcoma and neurofibrosarcoma respectively).

By far and away the commonest subcutaneous tumour arises from fat. This is the benign lipoma. Malignant tumours of fat (liposarcoma) are extremely rare.

LIPOMA

This is the commonest of all benign tumours. It usually arises in adults and although the sex distribution is equal, females are more likely to present to the surgeon for cosmetic removal of the lump. Lipomas may arise in any connective tissue, but are found especially in the subcutaneous fat, particularly around the shoulder and over the trunk. They do not occur in the palm, the sole, or the scalp, because in these areas the fat is contained within dense fibrous compartments. Occasionally multiple lipomas occur.

Diagnosis is rarely in doubt with this soft lobulated tumour (Fig. 18.13).

Treatment consists of excision of the lipoma if this is cosmetically troublesome.

Fig. 18.13. An enormous lipoma which has grown slowly to this size over many years. Note the dilated veins running over the tumour. Laboratory examination showed that it was completely benign.

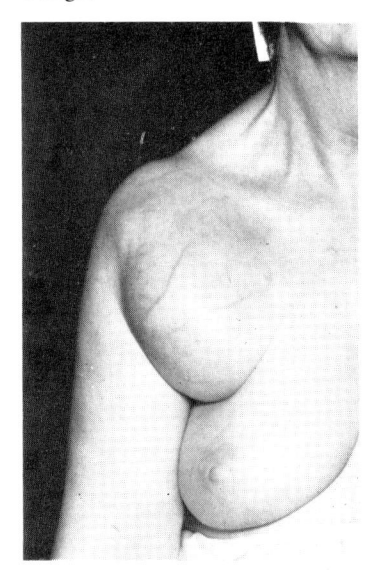

Chapter 19. Ophthalmology

The eye is exposed and vulnerable. Our whole lives are dominated by our sight, and the fear of anything that might lead to blindness is thus almost innate. Added to this, any blemish in the region of the eyes is especially disfiguring since it is so hard to conceal, and it is to the eyes that we look in judging our neighbour. In short, the care of the eyes and the control of eye disease is of paramount importance in nursing.

Anatomy

The *eyeball*, a sphere about one inch in diameter, lies suspended within the fat that fills the orbit; it is protected by the four converging bony orbital walls, but in front it is screened only by the upper and lower eyelids (Fig. 19.1). A third, vestigial eyelid can be seen, lying immobile in the inner angle, as a fold of conjuctiva (the 'plica semilunaris'), containing a pink nodule called the caruncle.

The *cornea*, about ten millimetres in diameter, is the transparent window of the eye, set like a watch-glass into the front of the *sclera*, the white wall which envelops the rest of the eyeball. Lining the under surface of the sclera is a sheet of supporting tissue, loaded with blood-vessels and with a variable amount of brown pigment, called the *uveal tract* (or 'uvea'); this layer is swollen at its front end by the two interior muscles of the eye that govern the focusing and the movements of the pupil; so that the uveal tract is composed of three sections: the main posterior part is called the *choroid*, further forward, where it incorporates the ciliary muscle, it is called the *ciliary body*, and further forward still it becomes the *iris*. The latter no longer clings to the wall of the eyeball, but lies as a flat surface

Ophthalmology

Fig. 19.1. Vertical section of eyeball within the orbit. (From *Medical Radiography and Photography*, Courtesy of Camille Hill Killan.)

1. Frontal Bone (orbital rim).
2. Orbicularis oculi muscle.
3. Cornea.
4. Anterior chamber.
5. Lens.
6. Iris root.
7. Ciliary body.
8. Ora Serrata (anterior edge of retina
9. Selera.
10. Choroid and retina.
11. Vitreous space.
12. Muller's muscle (involuntary; connecting L.P.S. and upper tarsal plate).
13. Tarsal conjunctiva.
14. Levator palpebrae superioris muscle.
15. Superior rectus muscle.
16. Optic nerve.
17. Inferior rectus muscle.
18. Inferior oblique muscle.

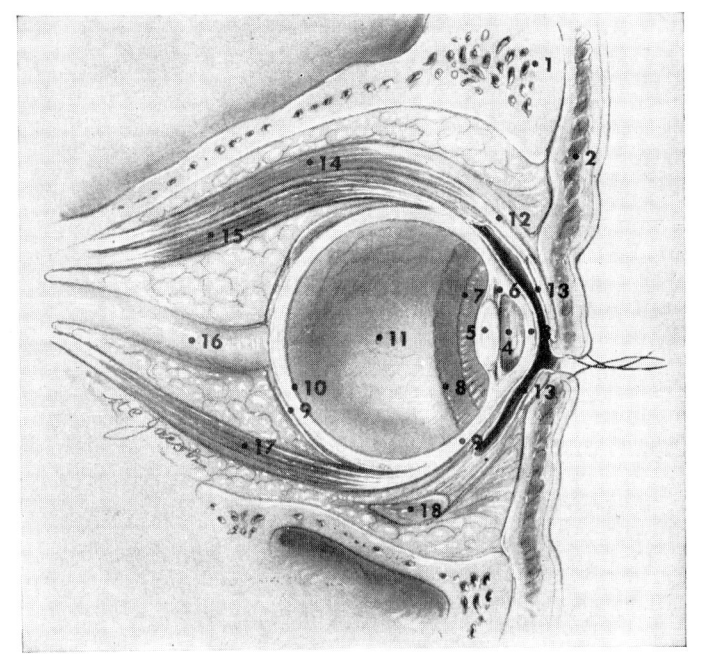

behind the cornea, having a central hole of adjustable size, the *pupil*; and it is separated from the convex cornea by a space, filled with clear liquid resembling the cerebro-spiral fluid called *aqueous humour*, and known as the *anterior chamber*; (the *posterior chamber* being the narrow space also filled with aqueous humour just behind the iris).

The *lens* consists of a clear, viscous substance enclosed within a thin elastic capsule. It is held in position directly behind the iris, by a suspensory ligament which tethers its outer rim to the encircling ciliary muscle; so that, when the latter contracts, the lens becomes more convex and thus focuses the eye for near vision. As age advances, the lens becomes stiffer and the ciliary muscle weaker, hence the increasing need to supplement the focusing with reading glasses in middle age (known as 'presbyopia').

The *retina*, which lines the inner surface of the choroid, is the equivalent of the film of the camera, since it records the image of the outside world, which is cast on it through the pupil, and brought into focus by the cornea and lens. It is a very thin transparent sheet, containing cells which can be bleached by light, as well as nerve cells, which register the specific areas that have been bleached. This information is passed up the optic nerves, (which form the stalk of the eyeball), and so back to register the visual image on the posterior lobes of the cerebrum. Finally, these crystallised cerebral images are adjusted by all our thought-processes and emerge into our consciousness as the 'percept', or the image we actually think we see.

As the images seen by each of the eyes need to be fused together, so that the brain receives only a single view of the outside world, both eyes must be kept in exact alignment; and this is achieved by a very careful co-ordination of the eye-movements in whichever direction the eyes are turned.

Rotation of the eye within the orbit is controlled by six muscles, which take their purchase from the bony orbital wall and insert into the eyeball. Four of them, the *superior, inferior, lateral and medial rectus muscles*, pass forwards directly from the apex of the orbit, enshrouding the optic nerve, to insert into the respective quadrants of the eyeball, about seven millimetres behind the corneal margin, and rotate the eye upwards, downwards, laterally and medially respectively. The *superior and inferior oblique muscles* assist in the vertical eye-movements, and take their effective origin from the front of the orbit (at its upper medial and lower medial angles) (Fig. 19.2). If the eyes fall out of alignment and point in different directions, they are said to 'squint'.

The exposed cornea is protected by the eyelids, each of which is

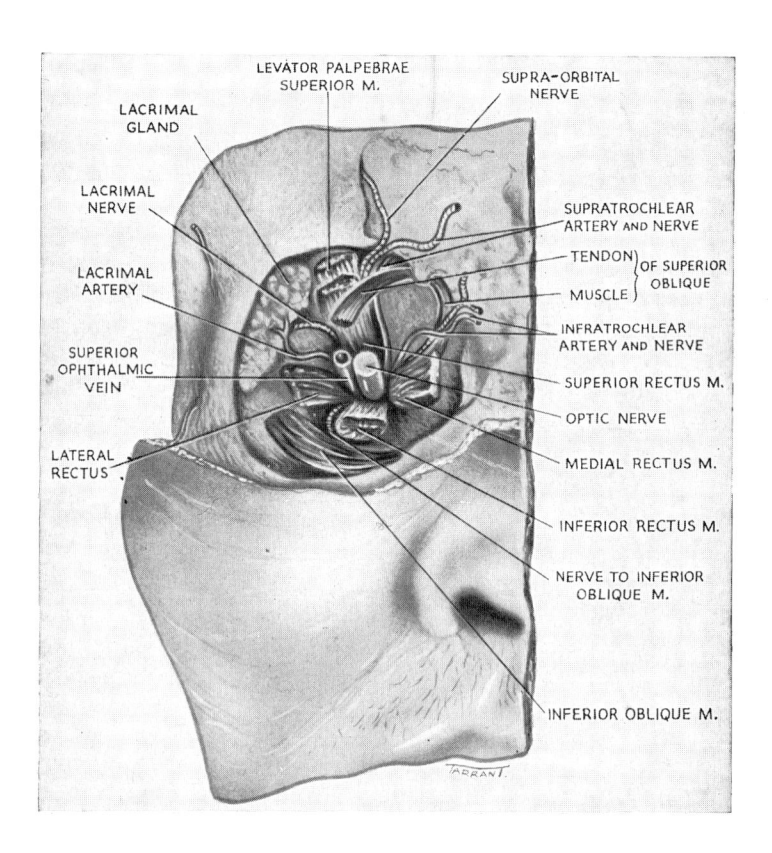

Fig. 19.2. Structures within right orbit, after removal of the eye.

stiffened by a fibro-cartilaginous *tarsal plate*, over which lies a horizontal band of muscle fibres (the orbicularis oculi) which closes the lids. The lids are opened by muscle fibres that sweep forwards to insert into their respective tarsal plates. Along the edges of each eyelid is a row of lashes, to provide further protection for the cornea; and, behind these, a row of openings (just visible to the naked eye) leading to the sebaceous *Meibomian glands*, which ramify within the tarsal plates, and secrete the grease which lubricates the corneal surface.

The surface of the cornea is kept clean by a flow of tears, which are secreted by the lacrimal gland. This is about the size of a large pea, and lies just beneath the overhanging upper-outer corner of the orbital rim (Fig. 19.2). The tears pass downwards and medially, and are drained away through the pin-sized openings of the lacrimal canaliculi at the medial ends of the lid margins (Fig. 19.3). These canaliculi run horizontally into a *lacrimal sac*, which nestles in a hollow of the underlying lacrimal bone, and thence the tears pass downwards (by a tear-duct or naso-lacrimal duct) into the lower meatus of the nasopharynx (hence the call to blow one's nose after weeping). There is normally a very gentle flow of tears throughout waking hours, augmented by a reflex flow if the eye is irritated or the emotions are sufficiently provoked, when the tears may spill across the lid margins.

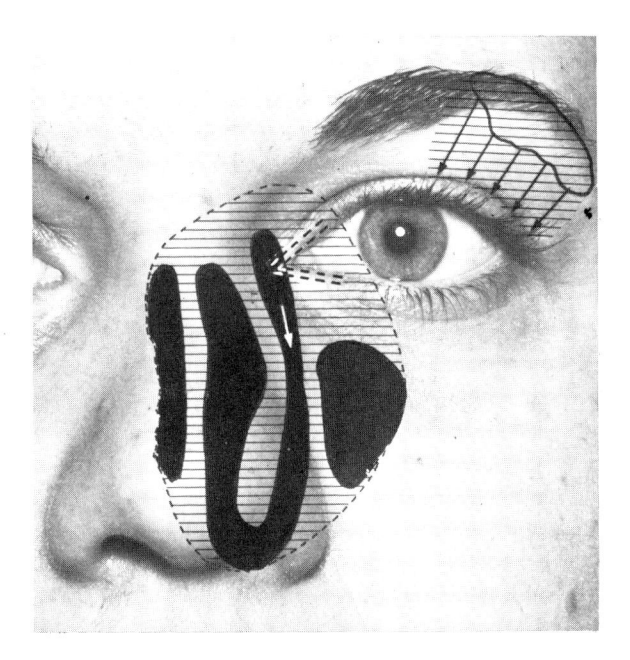

Fig. 19.3. The eyelids and lacrimal passages.

Examination

The *general examination* of the eye demands little beyond a good light, aided by a magnifying lens, to inspect the front of the eye, and an ophthalmoscope, for looking through the pupil and examining the posterior structures (the fundus of the eye). The light should be directed from the side to avoid dazzling the patient; and, if he is still reluctant to open his eyes adequately, the lids can be withdrawn gently by a finger (one lid at a time).

The *visual acuity* (Fig. 19.4) is then tested for each eye, first without glasses, and then with any distance-glasses he may possess. This is normally done by using letters of standard shape and size called Snellen's types, at a distance of six metres (to exclude all but a negligible amount of focusing). Vision is expressed as a fraction of the normal, the smallest letter usually visible without effort is thus '6/6'; if the patient can only see the letter twice its size, his visual acuity is '6/12'; while the largest letter usually displayed (ten times its size, and thus comfortably visible to the normal-sighted at sixty metres distance), designates a visual acuity of '6/60'. Still poorer vision is indicated by his capacity to count fingers ('C.F.'), see hand movements ('H.M.') and finally just to perceive light ('P.L.'). Near vision is similarly tested by a card bearing graded sizes of print.

The under surface of the upper lid can easily be inspected by *everting the lid* over a finger or glass rod (Fig. 19.5); this is most easily done by standing behind the patient, who is told to look at the floor, and then pulling the upper lashes forwards and upwards,

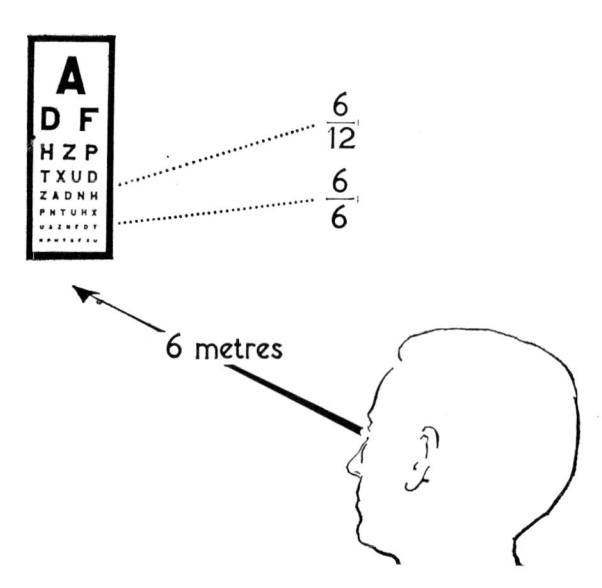

Fig. 19.4. Testing visual acuity.

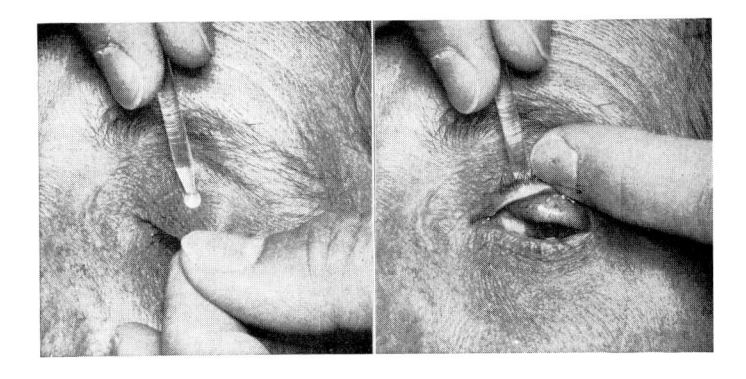

Fig. 19.5. Eversion of the upper lid.

so that the lid is rolled over the upper edge of its tarsal plate which is meanwhile pressed backwards by the forefinger of the other hand. (Foreign particles often become caught in the horizontal groove beneath the upper lid, and, when exposed in this way, can readily be whisked away).

The *visual fields* can be assessed by the perimeter (Fig. 19.6) which charts the position where a small white target first becomes visible

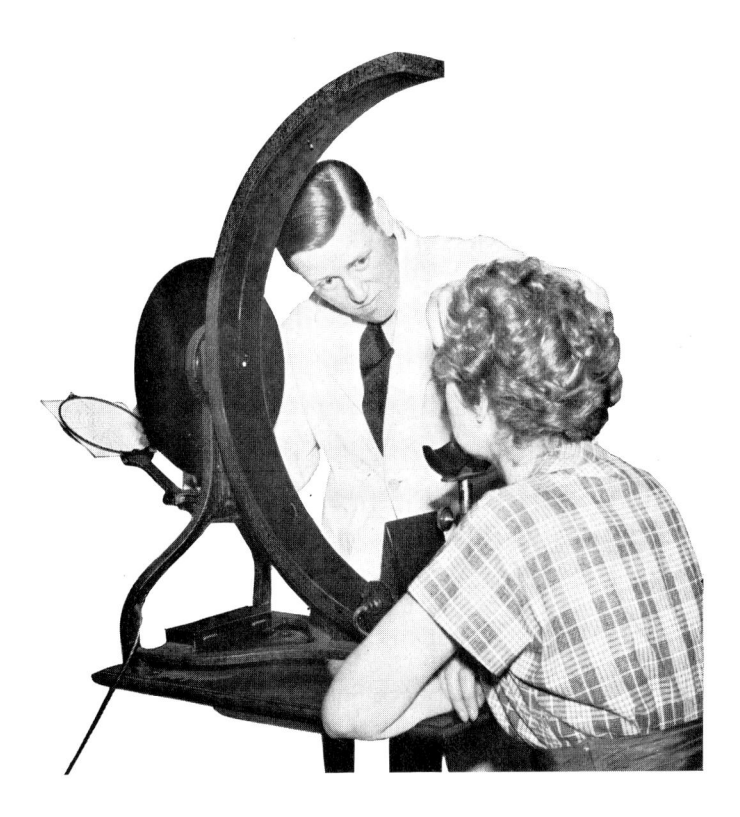

Fig. 19.6. Perimetry, using self-recording perimeter (Blaxter).

in each successive meridian, while the patient keeps his uncovered eye fixed on the hub of the instrument (cf. chart, Fig. 19.24).

Examination of the eye in small refractory children may require firm measures. The child should be wrapped tightly in a blanket, laid on a couch, with its head rigidly held between the assistant's hands. The eyelids can then be prised apart by simple retractors. If the fundus also needs inspection, the wandering eye may have to be secured by conjunctival forceps after local or general anaesthesia.

THE INFLAMED EYE

Conjunctivitis

The exposed surface of the eyeball, together with the under-surface of the eyelids, is covered by a thin mucous membrane called the *conjunctiva*; and this is condensed as a very smooth epithelium over the front of the cornea. Since this is exposed to all manner of injuries and infections, a *conjunctivitis* is the commonest form of eye-inflammation, comparable to simple mucosal inflammations elsewhere (like a 'cold' or 'sore throat'). Typically there is a generalised congestion of the superficial vessels, ('pink-eye' is the name sometimes used—Fig. 19.7), with a little watery discharge, which may become purulent in severe infections, and which tends to make the eyelids stick together on waking. The eye feels gritty, sensitive and uncomfortable. These conjunctivites may stem from a simple bacterial or viral infection, but are more often the sequel to allergies or external irritants, particularly the various cosmetics with which the female eye is belaboured, or the therapeutic lotions and ointments used.

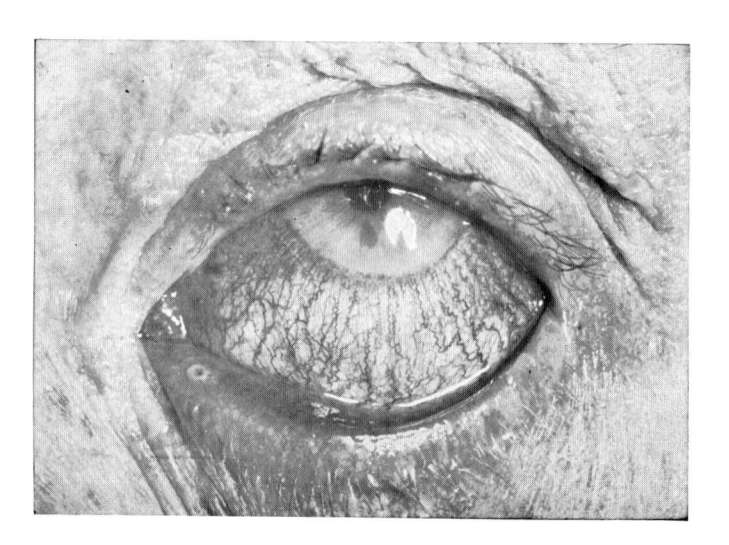

Fig. 19.7. Acute conjunctivitis, with secondary ectropion of lower lid, and eversion of lacrimal punctum.

Nearly all conjunctivites clear away within a week or so (like sore-throats), and treatment is barely necessary; but a broad spectrum antibiotic (such as chloramphenicol or neomycin) is justified if a frank infection is present. It should be remembered that by far the best and safest eye-lotion is a normal flow of tears (which contain their own antiseptic), and that most of the medicaments inserted into the eye do more harm than good. If the conjunctivitis persists, this may be due to the continued presence of an allergic irritant (such as pollens or cosmetics), or constant re-infection from a neighbouring inflammation, as in the lash roots (a *blepharitis*) or tear-sac (a *dacryocystitis*), or from a distortion of the lid margins (an *entropion* or *ectropion*).

Blepharitis

This is a very common eye-nuisance (Fig. 19.8), and generally is a sequel to a dry seborrhoeic skin (the Meibomian glands being simply enlarged sebaceous glands). Such patients tend to have reddish lid margins which become redder (and variably irritable) in smoky atmospheres, and when physical reserves are depleted (as after 'flu or a 'night-out'). The most effective treatment of this (as of simple allergic conjunctivitis) is the use of steroid drops, which will normally suppress the inflammation and therewith the symptoms, inserting these as often as necessary; they can be effectively combined with an antibiotic (e.g. prednisolone with neomycin drops) against any secondary bacterial infection. However, they must be used with caution, since they may promote the damaging corneal ulcers due to the herpes simplex virus, and they may also aggravate a simple glaucoma (although this is rare before middle age, by which time the

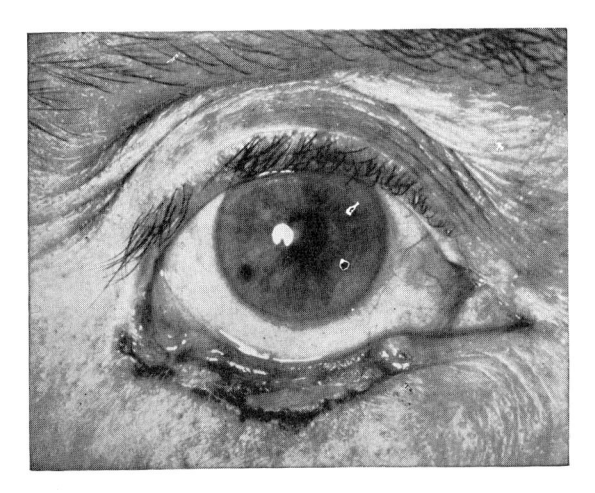

Fig. 19.8. Ulcerative blepharitis.

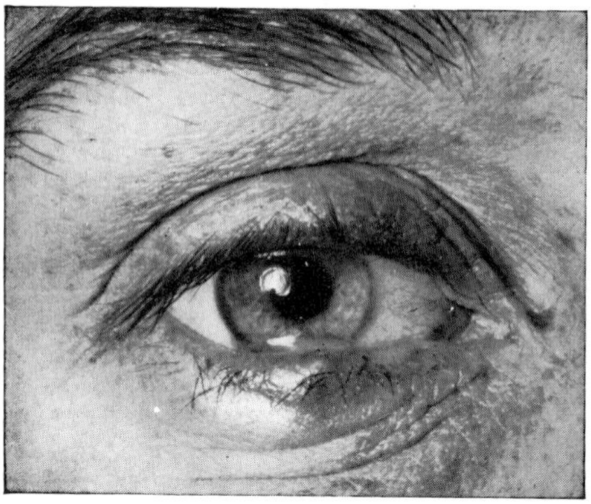

Fig. 19.9. External stye.

Fig. 19.10. Meibomian cyst.

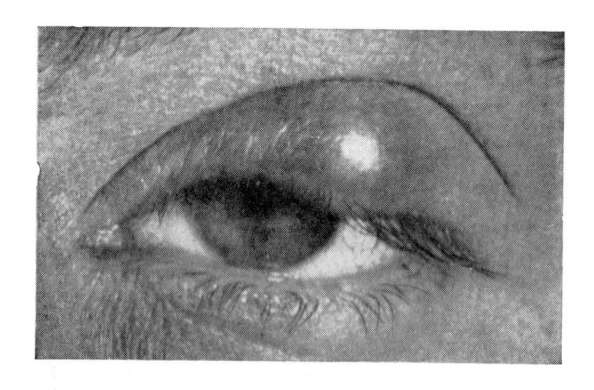

Fig. 19.11. Evacuation of meibomian cyst.

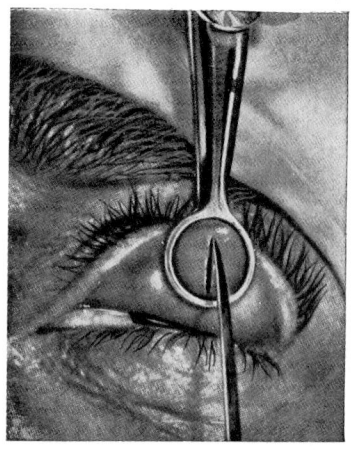

blepharitis is usually less troublesome). Such a blepharitis may lead to an accumulation of pus within an isolated eyelash follicle, an *external stye* (Fig. 19.9), or down a Meibomian gland, as an *internal stye*. Whereas the former (like any furuncle elsewhere) clears in a few days, irrespective of treatment, the Meibomian infection may leave a distended Meibomian cyst, (Fig. 19.10) which requires surgical evacuation (Fig. 19.11).

Dacryocystitis

This is also fairly common, especially in middle-aged women, infection having passed up the nasolacrimal duct from a nasopharyngitis. Very occasionally the inflammation is acute, causing a tender swelling medial to the inner angle of the eye. Far more commonly it simply produces a gradual obstruction to the drainage of tears, which increasingly dribble onto the cheek, particularly in cold winds.

The treatment of such a watering eye first entails syringing of saline through the lower canaliculus (Fig. 19.12). This shows whether there is a nasolacrimal duct obstruction, and in the early stages may in fact clear the blocked passage; astringent drops or lotions (such as zinc sulphate ½ per cent) may then help to reduce the watering. If the epiphora is sufficiently troublesome and has not yielded to several syringings, an operation may be justified; ideally this should be a dacryocystorrhinstomy (Fig. 19.13), fashioning a new opening between the sac and the middle nasal meatus, but in the old and feeble, especially where regurgitation of pus is the main trouble, a dacryocystectomy may suffice to ease the symptoms by simply removing the source of conjunctival re-infection. Probing the naso-lacrimal duct is of value only in the absence of established infection—as in infants when the duct has failed to open-up after birth.

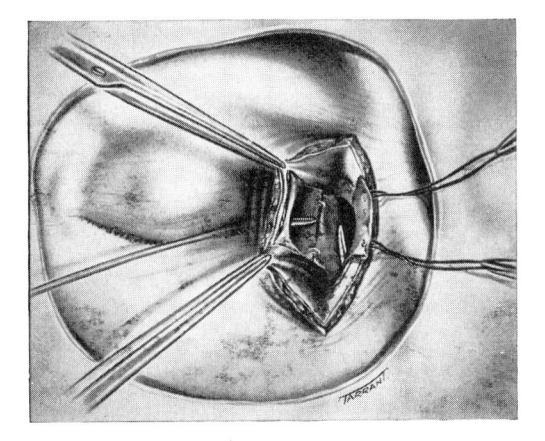

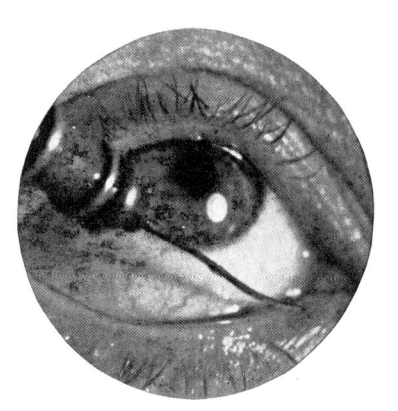

Fig. 19.12. Syringing the lacrimal sac.

Fig. 19.13. Dacryocystor-hinostomy.

Entropion

A rolling inwards of the lid margin can cause a conjunctivitis, since the in-turned lashes will then abrade the underlying conjunctiva and cornea. In tropical countries it is usually caused by scarring of the under-surface of the upper lid, as the sequel to a common and damaging infection called trachoma; but in temperate countries it is usually a spastic entropion of the lower lid, in people who are consistently screwing-up their eyes (Fig. 19.14). Both types require an operation; in the cicatricial entropion in order to straighten the buckled tarsal plate (an epilation of the ingrowing lashes will bring temporary relief), and in the spastic entropion to re-orientate the spastic fibres of the orbicularis muscle.

Fig. 19.14. Spastic entropion.

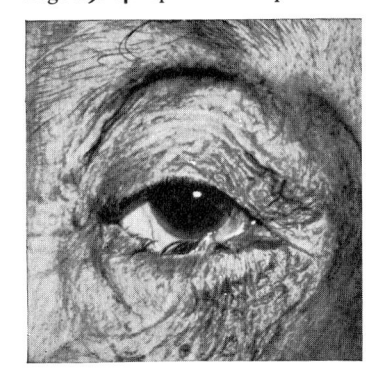

Ectropion

An outward rolling of the lower lid margin (Fig. 19.15), is conversely the sequel to a weakened orbicularis muscle, as after a facial palsy,

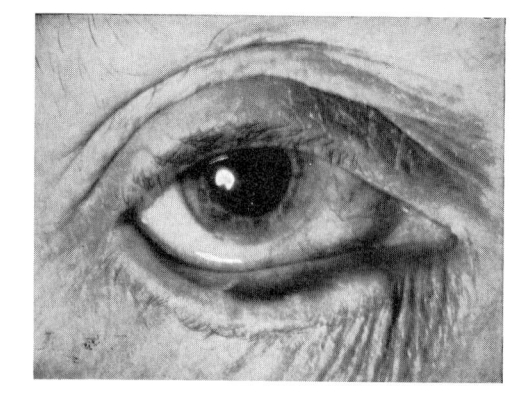

Fig. 19.15. Atonic ectropion.

Fig. 19.16. Corneal ulcer. (This ulcer, in the upper cornea, is so severe that pus has collected in the lower part of the anterior chamber).

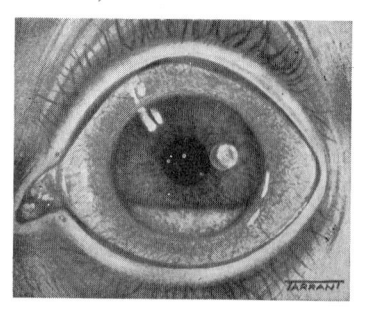

allowing a stagnant lake of tears to collect behind the lid. These soon become infected, causing a chronic conjunctivitis (which itself aggravates the entropion). Surgical re-ajdustment is again indicated.

A severe conjunctival infection may spread to involve the cornea, or the cornea may be directly abraded (as by an in-turned eyelash, a twig, or a foreign-body), provoking a *corneal ulcer* (Fig. 19.16). The pain is then more severe, the sight may be blurred, and the ulcer can sometimes be seen as a faint opalescence on the corneal surface; otherwise its presence can be made evident by inserting a drop of fluorescein, which turns the ulcerated area bright green. A little antibiotic ointment, followed by a firm pad to keep the upper lid splinted over the ulcer, will allow most simple abrasions to heal within a day or two. But some ulcers may be very slow in healing (especially the dendritic ulcer, caused by the herpes simplex virus); and if antibiotic or antiviral drops, atropine and a pad prove insufficient, cautery with carbolic acid may be needed, or even suturing together of the eylids or a corneal graft. When the ulcer is healed, a corneal scar remains, which, if it has been extensive, may impede the sight. Most corneal scars clear to a limited extent in time. But dense scars may persist and so reduce the vision that a corneal graft is justified—replacing a disc of the scarred cornea with a similar disc of cornea from a bequeathed eye (Fig. 19.17). Although technically exacting, this operation has become a straight-forward procedure in experienced hands, and a dramatic improvement in vision may be gained.

Inflammation of the inner eye

This usually involves the whole uveal tract; it is labelled a uveitis, or simply an iritis when only its anterior segment is apparently affected. The eye is again red and painful, but the pain is a constant

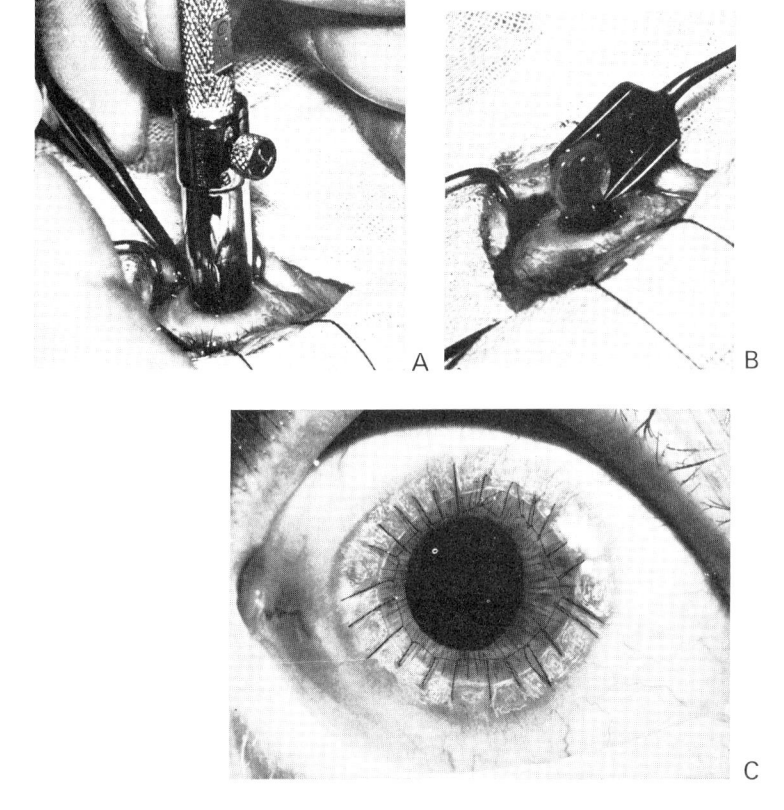

Fig. 19.17. Corneal graft (A) The disc of scarred cornea excised and replaced with a clear disc (B), which is sutured in place (C).

ache (not just the grittiness of a conjunctivitis) and the congestion is largely restricted to the blood-vessels around the cornea (nearest to the iris-root). The iris itself may be visibly affected, with festooning of the pupil (Fig. 19.18) where adhesions have tethered the pupil margin to the underlying lens. An iritis is serious, since any inflammatory exudate is retained within the eye, so impairing the vision; and this damage to sight may be permanent, if the inflammation is not checked—mainly by treatment with steroids (using hydrocortisone or prednisolone, as drops, ointment or tablets), supplemented by atropine, to keep the pupil dilated.

When the brunt of the inflammation falls on the posterior segment of the uveal tract, the choroid, there is no pain or congestion, but only a variable blurring of sight. Such a *choroiditis* is often unrecognised until, years later, the classical scars are noticed through the ophthalmoscope.

Uveitis may stem from many causes. It often is associated with rheumatism elsewhere in the body or generalised infections (as

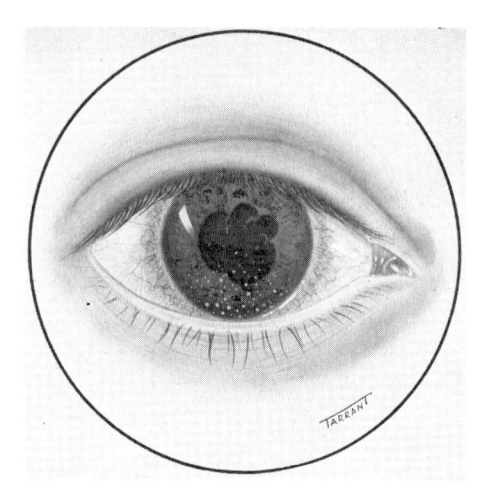

Fig. 19.18. Acute iritis.

syphilis or tuberculosis); but in the majority of cases no underlying cause can be found.

One other affection of the interior of the eyeball may cause a painful, red eye—the strangulated eyeball of an *acute glaucoma* (Fig. 19.19). Acute glaucoma is the sequel to a blockage to the flow of aqueous humour, so that it cannot escape from the eyeball into the veins outside, and the pressure within the eye rises till the eye becomes very hard. The vessels around the iris-root again become congested, but appearing dusky in colour (unlike the brick-red circumcorneal congestion in an acute iritis), and through the cornea the interior of the eye appears steamy and greenish (hence the word 'glaucoma'); and the sight is progressively blurred. Immediate treatment is necessary to relieve the pressure, by constricting the pupil with eserine or pilocarpine drops, by reducing the secretion of aqueous with Diamox tablets, and by sucking water out of the eye

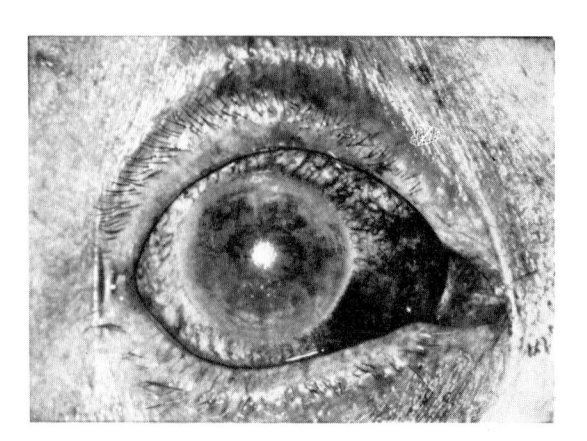

Fig. 19.19. Acute glaucoma.

through reducing the osmotic pressure of the blood with a draught of glycerol. Very occasionally the pressure remains high and a decompressing operation is needed.

FAILING SIGHT

Blindness in England is caused, in the main, by three diseases: cataract (23%), glaucoma (13%) and senile degenerations of the retina (27%). These are all diseases of the elderly which gradually erode the sight, but whereas cataracts can be remedied, glaucoma can only be arrested, and retinal degenerations ruthlessly progress. Sometimes the loss of sight is more rapid, as after a detachment of the retina or damage to the optic nerves (an 'optic neuritis' is usually the first evidence of disseminated sclerosis, or the nerves may be compressed by a brain tumour). Occasionally it happens suddenly, as the sequel to a thrombosis of the retinal vessels or a haemorrhage within the eye.

Cataract

The lens of the eye is transparent, but in old age it tends to become white (in the same way that the hair tends to become white), and some degree of lens opacity or 'cataract' is found in most people of over sixty, although in the vast majority of these it never progresses to the point where it materially interferes with sight. Very occasionally cataracts may form in younger age-groups, usually as the sequel to inflammation, injury (by concussion, penetrating wounds, noxious drugs or radiation) or sometimes as a congenital blemish.

Cataracts are the commonest cause of failing sight in old age. When advanced, they are easily observed as a grey opacity within the pupil; but in the earlier stages can readily be seen as an irregular silhouette with the ophthalmoscope, or in the beam of the corneal microscope (the 'slit-lamp') (Figs 19.20, 19.21). The only effective

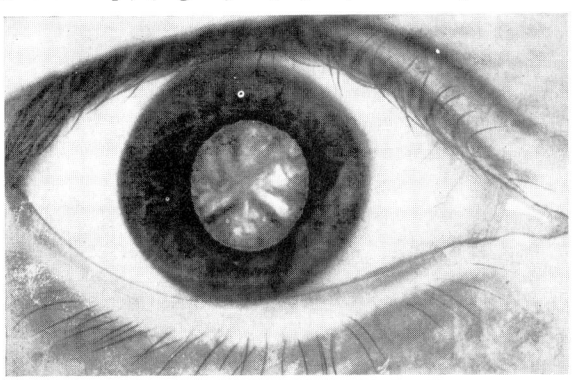

Fig. 19.20. Mature cataract.

Fig. 19.21. The wedge-shaped opacities of a peripheral cataract standing-out as a silhouette when viewed through an ophthalmoscope.

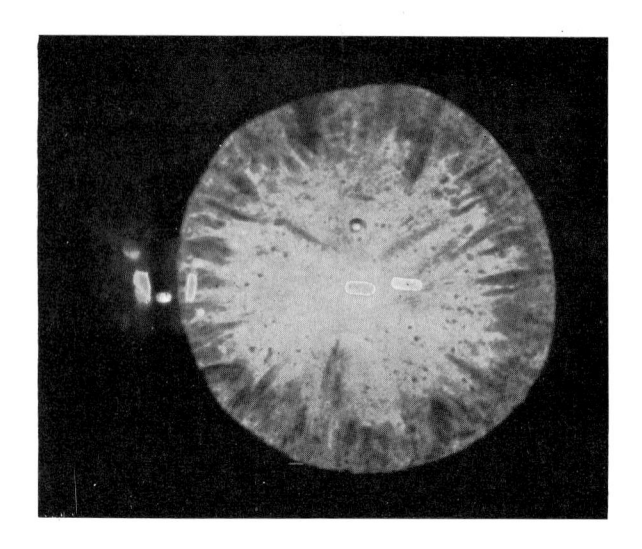

treatment for a cataract is to extract it by operation (Figs 19.22, 19.23), and this is justified if the sight has become so impaired that reading and close work are rendered difficult. After removal of a cataractous lens, the retinal image is necessarily out of focus unless a similar lens, in the form of spectacles or a contact-lens, is used as a replacement, and since these artificial lenses all introduce problems of their own (judgement of depth becomes difficult, the two eyes will not readily work in unison, the spectacle lenses are large and heavy, and the contact-lenses difficult to manage), an operation is rarely justified when only one eye is cataractous.

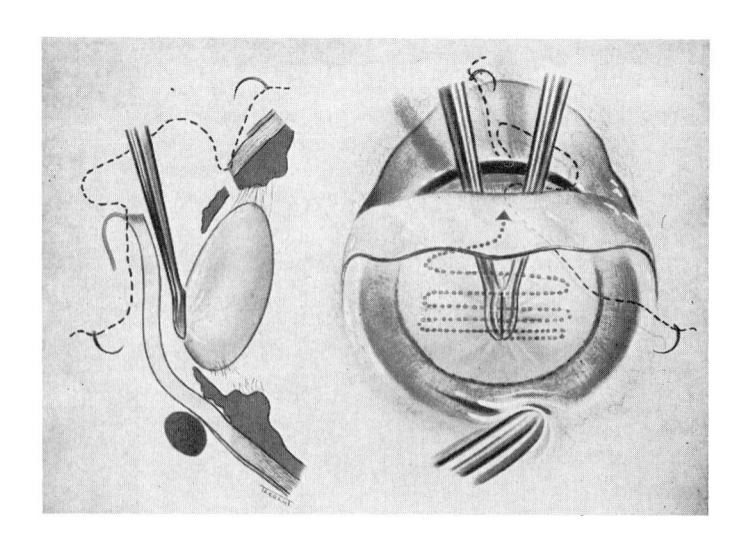

Fig. 19.22. Cataract extraction—the sutures are placed on the corneo-scleral incision, ready for closure, and the cataract lifted out by holding its capsule with forceps.

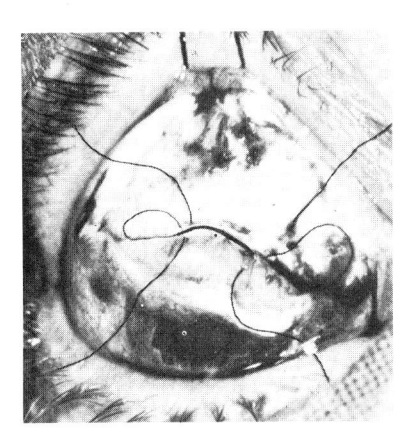

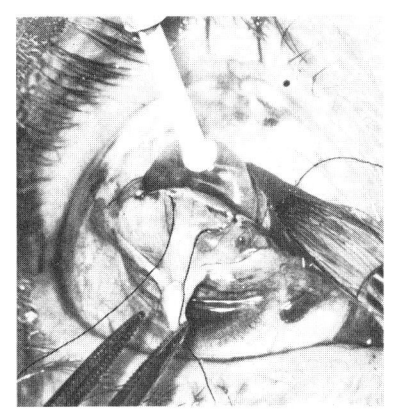

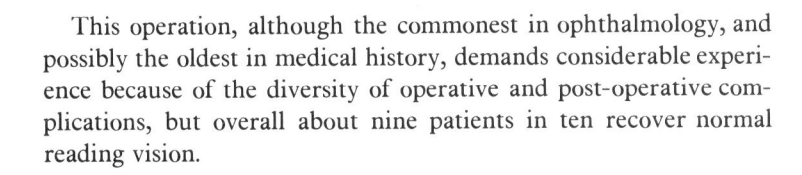

Fig. 19.23. Cataract extraction—the cataract can also be extracted by freezing it to the end of a probe.

This operation, although the commonest in ophthalmology, and possibly the oldest in medical history, demands considerable experience because of the diversity of operative and post-operative complications, but overall about nine patients in ten recover normal reading vision.

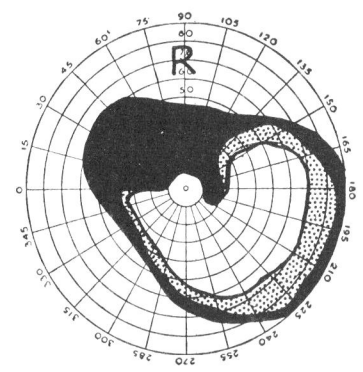

Simple glaucoma

After middle-age a silting-up of the spaces through which the aqueous percolates out of the eye may lead to a very gradual increase in the intra-ocular pressure; and in time the more vulnerable cells in the retina (those towards the retinal periphery) become destroyed, so that the sight is gradually whittled away. As this erosion of vision is mainly off-centre, the central vision remains unaffected until most of the 'visual field' has been irreparably lost, and the patient who can still read the smaller letters, may yet be unaware that his peripheral sight has gone. (Fig. 19.24.)

Simple glaucoma is usually diagnosed by the excavated appearance of the optic disc (the front-end of the optic nerve, where it lies exposed near the centre of the retina Fig. 19.25). This is often discovered on a routine check with an ophthalmoscope, and then confirmed by finding that the pressure is raised (through a pressure-gauge that rests on the cornea) and by plotting the field of vision with a perimeter (Fig. 19.6).

The pressure can normally be kept below normal (which should prevent further erosion of the visual field) by measures similar to those used in acute glaucoma Pilocarpine drops (usually 2%, t.d.s.), and Diamox tablets. (In some cases, where these still fail to arrest the field-loss, an operation (usually a sclerectomy) will allow the

Fig. 19.24. Field loss in acute glaucoma.

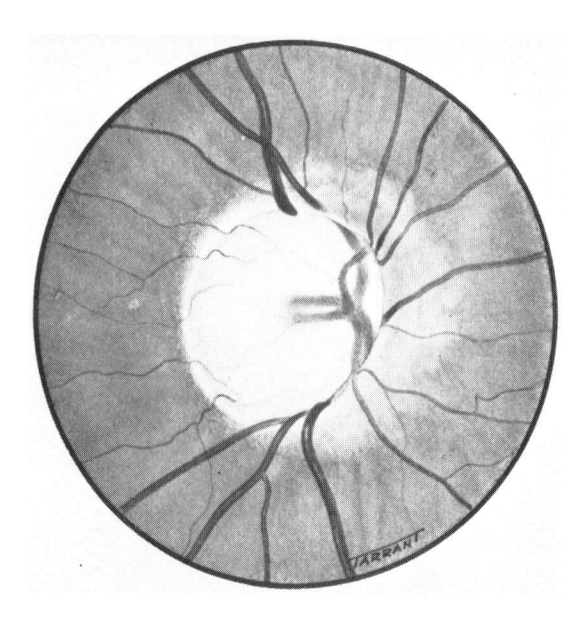

Fig. 19.25. Cupping of the optic disc from simple glaucoma.

acqueous to drain away more freely, through a hole in the sclera at the corneal margin, into the lymphatics beneath the conjunctiva (Fig. 19.26).

Retinal degenerations

The large majority are simply dystrophies, and the result of ageing in a very specialised tissue, where dying cells cannot be replaced; there is no effective treatment, but since most dystrophies only affect the central area (the macula), these old people can still get about quite well, although reading may be rendered impossible. Other degenerative changes are the sequel to advanced diabetes or hypertension, and a host of other disturbances to the retina and choroid are equally revealed through the ophthalmoscope (Fig. 19.27).

Retinal detachment

This is relatively common, and causes a dramatic loss of sight. It is the sequel to a tear in the retina, either following injury to the eye or certain degenerative changes, such as occur in high myopia (short-sightedness) (Fig. 19.28). The retina peels off the wall of the eyeball like torn wall-paper in a room, and the retinal cells will soon die as they become separated from their nutrient blood in the choroid, unless the retina is replaced by operation. This usually involves making a pleat in the overlying sclera, so that a fold of this

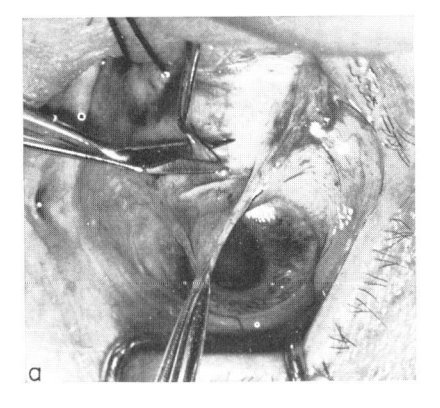

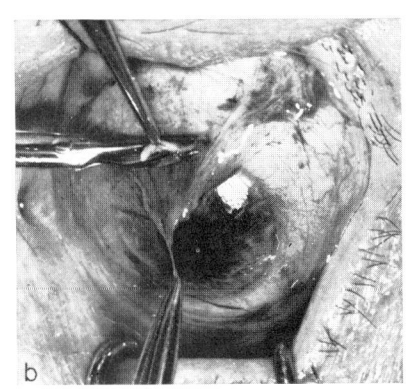

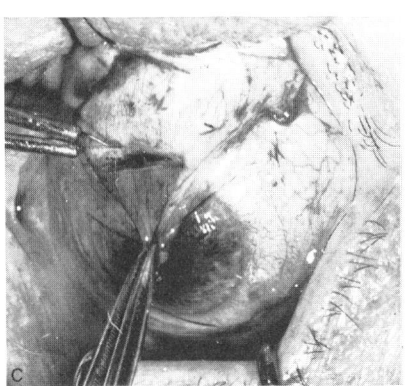

Fig. 19.26. Sclerectomy—a small piece of sclera is excised at the corneal margin, to allow the aqueous to escape beneath the conjunctiva.

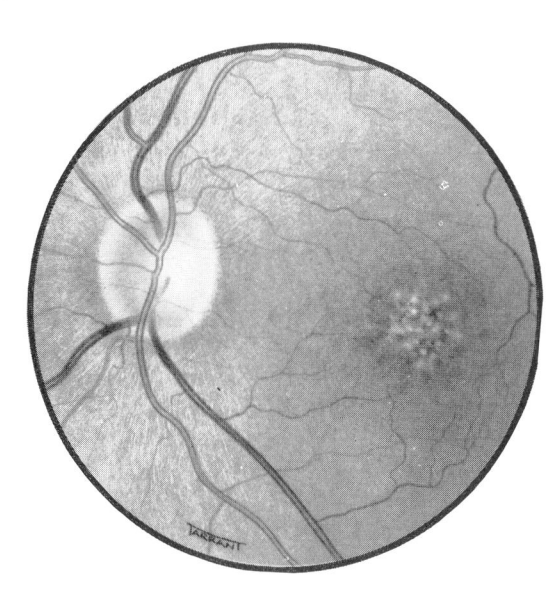

Fig. 19.27. The fundus in senile macular dystrophy.

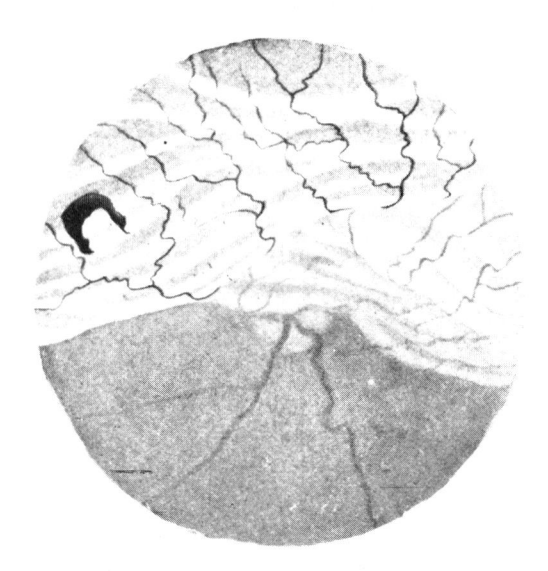

Fig. 19.28. Retinal detachment—the upper half of the retina has fallen forwards, following the large U-shaped tear.

Fig. 19.29. Retinal detachment—operation (a tight strap encircling the eyeball indents the sclera, and to this ridge the detached retina can be made to adhere).

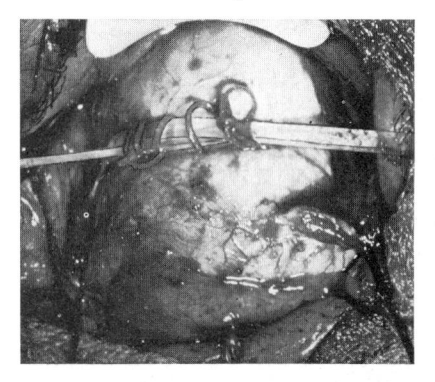

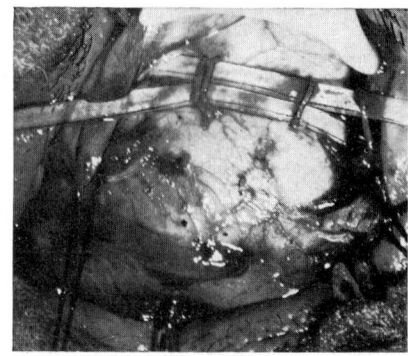

is pushed forwards to meet the detached retina, and then glueing these together by applications of a freezing-probe (Fig. 19.29). If treated early enough the majority of retinas can be replaced, although some loss of sight will be permanent.

Thrombosis of the central retinal artery or vein

These are both fairly common causes of sudden loss of sight, or of part of the sight if only one of the arterial or venous branches is involved, and they usually stem from cardiovascular degeneration in the elderly. Immediate treatment very occasionally clears an arterial occlusion (if from spasm or embolus), and a limited recovery is likely after a venous block.

Haemorrhages in the retina

These are common sequels to various blood disorders (hypertension, diabetes, anaemia, leukaemia, etc.) but the haemorrhages are usually small, and, unless involving the macular area, unnoticed by the patient. Any of these may erupt into the vitreous, leaving the eye almost completely blind, and clearance of such a haemorrhage may be slow and incomplete.

SQUINT

Our eyes are kept parallel by a complicated reflex, established during infancy, in the interests of single vision; but when they fall out of alignment they are said to 'squint'. Usually they deviate along a horizontal axis (so that the eyes converge or diverge) but occasionally there is a vertical squint, with one eye looking above its fellow.

The simplest form of squint is that due to injury to any of the twelve muscles that govern the eye-movements, or of the nerves that motivate them. The affected eye cannot then rotate into the direction of this paralysed muscle, and the squint is increasingly obvious on attempting to look in this direction. Such *paralytic squints* are thus commonly the sequel to head injuries (especially with facial fractures), or tumours and haemorrhages within the brain and they normally recover if the underlying damage is cleared. Thus all that is necessary in treatment is to cover the affected eye (usually by sticky paper over the appropriate spectacle lens) so as to prevent the double-vision that is inevitably provoked.

Much more frequently the squint starts in the first few years of life, when the child can no longer sustain the subconscious effort of holding the eyes straight under the stress of an illness (like measles), or of adaptation to an emotional situation (like the arrival of a younger baby). These are labelled *concomitant squints*, since the angle of deviation does not vary when the child looks in different directions. Once established, such squints tend to persist, since the vision of the squinting eye usually becomes suppressed (so as to avoid a tiresome double-vision), and the eye is then said to have become 'lazy'. Such childhood squints are usually convergent (Fig. 19.30), although divergent squints are not rare (generally arising in slightly older children).

Although in most children with 'cross-eyes', the convergence tends to become less marked in later childhood, such a natural cure is nearly always at the expense of spending the rest of their life with a lazy eye, in which full vision could have been restored (normally by sticking a patch over the spectacle lens of the master-eye and

Fig. 19.30. Convergent squint.

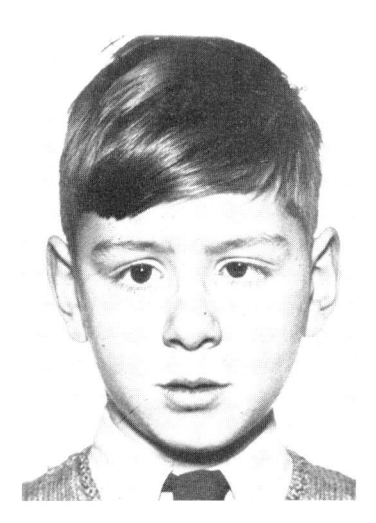

436
Chapter 19

Fig. 19.31. Convergent squint—occlusion of the master-eye by elastoplast on the spectacles.

Fig. 19.32. Convergent squint operation—recession of lateral rectus. The muscle is cut free from its insertion (A), and sutured to the sclera 5 mm. behind this (B).

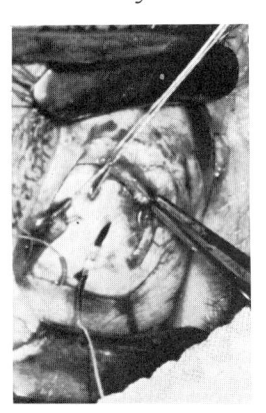

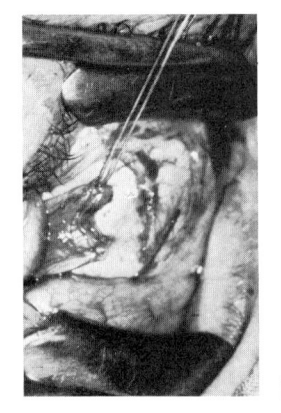

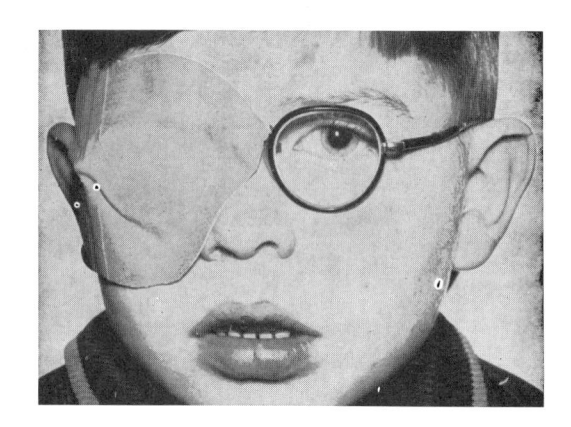

forcing the child to use the lazy eye (Fig. 19.31), if only this had been done in time—before the age of seven; for by the age of about ten, no further recovery of vision in the lazy eye can be anticipated.

The treatment of the childhood concomitant squint entails the use of spectacles if the child is sufficiently long-sighted, since correction of this long-sightedness often reduces the degree of convergence), then patching the master-eye, if its fellow is becoming lazy. Orthoptic exercises will thereafter help to build-up the child's capacity for using the eyes in unison (as an incentive for the eyes to stay straight). If the squint is still marked, an operation is needed to align the eyes, usually by recessing the medial rectus muscle (dividing the insertion, and sewing it to the sclera about 5 mm further back) and resecting the lateral rectus (excising about 5 mm of its length) (Figs. 19.32, 19.33). Such a straightening operation may be needed when only a few months old, if the squint is sufficiently gross and constant that the eyes cannot hope to be used in unison otherwise; and it can equally be done at any time of life purely for cosmetic reasons. But, because it is only during the first few years of life that a lazy eye can only be taught to see again and the eyes can only be taught to work in unison, all squinting children should be seen by an eye-doctor as soon as the squint is noticed.

SPECTACLES

Failing sight need not be a sequel to organic changes in the eyeball, but may just be due to one of the four so-called Refractive Errors which result in an out-of-focus image on the retina, and which can be requited by spectacles.

Presbyopia is simply the result of the natural weakening of our focusing power (from the ciliary muscle) as we grow older so that,

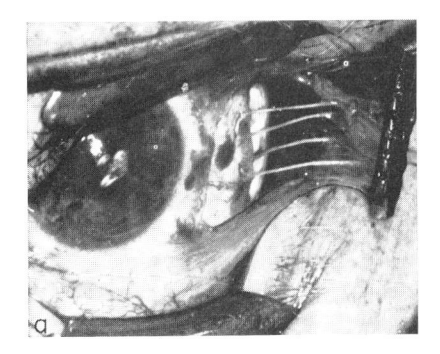

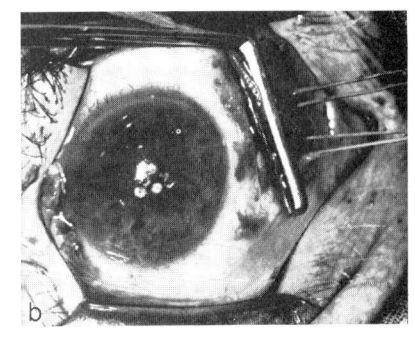

Fig. 19.33. Convergent squint operation—resection of medial rectus (the muscle is cut free from its insertion, and a segment of it, held in the clamp, is excised, before re-suturing).

by the age of about forty-five, the book must be held farther away from the eye than the normal reading-range. This can be compensated by weak convex spectacles, which will need to be strengthened a little every few years.

Sometimes the eyeball is rather shorter or longer than the normal: the short eyeball renders the eye long-sighted or *hypermetropic*, since some of the focusing power must be used-up in bringing the focus of the image forwards to the (abnormally forward-placed) retina. This leaves less of a reserve of focusing-power for near vision. Such patients will need the help of reading glasses before the usual age of forty-five (in other words, they have a premature presbyopia), and the effort of reading without glasses may cause eye-fatigue.

When the eyeball is too long, the eye is short-sighted or *myopic*, since, although near objects can be seen clearly, distant object can only be brought to a focus on the (abnormally backward-placed) retina by wearing a concave spectacle lens. Such myopes do not experience eye-fatigue, but simply have a blurred view of the distance unless they wear glasses. Myopia tends to run in families, and starts usually in later childhood, increasing in degree until growth stops: its progress is determined by one's heredity, and this cannot be influenced by wearing glasses, exercises, drugs, diet or any other fanciful remedies.

The eyeball is never a perfect sphere, and apart from being a little too long or short, a little flattening, labelled *astigmatism*, is almost universal. Only very occasionally is this enough to cause headaches or slightly blur the retinal image and so justify special correcting spectacles.

It must be emphasized that the vast majority of headaches bear no relationship to refractive errors, and also that the eyes themselves can never be damaged by uncorrected or wrongly-corrected refractive errors. Spectacle lenses can be darkened, like sun-glasses, and very occasionally a genuine photophobia justifies this, but the vast majority of dark glasses are sought in the hope of protecting a frail psyche or concealing a guiltful one from the harsh or revealing light of day.

PRACTICAL NOTES ON TREATMENT OF EXTERNAL DISEASES

1. Toilet to the eye

Use lint swabs, (folded, with the fluffy side inward) soaked in normal saline. The unaffected eye is cleansed first (there is often some 'sympathetic' discharge in the fellow eye, and this warns the patient what to expect when his tender eye is touched). The patient is told to close the eye gently ('as if in sleep') and the upper lids are wiped gently from the nasal corner outwards. The patient is told to open the eye, and the lower lid margins are wiped likewise; this is repeated until all discharge is removed. The swab must not touch the eye itself.

2. Instillation of drops and ointment

Careful check of label (this is often helped by coloured labels: Red = pupil-dilators, Blue = pupil-constrictors, Orange = antiseptics). Warn the patient that the drop or ointment is coming, and ask him to look upwards. Pull the lower lid gently down and insert into the 'gutter' behind it (but not onto the cornea) one or two of the drops (Fig. 19.34) or squeeze in a small strip of the ointment. Ointment has the advantage of lingering rather longer before the tears wash it all away, and so exerting its effect longer, and also of being mildly lubricating to a roughened conjunctival surface; but the ointment itself is sometimes irritating, and it makes the sight blurry for a few minutes. When treating themselves, some patients find ointment the easier to insert.

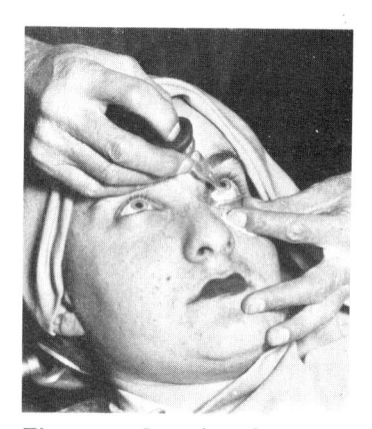

Fig. 19.34. Insertion of eye-drops.

3. Eye irrigation

This is rarely necessary, unless there is a frank discharge that needs clearance. Traditionally it is done by directing a stream of saline (or antiseptic) from an undine (Fig. 19.35) into the inner corner of the eye, and collecting it in a bowl or kidney-dish closely applied to the temple. For domestic use, an eye-bath is generally preferred; (routine bathing of the eye does not benefit the eye, and should normally be discouraged). When noxious chemicals have entered the eye, the head should be promptly submerged in a basin or pail of water, and the lids forcibly opened.

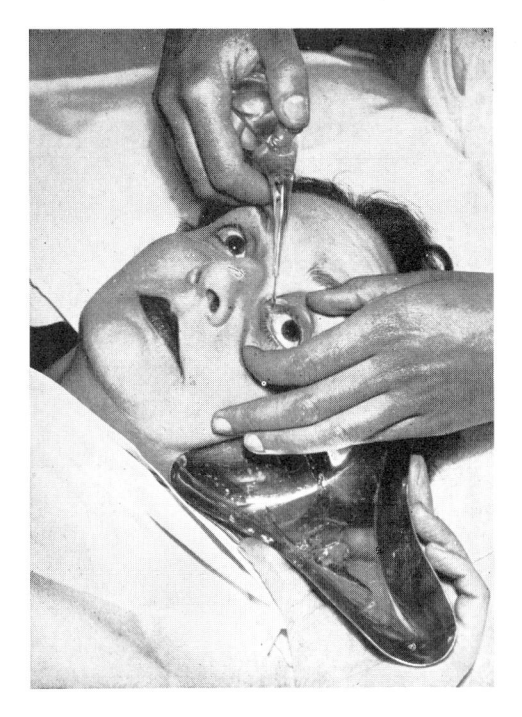

Fig. 19.35. Irrigation of the conjunctiva.

4. Removal of a foreign body

The patient should be recumbent or semi-recumbent, with good illumination. Examine, with a magnifying spectacle, to see if the foreign body is impacted on the cornea. If none is present, evert the upper lid, lest it is retained there (and whence it can readily be whisked away).

If there is an impacted corneal foreign body, insert a drop of local anaesthetic (e.g. amethocaine 1%). Attempt to dislodge it with twisted wisp of cotton wool. If (as is usual) this fails, excavate it with a fine, flattened needle. Insert antibiotic ointment and pad the eye. Refer the patient to an eye-surgeon unless the eye is white and comfortable by the following day.

5. Syringing of tear-ducts

Insert a drop of local anaesthetic (amethocaine 1%). The patient should be recumbent or semi-recumbent, and good illumination is needed. Expose the lacrimal punctum by everting the medial end of the lower lid with the left forefinger. Insert Nettleship's dilator gently, passing it vertically downwards for about 2 mm then directing it medially and twisting it slightly for a further few millimetres. Then withdraw it. Insert a cannula, fitted onto a 2 ml syringe, filled with saline. Inject the saline. If the duct is patent, the fluid will enter freely, and its passage into the nose is usually confirmed by a gulp from the patient. Otherwise, it may flow back along the lower lacrimal canaliculus or squirt out of the upper one.

NOTES ON MANAGEMENT OF MAJOR SURGICAL CASES

Pre-operative

The patient is admitted one to two days before operation to allow adjustment to hospital routine, general medical check (especially blood-pressure, urine, cough, etc.), and preparation of the eye. Some surgeons prefer the lashes to be cut (with fine scissors, smeared with Vaseline to catch the severed lashes), and preoperative cultures (via a sterilised platinum loop which gently scrapes the lower trough (fornix) of conjunctiva, behind the everted lower lid, and transfers the scraping to a blood-agar plate). Prophylactic drops are then inserted, usually chloramphenicol 0.5% t.d.s. to both eyes.

A mild aperient may be given on the day before operation, and a sedative on the previous night. On the morning before operation the patient has a bath, long hair is combed and plaited, and male patients are encouraged to shave.

Premedication for cataract surgery usually starts about an hour before the operation. If he is having a local anaesthetic, guttae cocaine 4%, adrenaline 0.1%, homatropine 1% and chloramphenicol 0.5% are usually instilled every few minutes for twenty minutes, and then at ten-minute intervals until the operation. The eye is meanwhile covered with a pad. If a general anaesthetic is used, the cocaine is omitted. Similar drops are normally used before operations for retinal detachments. For glaucoma surgery, the homatropine and adrenaline are normally omitted, and pilocarpine included. But there are many variations practised.

The eye requiring operation is usually marked with a cross on the forehead; and this is also indicated on a label (along with the patient's name and age) fixed to his wrist.

Post-operative care

The patient will normally be returned to the ward, having the eye covered by a pad, a stiff cartella shield, and a bandage; after a local anaesthetic, two or more pillows are normally permitted. The locker should be placed on the side of his uncovered eye and the nurse should also approach his bed from this side. Care is needed that the patient does not knock his bandaged eye, move around unduly, cough or vomit.

The first dressing is normally done on the following morning; drops of antibiotic solution (and, after cataracts, antropine) are instilled. Thereafter the patient may wish his own face and feed himself (under supervision). Smoking should be curtailed (there is an added fire-risk from smoking in bed, with one eye bandaged). Patients are usually allowed to sit out of bed during bed-making directly after the first dressing, although carefully avoiding stooping or sudden movements, and to use the bedside sani-chair on the third day; gentle walks follow about the sixth post-operative day, and all being well he may leave hospital a day or two later. Dark glasses are usually ordered after the eye-pad is discarded, since such eyes are light-sensitive, but these can be discarded as soon as the patient is comfortable without them.

After glaucoma operations the regime is similar but less exacting, and the patient usually leaves hospital within a week. After corneal grafts and detachment operations the stay may be more prolonged, and strict rest in bed (even in a specific position) may be required, especially in detachment cases, according to the site and extent of the detachment. After squint operations, since the eyeball has not been opened, only a few days hospital stay is needed, simply for toilet to the eye and antiseptic applications.

Chapter 20. Diseases of the ear, nose and throat

THE EAR

Anatomy and Physiology

The auricle or pinna is composed of cartilage, the closely adherent perichondrium, and skin. It is developed from six tubercles, and fistulae or other congenital abnormalities may occur if these tubercles fail to fuse.

The external auditory meatus, about one inch in length, is lined with skin which is supported by cartilage in its outer third and bone in its inner two-thirds.

The tympanic membrane or drum-head, commonly known as the 'ear-drum' (Fig. 20.1.) is composed of three layers—skin, fibrous tissue and mucous membrane—and is stretched across the medial end of the external auditory meatus.

The tympanic cavity, which contains the three ossicles—malleus, incus and stapes—communicates anteriorly with the nasopharynx via the *Eustachian tube* and posteriorly with the *mastoid antrum* and *air-cells* (Fig. 20.2). It is in close proximity to numerous anatomical structures including the facial nerve, internal carotid artery, sigmoid sinus and dura mater of the middle and posterior cranial fossae. Its detailed anatomy may be referred to in the standard anatomical text-books and, briefly, the function of its contents is to transmit vibrations of sound (which have been collected by the auricle and external meatus) from the tympanic membrane to the inner-ear or organ of Corti. This complex and incredibly difficult mechanical task is achieved with superb precision by the lever mechanism of the ossicles, the *malleus* moving with the tympanic membrane and in turn actuating the *incus*, whereby movement is imparted to the

Fig. 20.1. The normal tympanic membrane (left).

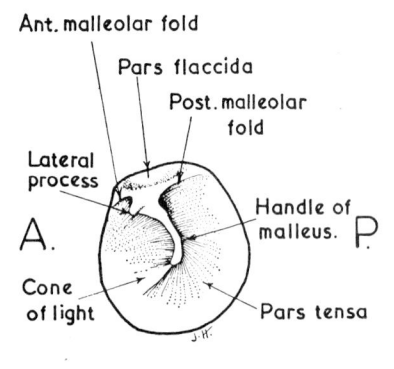

stapes, and thus eventually the fluids of the internal ear are set in motion, as the stapedial footplate is loosely sealed into the oval window.

CLINICAL EXAMINATION OF THE EAR

The ear is often examined in hospital clinics with the aid of the surgeon's head-mirror and small metal aural speculae into which may be fitted a pneumatic or Siegle's speculum—the latter enabling the examiner to vary the external air pressure on the tympanic membrane or drumhead and thus reveal small perforations. On the other hand the surgeon may choose to use an electric otoscope (auriscope) and certainly the latter is most convenient at the bedside.

Electric otoscopes require care and attention, and every effort must be made to ensure that the battery is well up to standard, the bulb is functioning and the speculum fits. Even then a poor view of the meatus and tympanic membrane may result, and in such cases the bulb holder may have become bent.

Assuming that a good instrument and a little tuition are available, a reasonably good view of the drum-head with its pearly lustre (Fig. 20.1) should be obtained without undue difficulty by the novice, though it is true that some external auditory canals are both narrow and tortuous and present problems to the most experienced observers.

Fig. 20.2. The tympanic cavity showing its relationship to Eustachian tube and mastoid cells. The tympanic membrane and malleus are indicated by broken lines.

Testing the hearing

Hearing tests range from the most simple to the most sophisticated, and in the first place many examiners make an approximate assessment of hearing acuity by asking the patient to repeat words which have been whispered or spoken at conversational level. Even in such a simple test as this precautions are necessary to avoid serious errors. The possibility of lip-reading must be excluded, and in the case of a patient with good hearing in one ear and moderate or severe deafness in the other, great care is necessary to exclude the better hearing ear from the test, not as one might suppose by blocking its canal, but by applying a continuous noise to it—in the clinic—by means of the Bárány noise apparatus (Fig. 20.3).

This important manoeuvre is known as masking and is used in different forms in many audiological tests.

Tuning fork tests are employed to detect not the degree but the type of hearing loss—Conductive or Perceptive. *Conductive deafness* being present when some disorder prevents sound waves reaching

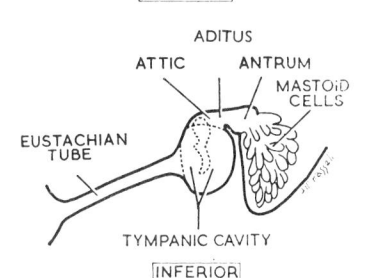

Fig. 20.3. Bárány noise apparatus.

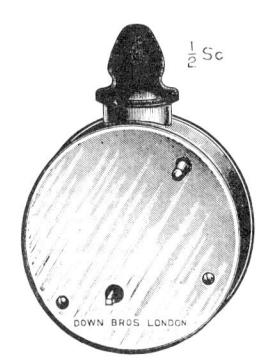

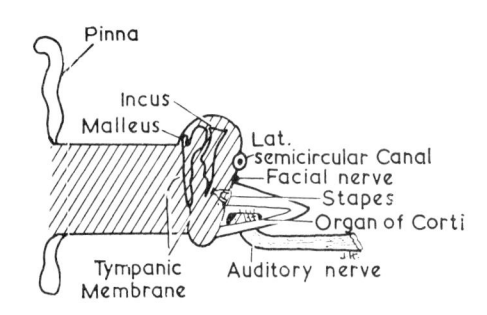

Fig. 20.4. Conductive deafness is caused by an abnormality of the external or middle ear (shaded).

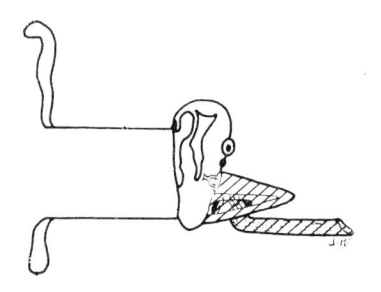

Fig. 20.5. Perceptive deafness is caused by an abnormality of the inner ear or auditory nerve (shaded).

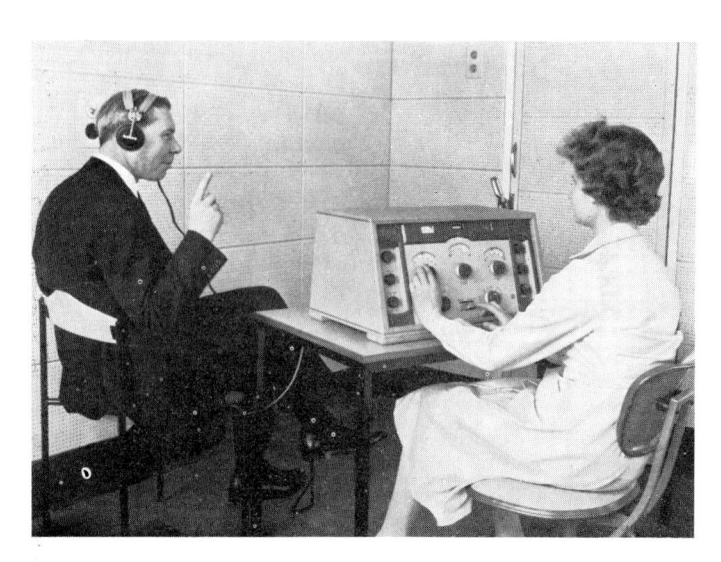

Fig. 20.6. Audiometry. The patient is signalling that he can hear a test tone.

the inner ear, (Fig. 20.4) and *perceptive deafness* signifying a disorder of the inner ear or auditory nerve (Fig. 20.5).

Examples of some of the causes of conductive deafness are wax, middle ear disease and otosclerosis and of perceptive deafness are Menière's disease, senile deafness and VIIIth nerve tumour.

In Rinne's test the tuning fork is normally heard better when it is held near the ear than when its base is applied to the mastoid process, though in conductive deafness the findings are reversed owing to the presence of some impediment to the normal magnification provided by the middle ear mechanism. In Weber's test the base of a tuning fork is held on the vertex and sound is heard in the more deaf ear in conductive deafness or the less deaf ear in perceptive deafness.

In pure-tone audiometry a series of tones ranging from 125 c.p.s (cycles per second) to 12,000 c.p.s. are fed into the patient's ear by means of a headphone (Fig. 20.6). The volume of these tones can be varied by the operator whose object is to discover the threshold at which the patient can only just hear any particular tone. By this

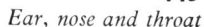

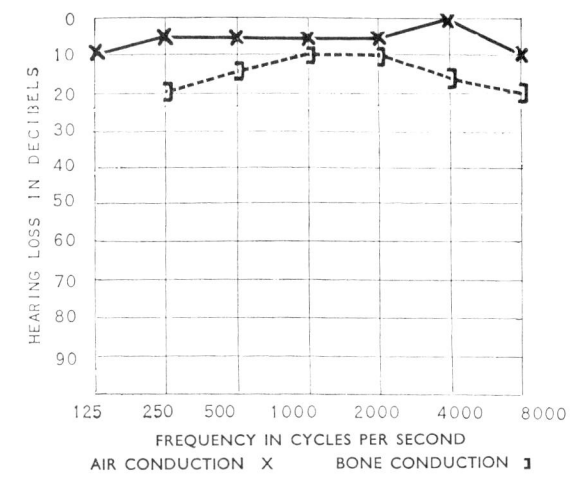

Fig. 20.7. Audiogram showing good hearing.

means a graph may be produced showing hearing loss by both air and bone conduction for a number of different frequencies (Figs. 20.7, 8 and 9). Such a graph is of great help in diagnosis and in estimating the degree of hearing-loss. Pure tone audiometry is practised widely, but in certain centres more sophisticated audiological methods such as speech, Békésy, impedance and evoked response audiometry are available.

Conditions of the auricle (pinna)

Congenital deformity may occur in the form of 'bat ears' in which the outstanding auricles are very unsightly and cause their owner to be the butt of much ragging in childhood. They are corrected surgically between the ages of four and six years. Other congenital anomalies are seen in the form of accessory auricle, fistulae around the ear or variations in the size of the auricle.

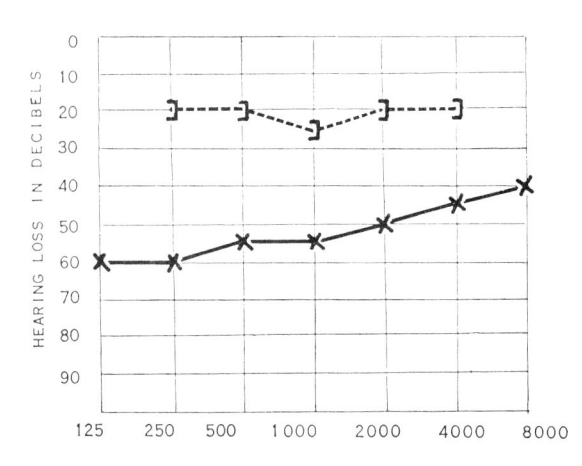

Fig. 20.8. Audiogram showing conductive deafness. Horizontal scale shows the frequency in cycles per second. Air conduction ×, bone conduction.

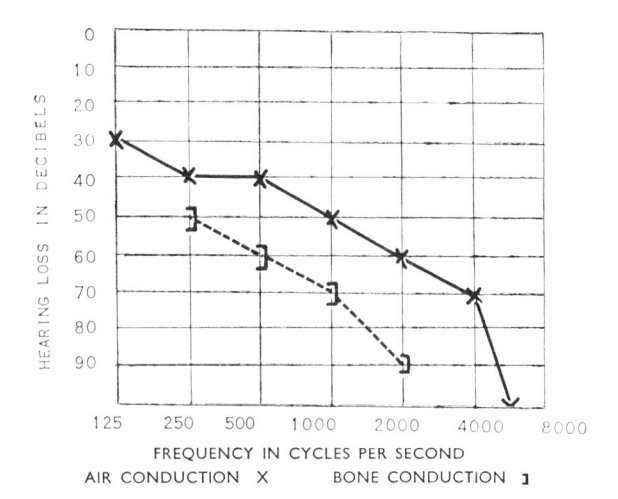

Fig. 20.9. Audiogram showing perceptive deafness.

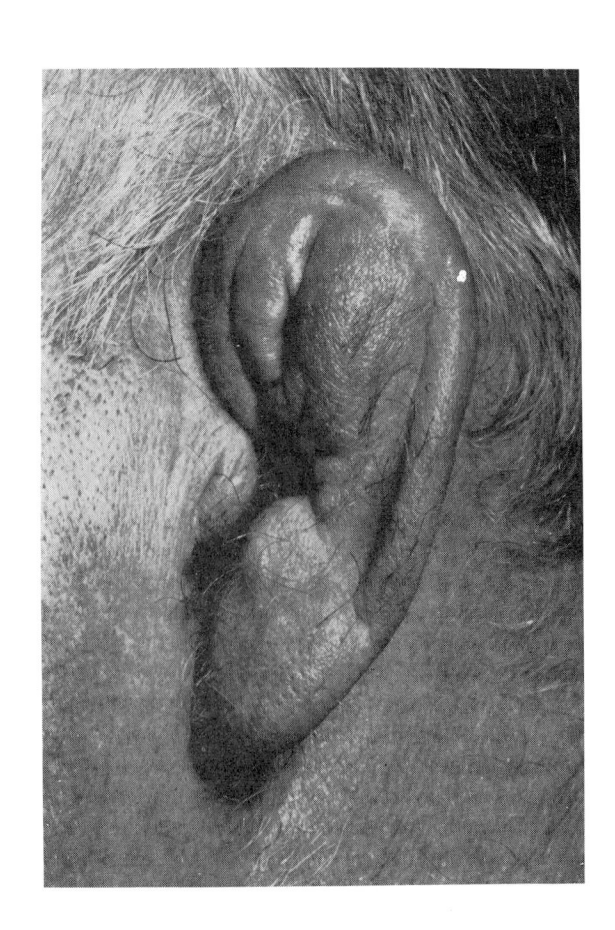

Fig. 20.10. Haematoma auris—needs careful treatment. A cauliflower ear may ensue.

Trauma not uncommonly occurs in football players or boxers and may result in a haematoma of the auricle (Fig. 20.10). Surgical drainage of the blood clot is required and a possible result of the trauma is a small shrivelled 'cauliflower ear'.

Tumours in the form of epithelioma or rodent ulcer occur sometimes on the upper edge of the pinna and are treated by surgical excision.

Conditions of the external auditory meatus

Congenital stenosis of the external auditory meatus is of course a condition calling for surgical relief in early childhood, if it is bilateral, on account of the serious degree of deafness associated with it.

Foreign body in the ear is a not uncommon problem in small children. The chief danger lies in clumsy attempts at removal by unskilled persons, (who may rupture the tympanic membrane), and if the child is in any way uncooperative it will probably be necessary to resort to general anaesthesia.

Ear syringing

Wax or cerumen is the normal secretion of the ceruminous glands situated in the outer part of the external meatus and may be troublesome if it forms a hard impacted mass. Ear-syringing (Fig. 20.11),

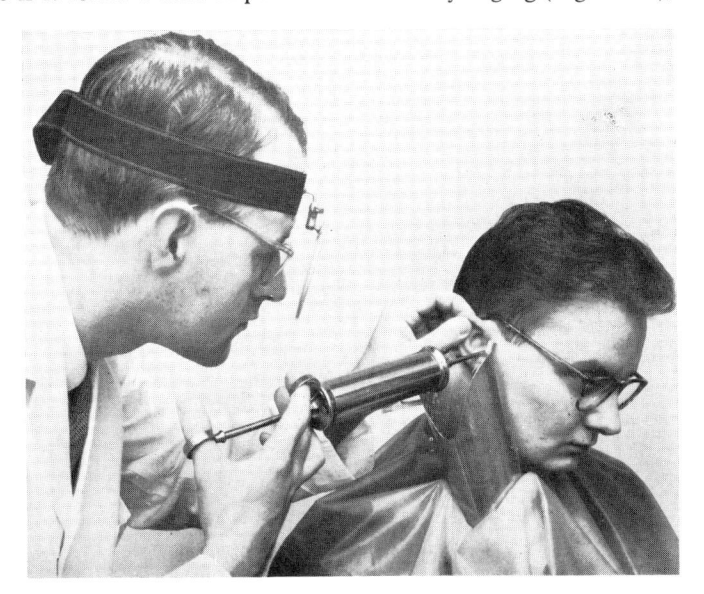

Fig. 20.11. Syringing an ear. Note that the surgeon is using a head-mirror and is drawing the auricle upwards and backwards in order to 'straighten' the external meatus.

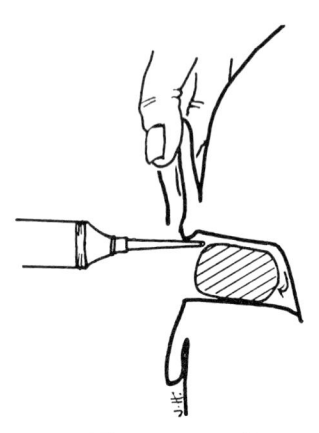

Fig. 20.12. Direct stream of solution along the roof of the external auditory meatus.

Fig. 20.13. Jobson Horne wool carrier. An invaluable instrument.

the usual method of removing wax, is an operation which almost any doctor or nurse is expected to carry out with skill, and attention must be paid to the following points:

1. *History.* Has the patient had a discharging ear? If any possibility of a dry perforation, do not syringe.
2. *Inspection.* If wax seems very hard always soften over a period of one week by using warm olive oil drops nightly.
3. *Towels.* Protect patient well with towels and mackintoshes. He will not be amused by having his shirt soaked.
4. *Lighting.* Use a head-mirror or lamp.
5. *Solution.* Sodium bicarbonate, 4–5 grammes to the pint, or normal saline, are ideal. Tap-water is satisfactory.
6. *Temperature.* This is vital. It should be 38°C (100°F). Any departure of more than a few degrees may precipitate the patient on floor with vertigo.
7. *Syringe.* A metal syringe is considered by some to be the most easily controlled, but others prefer rubber syringes of the Bacon type. In any case make sure that the nozzle is firmly attached to the syringe and is prevented from entering too far into the external meatus. Tympanic membranes have been ruptured by a deeply penetrating nozzle.
8. *Direction.* Direct stream of solution along roof of auditory canal (Fig. 20.12).
9. *Inspection.* After removal of wax, inspect thoroughly to make sure none remains. This advice might seem superfluous, but is frequently ignored.
10. *Drying.* Mop any excess solution from meatal canal. Stagnation predisposes to otitis externa.

Otitis externa is a diffuse inflammation of the skin lining the external auditory meatus and is characterised by irritation, scanty discharge and tendency to relapse. It has a predilection for certain persons, particularly those with a tendency to eczema and is not infrequently seen in Europeans visiting the tropics. There is usually a mixed infection with several types of microorganism, bacteria and fungi, and the bacteriology is investigated by submitting an aural swab for culture.

Aural toilet is carried out meticulously with the aid of the Jobson Horne wool carrier (Fig. 20.13) dressed with fluffed-out cotton wool, and following cleansing a dressing soaked in a solution such as 1.5 per cent hydrocortisone with neomycin is inserted with aural dressing forceps (Fig. 20.14) and left for 24 hours.

Following this initial treatment various medicaments in the form of ear drops may be advised and the patient is instructed to avoid scratching the ears and to prevent water from entering them. Repeated attention may be required.

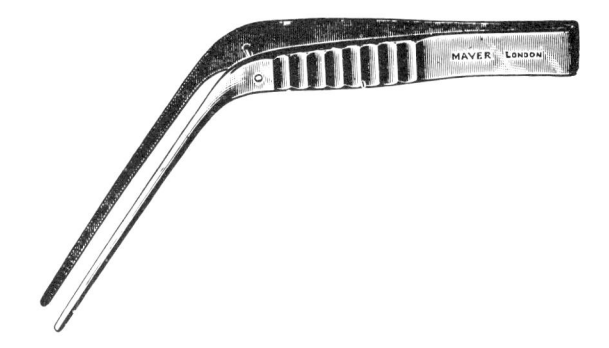

Fig. 20.14. Keen's aural dressing forceps.

Malignant disease of the external auditory meatus may be first manifested by a bloodstained discharge from the ear. Intractable pain may be a feature of this relentless affliction and treatment is by radiotherapy or radical surgery in which an attempt may be made to remove the entire ear and temporal bone.

Conditions of the middle ear

Acute otitis media is a common condition in childhood and is most frequently associated with acute tonsillitis, common cold, influenza, measles (and other infectious diseases of childhood), sinusitis and enlarged and infected adenoids. The infecting organisms are usually streptococci, pneumococci or staphylococci which arrive in the middle ear via the Eustachian tube.

The symptoms are earache and deafness and the temperature may be high. Examination reveals a red or bulging tympanic membrane and if treatment is delayed the membrane may burst with the release of pus (sometimes blood-stained). The ear-discharge (*otorrhoea*) may in fact be so profuse as to drip out of the ear.

Treatment varies according to the severity of the infection. In the mildest cases analgesics such as aspirin may suffice but in most cases antibiotics, such as penicillin, are necessary and occasionally—in the case of a persistently bulging tympanic membrane—myringotomy is required (Figs. 20.15 and 16). In this operation, which is

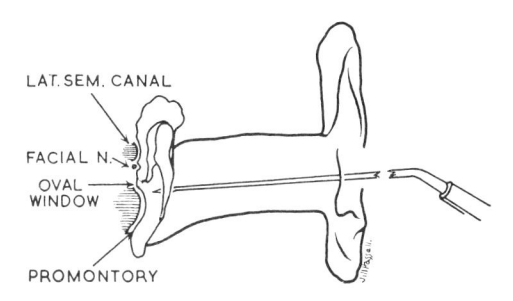

Fig. 20.15. Myringotomy. Coronal section of left ear.

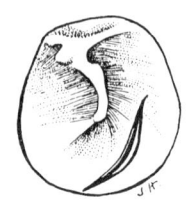

Fig. 20.16. Myringotomy. The extent of the incision.

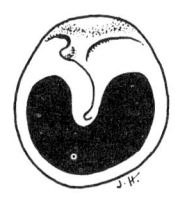

Fig. 20.17. A large central perforation as seen in the mucosal type of C.S.O.M.

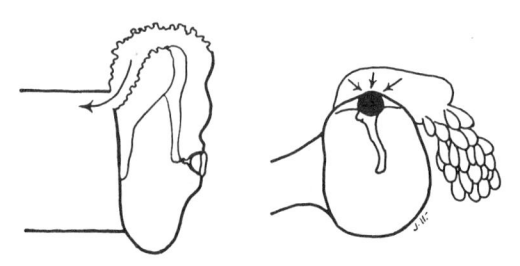

Fig. 20.18. A perforation in Schrapnell's membrane in the 'attic' type of C.S.O.M.

carried out under general anaesthesia, an incision is made in the tympanic membrane with a sharp and delicate knife known as a myringotome.

Chronic otitis media may ensue in some cases of acute otitis media which do not undergo complete resolution. This is particularly liable to occur if nasal or pharyngeal sepsis persists, or if lowered resistance, owing perhaps to malnutrition or anaemia, is present. In the so called *mucosal* type of infection there is mucoid discharge from a central perforation of the tympanic membrane (Fig. 20.17) and in the *bony* type of disease there may be purulent evil-smelling discharge from a marginal perforation (Fig. 20.18). The latter form of *chronic suppurative otitis media* (C.S.O.M.) is sometimes associated with the formation of cholesteatoma—an accumulation of epithelial debris—or with aural granulations. Serious complications of middle-ear infection are more liable to occur in the course of this type of infection than in the mucosal form.

Treatment consists in the first place of local toilet, the eradication of sepsis from the upper respiratory tract and attention to the general state of health. Aural toilet is carried out two or three times daily, ideally by skilled personnel using a Jobson Horne wool carrier. Obviously such attention can only be obtained in clinics but the intelligent patient can often be taught to mop the ear with orange sticks dressed with fluffed-out cotton wool. After the ear has been thoroughly cleaned, various preparations in the form of ear-drops may be instilled.

Operative treatment is indicated when the disease progresses in spite of conservative treatment or when the infection is likely to be associated with dangerous complications.

The most simple form of treatment is known as suction clearance which is carried out under a general anaesthetic and with the aid of the operating-microscope. In other cases various forms of mastoidectomy are employed. In the first place there is the *cortical* operation in which a post-auricular incision is made and the mastoid air-cells opened and drained. The tympanic membrane and ossicles however are left without interference and after recovery there may be little impairment of hearing. In *radical mastoidectomy*, which is employed in cases of more advanced disease, the incision may be post-auricular or endaural and the surgeon exenterates the mastoid cells and clears all diseased tissue from the antrum, aditus, attic and tympanic cavity together with remains of the tympanic membrane and ossicles, with the excepton of the footplate of the stapes.

In some cases the techniques of tympanoplasty are used in attempts to reconstruct the sound conducting mechanisms of the middle-ear by replacing the tympanic membrane with temporal fascia and by utilizing undamaged ossicles.

Complications of middle-ear infection

These are fortunately much less common than before the era of antibiotics but still occur from time to time and comprise the following (Fig. 20.19):

>Acute mastoiditis
>Meningitis
>Extradural abscess
>Petrositis
>Labyrinthitis
>Facial paralysis
>Lateral sinus thrombosis
>Brain abscess
>Subdural abscess

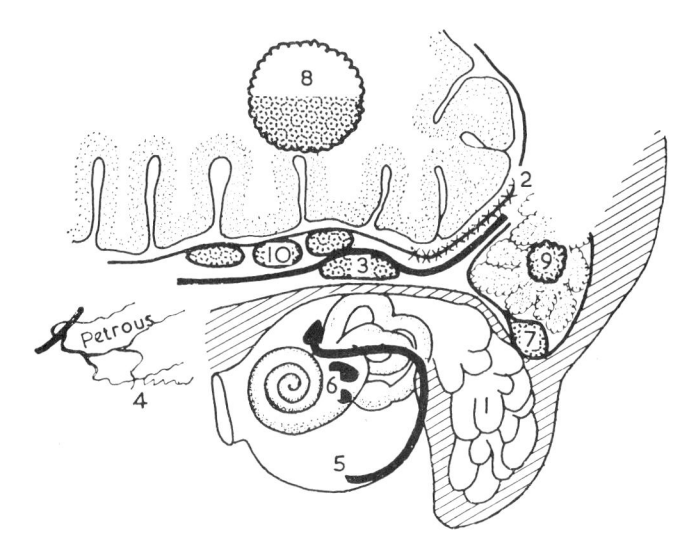

Fig. 20.19. The complications of middle ear infection. (1) Mastoiditis (2) Meningitis (3) Extradural abscess (4) Petrositis (5) Facial nerve paralysis (6) Labyrinthitis (7) Lateral sinus thrombosis (8) Temporal lobe abscess (9) Cerebellar abscess (10) Subdural abscess.

Acute mastoiditis is the result of extension of infection into the mastoid cells associated with bone necrosis and faulty drainage. There is persistent pain, pyrexia and sometimes swelling over the mastoid process. X-rays show loss of cell outline.

Meningitis is manifested by pyrexia, headache and neck rigidity. The C.S.F. shows characteristic changes and unless antibiotic treatment is given early and in adequate dosage other intracranial complications may ensue.

Extradural abscess or pus formation inside the skull but outside the dura mater sometimes occurs by direct extension from the mastoid cells and is characterised by severe pain.

Petrositis and Labyrinthitis are unusual, and as their names imply denote extension of infection from the mastoid to the petrous apex of the temporal bone and the labyrinth respectively. In the latter case there is, as one might expect, violent giddiness.

Facial paralysis may occur at any stage of middle ear or mastoid infection, acute or chronic, and when one considers the lengthy course of the facial nerve in the temporal bone and its close proximity to the middle ear and mastoid cells it is surprising that facial nerve paresis is not more common.

Lateral sinus thrombosis or thrombosis of the huge venous sinus which lies adjacent to the mastoid cells is of interest in that tremendous swings of temperature—often with rigors—are likely to occur.

Brain abscess and multiple subdural abscesses are the most sinister of all intracranial complications of middle ear disease. Nursing and medical personnel must be ever-watchful for such untoward symptoms as headache, apathy, drowsiness, malaise or nausea in patients suffering from any form of otitis media, for such patients may be quietly forming a brain abscess which will perhaps prove fatal unless recognised early.

The treatment of the various intracranial complications consists basically of antibiotics with, in some cases, mastoid surgery. Brain abscess, of course, calls for very special investigation including air-encephalography, angiography, electro-encephalography and radio-isotope studies and often neuro-surgical techniques, e.g. tapping through burr holes, are employed. (See page 137.)

Secretory otitis (glue ear) is frequently seen in young children and is undoubtedly due basically to inadequate Eustachian tube function. The Eustachian tube normally fulfils a most important role in that it enables the air-pressure within the middle-ear to adjust itself on swallowing to the external atmospheric pressure. If this function is interfered with—by, for example, enlarged adenoids, a partial vacuum forms in the middle-ear resulting in an effusion of fluid and resultant deafness.

Treatment is carried out under general anaesthesia. With the aid of the operating microscope a myringotomy is performed and the fluid which may be thin or viscous (glue) is sucked out. A grommet or Teflon tube (Fig. 20.20) is then inserted and the hearing usually returns to normal. The grommet functions as a 'stand-in' for the Eustachian tube by allowing equalization of air pressures on both sides of the tympanic membrane. Grommets often remain in place for several months and whilst in position it is customary for the medical adviser to render himself exceedingly unpopular by advising the grommets' young host not to enter the swimming pool.

Otosclerosis

This is a form of deafness which most commonly affects young females and is caused by fixation of the stapes in the oval window. There is a tendency for the deafness to occur in families and sometimes hearing loss is first noticed during pregnancy. Other symptoms are tinnitus, (ringing in the ears), and paracusis or the ability to

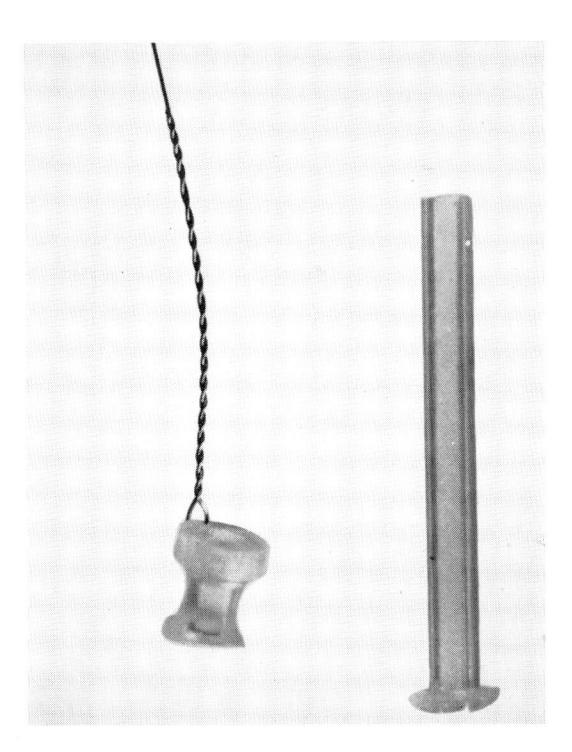

Fig. 20.20. Tubes inserted through the tympanic membrane for the purpose of ventilating the middle ear. A Teflon tube and a grommet with wire attached.

Fig. 20.21. A binocular operating microscope (in this case one of the Zeiss Otoscopes), is now being used for stapedectomy and for many other aural operations.

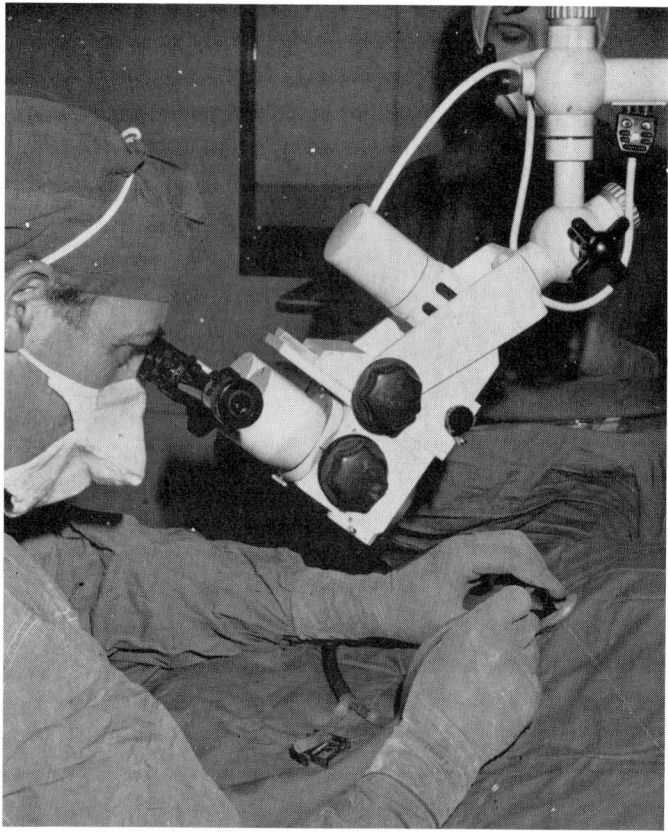

hear the spoken word more clearly in the presence of background noise. The diagnosis is confirmed by tuning-fork tests and audiometry, which show conductive deafness.

Treatment is by the operation of stapedectomy which is carried out with the aid of the operating microscope (20.21). Having reflected the tympanic membrane and opened the middle ear, the surgeon removes all or part of the fixed stapes replacing it with one of the forms of prosthesis shown in Fig. 20.22. One end of the prosthesis is fixed to the incus and the other end is able to move with some degree of freedom in the oval window thus forming the penultimate link in the vibrating chain—tympanic membrane—malleus—incus—prosthesis—organ of hearing (cochlea).

Earache (Otalgia)

Earache is associated with every inflammatory, and many other, conditions of the external ear and middle ear cleft, the most common *aural* causes of severe earache being furunculosis, acute otitis media and mastoiditis. Malignant disease of the external and middle ear may cause intractable pain and the victims of this appalling condition have sometimes been advised to undergo leucotomy in an attempt to control their suffering.

It is often forgotten that there are many causes of *referred otalgia*, i.e. the pain is felt as earache but the cause lies in some structure distant from the ear. These causes are obviously of great importance in diagnosis and are shown pictorially in Fig. 20.23. The conditions which most frequently give rise to referred otalgia are, impacted

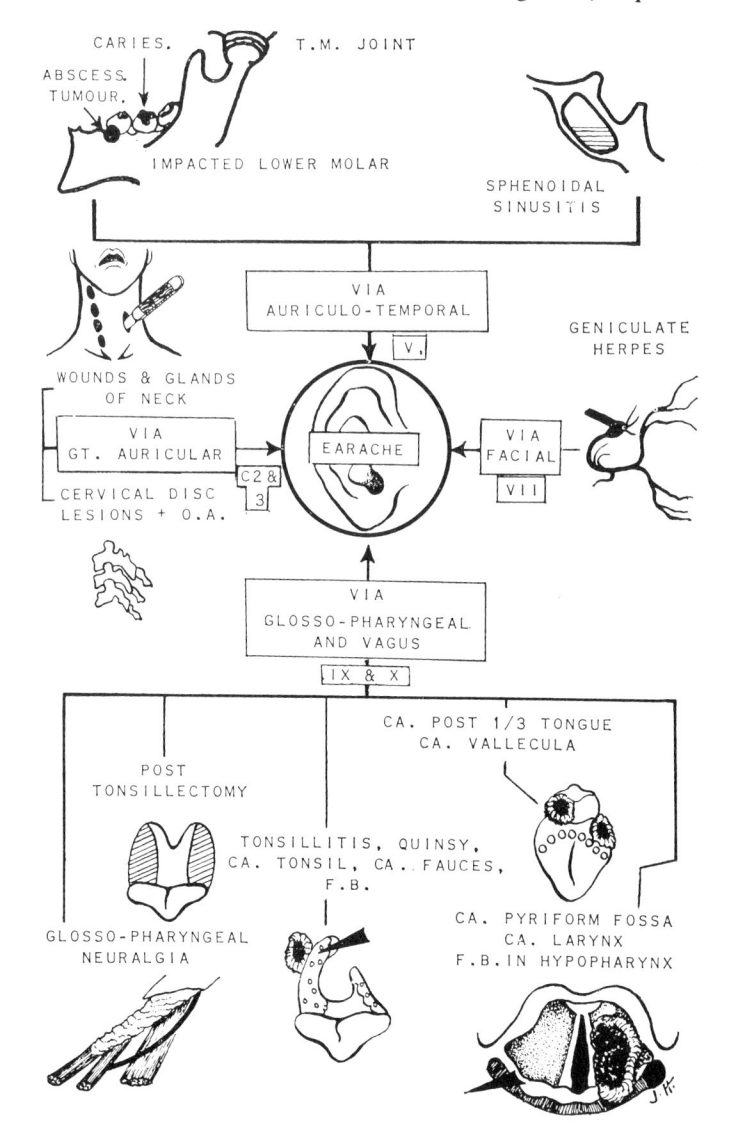

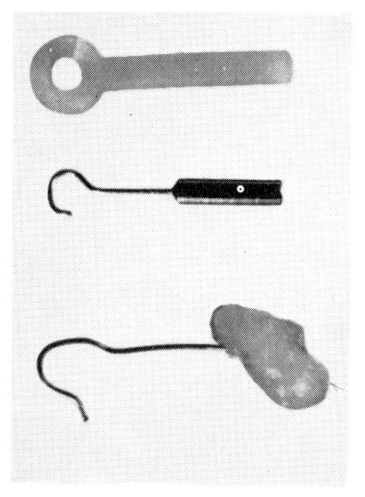

Fig. 20.22. Three forms of stapes prosthesis used in stapedectomy. From above down, Teflon piston, steel piston, fat and wire.

Fig. 20.23. Referred earache.

lower wisdom teeth, tonsillectomy (3rd–4th day post-operatively) temporo-mandibular joint disorders and malignant disease of the posterior third of tongue, vallecula, fauces, tonsil, lateral pharyngeal wall, larynx and hypopharynx.

THE NOSE, PARANASAL SINUSES AND NASOPHARYNX

Foreign body in the nose

Children between the ages of 1–4 years sometimes insert foreign bodies into one or both nostrils and even an intelligent child is unlikely to indicate that a foreign body is present owing to the fear of rebuke.

The rapidity with which symptoms develop depends to some extent on the nature of the foreign body, for example a vegetable object such as a green pea will soon produce a unilateral evil-smelling nasal discharge with excoriation around the nostril. On the other hand a more inanimate object, such as a small stone or glass bead, may remain in residence for weeks without upsetting its little host; eventually, however, a nasal discharge is likely to make its appearance.

Probably the chief danger lies in the attempts made by an unskilled person (e.g. grandma with a knitting-needle) to remove the foreign body, and such attempts, whilst very likely to push the latter yet deeper into the nasal passage, may even be the cause of a serious complication such as meningitis.

Always bear in mind the fact that a young child with a unilateral malodorous nasal discharge is very likely to be harbouring a foreign body, and expert attention is called for. In the case of a cooperative child the medical attendant may be able to extract the foreign body with ease but should the child be in any way refractory full general anaesthesia with an endotracheal tube is likely to be required.

Injuries of the nose

The nose is commonly injured in sport, traffic accidents and personal assault, and such injuries may result in lacerations of the skin, fractures of the nasal bones, deviation of the nasal septum or septal haematoma. *Epistaxis*, (nose-bleeding), may occur as a result of even the most minor nasal injury.

The nasal bones may be splintered into many fragments but provided no undue deformity is present no active steps to reduce the fracture are required. On the other hand a very simple fracture may result in the nose pointing markedly in one direction or the other or being squashed against the face, and if such unsightly deformity occurs, reduction under general anaesthesia must be carried out when local oedema has subsided (3–5 days). The surgeon is likely to employ Walsham's forceps (Fig. 20-24) and provided the operation is not delayed for more than about 10 days no great difficulty in mobilising the fragments should be encountered.

If however the patient seeks attention weeks, months or years after the injury a major surgical procedure, involving re-fracturing of the nasal bones, will be required in an attempt to restore his or her former beauty.

Epistaxis (Nose-bleeding)

The causes of epistaxis are numerous and are usually classified as *local*—'spontaneous', trauma, post-operative etc., and *general*—hypertension, atherosclerosis, abnormal conditions of the blood (e.g. anaemia, leukaemia) etc.

Spontaneous epistaxis is most common in children, adolescents and young adults and usually arises from *Little's area* of the nasal septum (Fig. 20.25). Patients often seek relief on account of the recurrent nature of this disorder which is embarrassing in its tendency to occur at the most unexpected and inopportune moments (e.g. when just about to propose marriage).

The problem is met by cauterising Little's area with some caustic substance such as a bead of fused silver nitrate or with galvano-cautery after the mucous membrane has previously been treated with a topical analgesic solution.

Epistaxis associated with hypertension or atherosclerosis usually arises far back in the nose and may be serious.

The method of arrest of epistaxis depends to some extent on the cause but in the first place *pressure and posture* is usually tried. The patient, in a sitting position with the head flexed slightly forwards, presses with his finger against the bleeding side of the nose for 10 minutes. The mouth is kept open, swallowing is forbidden, and a

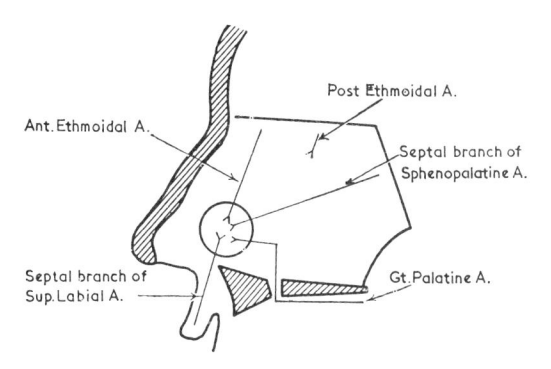

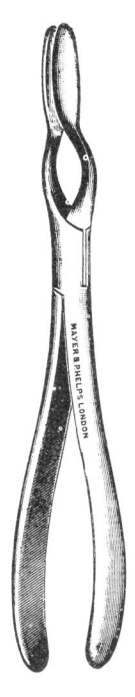

Fig. 20.24. Walsham's forceps.

Fig. 20.25. The blood supply of the nasal septum. Little's area is within the circle.

bowl—to receive dribble—is held under the chin. Epistaxis cannot always be treated with ease and security at home and elderly hypertensive patients should be regarded as candidates for hospital admission.

If pressure and posture fail to control the haemorrhage, resort has to be made to *anterior nasal packing*. The side which is bleeding is sprayed with a cocaine and adrenaline mixture (10 per cent cocaine, 1/1000 adrenaline, equal parts) and the nose is packed with ½-inch ribbon-gauze which may be soaked in a solution according to the surgeon's directions e.g. bismuth, iodoform, paraffin paste.

With Tilley's forceps (Fig. 20.26) the ribbon is first passed along the floor of the nose to the back in a loop, and then built up in successive loops from the floor upwards (Fig. 20.27). The pack may be left for 24 hours, or longer if the patient is under hospital supervision and antibiotic cover. An inflatable bag is sometimes used in lieu of a gauze pack.

When nasal bleeding is arising from far back in the nasal cavities or from the nasopharynx, *post-nasal plugging* may be necessary. The plug consists of a tightly compressed ball of gauze about the size of a small walnut firmly secured by stitches to the centre of a piece of tape about 2 feet in length. It is inserted via the mouth with the aid of a soft rubber catheter which has been previously passed along the floor of the nose and afterwards secured to the 'leading' end of the tape (Fig. 20.28). Once the plug has been inserted the

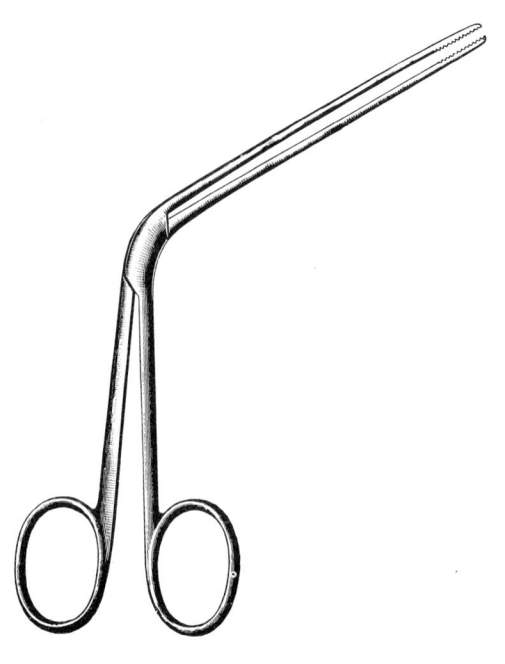

Fig. 20.26. Tilley's nasal dressing forceps.

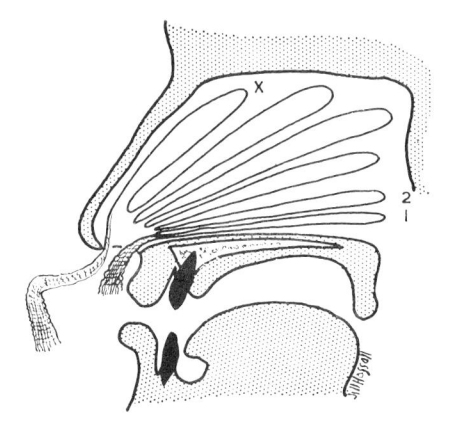

Fig. 20.27. Insertion of anterior nasal pack. 1 is the first loop, 2—the second, and X—the last.

leading end of tape is secured firmly to the side of the face with adhesive tape and the trailing tape emerging from the corner of the mouth is attached without tension.

Surgical methods e.g. ligation of the ethmoidal or maxillary arteries may have to be resorted to in an attempt to arrest epistaxis but such heroics are fortunately seldom necessary. At the same time epistaxis must always be treated with extreme respect as in some cases numerous blood transfusions are required and a fatal outcome has not always been avoided.

Disorders of the nasal septum

Deflected nasal septum, which is usually a result of trauma, is a common cause of nasal obstruction and in most cases may be corrected by surgery, with excellent results. In developmental cases a smooth S-shape deflection may be present but in the more common traumatic case there are sharp angular deviations or spurs.

The treatment is by the operation of *submucous resection* (S.M.R.) which is commonly carried out in adults but seldom in children,

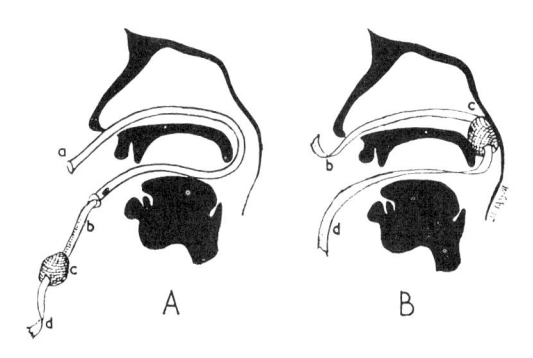

Fig. 20.28. Insertion of a postnasal plug (A) First stage (B) Second stage a. Catheter b. Leading tape c. Plug d. Trailing tape.

and the object of this delicate manoeuvre is to fillet out deflected cartilage and thin bone from between the two layers of muco-perichondrium (Fig. 20.29).

Surgeons vary considerably in regard to their preference of post-operative management and no single method of packing can be said to be 'right' or 'wrong'. One accepted method which has proved valuable over a number of years is to insert a glove-finger pack and a silastic splint in each nasal cavity at the conclusion of the operation. The packs are removed after 24 hours and the splints after 7 days.

Septal perforation is a troublesome complaint which may follow trauma, and very occasionally occurs post-operatively. It is associated with epistaxis and crusting in the nose and on rare occasions causes the patient to whistle softly with the nose on every breath.

Septal haematoma has already been mentioned as a possible result of trauma. Blood accumulates between the two layers of muco-perichondrium covering the septum and very severe nasal obstruction is caused. Surgical drainage may be necessary but in spite of every care a serious deformity of the nose may ensue.

Septal abscess forms, as might be expected, as a result of infection of a

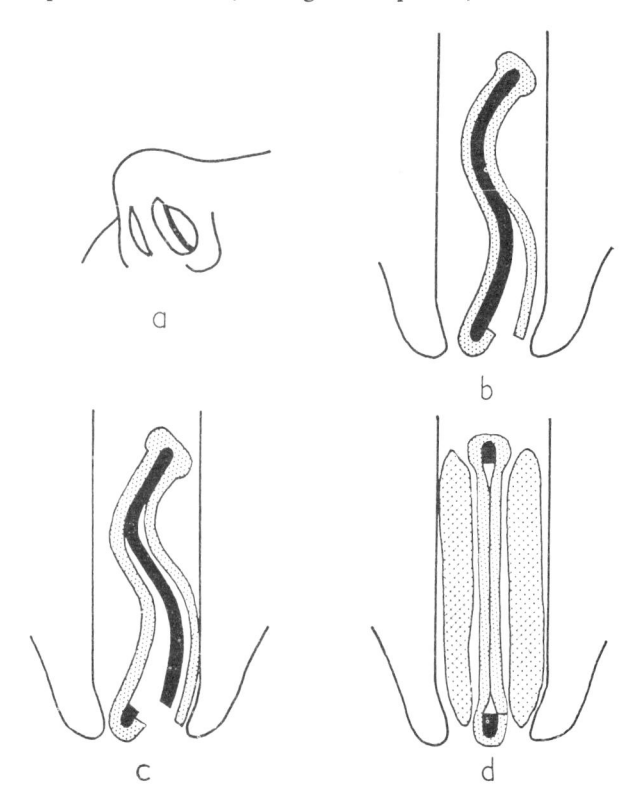

Fig. 20.29. Submucous resection of the septum. a. The incision. b,c,d. Diagrammatic transverse sections showing the separation of muco-perichondrium (stippled) from underlying cartilage and bone (black). In d, the packs (either side) have been inserted.

haematoma. It is likely to settle with adequate drainage and antibiotic therapy but in the pre-antibiotic era it was a sinister condition which might herald fatal cavernous sinus thrombosis.

Infections of the nose and sinuses

The nasal cavities and sinus mucosa are of course infected (usually by a virus) whenever we have a common cold or one of the upper respiratory infections which occurs in association with measles, German measles, etc. We do not, however, use the term 'sinusitis' unless there is in addition some form of obstruction to the sinus drainage, leading to specific symptoms. In the later stages of the common cold there is a secondary infection with bacteria causing a purulent nasal discharge for a varying number of days.

The correct treatment for the common cold is to keep warm, avoid contact with others, avoid antibiotics or local medicaments for the nose and throat, but take simple 'misery-relieving' preparations, such as soluble aspirin, in adequate quantity. Those unfortunate persons who are particularly liable to recurrent attacks of common-cold are often helped by a course of anticatarrhal vaccine administered at the end of the summer.

Acute maxillary sinusitis may arise during the course of a common cold or influenza, or it may occur as a result of diving or dental infection. The maxillary antrum becomes filled with pus, there is pain in the face and sometimes nasal discharge and obstruction. A tilted X-ray film may show a fluid level in the maxillary sinus (antrum) as shown in Fig. 20.30. Transillumination of the sinuses, in which the patient is seated in a blacked-out cubicle and has a bright light shone in the mouth, may demonstrate relative opacity of an infected antrum.

Treatment is by antibiotics such as penicillin, analgesics and the use of nasal decongestants such as 1–2 per cent ephedrine drops and in almost all cases the patient will, after a few days, have a very copious nasal discharge and lose his symptoms.

Chronic maxillary sinusitis used to be seen much more frequently in the pre-antibiotic era. The acute infection does not resolve and the patient continues to have a purulent nasal discharge associated with X-ray changes in the affected antrum. In such cases it is usual to carry out antrum puncture and lavage using a Lichtwitz trocar and cannula (Fig. 20.31). This minor procedure is usually carried out under local analgesia and once the surgeon has punctured the antrum via the inferior meatus of the nose, the sitting patient is instructed to lean forward over a bowl. Specimens for bacteriological investigation may then be aspirated and finally the antrum is

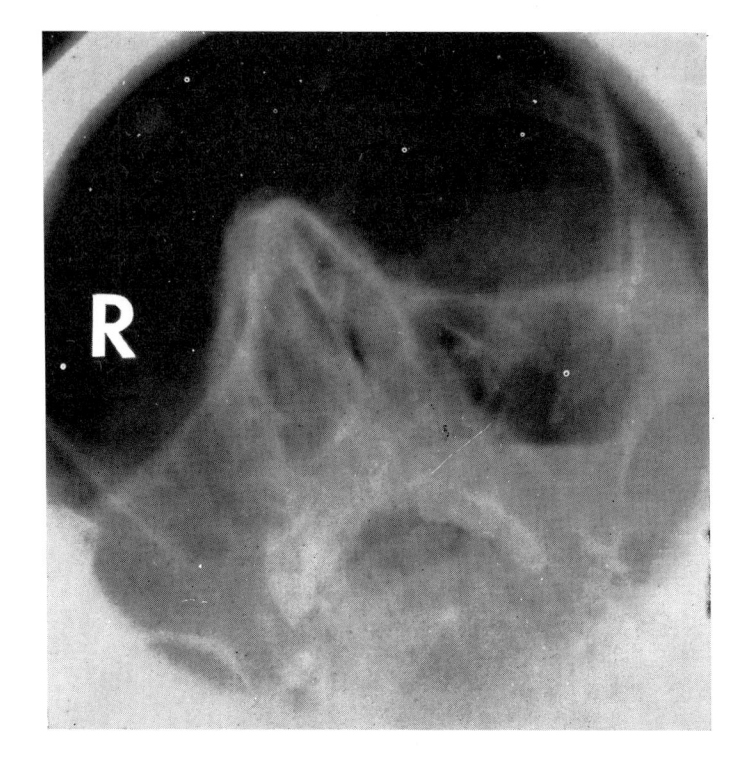

Fig. 20.30. X-ray of maxillary sinuses in tilted position. Note fluid level in left antrum.

irrigated with sterile normal saline by means of a Higginson's syringe.

Most surgeons prefer to carry out this manoeuvre under general anaesthesia if the patient is a child, and should this be necessary Walford's silver cannulae may be inserted and left in the sinuses for several days, during which time they may be irrigated frequently and painlessly (Fig. 20.32).

Sometimes the infection is particularly resistant and persists even after several 'wash-outs', in which case the next step in treating the adult patient may be the operation of *intranasal antrostomy*. In this operation an opening is made in the antro-nasal wall (under the inferior turbinate). In many cases the drainage opening will remain patent and enable the patient to wash out his own antrum with a curved (Rose's) cannula, after he leaves hospital.

There remain cases in which the membrane lining the antrum

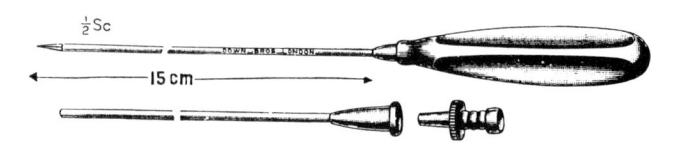

Fig. 20.31. Lichtwitz trocar and cannula.

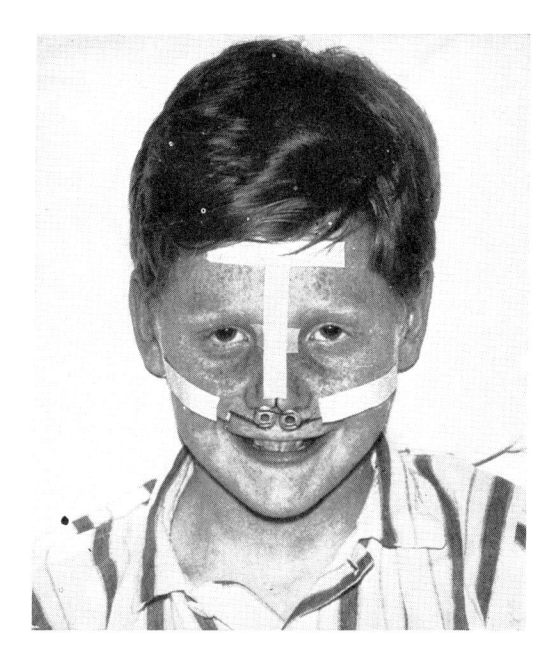

Fig. 20.32. Walford's silver cannulae have been inserted (under a short general anaesthetic) into the antra, which can now be irrigated painlessly several times daily.

is particularly unhealthy or for some reason it is necessary for the surgeon actually to look into the cavity—perhaps for the purpose of taking a biopsy. The operation of choice is the *Caldwell-Luc procedure*, sometimes known as radical antrostomy (Fig. 20.33) and in this case the maxillary sinus is approached via the buccal cavity.

Acute frontal sinusitis is fortunately much less common than maxillary sinusitis, though the predisposing causes (head-cold, influenza, diving, etc.) are similar. The pain is felt mainly over one eye and swelling over the affected area may occur. It is interesting to note that swelling of the face in maxillary sinusitis is hardly ever a feature, swellings of the face usually being of dental origin. X-rays are a valuable aid to diagnosis and resolution usually takes place with adequate antibiotic and decongestant treatment. It must be remembered however that, unlike maxillary sinusitis, frontal sinus infection is a potentially dangerous condition carrying the possibility of fatal complications (Fig. 20.34).

In some cases pain and swelling increase in severity when it may be necessary to drain the frontal sinus under general anaesthesia. An incision is made below the inner third of the eyebrow and the sinus opened with a hammer and gouge. Drainage tubes are inserted.

Recurrent and chronic infections of the frontal sinus may call for relatively minor procedures such as *submucous resection* of the nasal septum or *turbinectomy* in an attempt to improve drainage. On the

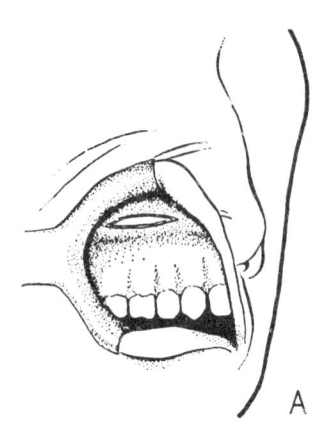

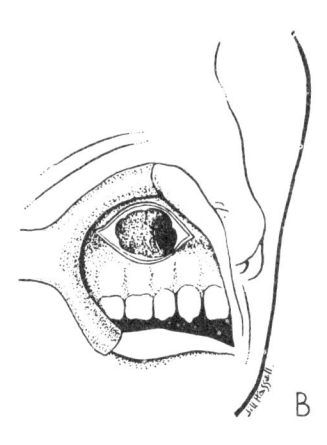

Fig. 20.33. Caldwell-Luc. A. An incision has been made in the mucoperiosteum of the right canine fossa B. A large window has been made in the anterior antral wall. An opening has also been made in the medial wall of the antrum providing free drainage into the nose.

Fig. 20.34. Complications of frontal sinusitis. 1. Osteomyelitis 2. Extradural abscess 3. Subdural abscess 4. Meningitis 5. Frontal lobe abscess. 6. Orbital cellulitis and abscess. 7. Cavernous sinus thrombosis.

other hand radical operations on the frontal sinus are very occasionally called for. These may be of the nature of *radical fronto-ethmoidectomy* in which a curved incision is made below the inner third of the eyebrow and carried down to a point medial to, and below, the inner canthus (Fig. 20.35). Diseased ethmoidal cells are cleared and a wide channel created to form a new fronto-nasal duct. An important practical point regarding the preparation for this operation is that the eyebrow should not be shaved, for if this is done the patient will present a lop-sided appearance for a very long time.

As an alternative to fronto-ethmoidectomy, *obliteration* of the sinus may be advocated. Techniques vary; some are directed to the removal of the anterior wall of the sinus, others to the raising of an osteo-plastic flap followed by the insertion of bone chips.

Tumours of the nose, sinuses and nasopharynx

Carcinoma of the maxillary antrum and ethmoids, which in its early stages gives rise merely to a persistent blood-stained nasal discharge and nasal obstruction, later will produce a grim clinical picture, including swelling of the cheek, epiphora (overflow of tears), proptosis, double vision, erosion into the mouth and severe facial pain (Fig. 20.36).

X-rays and biopsy are needed to confirm the diagnosis and treatment is usually a combination of surgery and radiotherapy. The surgery may be simply a large fenestration of the hard palate after which the patient wears an obturator built on to this upper denture. This enables him to speak and eat normally and also allows the surgeon to inspect the operative cavity afterwards. In some cases more radical surgery, e.g. total maxillectomy, or even exenteration of the orbit, will be necessary.

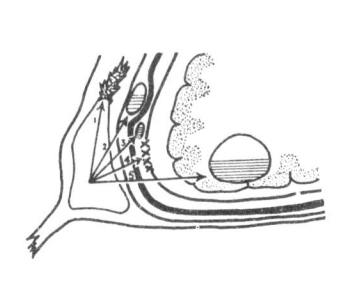

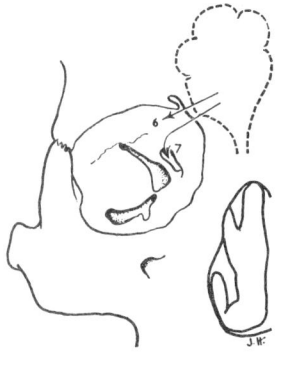

Carcinoma of the nasopharynx, though rare in Europeans, is common in some parts of the world—notably South China. It is responsible for early enlargement of the cervical lymph nodes and by virtue of the proximity of the nasopharynx to the base of the skull there is an amazing tendency to involvement of cranial nerves—the second, third, fourth, fifth, sixth, ninth, tenth, eleventh and twelfth may be affected. Other symptoms include deafness as a result of involvement of the Eustachian tubes.

Treatment is by radiotherapy.

Nasal polypi
Nasal polypi are common and are usually associated with allergy. they arise as a rule from the ethmoid sinuses, but a single 'antrochoanal' polypus has its origin in the lining-membrane of the maxillary sinus and passes back into the narrow aperture between the nasal cavity and the nasopharynx—the choana (Fig. 20.37).

It is customary to remove polypi in the E.N.T. clinic or consulting room using topical analgesia and a nasal snare (Fig. 20.38). On the other hand, if the patient is of a nervous disposition or has other nasal problems which require attention e.g. deviated septum or turbinate hypertrophy, it is far better for him to be admitted, in

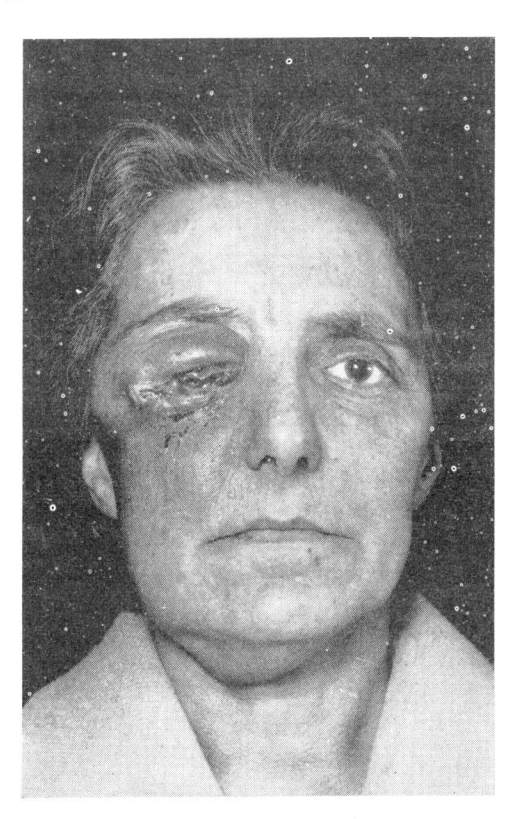

Fig. 20.35. Incision for radical fronto-ethmoidectomy.

Fig. 20.36. Carcinoma of the right maxillary antrum. The **orbit** has been invaded.

Fig. 20.37. Nasal polypi. A. Ethmoidal polypi hanging beneath the middle turbinate and obscuring the inferior turbinate B. A single antro-choanal polypus filling the nasopharynx.

Fig. 20.38. Nasal snare.

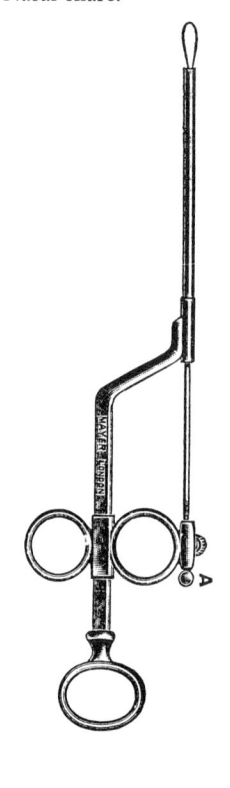

due course, to hospital for the various surgical manoeuvres required to be carried out under general anaesthesia.

Nasal catarrh

'Catarrh' is one of the commonest complaints of the Western World and embraces such symptoms as nasal obstruction, nasal discharge, post-nasal drip—with repeated clearing of the throat, sneezing and vague headaches.

The most common causes of nasal catarrh are vasomotor rhinitis, nasal allergy—with or without polypi, and deviations of the nasal septum. In days gone by a chronic sinus infection was fairly frequently to blame for catarrh but chronic infections of the sinuses are seen less and less, as a result no doubt, of antibiotics and improved living conditions.

Vasomotor rhinitis is not as its name might suggest—an infection, but a disorder affecting the blood vessels and mucus-secreting glands of the nasal mucous membrane. Thus the blood vessels may be dilated, causing congestion of the membrane and hence nasal obstruction, or the glands may secrete too much fluid causing excessive clear nasal discharge or *rhinorrhoea*.

Unhappily this condition is often made worse by the 'treatment' chosen by its victims i.e. the use of vaso-constrictor nasal drops and sprays, which are to be strongly condemned.

Cases of severe nasal obstruction resulting from turbinate hypertrophy are effectively treated by diathermy under general anaesthesia but the 'wet' cases in which rhinorrhoea is the most prominent symptom are more difficult to help. Treatment with drugs, such as piriton and imipramine, is to be preferred and psychotherapy is appropriate in some cases.

Nasal allergy likewise is associated with attacks of excessive watery rhinorrhoea, sneezing and sometimes increased secretion of tears. It may be *seasonal*, in which case it is caused by pollens, or it may be *perennial*, when the possible causes are numerous, the most likely one being the house-dust mite.

Allergic problems must first be carefully investigated by means of skin sensitivity tests and a course of hyposensitising injections is effective in some cases. In others, extensive precautions may have to be taken in order to prevent the patient from coming into contact with the allergen, e.g. the relegation of the unfortunate patient to carpetless, bare rooms in cases of house-dust allergy.

Choanal atresia

Choanal atresia is said to be present when one or both posterior openings of the nasal passages into the nasopharynx are occluded at birth by a bony or membranous stricture. Bilateral atresia is an exceedingly serious congenital deformity calling for prompt action if the newly-born infant's life is to be saved.

The baby will be unable to synchronize respiration and swallowing and may die from asphyxia or inanition unless the nursing or medical attendants recognize the problem and confirm the diagnosis by their inability to pass soft probes or catheters along the floor of the nose and into the nasopharynx and pharynx.

Once the diagnosis has been established no time is lost in removal of the obstructing membrane under general anaesthesia and the insertion of silastic tubes. Occasionally, tracheostomy is required and in any case choanal atresia calls for very expert nursing care.

Adenoids

The adenoids consist of a mass of lymphoid tissue situated on the posterior wall of the nasopharynx. In very young children much of the space may be occupied by adenoids but after the age of 7 or 8 years atrophy commences and by the time adult life is reached little or no adenoid tissue remains.

Some children suffer numerous set-backs as a result of large adenoids as the following list illustrates. Adenoid facies, a narrow nose and a perpetually open mouth; secretory otitis with deafness; recurrent attacks of acute otitis media with the possibility of serious impairment of hearing; chronic sinusitis; snoring, etc.

Treatment is by the operation of *adenoidectomy* and this is of supreme importance in cases where the ears and hearing are affected. In children under the age of 3–4 the operation is often performed on its own but in older children who have a history of recurrent tonsillitis, adenoidectomy and tonsillectomy are often combined. The operation is carried out under general anaesthesia with the patient in the 'tonsil' position (Fig. 20.39) and the adenoid pad or mass is removed with a special curette. After care is of great importance and is similar to that which applies to tonsillectomy.

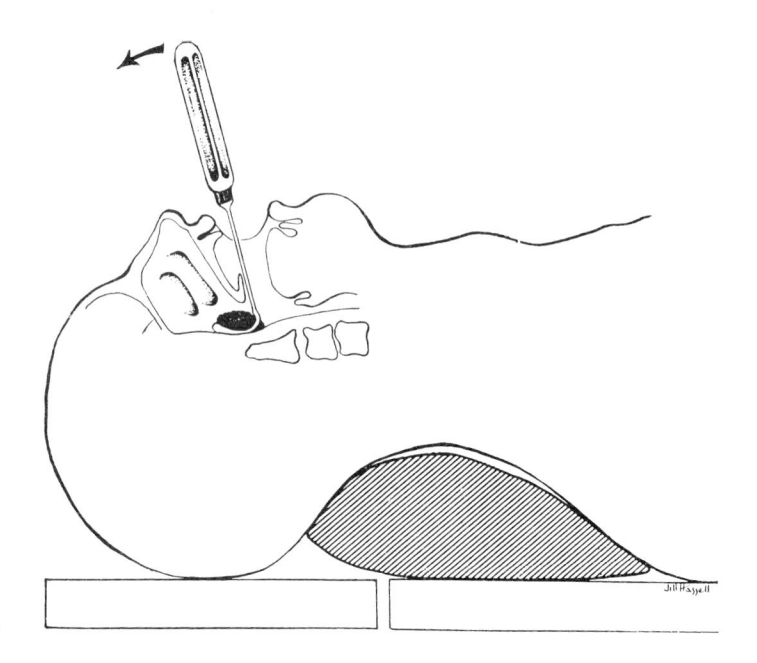

Fig. 20.39. Adenoidectomy. The curette is swept down the posterior wall of the nasopharynx.

THE TONSILS AND PHARYNX

Acute tonsillitis

Acute tonsillitis can occur at any age but is most common in children under 9. The symptoms consist of sore throat and dysphagia but very young children who do not know whereabouts the throat is to be found do not of course complain of sore throat. They just don't swallow anything. There may be earache, high temperature and a heavily furred tongue and often enormously enlarged and tender cervical lymph nodes. The tonsils are enlarged and may be covered with yellowish exudate, and sometimes present a speckled appearance, the so-called 'follicular tonsillitis'.

Swabs taken from the tonsils and cultured may disclose the presence of streptococci and treatment is with antibiotics, such as penicillin or ampicillin, rest, and aspirin mixtures. Disinfectant and antibiotic lozenges are of little value and may predispose to monilial infections.

The complications of tonsillitis include otitis media and quinsy. The former condition has been described.

Quinsy (Peritonsillar abscess) is a collection of pus arising outside the capsule of the tonsil and in close relationship to the soft palate. It is more common in adults than in children. The patient, already suffering from acute tonsillitis, becomes more ill and develops very severe pain and *trismus* (spasm of the muscles of mastication). He is thus unable to open his mouth or swallow and is consequently in a state of utmost misery. The quinsy may resolve with adequate antibiotic treatment or it may burst spontaneously into the mouth with immediate relief. On the other hand the medical attendant may decide to open it by making a small stab incision through the overlying palatal mucous membrane and inserting a pair of sinus forceps.

Pharyngeal ulceration

Ulceration and membrane formation may occur in the pharynx, buccal cavity or on the tonsils, and sometimes poses interesting and difficult problems for the diagnostician. The conditions responsible include such varied pathological processes as infectious mononucleosis (glandular fever), Vincent's angina, agranulocytosis, moniliasis (thrush), leukaemia, malignant disease and syphilis.

Tonsillectomy

Tonsillectomy is frequently indicated in cases of severe recurrent attacks of tonsillitis. One attack of quinsy is also a most important indication but other reasons for tonsillectomy such as focal sepsis are less certain. A commonly held fallacy is that large tonsils are of necessity unhealthy, but this is not so; the appearance of the tonsils is not regarded by specialists as being of particular significance when advising for or against tonsillectomy in any particular case but the frequency and severity of the attacks of acute tonsillitis undergone by the patient are all important in making a decision.

When the patient is admitted to hospital certain very important facts must be established. In the first place an attack of sore throat during the previous few weeks means that the operation may have to be postponed and secondly, if the question of abnormal bleeding or bruising tendency has not been already raised in out-patients, this matter must certainly be enquired about. If there is the slightest suspicion of such abnormality the patient must be fully investigated for haemorrhagic disorders. Simple tests for bleeding and clotting time are not sufficient.

The operation of tonsillectomy is almost always carried out under general anaesthesia. The 'guillotine' technique which calls for very great expertise and teamwork is employed in many centres with excellent results but it is probably true to say that the 'dissection' technique is more widely practiced.

The patient lies supine, the shoulders elevated on a small sandbag. A Boyle-Davis gag (Fig. 20.40) is inserted and the surgeon grasping the tonsil with special tonsil-holding forceps, then dissects it away from its bed using scissors or dissectors, and ulti-

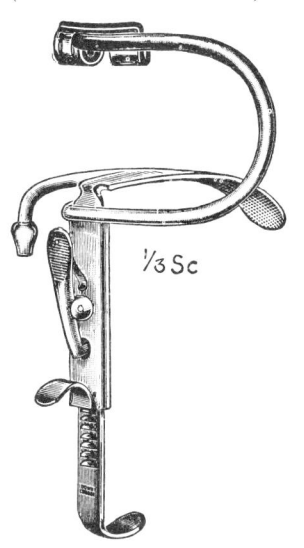

Fig. 20.40. Boyle-Davis gag. (Used in tonsil dissection).

mately a tonsil snare (Fig. 20.41) to sever its last attachments. He then spends some time arresting haemorrhage using, for example, Wilson's forceps (Fig. 20.42) and Waugh's tenaculum forceps (Fig. 20.43).

Post-operative care calls for experience, knowledge and a good deal of common sense, and the responsibility for post-tonsillectomy cases must never be delegated to inexperienced nurses. As soon as surgery is completed the patient is turned over into a semi-prone position, often with a pillow crosswise under the abdomen and lower ribs. This posture is of great importance in preventing the inhalation of blood or secretions and must be maintained until the reflexes return and the patient starts objecting to, and finally spits out, his metal or rubber airway. He now passes into a phase of post-operative sleep and even during this stage should be kept lying on the side and not allowed to roll over on to his back. It is most important during this phase that the patient should be allowed to sleep peacefully and, in the author's experience of over 30 years, visiting in the immediate post-operative period is not only undesirable but hazardous. The safety of the patient must come before emotional considerations.

On waking, his pillows may be restored to him, and bland fluids such as orangeade administered. In adults pain may be severe and pethidine or morphine are justified but one golden rule applies in this connection. *Sedative drugs must not be given unless the patient has fully regained consciousness.*

During the post-operative period the patient is watched with the utmost care and any untoward event, e.g. haemorrhage from the nose or mouth, swallowing movements or rising pulse rate must be reported immediately, so that necessary action may be taken without delay. Needless to say any degree of respiratory obstruction will call for instant restoration of the air-way by the attendant.

Complications include haemorrhage, which may be reactionary or secondary. Reactionary haemorrhage occurs within a few hours of operation and it may be stated with confidence that during this period the patient's life is entirely within the hands of the nursing staff for if haemorrhage is recognised and treated promptly it should not be dangerous, but if there is any tardiness in its recognition, or procrastination and delay in its treatment, it may be fatal.

If, in fact, any of the signs of haemorrhage mentioned above—e.g. bleeding from the nose or mouth, swallowing movements, or rising pulse rate—are present, medical advice is obtained *immediately*, and the exact treatment will depend on the surgeon's assessment. It is likely to consist of the administration of a sedative such as papaveretum, and this may be combined with the removal of blood clot from

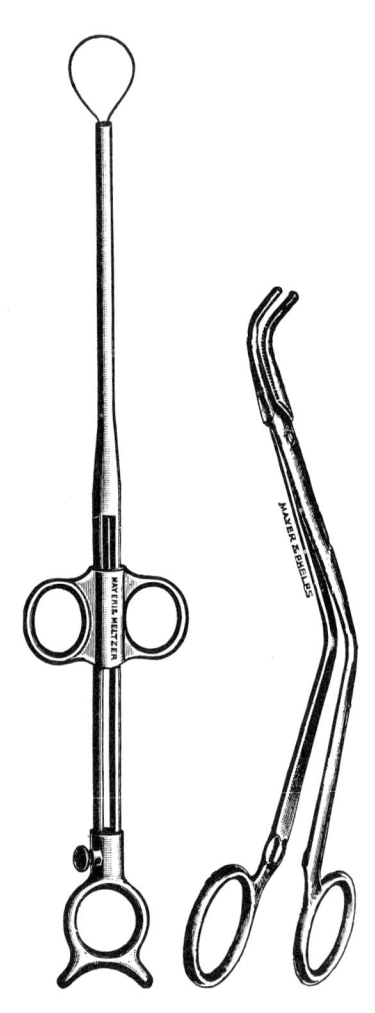

Fig. 20.41. (left) Eve's tonsil snare. (Used in tonsil dissection).

Fig. 20.42. (right) Wilson's tonsil artery forceps (Used in tonsil dissection).

the tonsillar fossa which is bleeding. Sometimes a swab soaked in 1/1000 adrenaline solution is applied to the area for a short time, but if haemorrhage continues the patient will be returned to the operating theatre for ligation of the bleeding point.

Secondary haemorrhage is uncommon but may occur between the fifth and tenth post-operative days. Parents of post-tonsillectomy children should always be warned of the possibility, and are advised to notify the doctor or hospital without delay if there is any bleeding in the mouth or from the nose. As a rule all that is required is re-admission to hospital and careful observation and sedation for a few days.

Otitis media sometimes occurs as a complication of tonsillectomy. Referred pain in the ears is present at some stage after almost every tonsillectomy, a fact which is so well known that the unwary may fall into the trap of disregarding the complaint of 'earache' and omit to report it to the medical attendant. Thus otitis media may be missed.

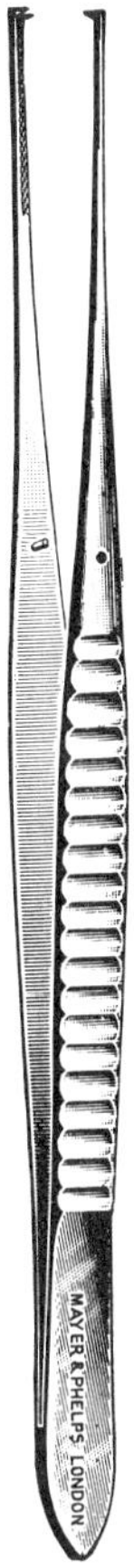

THE LARYNX

The larynx may be regarded as the specially adapted upper extremity of the wind-pipe. Its functions are primarily to protect the lungs and secondarily to produce sound, and speech. It is essential for these requirements—valve and voice-box—that its structure should be rigidly supported and this is achieved by the strong thyroid and cricoid cartilages which surround its lumen and are seen shaded in Fig. 20.44B. The vocal cords, which are not really cords but folds, extend antero-posteriorly and are normally examined with a laryngeal mirror (Fig. 20.44A).

A proportion of patients cannot tolerate the mirror touching the soft palate and it may be necessary for the laryngologist to apply a topical anaesthetic to the patient's palatal and pharyngeal mucosa. In some instances it is necessary to carry out an even more direct examination, with perhaps biopsy, and for this purpose a general anaesthetic is administered and a laryngoscope passed—*direct laryngoscopy*. It is now a routine matter to employ in addition the operating microscope—*microlaryngoscopy*.

Fig. 20.43. Waugh's tenaculum forceps. (Used in tonsil dissection).

Injuries of the larynx

The larynx may be injured by penetrating wounds, blows, hot or poisonous vapours, corrosive poisons or indwelling tubes (left for excessive periods).

Tracheostomy may be required as any injury of the larynx is likely to be accompanied by internal swelling—*glottic oedema*—and the

Fig. 20.44. A. View obtained in mirror at indirect laryngoscopy a. Epiglottis b. Vocal cord c. Vestibular fold (false cord) d. Interarytenoid region e. corniculate cartilage f. Cuneiform cartilage g. Pyriform fossa h. Vallecula.
B. Diagrammatic coronal section of the larynx showing the laryngeal sinuses between the vestibular folds above the vocal cords below.

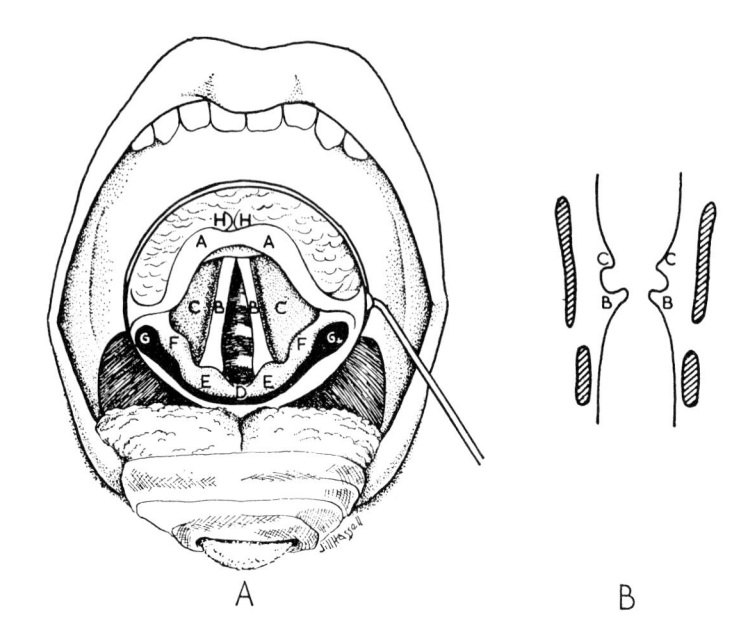

development of this sinister complication may result in asphyxial death unless prompt action is taken.

Infections of the larynx

Acute laryngitis is a not uncommon complication of upper respiratory infection and is predisposed to by shouting or excessive use of the voice, particularly if such an infection is present at the time. The voice becomes hoarse and may disappear completely and the most important part of the treatment is to ban the use of the voice by confining the patient to bed and prohibiting visiting. Bland inhalations of medicated steam such as Vap. Benz. or Pini are comforting, and reassure the patient that he has not been forgotten.

Acute epiglottitis is a localised infection, usually associated with H. influenzae, of the epiglottis, which becomes congested and oedematous. In the child the infection may kill within hours by respiratory obstruction and it is now thought that it may have been the cause of unexplained death in young children in the past.

A young child who develops stridor (noisy breathing) is in the shadow of death. Medical attention and hospital admission is required with urgency. Tracheostomy is likely to be necessary and ampicillin in heavy dosage often combined with steroids is employed in the treatment.

Laryngo-tracheo-bronchitis is also a serious condition of childhood and fraught with danger. Hospital admission with skilled nursing care, antibiotics, humidification oxygen therapy and occasionally tracheostomy will be required.

Laryngeal diphtheria is rarely seen in the British Isles thanks to immunization of the child population, but those of us who have seen it are not likely to forget its horror. The child is ill and presents the clinical picture of faucial diphtheria (membrane on fauces and tonsils). Stridor suggests the spread of membrane to the larynx and trachea and by the time this stage is reached even skilled treatment may not forestall death. Antitoxin and penicillin are administered in appropriate dosage and tracheostomy or intubation may be needed.

Chronic laryngitis is the term applied to those cases in which there is persistent hoarseness of voice perhaps as a result of habitual faulty voice production, over indulgence in alcohol or tobacco, or chronic upper respiratory infection.

Laryngologists never make a diagnosis of chronic laryngitis until all other causes of persistent hoarseness have been carefully excluded and in this connection it may be appropriate to mention that members of the medical and nursing professions should always be aware of the possible significance of hoarseness and advise an expert opinion when this symptom has been present for more than two or three weeks.

The reason for this golden rule is of course that carcinoma of the vocal cord (mentioned later) will perhaps cause no symptom other than hoarseness for many months and this type of malignant disease of the larynx is par excellence a form of cancer which, with early diagnosis and thorough treatment, can be completely cured in a high proportion of cases.

Tumours of the larynx

Benign tumours of the vocal cords occur rarely and cause hoarseness. They are removed at direct microlaryngoscopy and carefully scrutinised by the pathologist.

Carcinoma of the vocal cord, as already mentioned, causes hoarseness, and its presence is confirmed by laryngoscopy and biopsy. Early cases are given a full course of radiotherapy and carefully followed-up afterwards. Sometimes the disease fails to respond to radiotherapy, or, if diagnosis has been delayed, it may have spread within the larynx or trachea. In such cases *total laryngectomy* with or without removal of the cervical lymph nodes may be advised.

Removal of the larynx is a major procedure but owing to improved anaesthetic technique and modern antibiotics it is not associated with a high mortality as it was 30 years ago. Unhappily, like many other medical matters, it is bedevilled with popular fallacy, for example, that the patient will never speak again and become a permanent invalid unfit for any kind of work. In fact, the majority of patients, provided they possess 'guts', and are given good speech therapy and encouragement to use their new 'oesophageal voice' will be able to indulge in *any* occupation other than swimming; the latter being interdicted on account of the permanent tracheal stoma in the neck (Fig. 20.45).

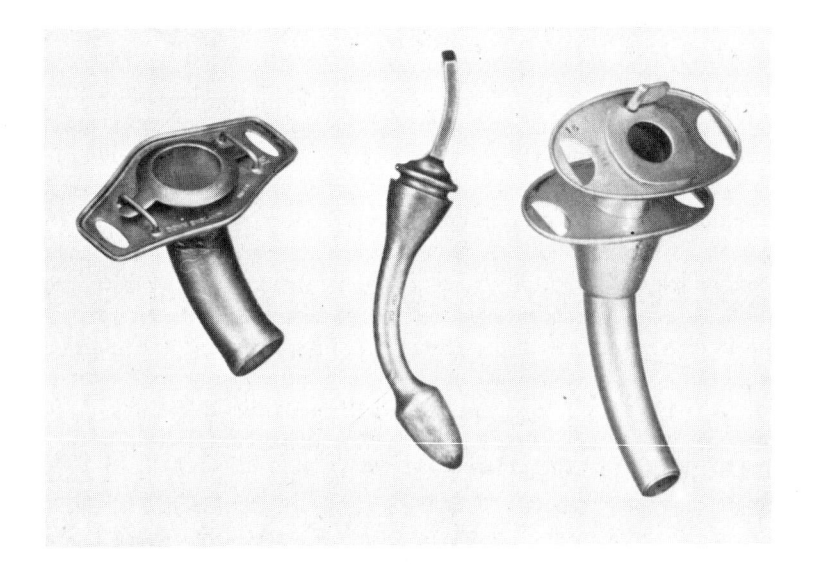

Fig. 20.45. Some patients after laryngectomy need to wear a Colledge tube (left). The central figure is its introducer, and on the right is a Moure-Lombard tube, which is used during the postoperative period when dressings might obstruct the orifice.

Stridor

Stridor or noisy breathing has already been mentioned in connection with acute epiglottitis and laryngeal diphtheria. It may be associated with many conditions including the congenital cysts and webs of the larynx (which if present are apparent in neonatal life) multiple papillomatosis of the larynx of childhood, general weakness of the larynx, foreign body, tumours or vocal cord paralysis. The noise may be maximal on breathing in—*inspiratory stridor* (most common in laryngeal cases); or it may be more apparent when the patient breathes out—*expiratory stridor* (often heard in asthmatic attacks).

In any case stridor is a danger signal and must never be passed over lightly. Some of the conditions which cause it are rapidly fatal unless relieved by skilled and speedy intervention.

Vocal cord paresis

Paresis, (weakness) or paralysis, (complete loss of function) of one or both vocal cords is caused by trauma or disease affecting the nerves which supply the vocal cord muscles, the recurrent laryngeal nerves.

The left recurrent laryngeal nerve is more commonly affected as it has a long course (into the thorax and back again to the larynx) and it may be involved in carcinoma of the bronchus or oesophagus, in enlargement of the mediastinal lymph nodes or following thoracic surgery.

In the neck either left or right recurrent nerve may be affected by surgery or carcinoma of the thyroid gland. If one vocal cord is paralysed the voice may be weak for a number of months though speech therapy can do much to improve matters. But if both cords are paralysed they move in to meet each other, as in phonation and the consequent reduction of the laryngeal airway is a matter of great danger. Tracheostomy may be necessary. The condition is often referred to as 'bilateral abductor paralysis' and some patients will continue to wear a tracheostomy permanently, speaking well with a K.C.H. speaking-valve in the tracheostomy tube. There have been devised several laryngeal operations (the most popular being Woodman's operation), for the purpose of drawing one of the vocal cords away from the mid-line and thus providing an airway and avoiding a permanent tracheostomy.

THE HYPOPHARYNX

The hypopharynx is that part of the pharynx which lies behind the larynx. It is in fact the upper part of the swallowing tube joining the back of the mouth or buccal cavity with the oesophagus, and because it is compressed between the cartilaginous box of the larynx (in front) and the cervical vertebrae (behind) it is slit-like in cross section. As there is more pressure on this flattened tube in its central part, most of our swallowed food and saliva goes down in the outer extremities sometimes known as the 'lateral food channels', but if we swallow a large hard object, for example a lump of undercooked potato, it has to occupy the central part of the food passage on its way down and pushing the larynx forwards causes considerable pain.

Foreign bodies

Fish, poultry and other bones (and sometimes unusual objects see Fig. 20.46) are often inadvertently swallowed, and in most cases scratch or tear the hypopharyngeal mucosa but pass down into the

Fig. 20.46. An object most commonly found on the chest wall, but in this unusual case firmly wedged in the cervical oesophagus. A *very* large oesophagoscope was required.

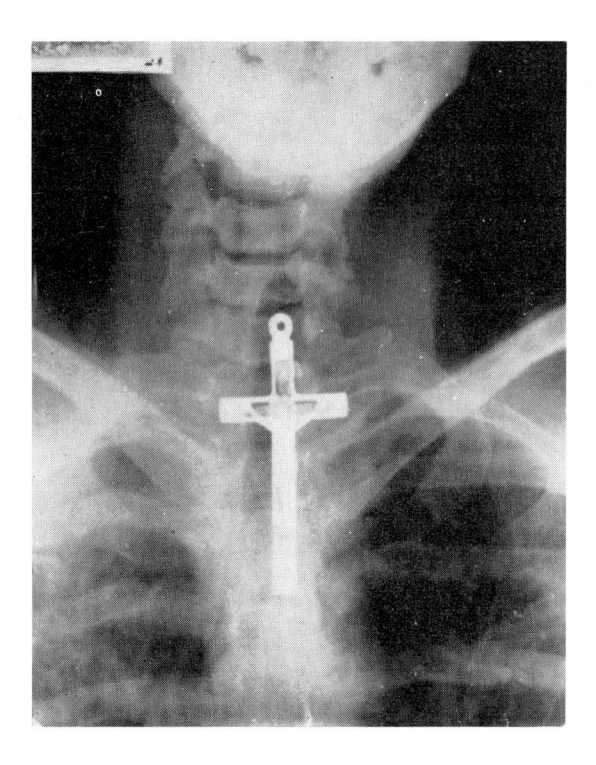

stomach and are eventually voided, occasionally causing consternation when reaching the anal canal. Sometimes, however, they become impacted in the hypopharynx or oesophagus, and unless removed may lead to perforation, parapharyngeal abscess or mediastinitis, and even fatal perforation of the aorta.

Patients who give a history of having swallowed a foreign body are x-rayed and even if no abnormality is disclosed, (many foreign bodies are radio-translucent), the patient is examined under general anaesthetic with an oesophagoscope.

Malignant disease

Malignant disease of the lateral food channel or its upper extremity —the pyriform fossa—occurs predominantly in men, and may reach an advanced stage over a number of months during which the symptoms and signs are seemingly relatively trivial e.g. slight discomfort in the throat and the appearance of a lump in the neck.

In women the disease is more commonly found in the lower and central part of the hypopharynx—the so-called post-cricoid region —and may be associated with a history of the Paterson-Brown Kelly syndrome extending over a period of several years. This syndrome, which was first described by Paterson and Brown Kelly in 1919 and again by Plummer and Vinson in America in 1940, is of interest and great importance as its early recognition and treatment may prevent the development of carcinoma at a later date.

The clinical picture is of dysphagia, soreness of the tongue, cracks at the corners of the lips, spoon-shaped finger nails and an iron deficiency anaemia. Webs and strictures may occur in the mucous membrane of the post-cricoid region and precede carcinoma.

Treatment in the premalignant stage consists of vigorous anti-anaemia measures with iron preparations such as ferrous sulphate or gluconate regularly each day, often combined with ascorbic acid. The patient is kept under surveillance.

The treatment of malignant disease of the hypopharynx may involve very major procedures, combining removal of the larynx, hypopharynx, oesophagus and cervical lymph nodes. How is the patient then able to swallow? The stomach is freed and brought up through the thorax to be anastomosed with the back of the tongue and oropharynx. Needless to say there are some patients whose general condition will not support such radical measures and others in whom the disease is so advanced as to render its recurrence likely, even after heroic surgery.

Hypopharyngeal diverticulum (Pharyngeal pouch)

Hypopharyngeal diverticulum or pouch is an uncommon condition affecting those in middle and later life. The mucous membrane herniates through the muscular wall of the hypopharynx, and over a period of months and years forms a sac, at first behind and later at the side of the oesophagus pressing upon it and causing dysphagia. Other symptoms may occur in addition to difficulty in swallowing—regurgitation of undigested food long after it has been swallowed—and strange gurgling noises in the neck, in fact one patient's wife told the writer that often when her husband swallowed it sounded as though the chain had been pulled.

The condition is investigated by means of barium swallow X-rays (Fig. 20.47) and oesophagoscopy, and treatment consists of regular dilatation of the oesophagus in the case of a small pouch giving rise to minimal symptoms, or excision via the neck in more advanced cases. Sometimes Dohlman's method is employed in very frail subjects. It involves the removal by diathermy of the thin wall between oesophagus and pouch and is carried out endoscopically, thus avoiding an open operation.

Fig. 20.47. Barium swallow demonstrating a pharyngeal pouch. A antero-posterior, B lateral view.

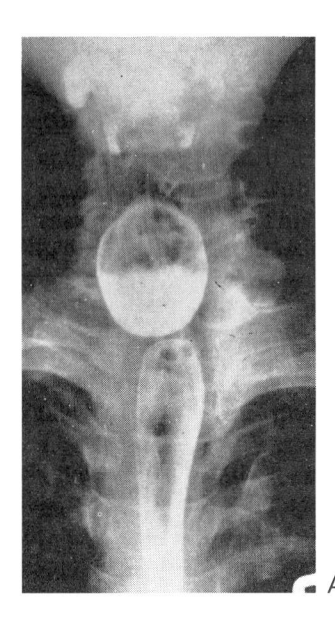

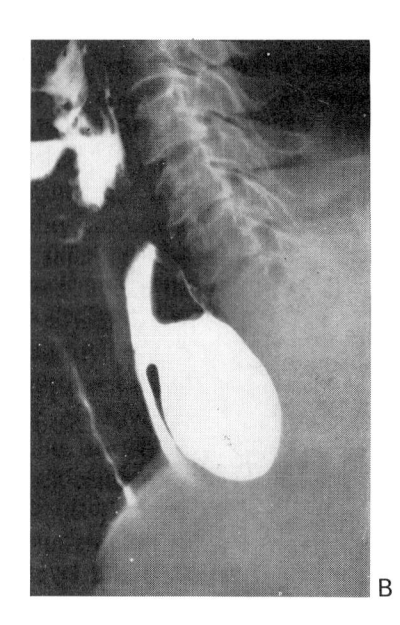

TRACHEOSTOMY

Tracheostomy, or the making of an opening into the trachea is an operation which has many, and very varied, indications. These may be classified as follows: (1) conditions causing upper respiratory obstruction, (2) conditions necessitating protection of the lungs and (3) conditions causing respiratory insufficiency.

Upper respiratory obstruction includes such conditions as congenital stenosis, foreign body and trauma of the larynx, infections such as acute epiglottitis, laryngo-tracheo-bronchitis and diphtheria, malignant disease of the larynx and bilateral recurrent nerve paralysis. All these conditions are fairly obvious causes of severe respiratory obstruction and tracheostomy may be required with varying degree or urgency in an attempt to restore the airway and save life.

Protection of the tracheo-bronchial tree is perhaps a less obvious reason for tracheostomy but it is, in fact, often required in such conditions as coma due to barbiturate poisoning, head injuries, cerebral vascular catastrophes, neurological and traumatic conditions, and in other circumstances where inhalation of secretions may constitute a risk of drowning.

Respiratory insufficiency may occur in pulmonary disease, severe chest injury and of course in many of the conditions mentioned above such as coma, when tracheostomy is not only necessary to prevent inhalation of secretion but to provide a means of carrying out intermittent positive pressure respiration (I.P.P.R.) using a respirator.

Technique of tracheostomy

In past years tracheostomy was almost always performed under local analgesia but today it is more often carried out under a general anaesthetic after preliminary intubation.

The patient lies supine with the head hyperextended over a small sandbag placed under the neck. The surgeon may infiltrate the incisional area with 0.5 per cent Lignocaine and he may choose to make either a transverse collar, or a vertical incision over the trachea. He then dissects down between the small strap muscles and, clearing several layers of fascia, divides the isthmus of the thyroid gland and makes a window in the tracheal wall through which he inserts a tracheostomy tube (Fig. 20.48).

Tracheostomy tubes

The standard form of tracheostomy tube is of silver and there are several excellent patterns, e.g. the K.C.H. tube (Fig. 20.49) and the

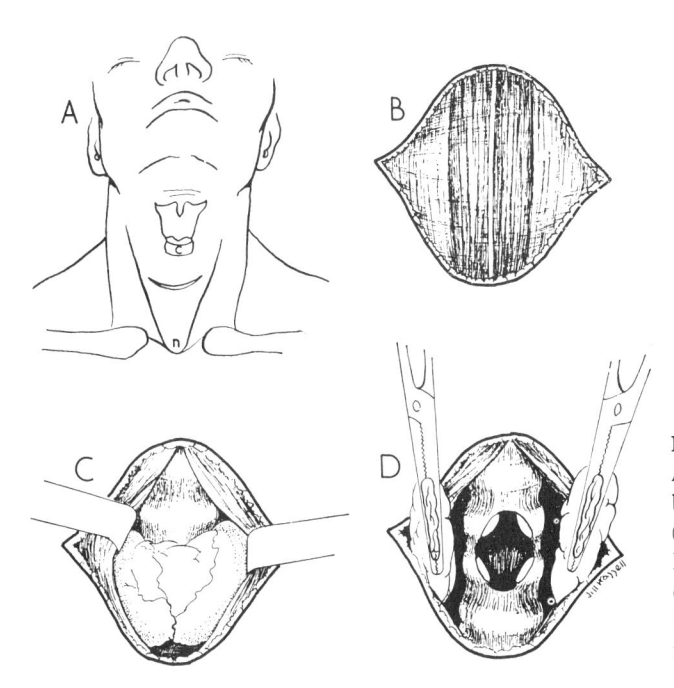

Fig. 20.48. Tracheostomy. A. The incision is midway between the cricoid cartilage (c) and suprasternal notch (n) B. The investing layer of fascia covering the pretracheal muscles C. The thyroid isthmus D. The tracheal window.

Fig. 20.49. The K.C.H. or Negus tracheostomy tube. From left to right: introducer, outer tube, inner tube with 'speaking valve' and open inner tube.

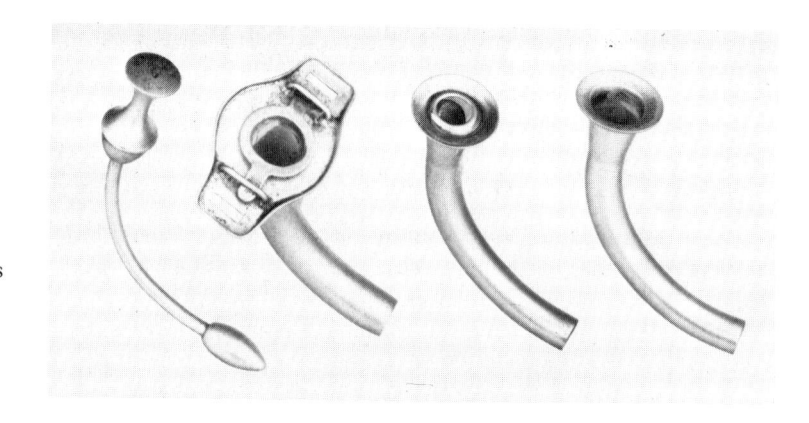

Durham or lobster-tail tube (Fig. 20.50). When intermittent positive pressure respiration is necessary, or when the lungs are at risk from inhaled secretions some form of cuffed tube is essential (Fig. 20.51). In infants a most suitable tube is the 'Great Ormond Street' pattern (Fig. 20.52).

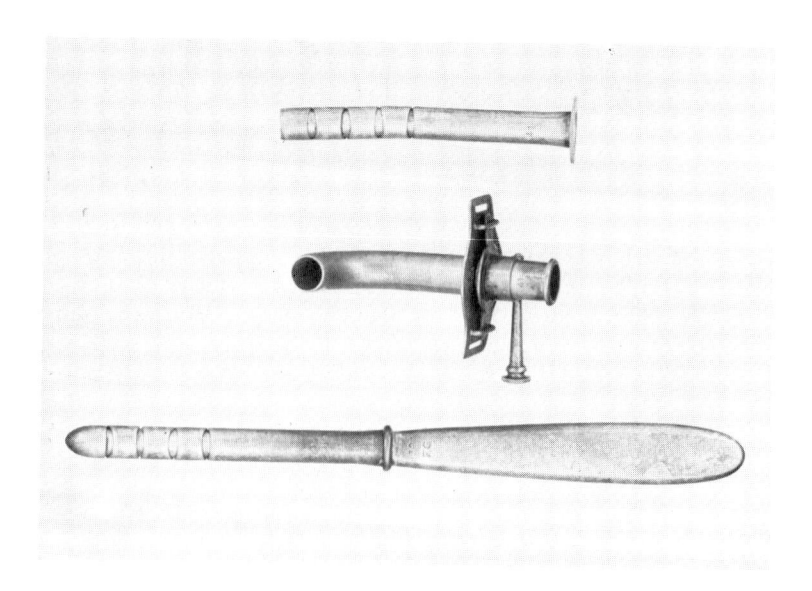

Fig. 20.50. The Durham tracheostomy tube (centre). Above is the 'lobster-tailed' inner tube and below—the introducer.

After care in tracheostomy cases

Tracheostomy cases demand the most dedicated and skilled nursing care, and any lapse of attention or thoughtless action on the part of the attendant nurse may have a catastrophic result.

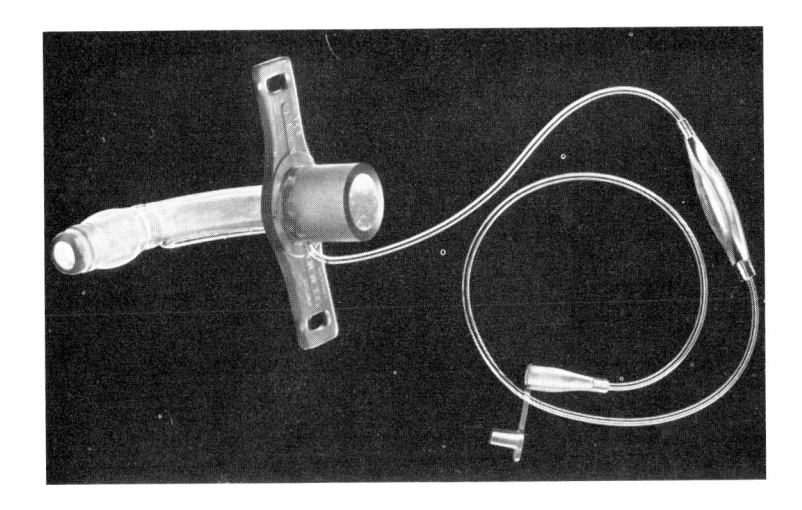

Fig. 20.51. A cuffed Portex tracheostomy tube.

Fixation of the tracheostomy tube is a matter of basic importance. The tapes securing the tube must not be too loose or too tight.

Aspiration must be performed regularly, using a sterile catheter attached to the sucker. Disposable gloves are employed and up to 1 ml of 5 per cent sodium bicarbonate solution may be run into the trachea if the secretions have become very tenacious.

Humidification of the inhaled air is essential for some days or even weeks after the establishment of a tracheostomy. The main function of the nose is to moisten and warm inhaled air and condition it so that it does not cause too traumatic an impact on the delicate mucosa of the pulmonary alveoli. The tracheostomised patient's nose has been bypassed, so humidification is necessary and constitutes a large subject in itself. There are several elaborate humidifiers available and these have largely replaced the steam-kettle of former days.

Tube-changing constitutes no problem when a silver tube with inner fitting is being employed. It may be necessary at first to remove the inner tube once or twice every hour for cleaning and sterilizing but at a later stage this manoeuvre may be carried out less frequently.

In the case of plastic tubes which have no separate inner lining, the whole tube may have to be removed if it becomes occluded with tenaceous secretions. This is a matter for experienced medical staff. In their absence complete blockage of the tube will require immediate action. Courage and resolution are necessary—the tube is removed and the track leading down to the opening in the trachea held open with a tracheal dilator until assistance arrives.

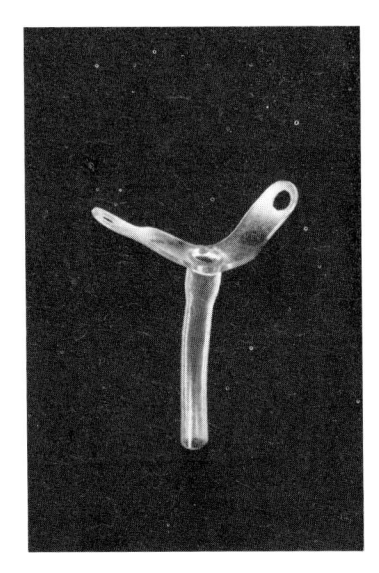

Fig. 20.52. Great Ormond Street pattern tracheostomy tube.

Chapter 21. Fractures

Trauma is the modern epidemic and a large percentage of the injuries seen in the Accident and Emergency departments of our hospitals are due to road accidents. Many details of the injured patient have been described in the previous chapters (skull fractures, Chapter 10; abdominal trauma, Chapter 14) and the systemic changes seen in the patients with multiple injuries and shock have been discussed in Chapter 3.

CARE OF THE INJURED PATIENT IN THE ACCIDENT DEPARTMENT

When a person injured in a road traffic accident is brought into the Accident Unit it is important to examine the patient's body as a whole. The Ambulance Staff always indicate the main injuries, but frequently fractures or soft tissue injuries are not immediately apparent. It is always useful to obtain information as to the cause of the accident to help both the nursing and the medical staff to assess the damage. Whilst the nurse on duty is summoning the Casualty medical staff to the injured person's assistance, she should make sure that (1) there is an adequate airway, (2) the position of the unconscious patient is correct. Ideally, he should be positioned on his side (Fig. 10.13), especially if he is vomiting, to prevent aspiration and further respiratory obstruction. (3) the shocked patient should be put into a head-down tilt position to maintain the blood pressure and stimulate blood circulation to the vital centres, and to assist venous return from the lower limbs. (4) excessive bleeding must be stopped by local pressure on the wound or by elevation of the limb. (5) the nurse should make her own assessment of the skeletal injuries

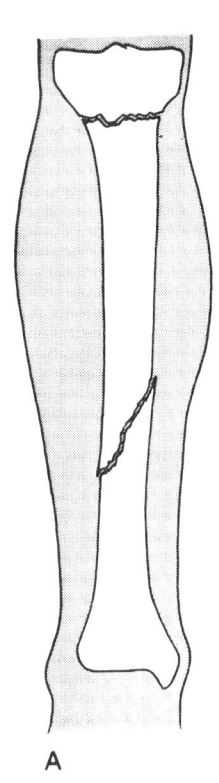

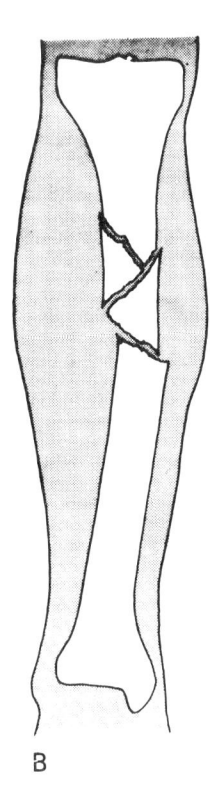

Fig. 21.1. Simple fractures of different types. A Undisplaced transverse and oblique fractures; B Comminuted displaced fracture with many fragments.

Fig. 21.2. A compound fracture. The overlying skin is broken.

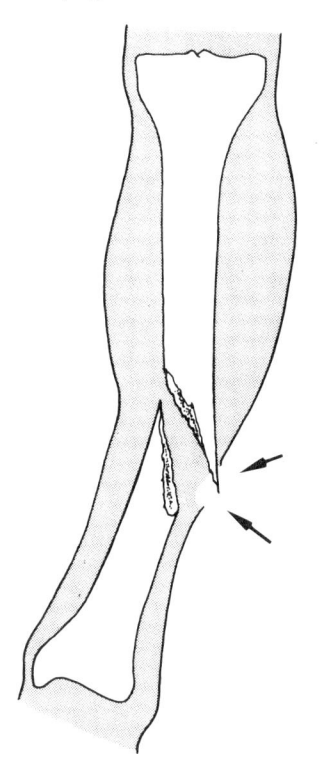

in order to prevent further damage and to plan appropriate splints and plasters. When these essential procedures are completed the patient's fracture treatment may be planned.

FRACTURES

A *fracture* is a break in the continuity of a bone. There are many types of fracture (Fig. 21.1) but from the practical and treatment point of view they should divided into:
1. *Simple or closed fracture* where the bone is broken but the overlying skin remains intact.
2. *Compound fracture* where there is a wound in communication with the break contaminating the bone and producing the possibility of infection (Fig. 21.2).

Greenstick fracture (Fig. 21.3)

In the immature skeleton of a child the bone frequently bends, fracturing one cortex of the bone, but leaving the other intact. A green twig of a tree breaks in a similar fashion, hence its name.

Pathological fracture (Fig. 21.4)

The skeleton may be infiltrated with secondary deposits from various carcinomas arising especially from the breast and lung. The bone is weakened at these sites and pathological fractures may result (see Fig. 15.23). Similar fractures may occur through benign tumours, the weak bone of osteoporosis and osteomalacia, and the bone disease of Paget.

Joint dislocation is the total separation of the two bones which articulate together (Fig. 21.5). The retaining ligaments are completely ruptured.

Joint subluxation is the partial and incomplete separation of these two bones with only partial rupture of the ligaments and the joint capsule (Fig. 21.6).

The dislocation or subluxation may become recurrent and a fracture may complicate this injury.

Fracture Healing

Fracture healing depends upon a good blood supply and an adequate diet providing vitamins, protein and calcium salts. The process which heals bones is slow and the re-modelling which follows takes many months. (Figs. 21.7, A & B). The blood present around the fracture site at the time of injury soon clots and then organises, with infiltration of granulation tissue. Calcium salts are laid down

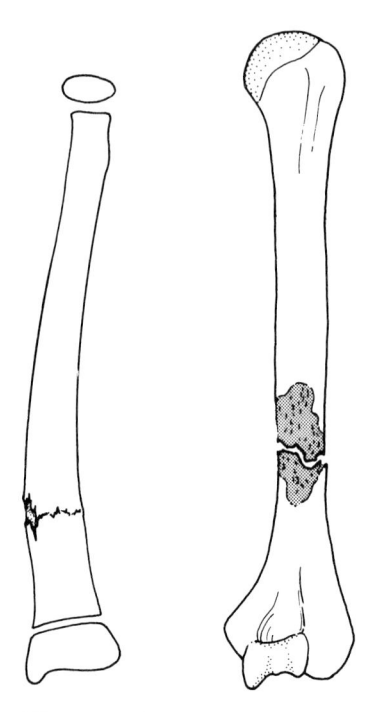

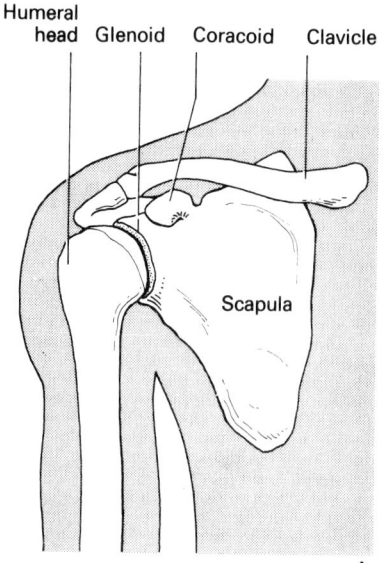

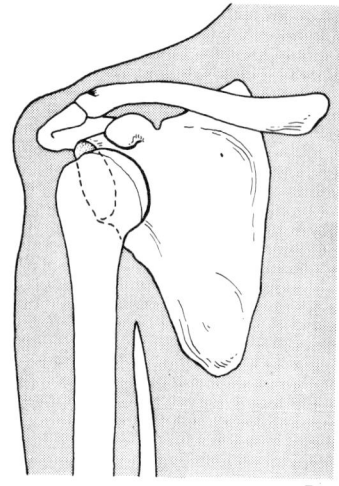

Fig. 21.3. A greenstick fracture of a child's radius.

Fig. 21.4. A pathological fracture through a tumour deposit.

Fig. 21.5. A The normal shoulder. B Anterior dislocation with the humeral head out of socket.

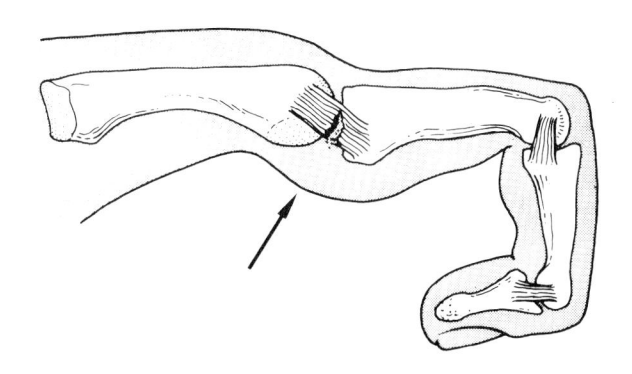

Fig. 21.6. Subluxation of a finger joint.

and at this stage a fluffy shadow around the fracture site will be seen on X-ray; this is called *callus*. Bone forming cells called osteoblasts then move in to the granulation and fibrous area and true bone is laid down between the bone ends and beneath the periosteum. Eventually subperiosteal new bone completely bridges the gap between the bone ends and re-modelling continues to strengthen the repair over the next few months.

Complications of fractures

These may be divided into early, intermediate and late.

Early
1. *Haemorrhage.* Excessive bleeding may shock the patient and in multiple fractures blood transfusion is essential to restore blood volume.
   The blood loss in major fractures is greater than one would expect and average quantities are:
   a. Femoral shaft fracture, 1.0–1.5 litre (i.e. equivalent to 2 to 3 units of transfusion blood).
   b. Tibial shaft fracture, 0.5–1.0 l.
   c. Major pelvic fractures 1.0–2.0 l.

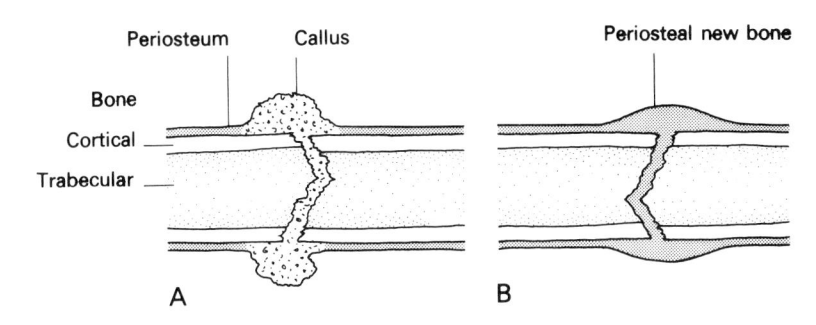

Fig. 21.7. Fracture healing and remodelling.

2. *Damage to large vessels.* In the supracondylar fracture of the child's humerus the sharp spike of bone may pierce the brachial artery (Fig. 21.8).

3. *Nerve Damage.* The radial nerve winds around the back of the humeral shaft and may be damaged by fractures at this site. The result is a wrist drop with the extensor muscles of the forearm losing their innervation.

4. *Damage to viscera.* The lung may be penetrated by a rib fracture and the bladder and urethra pierced by fractures of the pelvis.

Intermediate

Fat embolism. In every fracture of a long bone the fat laden marrow cavity is disturbed and fat globules escape into the circulation. In a very small number of injured patients with multiple fractures the fat globules produce widespread areas of ischaemic damage. The brain is affected, with the patient becoming confused and later unconscious. The lung becomes consolidated and fine petechial haemorrhages are seen in the skin and the conjunctiva. The severe fat embolism syndrome is frequently fatal but vigorous treatment designed to avoid hypoxia and lung hypoventilation together with the addition of anticoagulants is frequently successful.

Pulmonary embolism. See Chapter 2.

Metabolic changes. In the injured patient salt and water is retained in the body for the first 48 hours. After this period excessive potassium

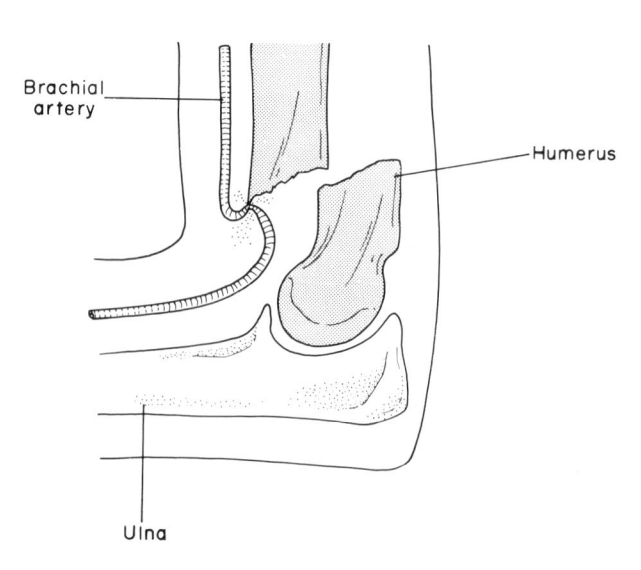

Fig. 21.8. Supracondylar fracture above the elbow with arterial damage.

excretion becomes a problem resulting in electrolyte and fluid inbalance. The management of fluid and electrolyte change is outlined in Chapter 2.

Late

Delayed union. In the lower limb 12 weeks is the average time required for the union of fractures strong enough to allow weight bearing. In the upper limb weight bearing is not a problem and the fractures are usually united satisfactorily to allow full function after 6 weeks. If union is seen to be progressing but is delayed beyond these times then it should be considered a 'delayed union'.

Non-union. The fracture remains unhealed and is painful and mobile. The limb functions poorly and eventually a false joint may develop at this non-union site.

Fracture healing may be disturbed by many processes. Essentially these fall into three groups:
1. Inadequacy of the blood supply. The lower shaft of the tibia is particularly vulnerable, and this is a site commonly affected by non-union.
2. Lack of immobilisation. The limb long bones unite faster if they are immobilised by either external plaster or internal fixation devices. Constant movement of the long bone results in a non-union state.
3. Interposition of soft tissues. In femoral shaft fractures muscle may be interposed between the bone ends and this usually results in non-union.

Mal-union. A very displaced fracture may well unite but it will produce deformity or angulation which if severe will interfere with function. Fractures cannot always be reduced anatomically but it is important to correct the alignment. The displaced but well aligned fracture will always remodel satisfactorily but the malaligned bone shown in Fig. 21.2 always produces deformity however well the remodelling process continues.

PRINCIPLES OF FRACTURE TREATMENT

1. Reduction

A fracture is frequently displaced and needs to be repositioned in good alignment with adequate bone contact. The bone ends may be manipulated to achieve this result, usually under a general anaesthetic. Traction on the peripheral part of the limb is necessary to disimpact the bone ends from one another before manipulation is successful. The reduction of most fractures is possible by closed methods of manipulation through the skin, but difficult fractures may require open operation to restore satisfactory position.

2. Fixation

The fracture is held in this reduced position by an external plaster of Paris cast or by internal metal fixation devices. Plaster casts must be carefully applied with soft padding protecting the skin. The plaster is manufactured in rolls which are soaked in tepid water and applied as bandages. The cast must be firm, but not tight, and should be moulded around the fracture site. If the cast immobilises the joint above and below the bone which is fractured then adequate control of the break is possible (Fig. 21.9.)

Dangers of plaster casts

If a tight plaster is applied to an injured limb, continued swelling of the tissues against the rigid cast may occlude the peripheral blood supply. The first signs of this compression are pain and swelling of the periphery with cold and pale skin. The fingers or toes then become numb and anaesthetic, and peripheral gangrene due to tissue death may occur. Any patient who has a plaster applied must be given instructions to ensure that he returns to the hospital or to his doctor if any of these worrying symptoms or signs develop. The orthopaedic surgeon ensures against this catastrophe by applying only a plaster backslab if considerable swelling is expected, or by splitting the plaster to allow expansion. A plaster must be padded adequately by application of thin rolls of cotton wool. This protection will usually prevent pressure sores where the plaster is liable to rub over bony prominences.

Sustained traction

Fractures of the shaft of the femur are surrounded by large muscle masses and it is initially difficult to reduce the fracture by simple manipulation. They are almost impossible to control by external plaster fixation. Strong traction, however, will align and reduce the fracture adequately and if the pull is maintained on the peripheral part of the leg the immobility will be adequate to allow the bones to unite. Skin traction, (Fig. 21.10) will satisfactorily hold a limb in the correct position, but as 10 lbs. is the maximum which can be applied continuously, it is not enough to reduce the femoral

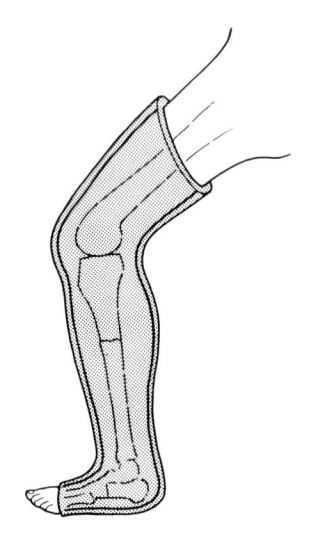

Fig. 21.9. A tibial fracture is immobilised by a plaster cast from foot to mid thigh.

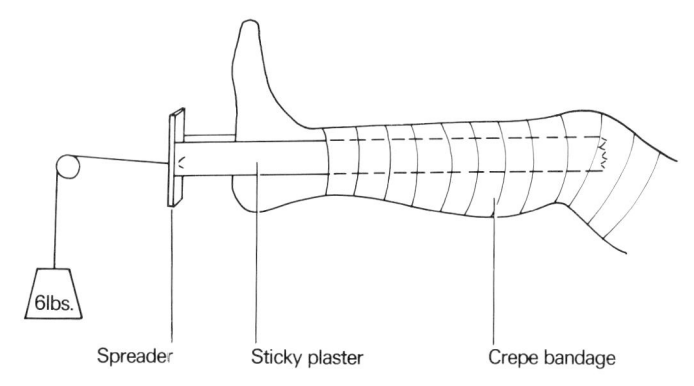

Fig. 21.10. Skin traction.

fracture. Skeletal traction is necessary with a metal Steinmann's pin drilled through the bone of the upper tibia (Fig. 21.11). Twenty pounds can be comfortably applied to this pin and this weight is usually more than enough to maintain most fractures in good position.

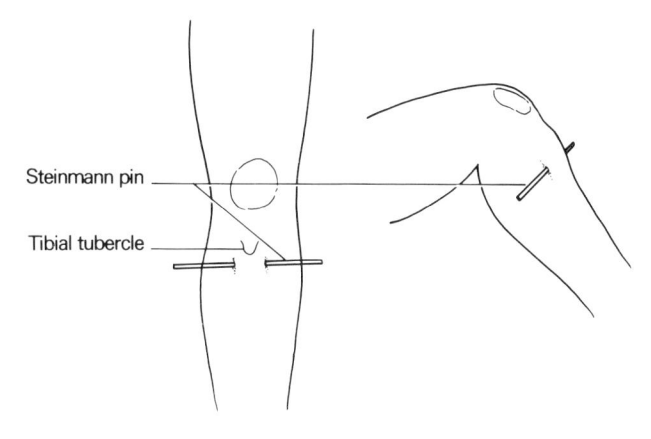

Fig. 21.11. A Steinmann pin through the upper tibia enabling skeletal traction to be applied to a femoral fracture.

Internal fixation

The fracture may be stabilised with a plate and screws (Fig. 21.12) or a metal rod through the medullary canal (Fig. 21.41).

3. Rehabilitation

If a limb is put into a plaster of Paris cast the joints which are not immobilised must be exercised regularly and effectively. Sometimes the help of a physiotherapist is required, especially if the limb is swollen and painful.

It is important to remember that the shoulder frequently becomes stiff if an arm plaster is applied. Similarly, the knee may become a problem in a below knee plaster applied to immobilise an ankle

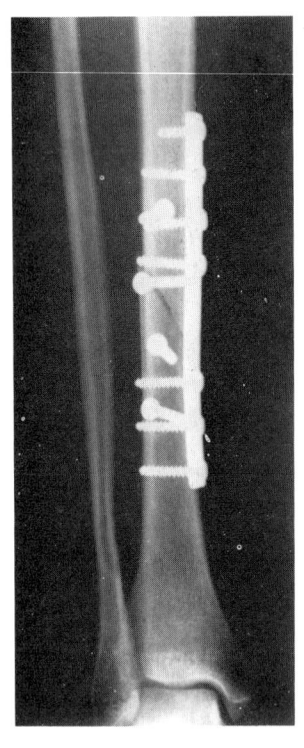

Fig. 21.12. Internal fixation of a fracture by means of a plate and screws.

fracture. If the patient is in bed with skeletal traction to immobilise a femoral fracture then the nurse or physiotherapist must make sure that all joints are regularly mobilised, the chest is exercised and the patient is turned regularly to avoid the complications of a deep vein thrombosis and skin pressure problems.

PRINCIPLES OF TREATMENT OF A COMPOUND FRACTURE

The open or compound fracture is a potentially dangerous situation for infection may complicate the injury. If the bone becomes infected the resulting osteomyelitis may be resistant to treatment (page 526), and the bone union is severely delayed.

The patient with a compound fracture must be given tetanus prophylaxis and must be put on the appropriate antibiotic. Tetanus toxoid 0.5 ml is given routinely subcutaneously. Anti-tetanus serum is only rarely given (see page 12) in those wounds which are grossly contaminated. Penicillin 500 mg q.d.s. and ampicillin 250 mg q.d.s. is a satisfactory combination to use and should be continued for seven days. The wound is cleaned and dressed in a sterile fashion in the Accident and Emergency department and arrangements are made for exploration of the wound—usually under a general anaesthetic. At operation it is essential to remove dirt and debris from the wound and to excise the wound edges. All crushed and contaminated fat and muscle are removed and all crevices of the wound are explored and carefully debrided. After this careful wound excision and clearance the surgeon will suture the wound if he is certain of its cleanliness and if the wound edges will come together without tension. However, the grossly contaminated wound or one in which much skin and tissue is removed so as to make closure impossible will be left open and packed with a paraffin tulle-gras dressing.

The fracture is treated by reduction in the usual way and then stabilised by means of external plaster or by traction. It is important to avoid internal fixation initially for the metal may act as a nidus for infection. When the wound is well healed it may be possible to fix the fracture if necessary by some internal means as described above.

FRACTURES AND DISLOCATIONS IN THE UPPER LIMB

The clavicle

This bone is usually fractured by falls on to the outstretched hand. It is frequently severely displaced but it rapidly unites with conservative treatment.

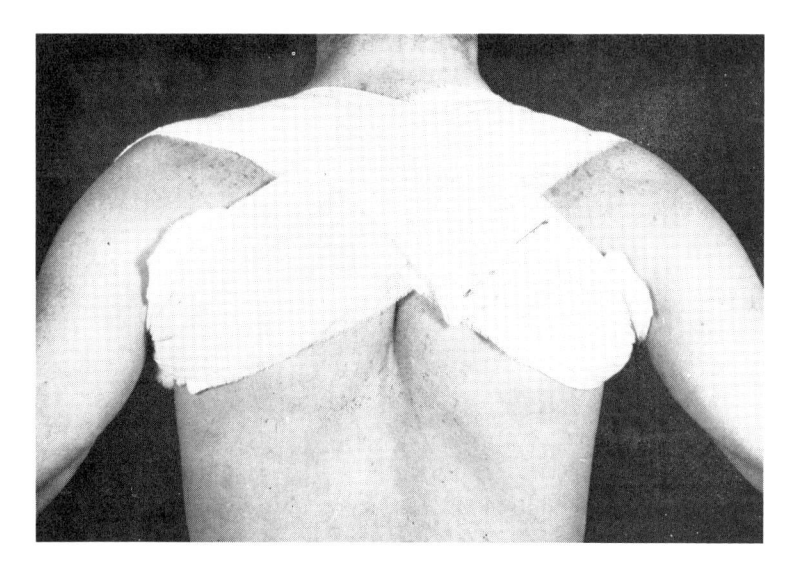

Fig. 21.13. Figure-of-eight bandage to brace the shoulders in fracture of the clavicle.

Treatment

A figure of eight bandage applied as in Fig. 21.13 will brace back the shoulders, will tend to reduce the displacement and will hold the fracture comfortably. It is important not to apply the bandage too tightly, for pressure in the axilla will then become a painful problem. After a week or two in this bandage a simple sling will be required until the shoulder is comfortable enough to be mobilised.

Acromioclavicular separation (Fig. 21.14)

A direct blow to the shoulder whilst playing rugby is often responsible for this injury. There is tenderness and swelling at the

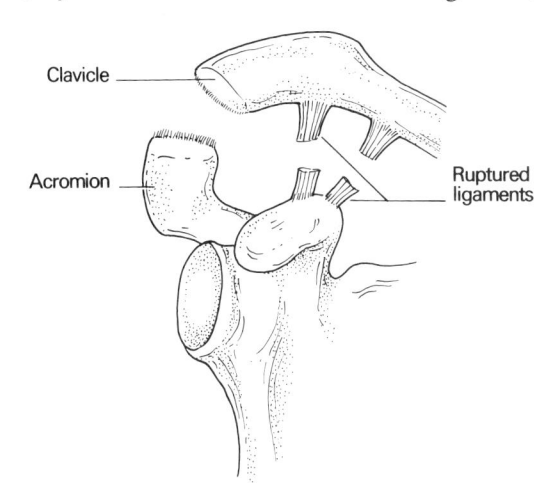

Fig. 21.14. Acromio-clavicular separation.

joint site and if there is wide separation of the two bones the lateral portion of the clavicle will be easily felt beneath the skin.

Treatment

Most separations are minor and will repair satisfactorily. A simple sling is applied until the shoulder is comfortable enough to be mobilised. If there is wide dislocation of the joint as shown in Fig. 21.14 internal fixation with a screw from the acromion to the clavicle will be necessary.

FRACTURES OF THE UPPER HUMERUS

The great tuberosity

Direct falls on to the shoulder may crack the great tuberosity, (Fig. 21.15). Although this would appear a very minor injury the shoulder function may be interfered with for the tendon and ligaments constituting 'the rotator cuff' are damaged.

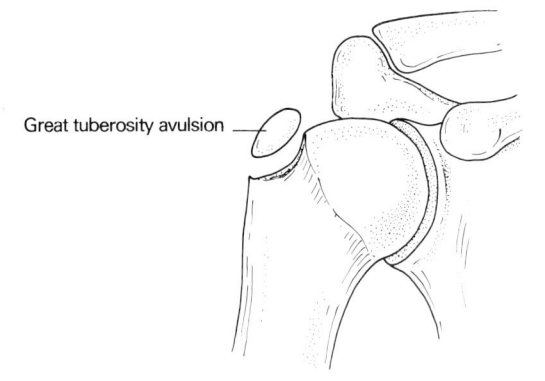

Fig. 21.15. Avulsion fracture of great tuberosity of the humerus.

The surgical neck of the humerus (Fig. 21.16)

Again, falls on to the outstretched hand will fracture this site beneath the humeral head, especially in the elderly patient. Pain, bruising and extreme tenderness will be present around the shoulder, and joint function is grossly limited. Most fractures in this region are impacted with the shaft fragment tightly and stably thrust into the head of the humerus.

Treatment

The great tuberosity and the impacted humeral neck fractures should be rested in a simple arm sling until comfortable. The physiotherapist will then be asked to mobilise the shoulder at the

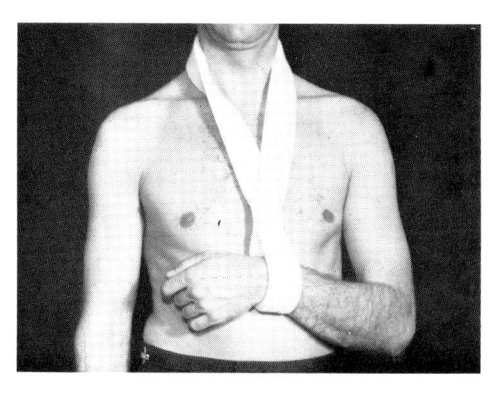

Fig. 21.16. Fracture of surgical neck of humerus.

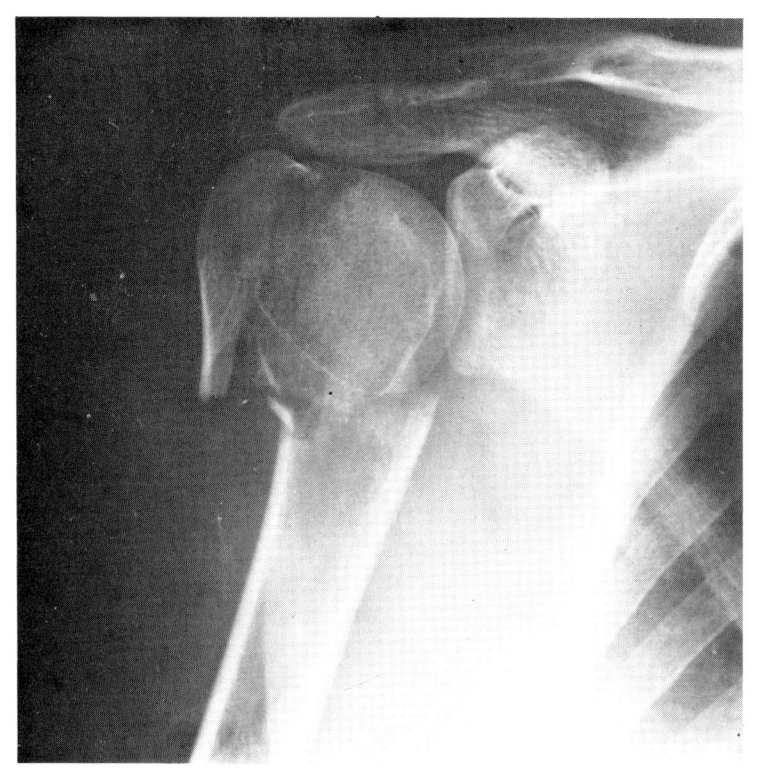

earliest moment to prevent joint stiffness. The upper humeral fragments may be unstable and displaced, in which case open operation to reduce and internally fix the fractures with a nail may be required.

The shaft of the humerus

This fracture is frequently very displaced but rapidly comes into good alignment with a simple collar and cuff sling (Fig. 21.17). The radial nerve winds around the posterior aspect of the humerus

Fig. 21.17. Collar and cuff sling.

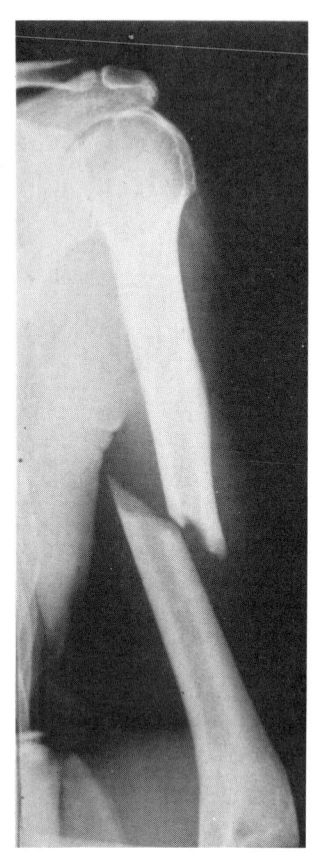

Fig. 21.18. Humeral shaft fracture.

in this mid-shaft region and may be damaged in fractures at this site (Fig. 21.18). A dropped wrist develops if the radial nerve is divided or more commonly pressurised by this injury. However, the paralysis is usually temporary.

Treatment

If the patient is sat up and allowed to stand erect with the arm in a collar and cuff sling, the pull of gravity will tend to reduce and align the fracture. A plaster 'U loop' may be added to give greater stability, but the point of the elbow must be left hanging free.

Shoulder dislocation

Rotational forces on the shoulder in falls and in sports injuries may dislocate this joint. Most of the dislocations are anterior but rarely the displacement of the humeral head is posterior or inferior. The shoulder joint may be considered a ball and socket joint, but as seen in Fig. 21.5 the glenoid socket of the scapula is very shallow and is deepened by a fibrous ring, called the labrum. In the anterior dislocation of the shoulder joint the labrum or capsule (or both) is torn severely anteriorly. If it repairs poorly then recurrent dislocation through this weakened area may occur.

Treatment

Traction is applied to the arm and with a sustained pull relocation is usually possible. The method described by Hippocrates—the Greek father of medicine—in the 4th Century B.C. is still considered the best. The surgeon's foot is placed in the axilla and this acts as a counter pull to the arm traction.

The supracondylar fracture

This particular injury proves to be the most troublesome fracture in the child because of the vascular complications which may ensue. The distal condylar fragment is displaced posteriorly and the sharp spike of the upper fragment irritates or in a few cases actually lacerates the brachial artery (Fig. 21.19). The pressure of haematoma and the vessel irritation may close the lumen of the brachial artery at this site and unless it is re-opened a pulseless and bloodless forearm and hand will result. The end result of this avascular periphery will be a Volkmann's contracture, in which the dead and fibrosed forearm muscles produce clawed and contracted fingers, and the death of the peripheral nerves will produce anaesthesia and trophic ulcers (Fig. 21.20).

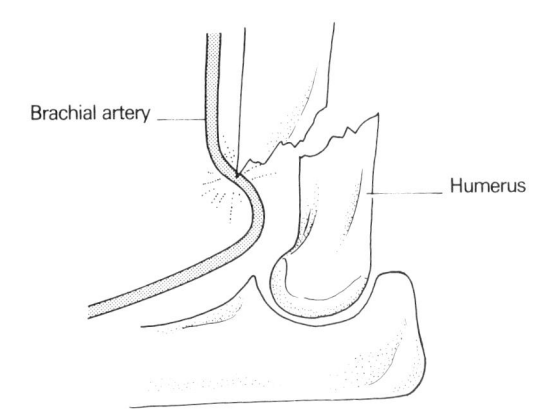

Fig. 21.19. A supracondylar fracture with vascular injury.

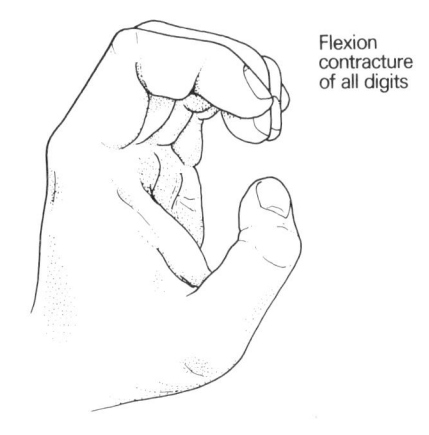

Fig. 21.20. Volkmann's contracture of the hand.

Treatment

When the child is first admitted to the Accident Unit the nurse should feel for the radial pulse. If it is absent, reduction of the fracture should be undertaken without delay. Under an anaesthetic the fracture is manipulated to a reduced position and a well padded backslab of plaster is applied with the elbow at a right angle. The reduction of the fracture usually restores the circulation but if it fails the brachial artery must be explored and decompressed. In a few cases arterial repair or grafting is necessary to restore the blood flow.

Dislocation of the elbow (Fig. 21.21)

Falls on to the hand are again usually responsible for this injury with the forearm dislocating posteriorly on the humerus.

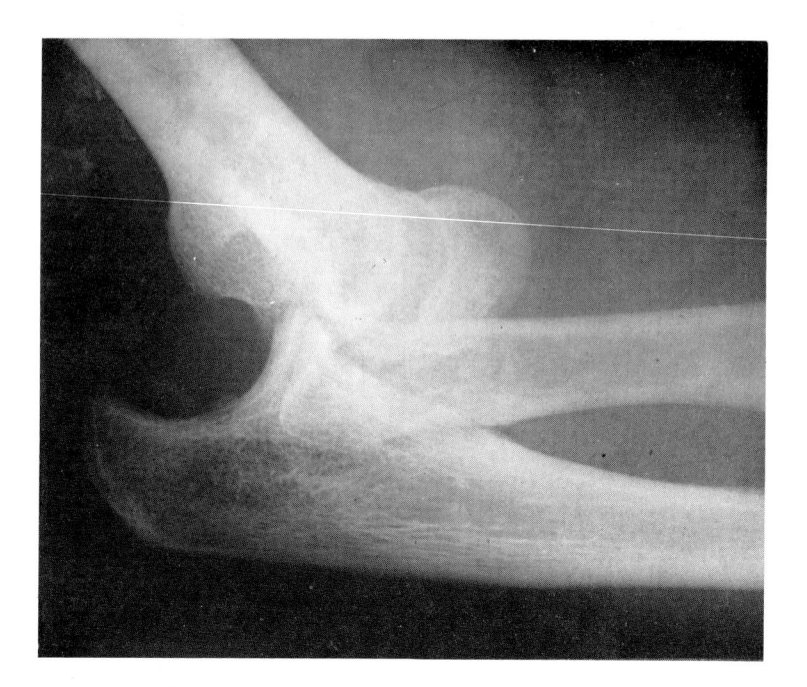

Fig. 21.21. Posterior dislocation of elbow.

Treatment

Manipulation of the joint under an anaesthetic with traction on the forearm will easily reduce the dislocation. The elbow must be rested in a sling or a backslab, for an irritable elbow joint which is not rested following an injury reacts by producing joint stiffness. This is due to scarring or even calcification and ossification of the capsule (a condition called myositis ossificans).

The olecranon

The upper ulna is fractured by a direct blow or a fall on to the point of the elbow. The olecranon receives the insertion of the triceps muscle and this bone fragment pulls away from the ulna by the action of this muscle. Operative fixation is required for restoration of the normal anatomy and elbow function, and the screw fixation shown in Fig. 21.22 is effective.

The radial head

The radial head articulates with the humerus and the ulna at the elbow joint and fractures of this bone may interfere with rotation of the forearm.

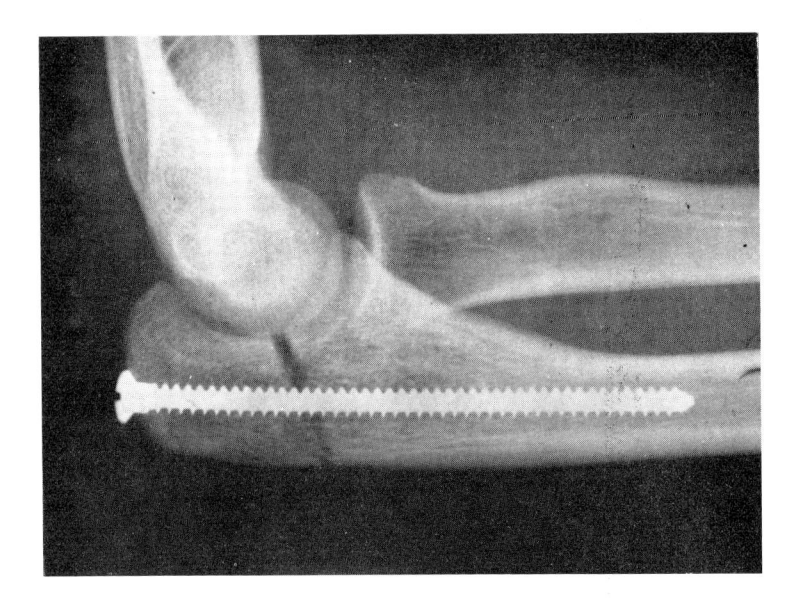

Fig. 21.22. Fracture of the olecranon—internal fixation with screw.

Treatment

Minor displaced fractures are allowed to unite by resting the elbow in a sling for three weeks. If a substantial portion of the radial head is avulsed then it is best to remove the fragment and excise the damaged head remnant. If an irregular radial head fragment remains there is a risk of subsequent osteoarthritis in the elbow joint. The radial neck is still retained in an annular ligament and rotation persists.

Colles' Fracture

This fracture is the commonest seen in the Accident and Emergency departments and is again sustained by a fall on to the outstretched hand, usually in elderly ladies. It is an impacted fracture of the lower radius within an inch of the joint line. The distal radial fragment is displaced and rotated posteriorly and the ulnar styloid is sometimes fractured and separated. The patient complains of pain and tenderness in the wrist, and there is frequently such displacement that a deformity, similar to a dinner fork, is noted. (Fig. 21.23).

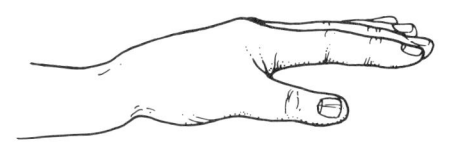

Fig. 21.23. Colles fracture with displacement produces a 'dinner fork' deformity.

Treatment

The fracture must be reduced in all but the elderly or those in poor general health in whom operation is contraindicated. A general anaesthetic is usually advisable but local regional anaesthesia may be undertaken.

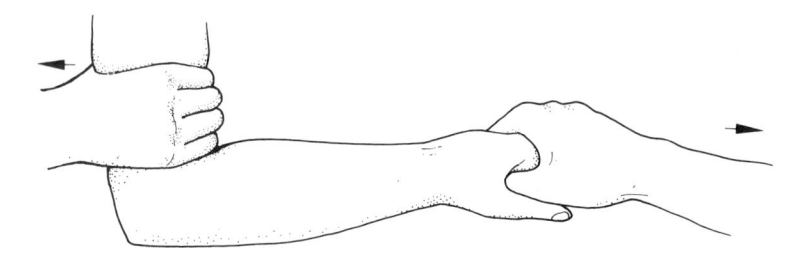

Fig. 21.24. Reduction of a Colles fracture by traction.

Fig. 21.25. Back-slab applied to the wrist following reduction of a Colles fracture.

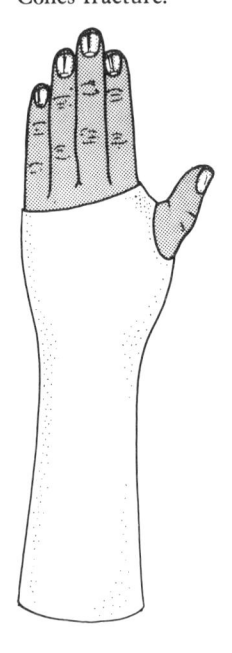

Technique of Reduction The impacted fragment can be disimpacted by traction, (Fig. 21.24). The radial fragment must then be manipulated so that the joint surface of the wrist joint comes into the correct alignment. A plaster backslab is then applied to maintain position (Fig. 21.25). A full plaster is not advisable at this stage for the wrist will continue to swell after reduction and pain and decreased circulation will result. Following the manipulation the fracture position is checked on X-ray and the patient should be seen again in 3 to 4 days to again check the position and to complete the plaster. Further check on X-ray is advisable at about the tenth day, for after this it will be very difficult to alter the fracture position if slipping should occur. The plaster is retained for approximately 6 weeks and the physiotherapist then mobilises the stiff wrist joint.

A Smith's fracture is a reverse Colles and its treatment is by manipulation in the reverse direction.

Scaphoid fracture (Fig. 21.26)

This small bone of the carpus is fractured in falls on to the wrist and hand. It often heals with difficulty and if it remains ununited the proximal fragment may collapse due to an inadequate blood supply. This complication is called *avascular necrosis* and results in osteoarthritis of the wrist. Diagnosis is by clinical examination of the wrist, for there is pain and tenderness on the radial side. The fracture does not always show up on the first X-ray examination, but if a scaphoid fracture is suspected a plaster cast must always be applied. Ten to 14 days later a re-X-ray will demonstrate the break

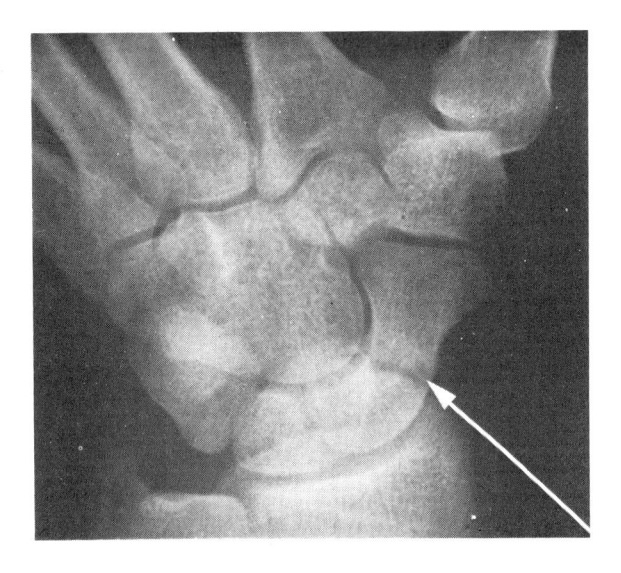

Fig. 21.26. Fracture of the scaphoid bone.

for the fracture line will be more obvious. A plaster cast is retained initially for 6 to 8 weeks, but if it remains ununited internal fixation with a small screw or bone graft will be necessary.

Fractures of the fingers and thumb

Fractures of the metacarpal necks are common and are nearly always the result of a 'hard punch'. The knuckle may be a little flattened by displacement at the fracture site but union rapidly occurs. A useful axiom in the treatment of fractures of the hand is to 'forget the fracture and exercise the joint' and there is no exception in metacarpal fractures. The fracture-dislocation of the base of the thumb metacarpal is called a *Bennett's Fracture* and a wire piercing the skin and traversing the fracture is frequently required for its fixation (Fig. 21.27).

The phalanges of the fingers are often fractured in crush injuries of the hand. They unite quickly and it is again essential to encourage the early movement of the small joints of the injured digit. A useful method of splinting the finger to avoid the stiffness that a plaster or metal splint would produce is to strap one finger to the next and to encourage movement of both together (Fig. 21.28).

A mallet finger deformity (Fig. 21.29) occurs when the terminal phalanx is stubbed on a cricket ball or other hard object. The extensor tendon is torn from the distal phalanx and frequently a fragment

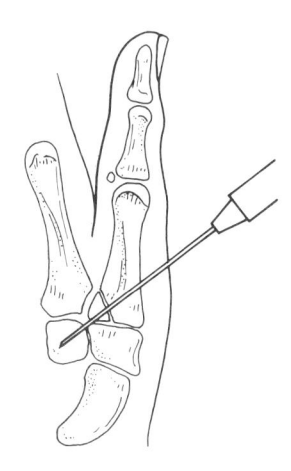

Fig. 21.27. Bennett's fracture being internally fixed by a percutaneous wire.

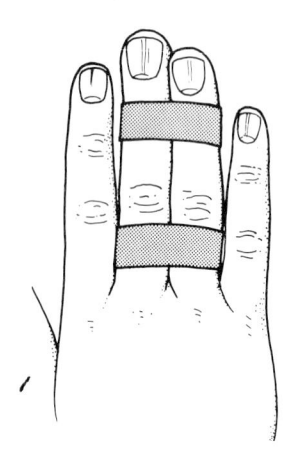

Fig. 21.28. Splintage of two fingers together.

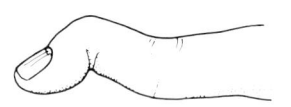

Fig. 21.29. Mallet finger deformity.

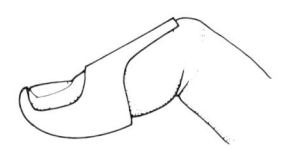

Fig. 21.30. Mallet finger splint.

Fig. 21.31. Posterior dislocation of the hip.

of bone is avulsed. To restore active extension to the terminal phalanx a mallet finger splint (Fig. 21.30) should be applied for one month.

FRACTURES AND DISLOCATIONS IN THE LOWER LIMB

Hip joint dislocations

Hip joint dislocations are seen commonly in major car accidents. The most common type is the posterior dislocation which may also be associated with a fracture of the acetabulum. The femoral head may dislocate centrally, fracturing the acetabulum as it enters the pelvis, but only rarely does the femoral head come out anteriorly.

Posterior dislocation of the hip

This is seen in front seat passengers when injured in a car and not wearing safety belts. The knee hits the dashboard and a violent force is transmitted along the shaft of the femur to the hip where the femoral head is forcibly dislocated posteriorly (Fig. 21.31).

Treatment

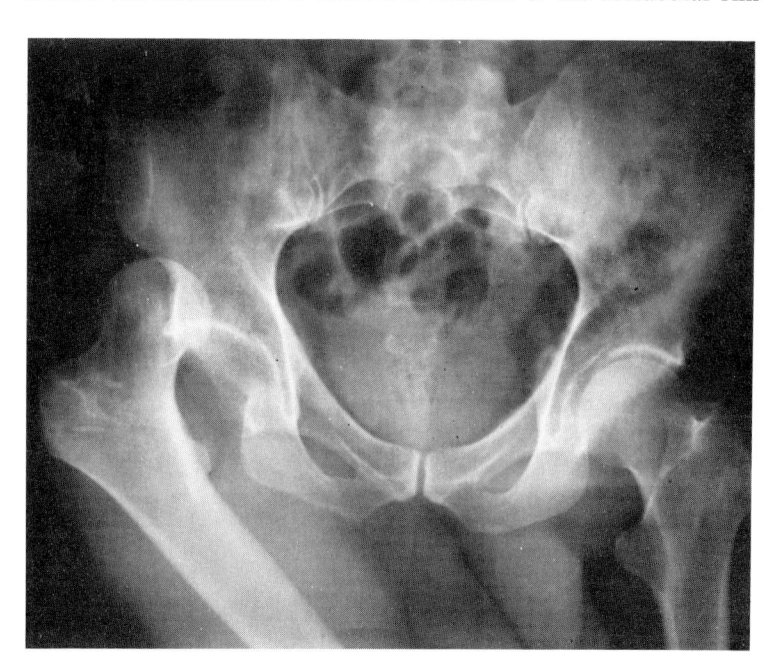

Under a general anaesthetic strong manipulation is required to reduce the dislocation. If there is a fracture of the acetabular rim making the reduction unstable, internal fixation of the bony fragment may be required. The limb should be immobilised in traction for 6 weeks post-reduction to allow the capsule to heal and to restore and maintain the blood supply to the femoral head.

Central dislocations

Pedestrians struck by a vehicle on the lateral side of the hip region may sustain this injury; the femoral head and neck are driven into the pelvis through the acetabulum. Multiple fractures of the pelvis may be sustained.

Treatment

Strong skeletal traction is required to bring the femoral head back into its original position.

Fractures of the femoral neck

These are common fractures seen in the elderly patient, especially female. It occurs in patients with soft osteoporotic bones and may follow relatively minor trauma. The mortality is high, for the patient is elderly and often has associated general health problems which complicate the treatment. The patient's immobility may lead to early bronchopneumonia, congestive heart failure and pulmonary embolism. With many old people it is not the treatment which is the problem, but the aftercare and return to independence. These patients frequently live on their own and after such an injury they require a period of support which a keen and enthusiastic family may be able to give. However, this responsibility may be shunned by relatives and the patient's retention in a geriatric hospital or other rehabilitation unit puts a severe strain and burden on the hospital and social services.

Fractures of the femoral neck are described according to their anatomical position (Fig. 21.32):
1. Subcapital
2. Transcervical
3. Trochanteric
4. Subtrochanteric

It should be noted from Fig. 21.32 that fractures affecting the neck proper occur within the capsule of the hip joint, and the blood supply to the femoral head, which runs along the femoral neck, is disturbed. In neck fractures where there is considerable displacement, this major complication of *avascular necrosis* of the femoral

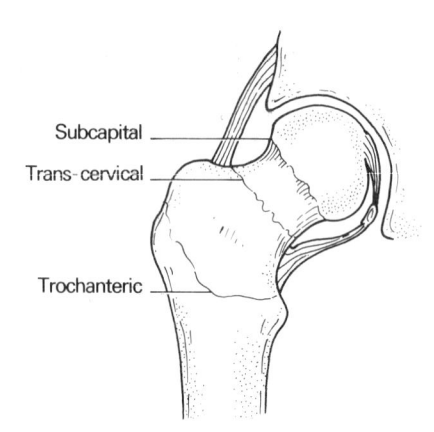

Fig. 21.32. Sites of femoral neck fracture.

head is very high. Avascular necrosis results in collapse of the head and severe osteoarthritis of the hip ensues. This is a disastrous complication (Fig. 21.33).

Fractures affecting the trochanteric and subtrochanteric region are outside the capsule and the blood supply to the femoral head is never interfered with. These fractures, therefore, unite without avascular necrosis.

Some fractures of the femoral neck may unite without operation, but the mortality is high, for the patient may develop pneumonia, urinary tract infection, deep vein thrombosis and pressure sores. It is important, therefore, to stabilise the fracture of the hip joint by appropriate surgical means using internal fixation to allow the patient to get up rapidly and to avoid these severe complications.

Clinical features

Most of these fractures occur in falls in the home and as mentioned previously the trauma involved may be very minor. The elderly patient tripping over a carpet or mat may fracture the femoral neck with the rotary forces applied. The hip is painful and the patient is frequently unable to get up. If the fracture is impacted, reasonable function may be maintained and walking on the hip is possible. In most cases, however, pain and instability is such that the patient has to call for help and is brought to the Accident and Emergency department by ambulance. The affected limb is short, adducted and externally rotated, as shown in Fig. 21.34. Any attempt to move the limb is painful and strongly resisted by the patient. Any elderly patient who has a painful hip following a very minor injury should always be suspected of having this fracture, for although initially it may be impacted and stable, spontaneous loosening at the fracture site may occur and the fragments may become unstable.

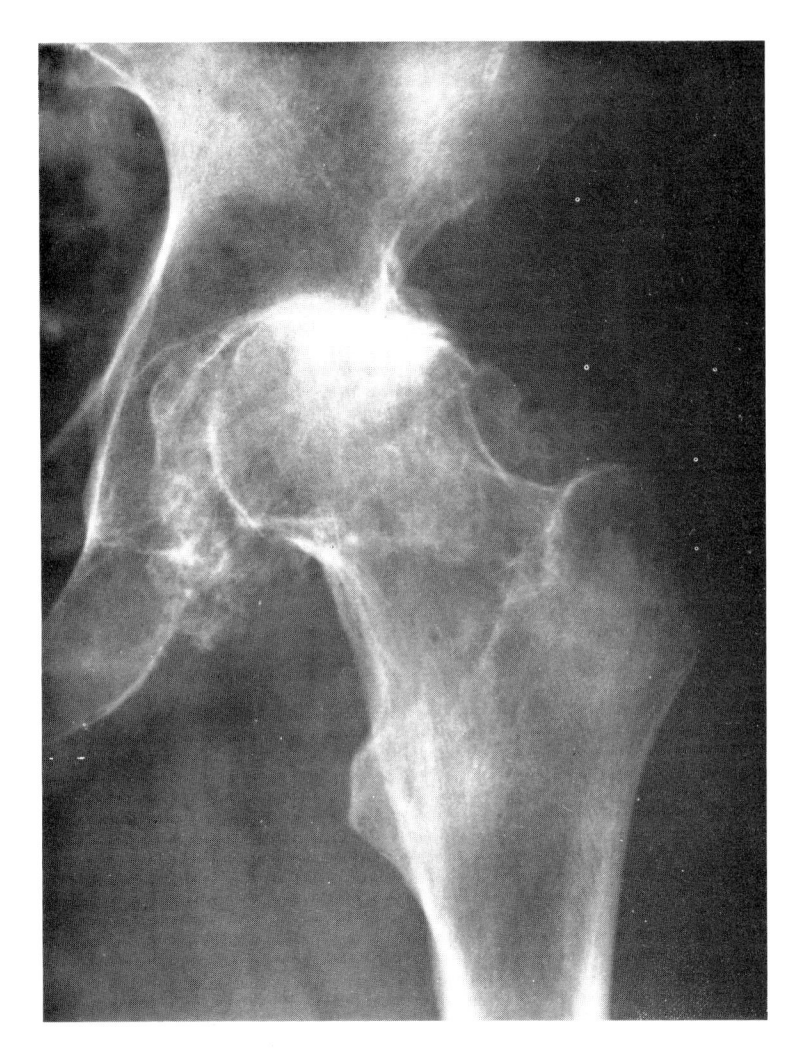

Fig. 21.33. Avascular necrosis of the femoral head. Note the densely sclerotic bone.

Fig. 21.34. Position of the leg after left femoral neck fracture.

Treatment

(a) *Subcapital and transcervical fractures (the intracapsular fractures).* If the fracture is impacted and with only very minor displacement internal fixation with a tri-fin nail is undertaken. The correct position is obtained with a guide wire under X-ray control and a Smith–Petersen nail is inserted over this guide wire to immobilise the head on the neck of the femur (Fig. 21.35).

Fractures of the femoral neck which are so displaced as to cause disturbance of the blood supply to the femoral head will be complicated by avascularity of the head with resulting collapse and osteo-arthritis of the hip joint.

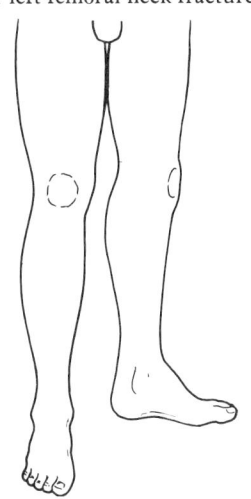

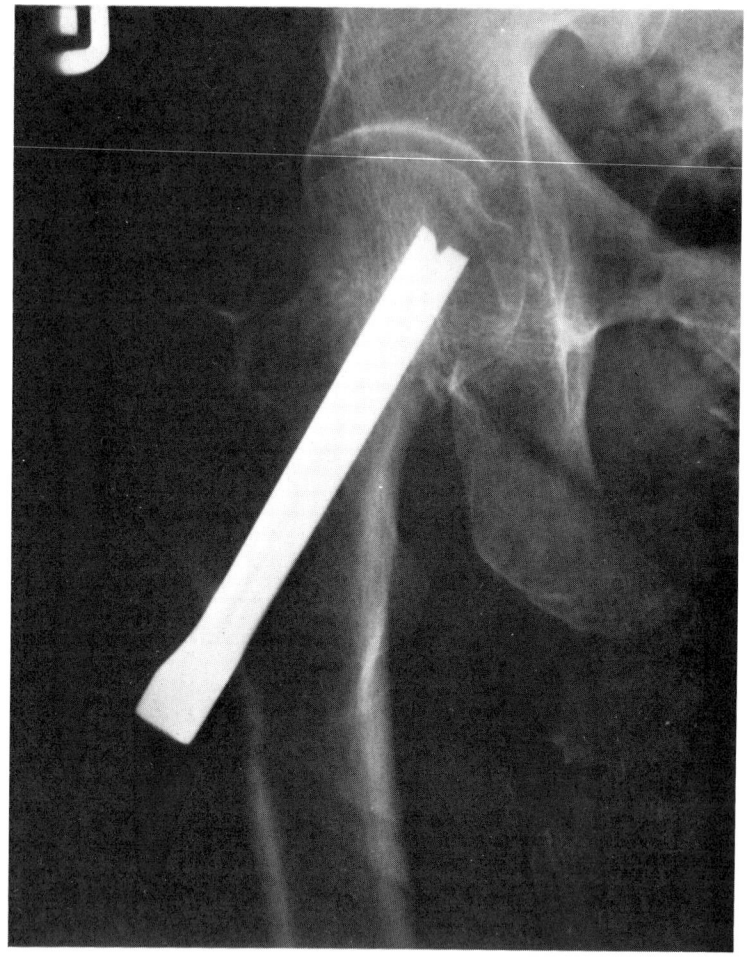

Fig. 21.35. Nail fixation of a sub-capital fracture.

In most elederly patients the head is excised, the neck trimmed and a replacement prosthesis of a Thompson or Austin Moore type is inserted (Fig. 21.36). The Thompson prosthesis is often seated in acrylic cement in the upper femoral neck and shaft for added stability.

(b) *Trochanteric and subtrochanteric fractures of the femoral neck.* Fractures at this site unite satisfactorily for much of the bone is cancellous with good healing properties and the blood supply to the femoral head is not disturbed. Internal fixation of the fracture is satisfactorily carried out with a pin and plate (Fig. 21.37). The pin is inserted into the femoral neck and head over a guide wire inserted with X-ray control and the plate is attached to the pin by means of a bolt, and to the upper femoral shaft by means of multiple screws.

Fig. 21.36. Thompson replacement of femoral head following sub-capital fracture.

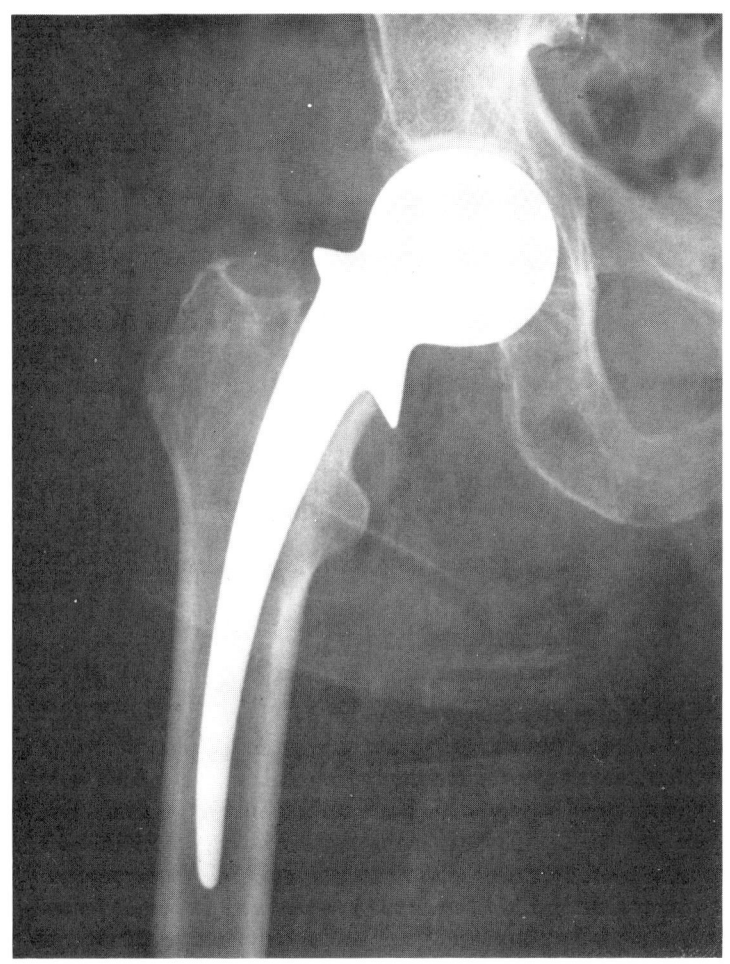

The post-operative management of the patient following hip surgery.

Patients who have had their fractures internally fixed are sat up out of bed the next day if possible. Walking with support—guided by the physiotherapist—is encouraged as soon as the patient is able to co-operate. When a pin or a pin and plate is inserted only partial weight bearing is allowed on the appropriate limb until the fracture has united at approximately the third post-operative month. Until that time frame or crutch support is advised. If the patient has had a prosthetic replacement of the femoral head, rest in bed for two or three days is advisable, with the hip abducted by means of appropriate pillows, or light skin traction. Abduction of the hip is important following this operation for dislocations can occur and this complication is avoided by keeping the legs wide apart during

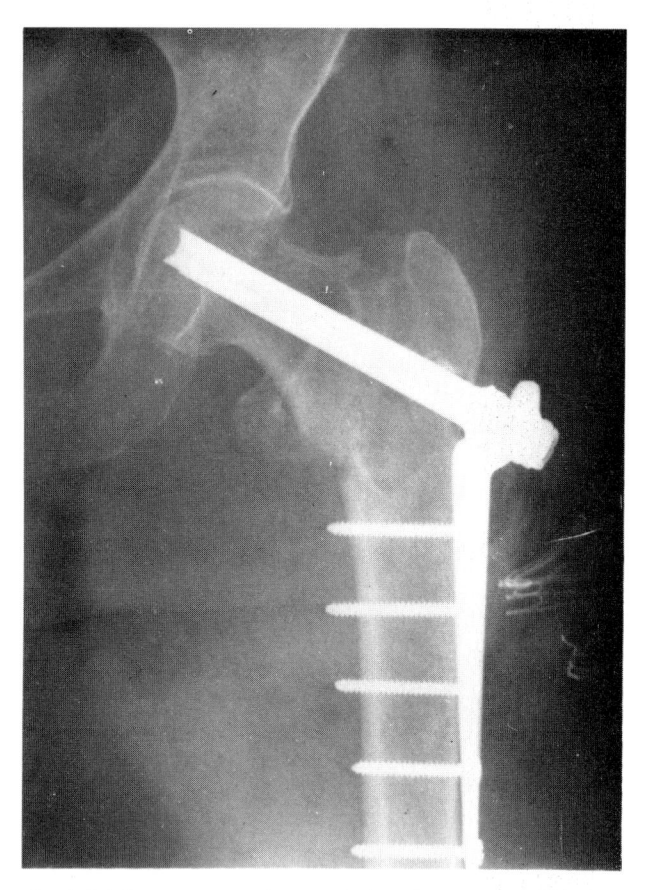

Fig. 21.37. Pin and plate fixation of a trochanteric fracture.

the initial post-operative period. When muscle control is regained two or three days post-operatively the physiotherapist may get the patient up and walking. The minimal support of sticks is all that is required.

Fractures of the femoral shaft

This is a common fracture seen in all age groups and is sustained in road traffic and industrial accidents and falls from a height. The fracture is frequently associated with other injuries and the patient is often in a shocked state when admitted to the Accident and Emergency department. In the absence of any other injury a fracture of this large bone will produce considerable blood loss. The thigh becomes swollen and tense, and two to three bottles of blood (1.0 l–1.5 l) are lost into the muscles and soft tissues of the thigh. The hypovolaemia resulting from such a fracture may surgically shock the elderly patient and so steps must be taken on admission to **restore the blood volume with appropriately cross matched blood.**

Treatment

Traction is the secret of both reduction and fixation of this fracture. In the child a simple Gallow's traction apparatus (Fig. 21.38) is adequate, and after 4 to 5 weeks the fracture is stable enough for mobilisation to begin.

In the adult strong traction is required to align and reduce the fracture and to keep it fixed in such a position that union will occur. Skeletal traction is required, for weights of between 15 and 20 pounds are not uncommonly necessary. A Steinmann's pin is placed through the upper tibia under a local or general anaesthetic to attach the main traction weight (Fig. 21.39). The body itself acts as a counter-traction with the head end of the bed lowered. The alignment of the fracture and the management of this painful and unstable limb is aided by a Thomas' splint with a knee flexion piece; the whole apparatus being balanced by multiple weights (Fig. 21.40). In many units a simple pillow beneath the thigh is used to maintain the position of the fracture whilst traction is continued, dispensing with the Thomas' splint. Three months in traction are necessary and

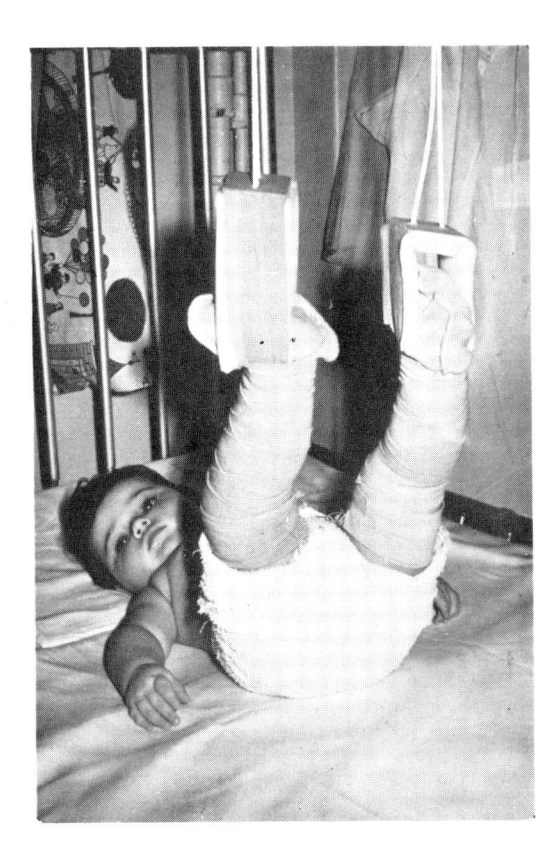

Fig. 21.38. Gallow's traction.

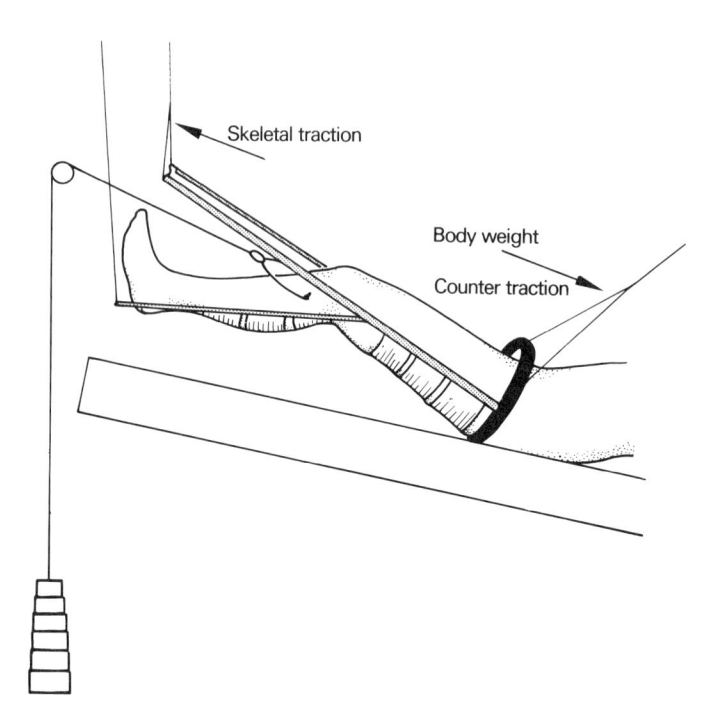

Fig. 21.39. Skeletal traction apparatus for femoral shaft fracture.

Fig. 21.40. Thomas' splint.

during this time it is vital that the knee is kept mobile. The patient's pressure areas are dealt with adequately and the general exercise and rehabilitation of the patient is started as soon as possible after the accident.

Most femoral shaft fractures are adequately treated by conservative means. If attention is paid to the rehabilitation of the patient and the mobilisation of the knee in particular, no disability will result.

Internal fixation with an intramedullary rod is undertaken in the following circumstances:

1. Where it is impossible to reduce the fracture due to soft tissues and muscle being interposed between the bone ends.
2. In a pathological fracture where metastasis to the femoral shaft has occurred from a carcimona elsewhere.
3. In multiple injuries, where the tibia, femur and perhaps other bones are fractured. It is impossible to mobilise the knee adequately if multiple fractures in one limb are treated conservatively.
4. If the patient is very elderly and will not tolerate 3 months in traction in bed.

Intramedullary nail fixation of this fracture (Fig. 21.41) has the great advantage of speedy mobilisation and allows full weight bearing, but it should always be remembered that a very small percentage become infected and if an intramedullary nail is present the whole femoral shaft may be involved.

The supracondylar fracture

This is a common fracture in elderly people. It is treated usually conservatively by similar means to the femoral shaft fracture with skeletal traction and an adequate pad beneath the knee to lift up the distal fragment, but again internal fixation with a blade plate (Fig. 21.42) may be necessary.

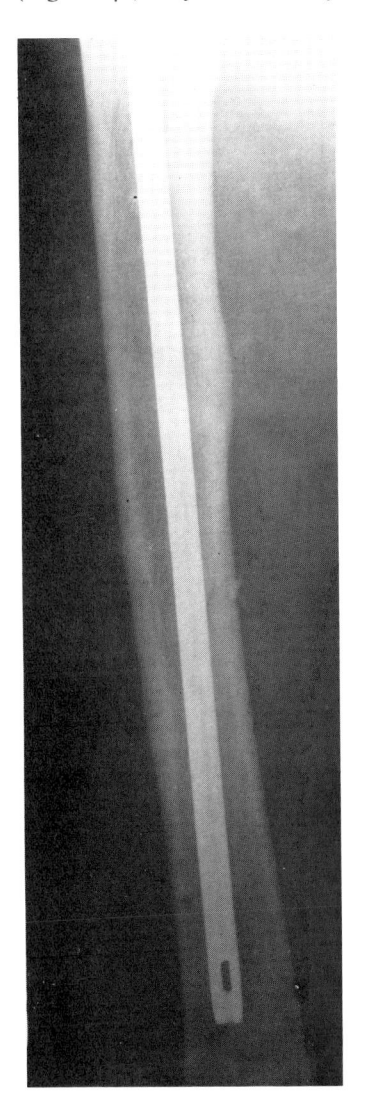

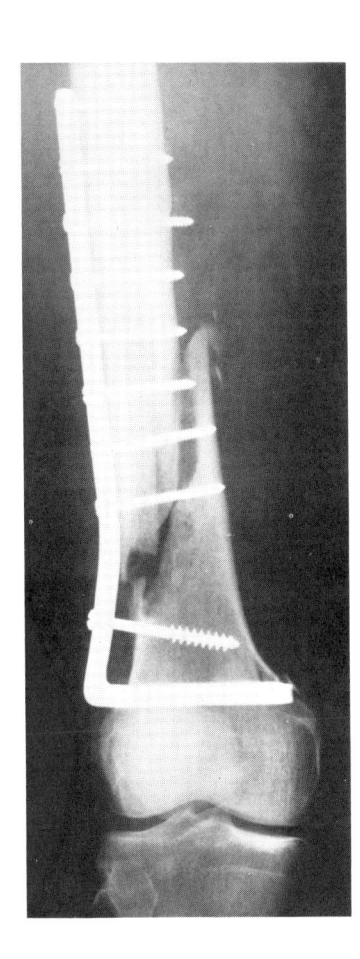

Fig. 21.41. (LEFT) Intramedullary nail for a femoral shaft fracture.

Fig. 21.42. (RIGHT) Internal fixation of a supracondylar fracture with a blade plate.

Patellar fractures

A transverse fracture is sustained when the knee is struck anteriorly and the pull of the large thigh muscles—the quadriceps—cleanly separates the bone into two fragments. If the fragments can be brought together anatomically they may be fixed by means of a screw (Fig. 21.43) or by an encircling wire. A comminuted fracture with multiple fragments (Fig. 21.44) cannot be replaced and so excision of the patellar portions is undertaken and the surrounding torn capsule is repaired.

Fractures of the tibia

This bone is commonly fractured and as its medial surface is subcutaneous it is the most frequently compound fracture seen. It is this latter aspect, together with the relatively poor blood supply of the bone in the lower portions of the tibia, which make it such a difficult injury to treat. In most cases, a simple tibial fracture can be put straight and into good position under a general anaesthetic. The alignment and replacement can be adjusted by manipulation and with a well padded good fitting plaster of Paris cast the fracture will unite satisfactorily in 3 months. The plaster should stretch from the toes to the upper thigh region to adequately immobilise the knee

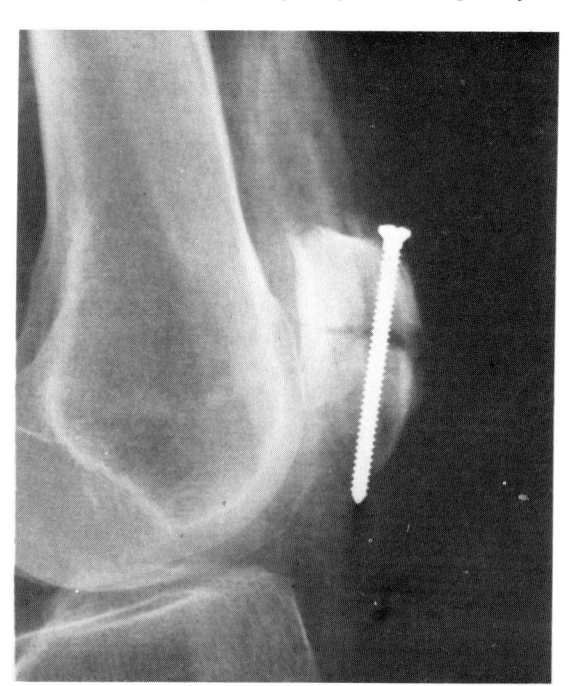

Fig. 21.43. Patellar fracture fixed by means of a screw.

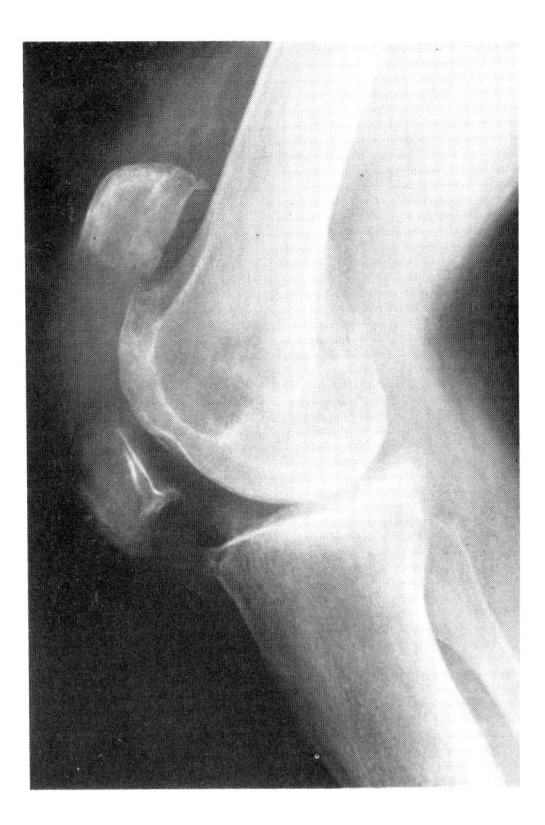

Fig. 21.44. Comminuted patellar fracture.

and the ankle joints. If the fracture is compound the treatment regimen outlined on page 490 is undertaken. If the tibial fracture is very comminuted and shortened, traction is undertaken with a skeletal Steinmann's pin inserted through the calcaneum.

Many tibial fractures are unstable and this is particularly so in the short oblique fracture, where it is often impossible to stabilise and maintain the position by manipulation. It may be decided in these cases to fix the bone internally with a plate and screws which will hold the position accurately and stably (Fig. 21.12). The stability of internal fixation is increased by a compression plating technique whereby the bone ends are compressed together by the device shown in Fig. 21.45.

POTT'S FRACTURE (Fig. 21.46).

A Pott's fracture is a fracture dislocation of the ankle joint. It is most commonly caused by the patient falling or stumbling, thus rotating the foot externally and forcing it backwards.

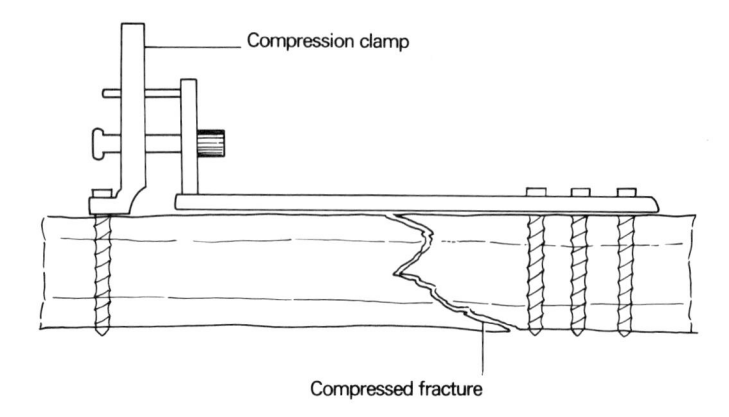

Fig. 21.45. Compression plating technique.

Grade I Pott's fracture. The fibula is fractured on the lateral side of the ankle and a spiral break is present. The talus bone, which is retained in the ankle joint mortice by the medial and lateral malleoli, may shift laterally at the time of this fracture dislocation.

Grade II Pott's fracture. With a greater external rotation and posterior force on the foot, the lateral and medial malleoli may both fracture. Frequently the talus shifts and accurate reduction of both bones is necessary. As both sides of the joint are unstable, internal fixation may be required.

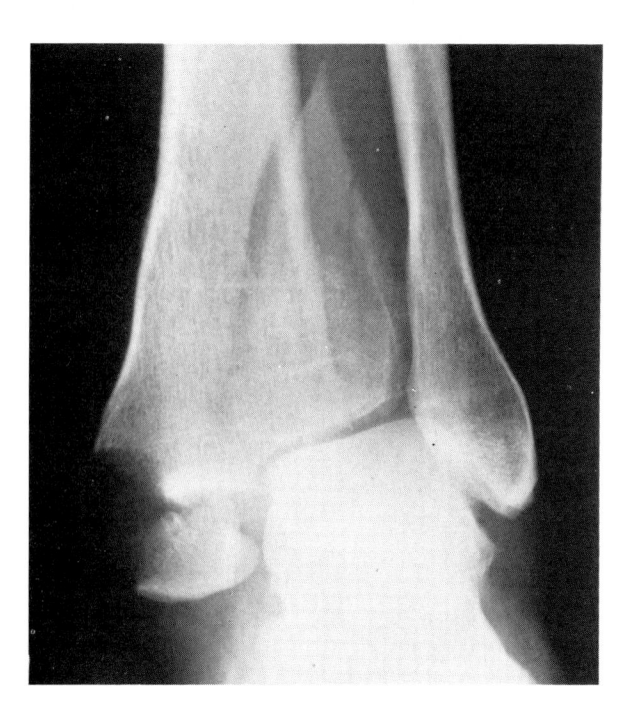

Fig. 21.46. Pott's fracture-dislocation of ankle.

Grade III Pott's fracture. The force applied to the ankle joint is sometimes so great that the posterior lip of the tibia is also avulsed. The talus then shifts laterally and posteriorly and the displacement may be so great that the blood supply to the foot is occluded.

Treatment

Grade I Pott's fracture may be treated conservatively by manipulation of the lateral malleolus into a good position. The plaster is applied below the knee with the foot at right angles for 6 to 8 weeks and only in the latter part of this period is weight bearing allowed. In a Grade II fracture, the instability may be such that both the medial malleolus and sometimes the lateral malleolus requires fixation (Fig. 21.47). Grade III fractures always require internal fixation for they are very unstable.

FRACTURES IN THE FOOT

The calcaneum or heel bone is often fractured in falls on to the feet. If the patient falls from a great height not only are the heel bones damaged but frequently a crush fracture of one of the upper lumbar

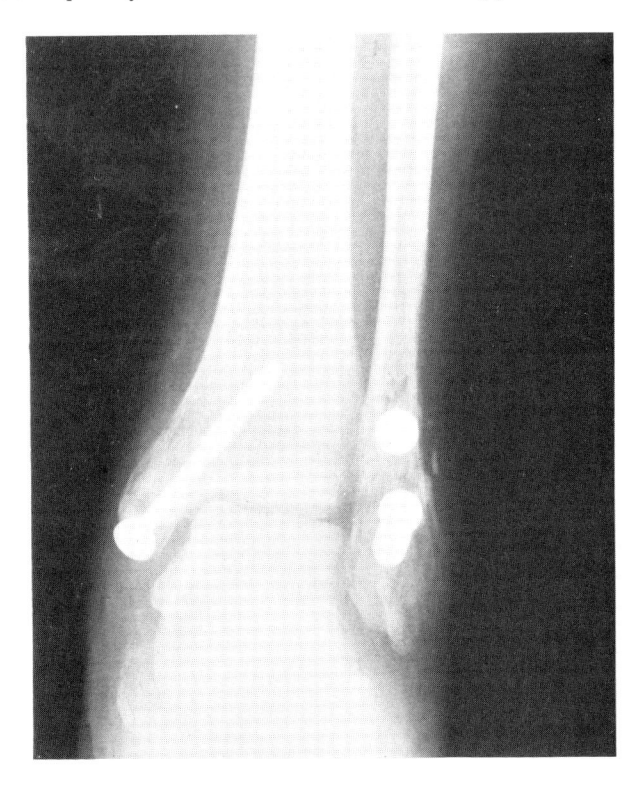

Fig. 21.47. Internal fixation of a Pott's fracture.

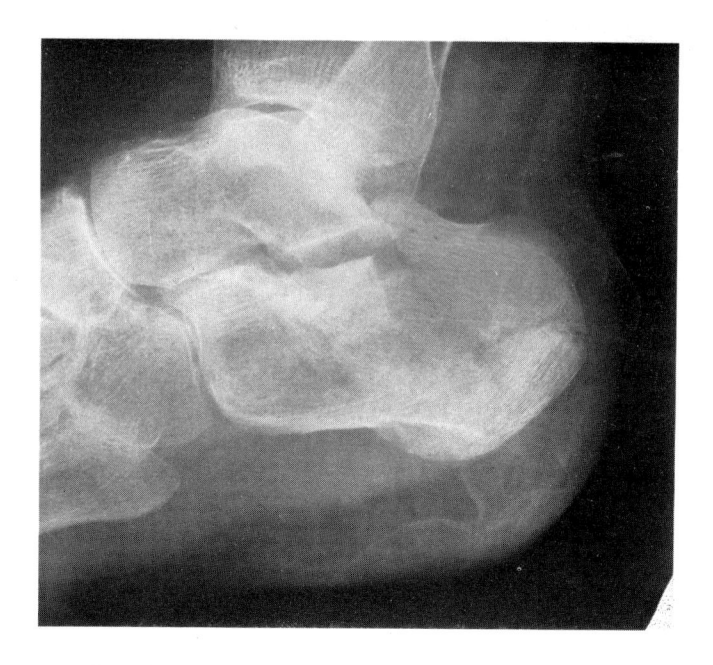

Fig. 21.48. Fracture of calcaneus.

Fig. 21.49. Flexion injury of the neck producing fracture-dislocation. Note the complete transection of the spinal cord.

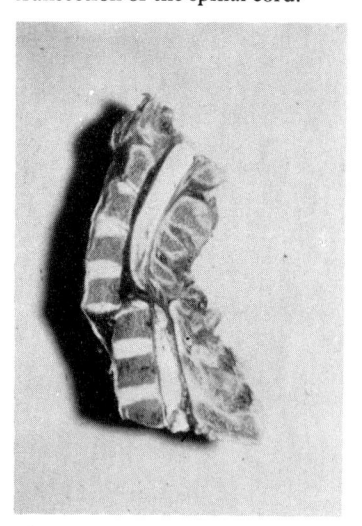

vertebrae is sustained. The calcaneal fractures which do not involve the subtalar joint are treated by initial plaster cast or by elevation. The foot is mobilised as soon as comfort will allow. Fractures involving the subtalar joint (Fig. 21.48) are more serious for inversion and eversion of the foot will be interfered with, and further operative treatment will be required to arthrodese the joint.

Metatarsal and phalangeal fractures

These injuries are troublesome for they cause great pain on weight bearing. The patients recover faster if weight relief is given by temporary crutches or sticks but the foot must be kept as mobile as possible.

SPINAL INJURIES

Cervical spine

Serious neck injuries are most commonly sustained in road accidents, diving in shallow water and, rarely, in Rugby Football. Head injuries are frequently associated and it is the acute flexion of the neck which does the damage (Fig. 21.49). A patient complaining of a painful and stiff neck after a fall or a road accident of this type should be suspected of having a cervical spine injury, which may be potentially dangerous. If it is possible to lie the patient on his back this will bring the cervical spine into an extended position and this is the safest way to transport him. If, however, the patient is unconscious or there is some other contra-indication to the supine position the neck must be steadied gently by the first aid attendant whilst the patient is transferred to an Accident and Emergency department.

Many cervical spine injuries are stable with the spinous process fractured or the vertebral body crushed. In these instances a simple collar is the only requirement and this together with adequate rest and analgesics will allow the fracture to unite with good restoration of cervical spine movements.

It is the unstable dislocation or fracture-dislocation which is dangerous for the spinal cord may be damaged, producing either death or paraplegia.

Treatment of the unstable cervical fracture dislocation

This fracture, like all others, must be reduced and here again traction in an extended neck position is the answer. Skeletal traction must be used, for any other method of applying a pull to the neck is unsuccessful and extremely uncomfortable. Crutchfield tongs are inserted with spikes which pass through only the outer table of the skull. Traction of 20 to 30 pounds may be required to reduce the fracture dislocation of the cervical spine (Fig. 21.50). Traction for approximately 6 weeks is required and during this time the patient is best nursed on a circle electric bed (Fig. 21.51) or a Stryker frame which will allow the turning of the patient without disturbing the traction or the position of the cervical spine. If the cervical spine is found to be stable at the end of this 6 weeks' period a plaster collar may be applied for a further 6 weeks. If the cervical spine still remains unstable at the end of the 6 weeks, fusion of the unstable segments should be undertaken by means of either an anterior approach with insertion of graft into the damaged vertebral bodies, or by a posterior approach in which the spinous processes are wired together and strut grafts are applied along the laminae of the vertebrae (Fig. 21.52).

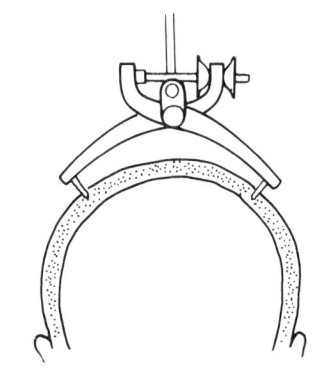

Fig. 21.50. Crutchfield tongs.

Thoracic spine

Thoracic vertebral bodies are frequently crushed in flexion injuries in the elderly osteoporotic patient. There is initial pain and tenderness and there may be some difficulty in rehabilitation of the patient. This fracture is stable and requires no more active treatment than extension exercises and active mobilisation as soon as the patient is comfortable.

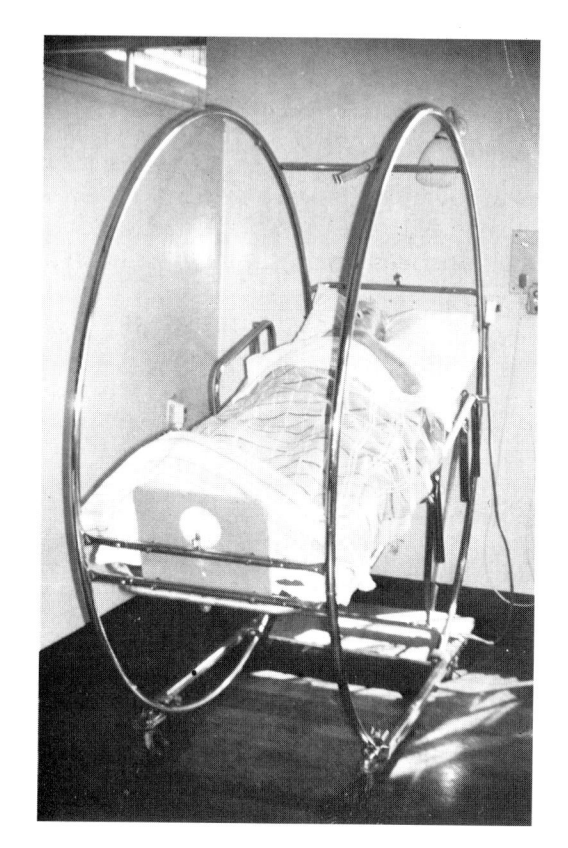

Fig. 21.51. Circle-electric bed.

Fig. 21.52. Posterior cervical fusion.

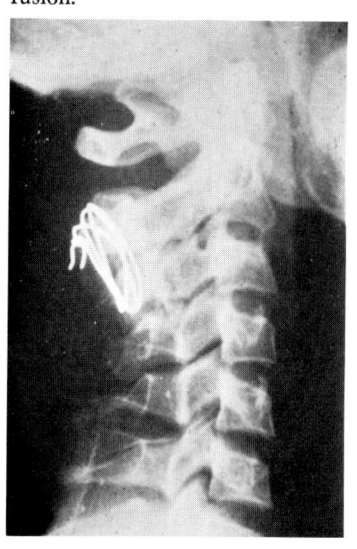

Lumbar spine

Fractures in this region may again be stable or unstable. If they are stable the same principles apply, with bed rest and analgesics being given until the patient is comfortable. Active mobilisation with particular emphasis on extension exercises are given as soon as possible.

Unstable fracture dislocations of the lumbar spine

This is a serious injury for damage to the cauda equina may occur at time of injury or later if the first aid measures have not prevented further movement at the fracture site. The patient must be treated with great care at the site of the accident and also whilst being transported to the hospital. If he is to be carried on a stretcher it is best to do so lying on his front for the extended position of the spine will tend to prevent further shift and dislocation.

Neurological signs of paralysis and anaesthesia in the lower limbs together with bladder paralysis indicates damage to the nerve roots in the cauda equina. The patient must be nursed as described above on a circle electric bed or a Stryker frame. The nursing areas of particular importance are:

1. Pressure areas. Frequent turning and attention to pressure points must be made.
2. The bladder. Catheterisation is undertaken initially but later regular expression of urine may be made by pressure on the lower abdomen. A urinary antiseptic must be given e.g. sulphadimidine 0.5 gm q.d.s.
3. The chest. The avoidance of chest infection is important. Frequent deep breathing exercises are encouraged.
4. Rehabilitation. When the initial problems of the paralysed patient are over, the nurse will be part of the team which will undertake the rehabilitation programme. The eventual outcome will depend upon the neurological level of paralysis, but with the help of the physiotherapist, physical medicine consultant, appliance maker and social worker the patient should be able to return to a suitable job and lead a reasonably happy and useful life.

Operative treatment

Internal fixation of the unstable fracture dislocation of the lumbar spine may be necessary. The patient who has minor neurological signs but an unstable injury would benefit from this procedure. The spine is explored posteriorly and fixation plates and bolts hold the spinous processes in good position (Fig. 21.53). Bone grafts are laid along the exposed areas and will allow the unstable segments to solidly fuse together.

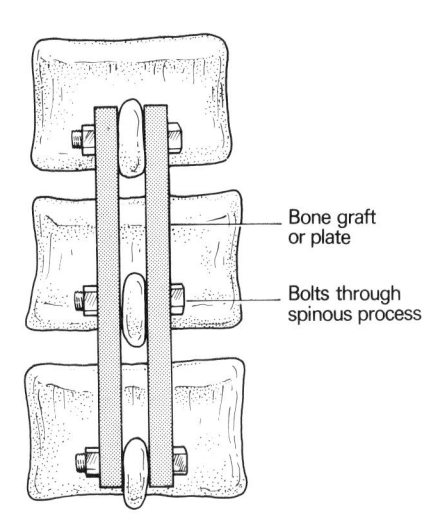

Fig. 21.53. Posterior fusion of lumbar spine.

518
Chapter 21

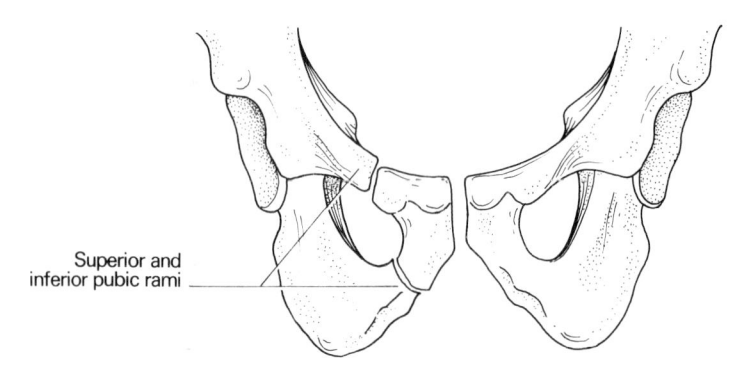

Superior and inferior pubic rami

Fig. 21.54. Fracture of the pubic rami.

Fig. 21.55. Major pelvic ring fractures.

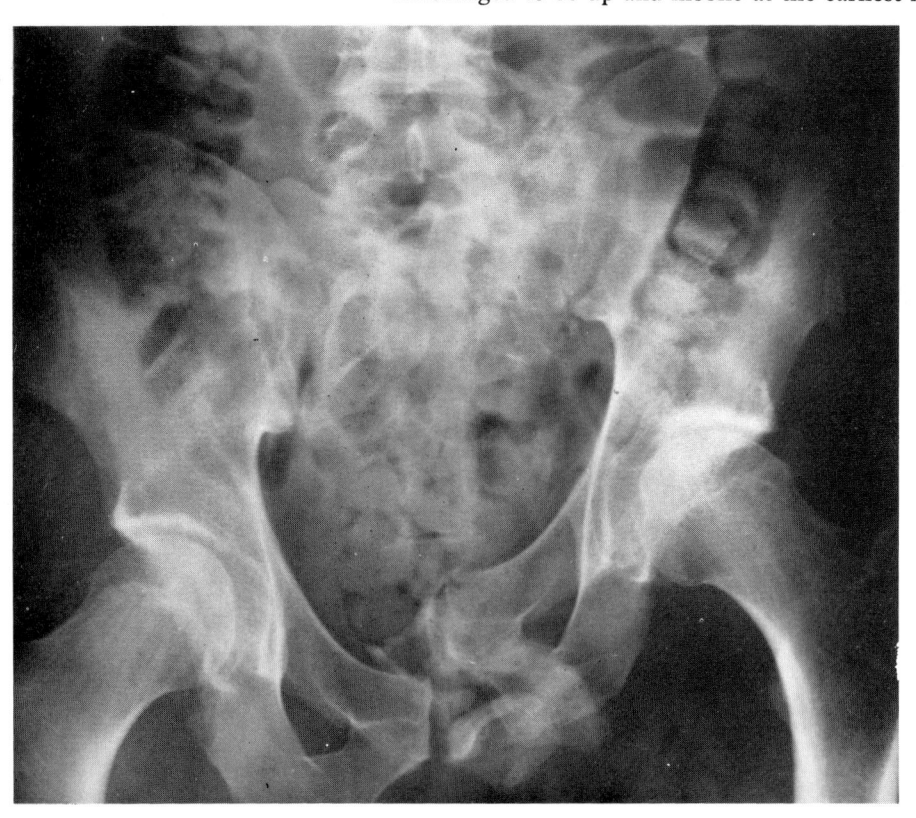

PELVIC FRACTURES

Fractures of the pelvic ring are common and may be sustained by both minor falls and by major crushing injuries. Minor fractures of the pubic rami (Fig. 21.54) occur commonly in the elderly and osteoporotic patients and cause enough pain to prevent walking for a few days. No specific treatment is necessary but the patient must be encouraged to be up and mobile at the earliest moment.

Crushing injuries which are sustained frequently in road traffic accidents may disrupt the pelvic ring by producing fractures in two or more places (Fig. 21.55). A prolonged period of bed rest is required and often traction to one or both lower limbs is helpful to re-position the fragments.

Complications

1. Haemorrhage. Much of the pelvic bone is cancellous and bleeding from fractured areas may be enormous. Several bottles of blood may be required to restore the blood volume following an injury of this type, and the retroperitoneal haematoma which develops may be equivalent to the size of a 30 week pregnancy.
2. Damage to pelvic viscera. The bladder, and more particularly the urethra, may be damaged by anterior pubic fractures especially in those cases in which a segment is pushed backwards. Any attempt at catheterisation following a pelvic injury must be carried out in the operating theatre if the possibility of urethral or bladder damage is expected. (See pages 342 and 347).

Chapter 22. Orthopaedics

Orthopaedics means literally the 'straight child' (orthos and pais in Greek) and the first part of this chapter will be devoted to deformities and diseases of childhood. Orthopaedic surgery covers a wide range of deformities, diseases and ailments of the locomotor system and especially those affecting the limbs, bones, muscles and joints. It is a speciality which is closely connected with the trauma described in Chapter 21 and orthopaedic surgeons usually deal with both injuries and elective orthopaedic problems.

PAEDIATRIC ORTHOPAEDICS

There are many congenital deformities, some single and others complex and multiple, which affect the locomotor system. In most the aetiology is unknown but recent advances in genetics indicate that some are due to abnormalities of the chromosomal composition of the cells. Disease in pregnancy such as rubella may produce abnormalities and the administration of thalidomide to pregnant women during the late 1950s and early 1960s produced a large number of skeletal deformities. Most of the common problems discussed in this section are of unknown aetiology.

CONGENITAL DISLOCATION OF THE HIP (C.D.H.)

This serious abnormality affects girls more frequently than boys (6:1) and the incidence in most of the United Kingdom is approximately 3 per 1000 live births. There is a definite familial incidence and its occurrence is high in certain races such as the North Italians and also the North American Indians. The babies born by breech delivery are especially at risk and the underlying anatomical abnormality is most probably laxity of the hip joint ligaments.

Diagnosis

It is important to diagnose the condition in the early neonatal period for treatment may be fully corrective if started at this early stage. Unstable hips are diagnosed by clinical means and not by X-ray for the joint is too immature skeletally. It is important that the midwife and paediatrician examine the hips of all babies born, for delayed diagnosis may complicate treatment seriously.

If there is a full dislocation the limb will be shorter and abduction of the hip will be limited. Abduction of the hips, as shown in Fig. 22.1 will produce a clunk and a movement of the head of the femur when the hip rides in and out of socket. This is called Ortolani's click test. If the pelvis is steadied with one hand and the suspicious hip manipulated as shown in Fig. 22.2 again a clunk with movement indicates a subluxation or full dislocation of this unstable hip (Barlow's test).

If diagnosis is not made by the medical attendants in the neonatal period then the mother sometimes notices shortening and the absence of full movement of the hip at six months of age. More frequently it is not until the limp is noted at about 16 months that diagnosis is made. By this stage the radiological appearance is very abnormal (Fig. 22.3).

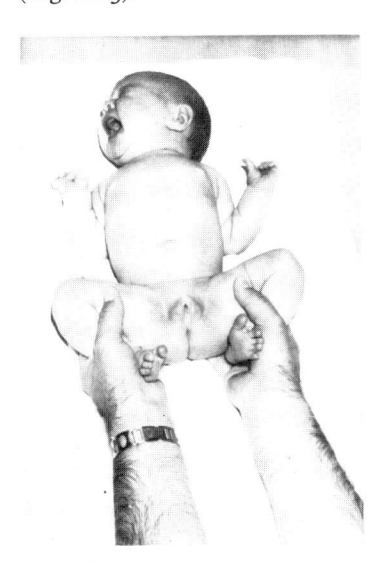

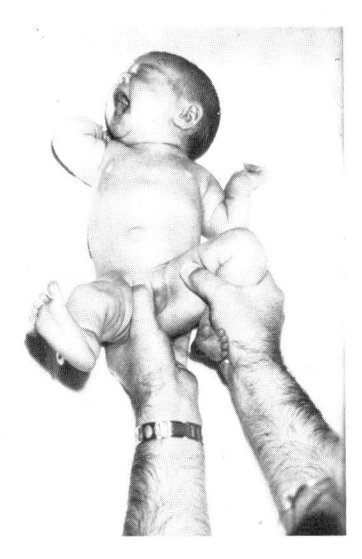

Fig. 22.1. (LEFT) Ortolani's test for hip instability.

Fig. 22.2. (RIGHT) Barlow's test. The pelvis is fixed and the hip is abducted.

Fig. 22.3. Congenital dislocation of the hip. The femoral head is displaced from the shallow acetabulum.

Treatment

In the neonatal period the application of an abduction splint for 6–8 weeks may be all that is necessary (Fig. 22.4). After 3 months of age, abduction of the hips and their retention in this position by a frog-style plaster (Fig. 22.5) allows the normal growth of the acetabulum to deepen the socket around the femoral head.

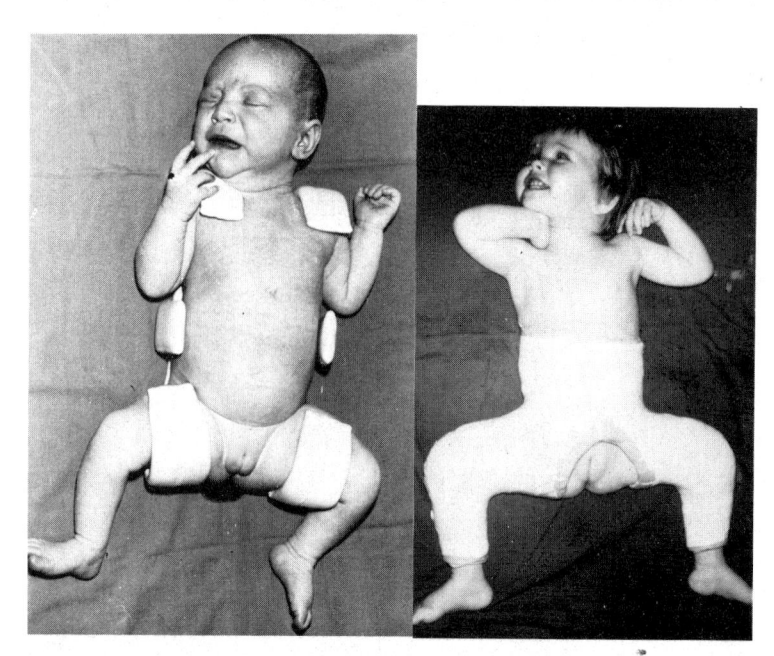

Fig. 22.4. Abduction splint.

Fig. 22.5. 'Frog' abduction plaster.

Conservative treatment is usually satisfactory until the age of one year but after this time operative treatment is usually necessary. If the hips are tight, abduction traction is applied slowly and increasingly from the neutral position to the fully separated position (Fig. 22.6). A plaster cast will then retain the reduced position and this is maintained until the socket is deepened enough.

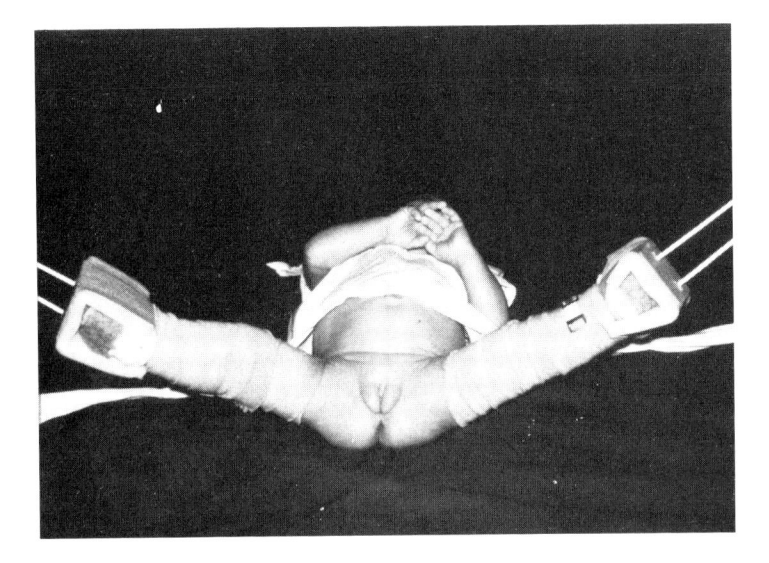

Fig. 22.6. Abduction traction.

After the age of one year operative treatment may become necessary to reduce the dislocation. Tight capsular and other obstructing structures are removed to enable the deeper setting of the femoral head. To give greater stability upper femoral osteotomy or pelvic osteotomy (Fig. 22.7) may be necessary. Meticulous follow-up of the child with a congenital dislocation or dysplasia of the hip will be necessary until skeletal maturity occurs.

Fig. 22.7. Salter's pelvic osteotomy to deepen acetabular socket.

The untreated or, even worse, the inadequately treated hip dislocation will lead to gross hip deformity and osteoarthritis in later life.

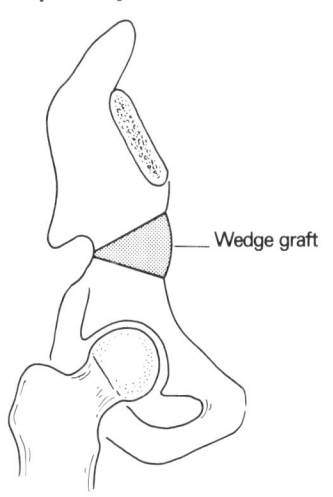

CONGENITAL CLUB FOOT (Talipes Equino-Varus, T.E.V.)

The term talipes refers to any foot and ankle deformity. The deformed foot is in equinus (plantar flexion), varus (with the soles turned in) and the forefoot ia adducted (twisted towards the mid-line). The whole deformity is illustrated in Fig. 22.8.

The club foot is a difficult deformity to treat successfully. It is commoner in boys (3:1) and occurs in its full form in approximately 2 per 1,000 live births. Its minor forms are more common.

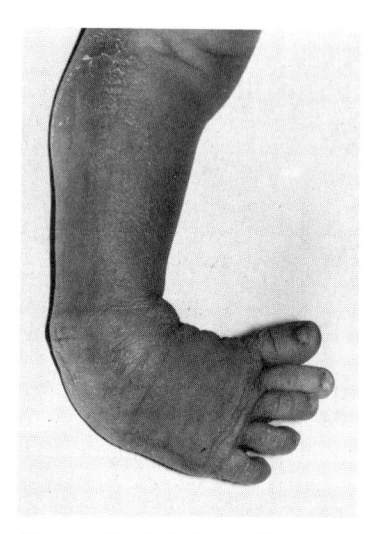

Fig. 22.8. Club foot (talipes-equino-varus).

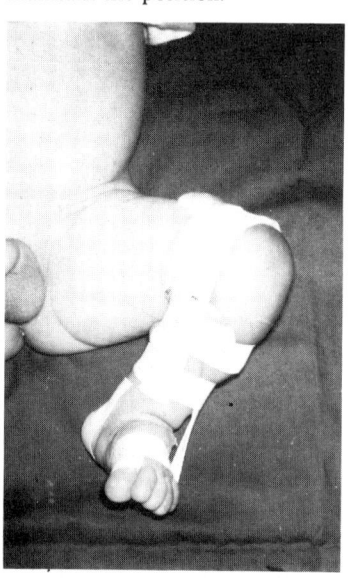

Fig. 22.9. The foot is strapped to maintain the position.

The club foot deformity may be due to a neurological abnormality such as spina bifida or later acquired in poliomyelitis but most of the babies seen with this abnormality have a congenital talipes equino-varus, of unknown aetiology.

Treatment

Early treatment is again important, and manipulation should be started by the surgeon or the physiotherapist on the first day of life. The soft tissues later become more contracted and difficult to stretch and eventually a secondary bone deformity develops.

Very regular stretching and manipulation is essential for success. The varus heel must be stretched outwards and the equinus foot must be manipulated upwards to the neutral position. The inturned forefoot is corrected and strapping is then applied to maintain the position (Figs.s 22.9 and 22.10).

In approximately half the babies the foot may be corrected without operation. After 6–8 weeks of meticulous manipulation a decision can be reached as to whether conservative treatment will be successfull or not. If surgical assistance is necessary it is best to release the deformity at this early stage. Releasing the tight Achilles tendon posteriorly will be sufficient in some but in the others more extensive surgical release will be necessary.

SPINA BIFIDA & MYELOMENINGOCELE

This is a relatively common deformity (2.5 per thousand live births) and occurs when the posterior elements of the spine fail to form and allow the meninges, spinal cord and nerve roots to prolapse through to the body surface (Fig. 22.11). The lumbar region is most commonly involved but it can occur at any spinal level.

Hydrocephalus occurs in 80% of these children and the head swells progressively due to enlargement of the brain ventricles filled with excessive cerebro-spinal fluid under high pressure.

Treatment

Babies with this condition pose a severe moral and ethical problem for the obstetrician and paediatrician. Many of the children will develop severe disturbances of intellect, abnormalities of the urinary tract and paralysis of the lower limbs. The prognosis is worst if the myelomeningocele is high in the spine and covers many segments.

If the defect is not closed many will die of a meningitis. The child with a surgically closed defect will usually require insertion of a

Spitz-Holter valve to drain the cerebro-spinal fluid from the ventricles to the right superior vena cava and right atrium of the heart. This drainage of cerebro-spinal fluid will prevent hydrocephalus from developing (see page 134).

Bladder paralysis and subsequent problems of the urinary tract are often treated by the formation of an ileal loop bladder. Paralysis of the lower limbs is managed by appropriate calipers and braces (Fig. 22.12) but in some children stability and rebalance of musculature is achieved by muscle and tendon transpositions.

The lower limbs may be anaesthetic and the paralysis may be so severe that many children take to a wheelchair in later life.

SCOLIOSIS

Scoliosis is a lateral curvature of the spine (Fig. 22.13). The scoliosis may be postural when there is a sciatica and where there is no fixed anatomical abnormality. A true structural scoliosis with a fixed deformity is due to either congenital or acquired causes:

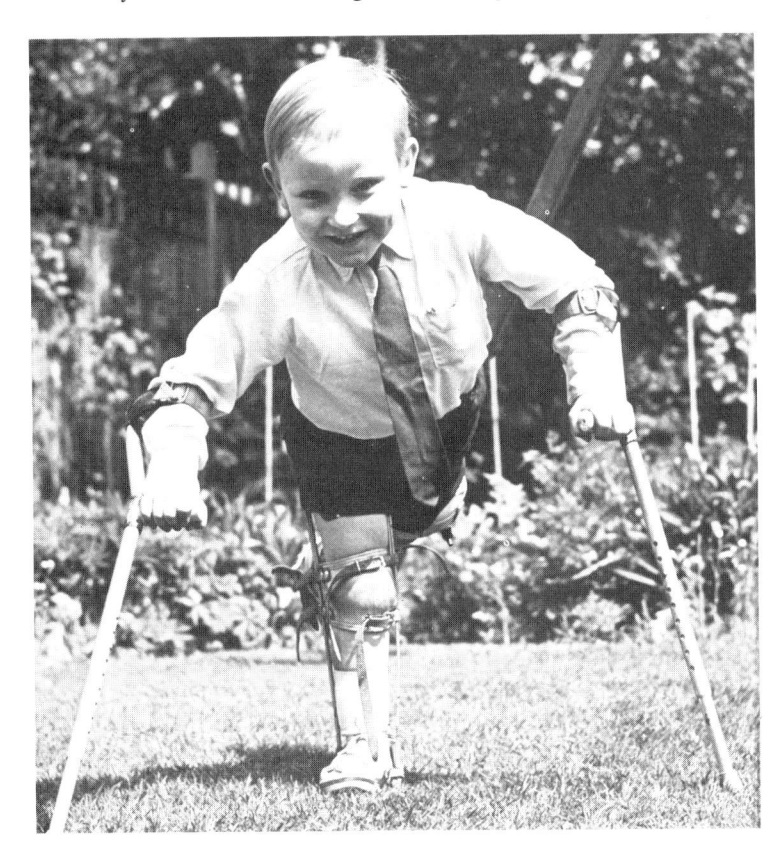

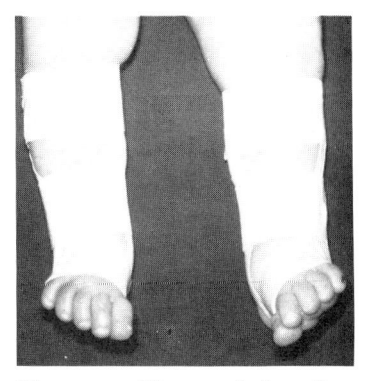

Fig. 22.10. The completion of successful conservative treatment.

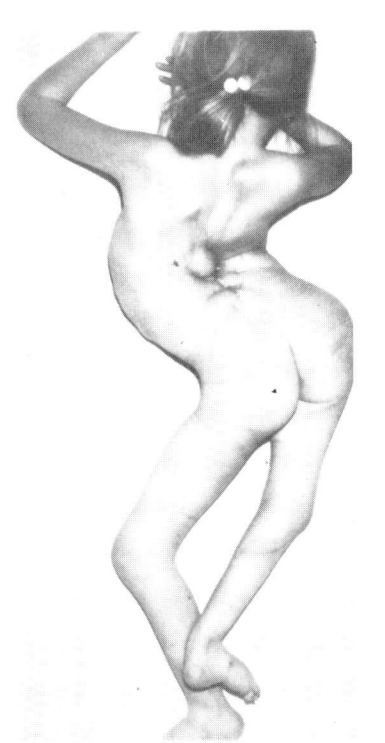

Fig. 22.11. Spina bifida and myelomeningocele.

Fig. 22.12. Caliper and brace to stabilise paralysed lower limbs.

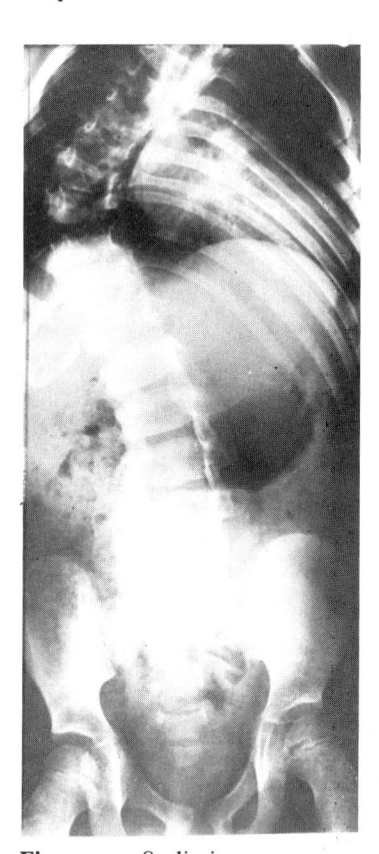

Fig. 22.13. Scoliosis.

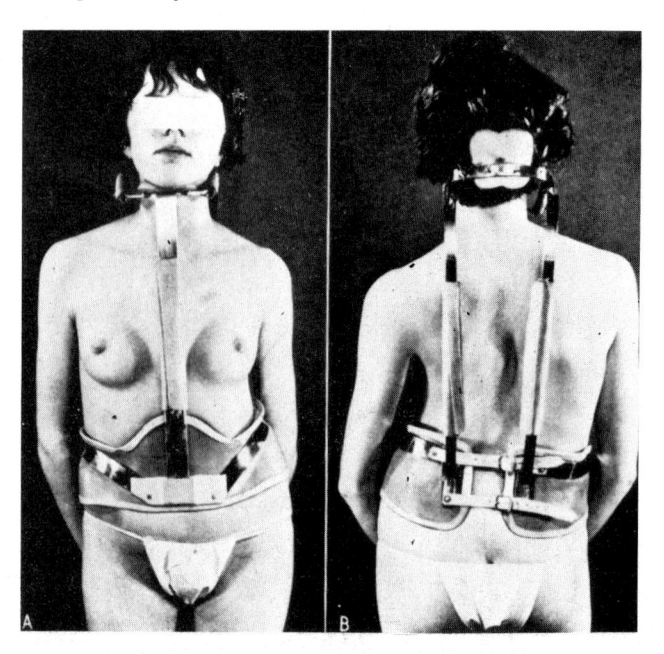

Fig. 22.14. Milwaukee brace to hold the scoliotic spine.

Congenital scoliosis occurs where there are abnormalities of the structure of a vertebral body or a spinal segment.

Paralytic—poliomyelitis or other neurological problems produce inbalance of spinal musculature.

Idiopathic—This is the commonest variety and has no known cause. The curve may increase and may be associated with rotation of the chest cage, producing an unsightly rib hump. The severe scoliosis will produce a decrease in the lung function.

The management

When the skeleton is mature the curve will cease to progress. In children below 10 years of age with a progressive scoliosis a brace must be worn (Fig. 22.14).

Operation is necessary over the age of 10 when the type of scoliosis curve is known to be progressive. A period of stretching in a halo-pelvic traction apparatus may be required pre-operatively (Fig. 22.15) and at operation spinal fusion is carried out, sometimes associated with a Harrington distraction rod (Fig. 22.16).

OSTEOMYELITIS

Bone infection, or osteomyelitis, may affect any part of the skeleton. The child is more frequently affected than the adult but no age is exempt. It may be acute or chronic.

Acute osteomyelitis

Pyogenic organisms such as the staphylococcus, streptococcus, pneumococcus, meningococcus, and more rarely the gonococcus and E. coli spread by the blood stream from an infected focus, such as a boil, to the metaphyseal area of a bone (Fig. 22.17). Pus soon forms and bursts out through the cortex of the bone to lie beneath the periosteum. The pressure of pus cuts off the blood supply to some areas of the bone; this dead necrotic bone is called a *sequestrum* (Fig. 22.18).

Clinical features

Pain rapidly becomes intense and the child becomes pyrexial and ill. Local signs of inflammation soon become apparent over the infected bone with increased heat, swelling, redness and tenderness. The diagnosis is made from the above symptoms and signs and a blood culture usually grows the infecting organisms. X-rays are not helpful in the first week but during this time it is important to make the diagnosis. Later a periosteal reaction is seen on X-ray and bone destruction in the metaphyseal region becomes apparent. A sequestrum is seen in the later stages as a dense sclerotic area (Fig. 22.19).

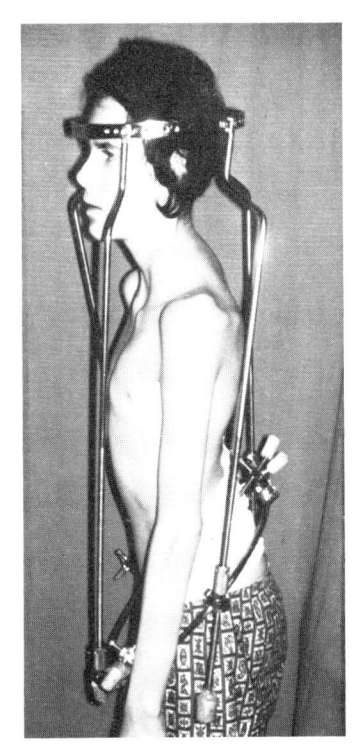

Fig. 22.15. Halo-pelvic traction.

Treatment

Antibiotics alone may be successful in the earliest stage. A large dose of cloxacillin and ampicillin together (adult dose 500 mg and 250 mg q.d.s. respectively) is given. When the blood culture is known, the appropriate single antibiotic can then be prescribed. If the temperature and local signs are not reversed within the first 48 hours of this medication operation is indicated.

The bone is exposed at the site of maximum inflammation and the periosteum is incised. Pus is sometimes found beneath the periosteum but failing this the bone is drilled and pus may be found within.

Chronic osteomyelitis

This may follow an acute osteomyelitis with pyogenic organisms. Infection with tubercle bacilli may produce a chronic osteomyelitis and Pott's disease of the spine is a good example (Fig. 22.20). The tubercle bacilli becomes established in the disc space and spread into the vertebral bodies on either side. The wedge-shaped collapse of the vertebral bones produces an angular kyphosis of the spine, usually

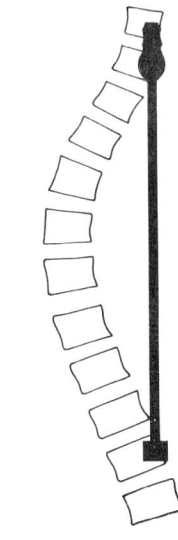

Fig. 22.16. Harrington rod correcting scoliosis at the time of spinal fusion.

Fig. 22.17. (LEFT) Osteomyelitis. Infection arises in the metaphysis of the bone.

Fig. 22.18. (RIGHT) Continued infection produces a necrotic sequestrum.

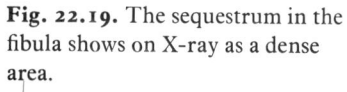

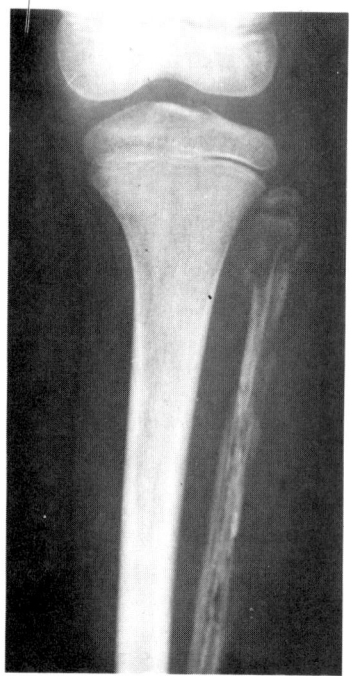

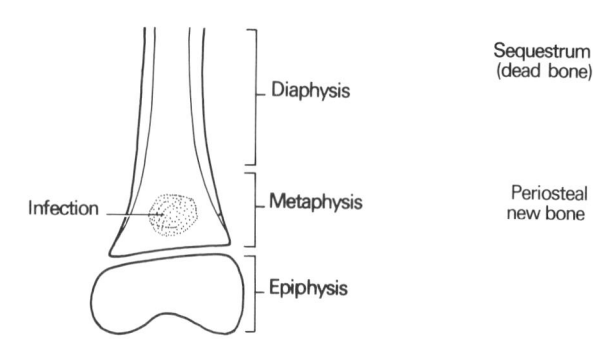

Fig. 22.19. The sequestrum in the fibula shows on X-ray as a dense area.

in the thoracic region. Pus may spread from the bone as a cold abscess compressing the spinal cord (Pott's paraplegia) or it may present in the groin as a psoas abscess.

SEPTIC ARTHRITIS

A joint may be affected with organisms similar to those found in osteomyelitis. Children are again particularly affected and the hip joint is the most common site of neonatal infection (Tom Smith's disease). The infection is blood-borne but in a few cases of septic arthritis of the knee a penetrating wound may be the cause of bacterial entry.

Clinical features

Pain and loss of function of the infected limb develops at an early stage. The child rapidly becomes ill and feverish and a blood culture may reveal the infecting organism. X-rays may show excessive distention of the joint cavity, and at a later stage erosion of the joint surfaces becomes apparent (Fig. 22.21).

A final diagnosis is made by aspirating the joint with a needle and syringe and if pus is present the joint must be opened and adequately drained under a general anaesthetic. Long-term antibiotics will again be required.

OSTEOARTHRITIS

All joints wear over the years. In some patients however, the wear and tear process is excessive and the joint becomes painful, stiff and eventually deformed. This process is now called degenerative joint disease or osteoarthrosis (osteoarthritis). It should be noted that there is no true inflammation but purely a degeneration of the articular cartilage. Eventually the cartilage wears away completely, leaving bone to articulate with bone. Secondary changes now occur with spurs of new bone forming around the joint margins (osteophytes), thickening of the bone ends (sclerosis), and cysts developing beneath the joint surface (Fig. 22.22).

Aetiology

Joints which have been previously damaged by infection or trauma develop a secondary osteoarthritis at an early stage. Primary or idiopathic osteoarthritis develops as a degeneration of the joint surface but the cause is unknown.

Clinical features

The first symptom is a little pain or ache after exercise in or around the joint affected. The disease is variably progressive and there are frequently exacerbations and remissions in the symptoms. The pain

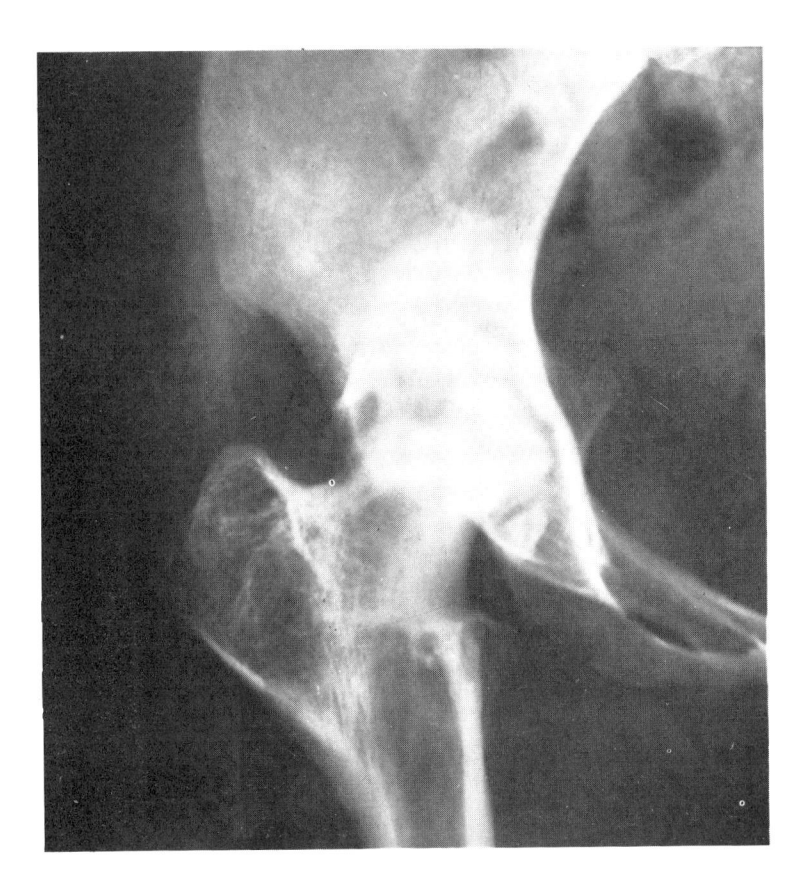

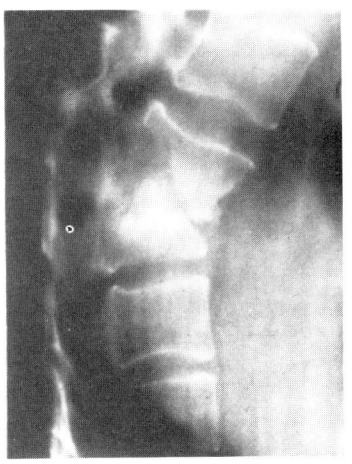

Fig. 22.20. Pott's disease (tuberculosis of the spine).

Fig. 22.21. Erosion of the joint surface in a septic arthritis.

may increase and may become particularly troublesome at night. Stiffness increases as the range of joint movement decreases and contractures eventually deform the joint and the limb.

Treatment

Osteoarthritis of the hip is the most common large joint affected and this will be used as an example to illustrate the range of therapy available.

1. *Medication.* Simple aspirin is useful to control the pain. Phenylbutazone 100 mg t.d.s. may be more effective in decreasing pain and stiffness.

2. *Support.* A stick is useful to decrease the weight put upon the affected hip.

3. *Physiotherapy.* Increasing the range of movement and strengthening of the musculature around the joint will always be beneficial. Exercise in a pool (hydrotherapy) may be particularly effective.

4. *Operative treatment.* If the above conservative measures are no longer effective the orthopaedic surgeon may consider one of the following procedures advisable:

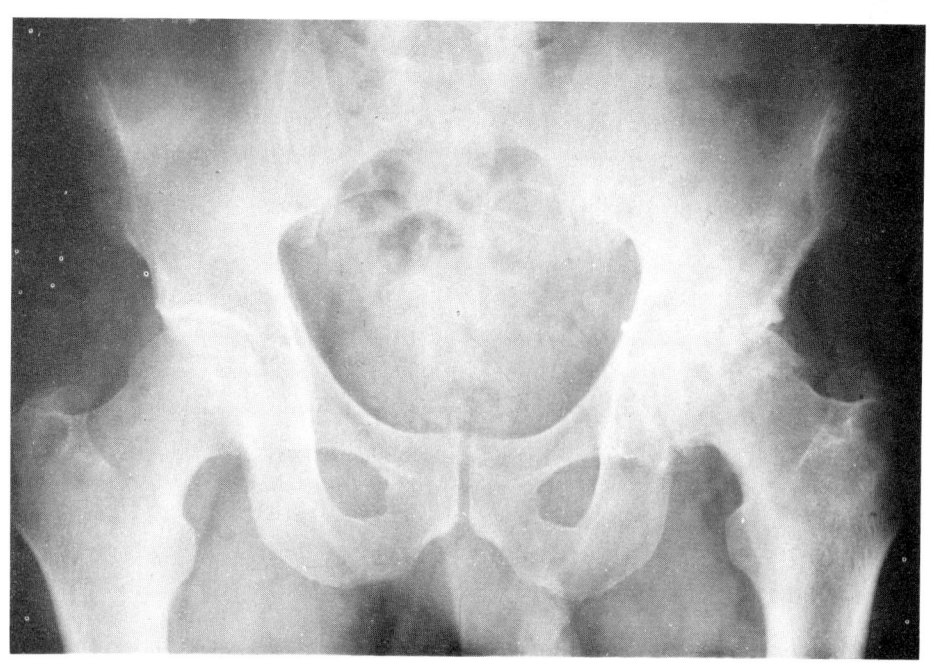

(i) *Trochanteric osteotomy*—Pain may be dramatically decreased by dividing the upper femur and repositioning the head and neck as shown in Fig. 22.23. A new articular area is brought into the

Fig. 22.22. Osteoarthritis of the left hip.

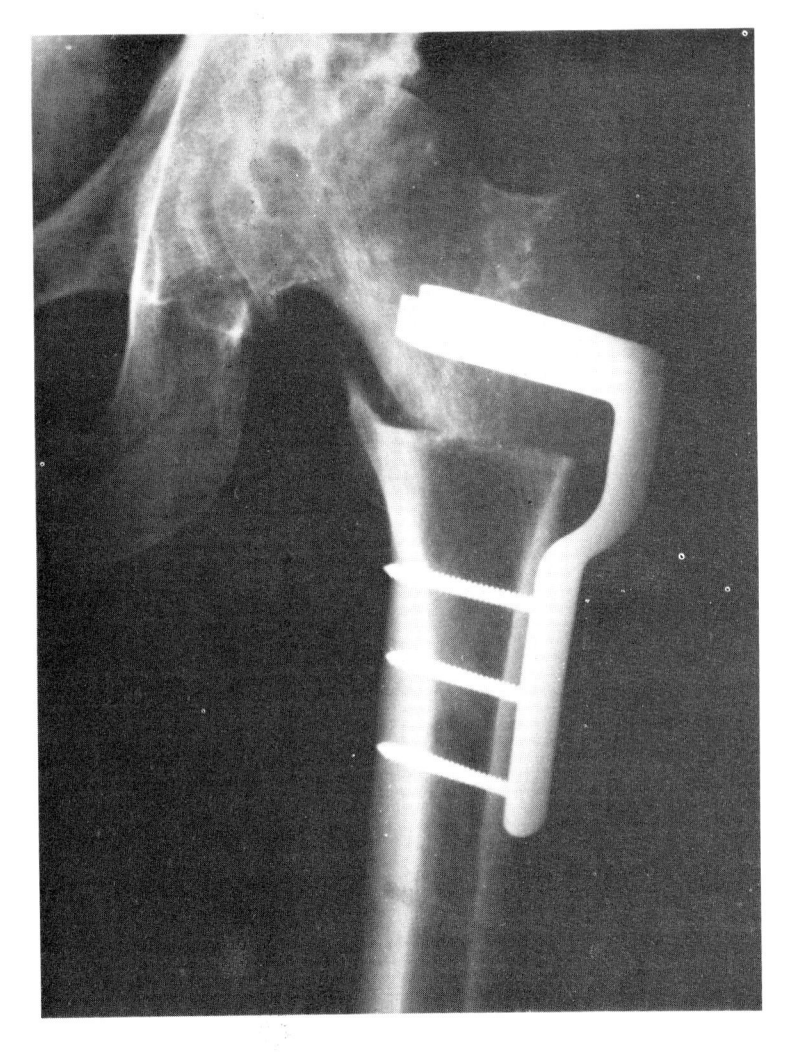

Fig. 22.23. Trochanteric osteotomy fixed with a blade plate.

acetabulum and the fracture healing process remodels the diseased bone of the femoral head. The operation is most effective in the osteoarthritic hip joint where there is considerable pain but still a good range of movement. The osteotomy is only successful in relieving the symptoms in two-thirds of the patients operated upon.

(ii) *Total hip replacement arthroplasty*—When the destructive arthritic changes are very severe, replacement of both surfaces of the joint becomes necessary. The head and neck are removed, the acetabular cartilage is excised and the socket deepened. A plastic acrylic cement substance is used to seat firmly the metal or polyethylene components of the new joint. There are many types of total replacement arthroplasty but they fall into two categories: (1) the

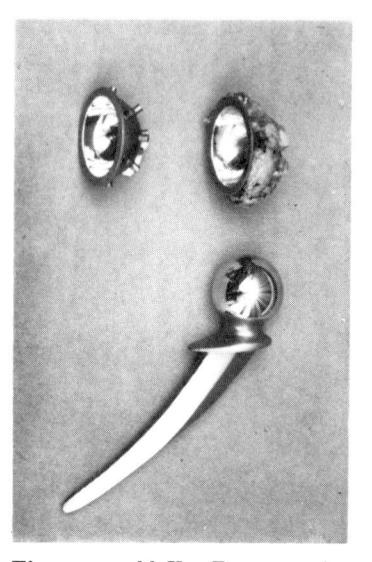

Fig. 22.24. McKee Farrar total hip replacement.

Fig. 22.25. Charnley total hip replacement.

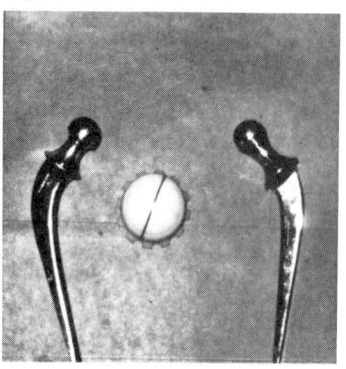

metal to metal bearing prosthesis typified by the McKee Farrar model (Fig. 22.24), (2) the metal to high density polyethylene bearing prosthesis of the Charnley type (Fig. 22.25).

These replacement arthroplasties are very successful in returning mobility and comfort to the joint. Complications are few but dislocation may be a problem if the components are not angulated correctly. Infection will always be disastrous and steps must be taken to keep this complication as low as possible.

(iii) *Arthrodesis*—Arthrodesis means the elimination of the joint articulating surfaces and fusion together of the two bones. Arthrodesis produces a painless, stable situation but there is, of course, no mobility. A hip may be arthrodesed in the young person and is usually carried out in the osteoarthritic hip which develops secondary to previous trauma or infection. It is impossible to arthrodese both sides.

RHEUMATOID ARTHRITIS

Rheumatoid arthritis is an inflammatory disease of joints which affects both young and old. There is also a juvenile type called Still's disease.

The first site of this disease is in the synovial membrane lining the joint. This membrane becomes inflamed and thickened and gradually proliferates to eat away the surrounding ligaments and articular cartilage of the joint surfaces. It affects peripheral small joints initially but later the larger weight-bearing joints may become affected.

Treatment

The treatment of rheumatoid arthritis is essentially medical but surgery may have a small part to play. Rest is important in the acute phase and medicines are given to prevent pain and inflammation. Aspirin, 300–600 mg several times each day and phenylbutazone, 100 mg t.d.s. are commonly used. The physiotherapist is an important member of the team treating the patient with this disease for she will help to preserve the mobility and strength of the joints. The occupational therapist will also give good advice as to the aids which may be helpful to the disabled person.

Surgery has a small but important part in the management of the patient with rheumatoid arthritis. Frequently very small surgical procedures have great benefit and such operations as repair of ruptured tendons, release of trigger fingers or release of carpal tunnel syndromes, may help the patient greatly.

Rheumatoid disease may so destroy joints that surgical replacements may become necessary. At the hip the total replacements are very successful. The knee is a difficult joint to replace but a hinge-type prosthesis is indicated in some, and a condylar type replacement of the joint surfaces in others (Fig. 22.26).

Arthrodesis of the knee produces a stable, painless, but fixed joint but again this can only be performed on one side. The hand becomes grossly deformed by rheumatoid disease (Fig. 22.27) but the patients may retain remarkably good function with destroyed joints. There is an indication to replace the metacarpal-phalangeal joints with silastic hinges in some but it should be stressed that the indication for joint surgery of this type is gross limitation of function (Fig. 22.28). The poor appearance of the hand does not constitute an indication for surgical intervention.

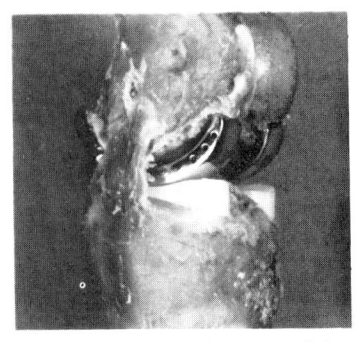

Fig. 22.26. Westminster condylar replacement of the knee. The femoral surfaces are replaced with metal and the tibial surfaces with polyethylene.

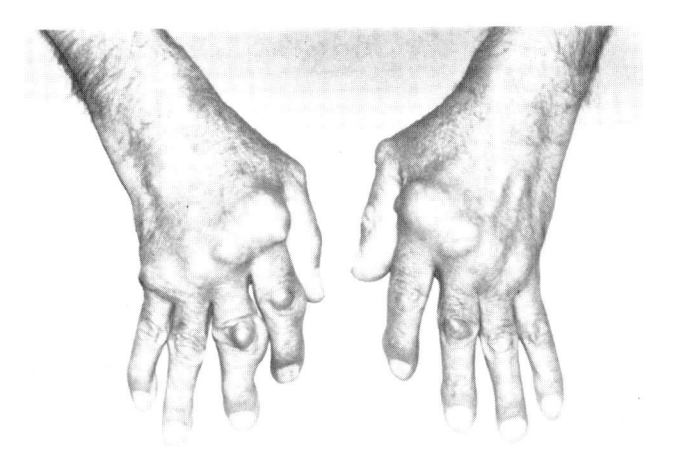

Fig. 22.27. (LEFT) The hand affected by rheumatoid arthritis.

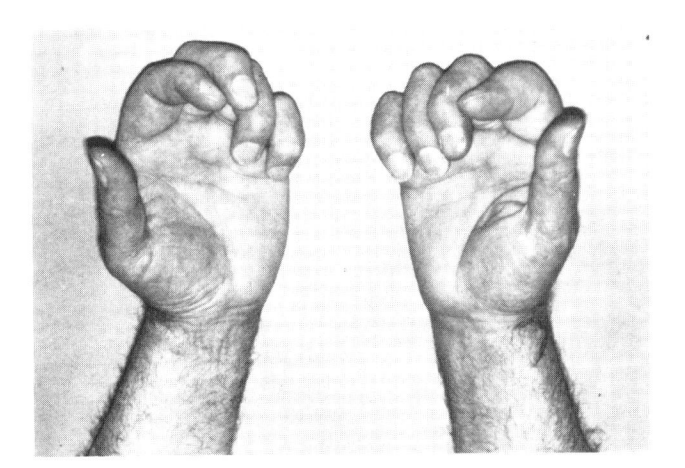

Fig. 22.28. Rheumatoid hand with an extremely poor grip.

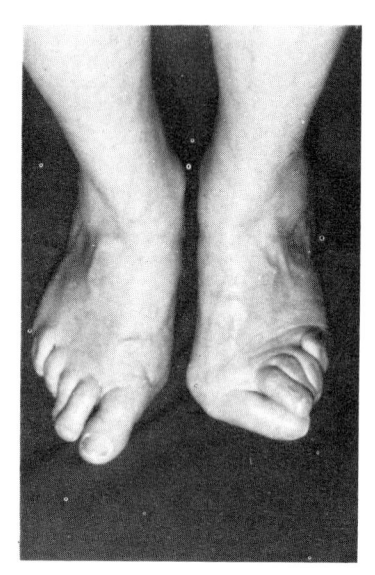

Fig. 22.29. The right forefoot has been treated by excision of the metatarsal heads.

The toes frequently become very deformed and dislocated on the metacarpals. Excision of the metatarsal heads will restore the shape and comfort of the foot (Fig. 22.29).

BONE TUMOURS

Tumours affecting the skeleton are either benign or malignant. Malignant tumours are primary when they originate in bone or secondary when they have spread to bone from a tumour in another organ. The most common bone tumour which is seen is a secondary deposit (Fig. 22.30). The tumours which particularly spread to bone

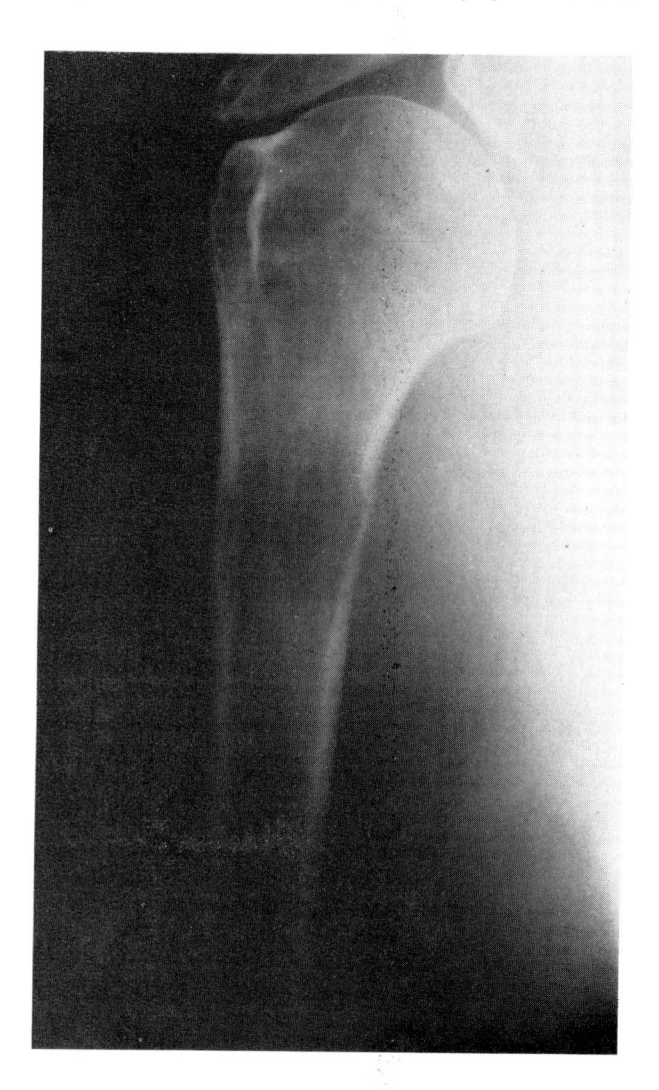

Fig. 22.30. A metastasis in the humerus. The primary was a carcinoma of the lung.

are carcinomas of the breast in the female and bronchus in the male. The prostate, kidney and thyroid when affected by cancers may all spread to the skeleton.

BENIGN TUMOURS

1. *Osteoma*—this produces a bony lump called an exostosis. It is frequently found in the child as a single lesion but in the condition called diaphyseal aclasis multiple exostoses are seen (Fig. 22.31).

2. *Chondroma*—these cartilage tumours develop within or upon the surface of bone. They frequently present as pathological fractures in the bones of the hand (Fig. 22.32).

3. *Fibroma*—these are frequently seen in X-rays of children's long bones. They usually disappear at the time of skeletal maturity but large areas of fibrous dysplasia may sometimes persist in the bone shaft (Fig. 22.33).

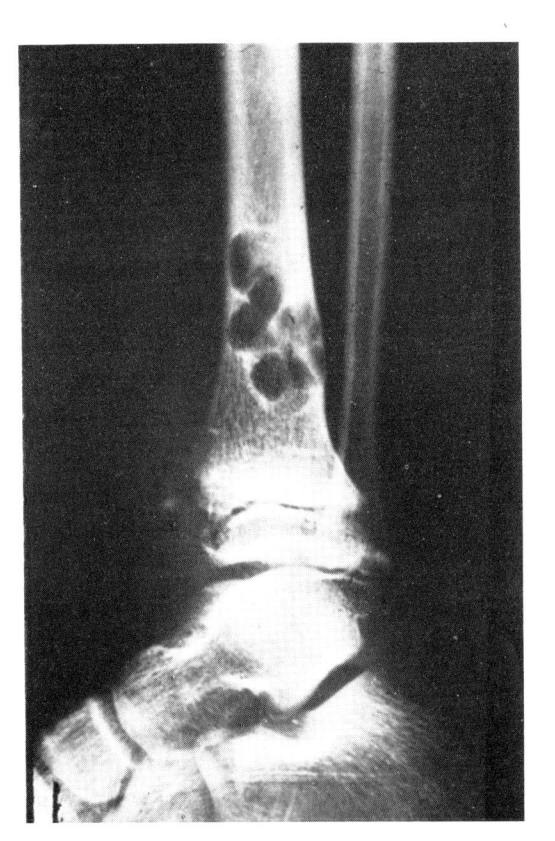

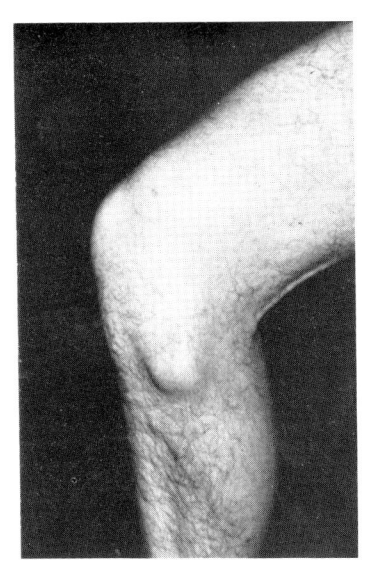

Fig. 22.31. An upper tibial exostosis.

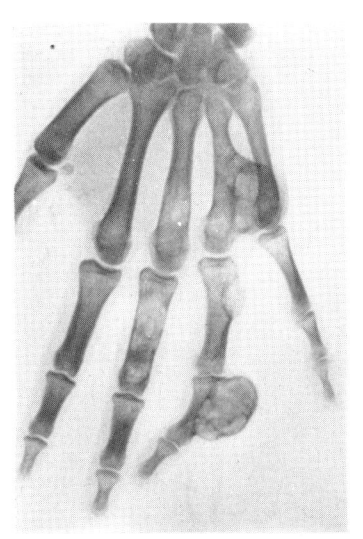

Fig. 22.32. Chondromas of metacarpals and phalanges.

Fig. 22.33. Fibroma.

GIANT CELL TUMOUR (Osteoclastoma)

This is a primary bone tumour which affects the mature skeleton, particularly in the upper tibia and lower femur. The epiphyseal area of the bone is affected and a tumour mass may approach the joint surface. It may remain benign and treatment consists of simply curetting the tumour from the bone. It may be locally recurrent and now more radical measures may have to be undertaken. It may be fully malignant with a production of distant metastases.

Wide local excision of the more aggressive giant cell tumour may be necessary and the neighbouring joint may require replacement with a total prosthesis.

MALIGNANT BONE TUMOURS

2. *Osteosarcoma*—This is a very malignant primary bone tumour which affects young people between the ages of five and twenty-five. It is also seen in the elderly patient and occurs in an area of Paget's disease of bone. Most osteosarcomas develop de novo without known cause but a few may follow radiotherapy to the skeleton.

Clinical features

The osteosarcoma is a very rare tumour and diagnosis is frequently delayed. A lump in relationship to the knee is the most common presenting sign and the swelling may become acutely inflamed and may be mistaken for a bone infection or a joint injury. The X-rays shows much new bone together with bone disruption, as illustrated in Fig. 22.34. The definite diagnosis can only be made on biopsy and a very careful examination of the patient clinically, radiologically, and by bone gamma-scan will be necessary to exclude distant metastases. The tumour rapidly and aggressively metastasises to the lungs and this is the reason for not advising radical amputation of the limb at an early stage.

The tumour is irradiated with a high dose of deep X-rays and then careful follow-up is undertaken over the next 6 months. In many cases metastases will develop during these months but in some no spread will be detected.

At the end of the 6 month period the patient is again carefully reviewed and if there is certainly no evidence of lung or distant metastases then the amputation of the limb will be performed. This treatment programme will eliminate much unnecessary suffering for the amputation of a limb will be avoided in a child who develops metastases after just a few weeks or months. In spite of this treatment regimen the 5 year survival rate still remains at 25%.

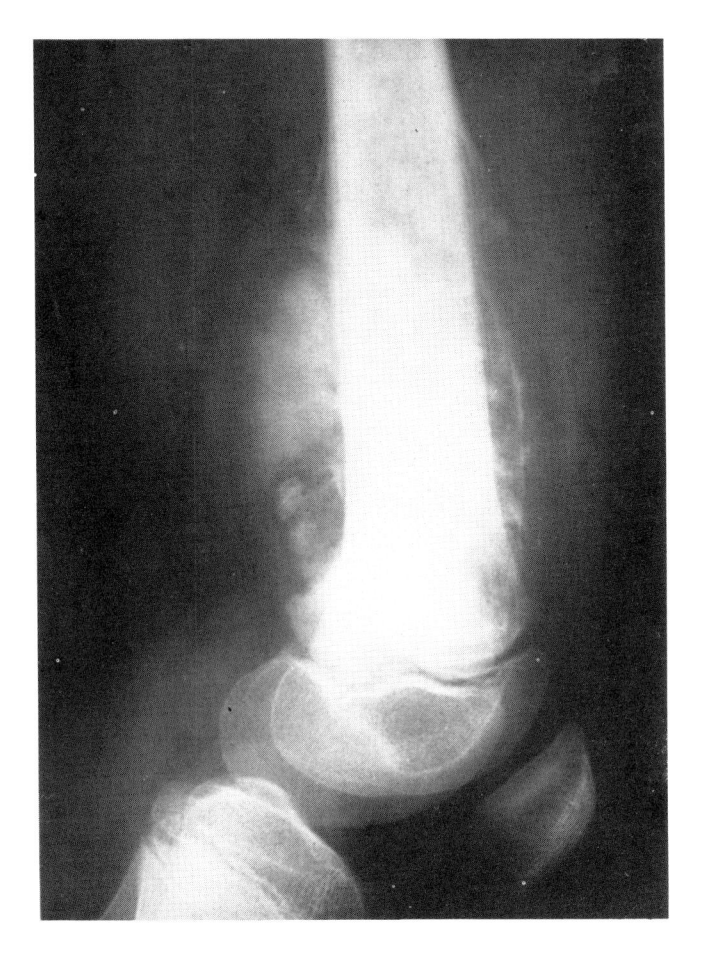

Fig. 22.34. Osteosarcoma of the lower femur.

2. *Chondrosarcoma*—This is a malignant cartilage tumour which usually requires radical amputation for its treatment. It is not quite so malignant as the osteosarcoma but the survival rate is again poor.

3. *Ewing's sarcoma*—This is another very malignant tumour affecting the mid-shaft region of the long bones of the child. Radiotherapy is the treatment of choice but the mortality is extremely high.

NEUROLOGICAL CONDITIONS PRODUCING DEFORMITY

1. **Poliomyelitis**

This is now a rare condition in Western countries but it is still seen in less developed areas of the world. A virus infection affects the anterior horn cells of the spinal cord and produces a flaccid paralysis of the limbs.

The principles of treatment are to maintain the stability and balance of the limb by:
(i) using calipers to brace the limb.
(ii) joint stabilisation operation such as foot or wrist arthrodesis.
(iii) tendon transfers to make good use of the remaining muscles in a paralysed area.

2. Hemiplegias

Cerebro-vascular accidents frequently leave the patient with a hemiplegia. The muscles are spastic and the joints become deformed. Full rehabilitation of the patient is necessary and joint abnormalities may be helped by the lengthening or division of tight tendons. Calipers are again often useful for support.

3. Cerebral palsy

Birth trauma may produce a spastic paraplegia. The child may be of normal intelligence but there is often some associated mental handicap. Spasticity of the muscles of the limbs produce gross problems of function and the joints may become deformed. Treatment in a special spastics centre is ideal for there are particular educational needs and the physiotherapist will be able to continue long-term treatment. Surgery has only a very small part to play in the treatment of these disabled children but simple measures such as the lengthening of tendons and the release of contractures may assist the balance and the walking ability.

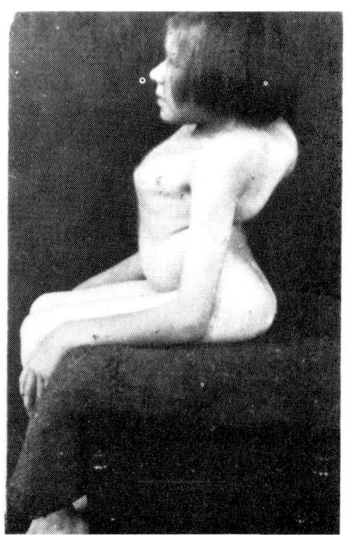

Fig. 22.35. A thoracic spine kyphosis.

BONE DISEASES

Osteoporosis

A decrease in the protein part of the bone matrix produces a decrease in the bone strength. It occurs especially in the elderly and is associated with the post-menopausal state in the female. It is exacerbated by a poor diet. The decrease in bone strength allows crush fracture to occur in the vertebral bodies and the spine becomes slowly kyphotic (Fig. 22.35). Hip fractures are common in the elderly female suffering from osteoporosis.

Osteomalacia

This occurs when there is a decrease in the mineral content of bone and may be associated with kidney disease and steatorrhoea syndromes. Pathological fractures are common.

Rickets

This is a disease seen in the child and is again characterised by a defect in the mineral content. The most common cause throughout the world is a deficiency of vitamin D in the diet but again kidney and alimentary disease may be responsible. The child affected becomes progressively ill and the bones become bowed and deformed. Growth decreases and the ends of the long bones become widened (Fig. 22.36).

Treatment with extra vitamin D is essential and where there is deformity in the more established case bone division and realignment may be necessary.

Fragilitis osseum (osteogenesis imperfecta)

This is an abnormality of primitive mesoderm tissue. It is characterised by soft bones with multiple fractures (Fig. 22.37) and the sclera of the eyes is frequently blue. There is a congenital type in which multiple fractures are present at birth and a tarda type in which the disease is not so progressive. Deformity follows multiple fractures, and treatment by internal fixation is necessary.

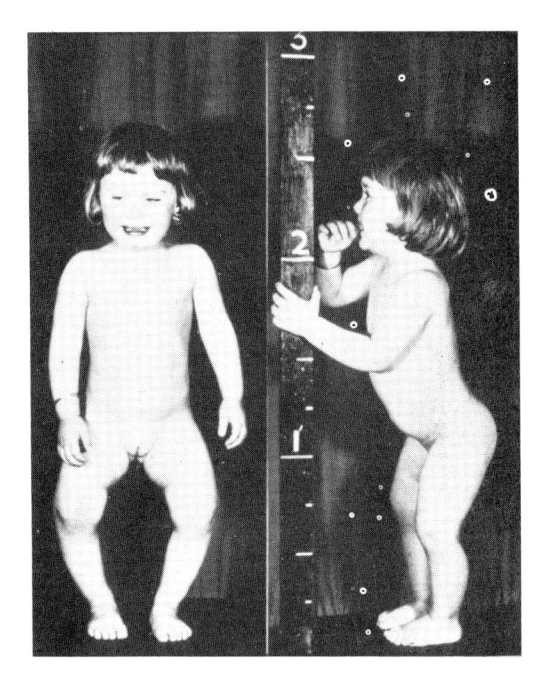

Fig. 22.36. Rickets. The bones become bowed and their metaphyses widened.

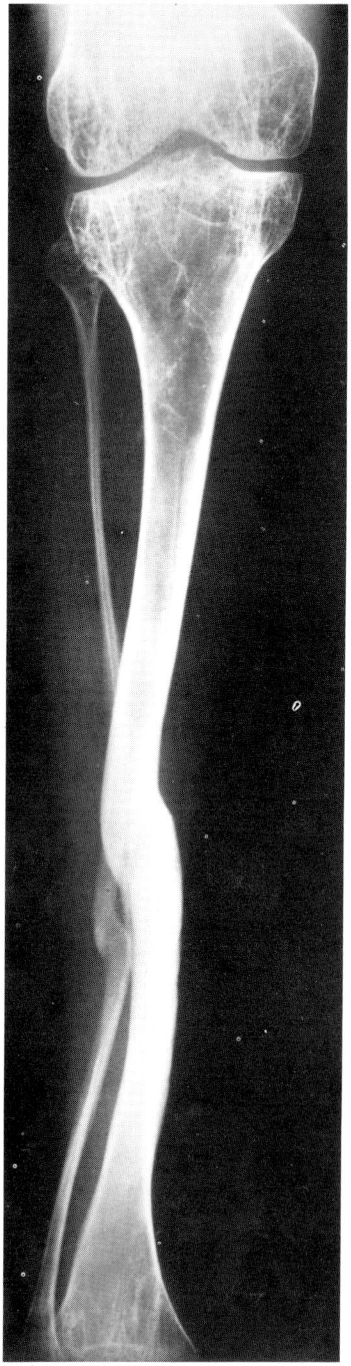

Fig. 22.37. Fragilitas ossium. Multiple fractures produce severe deformity.

PERIPHERAL NERVE LESIONS

Carpal tunnel syndrome

The median nerve runs through a closed tunnel at the wrist. The nerve may be compressed by rheumatoid disease or a Colles fracture but in many cases the cause of this nerve compression syndrome is unknown. It frequently affects the middle aged female and produces pain and numbness in the thumb, index and middle fingers. The syndrome sometimes is seen in the pregnant woman where there is swelling and oedema of the extremities.

The symptoms awaken the patient in the early morning and as the compression progresses the muscles of the thenar eminence become wasted and paralysed. The condition is simply treated by dividing the carpal ligament at the wrist, relieving the pressure on the median nerve.

Ulnar Neuritis

The ulnar nerve lies in a groove along the medial side of the elbow where it may be compressed by arthritic changes in the elbow joint. The patient experiences pain and tingling and then numbness in the distribution of the ulnar nerve (i.e. the little and ring fingers). As the compression progresses the small muscles of the hand become paralysed and a claw hand develops (Fig. 22.38). The ulnar nerve must be decompressed by its release from the ulnar groove behind the medial epicondyle at the elbow and its transposition to the anterior aspect of the joint.

PERIPHERAL NERVE INJURIES

Division of the median nerve usually occurs at the wrist and is frequently seen in the child who falls carrying a milk or lemonade bottle. The median nerve laceration produces anaesthesia and muscle paralysis as outlined in the median nerve compression syndrome above. The ulnar nerve is again frequently lacerated at the wrist and produces anaesthesia of the ulnar two fingers and paralysis of all the intrinsic muscles of the hand with the production of a weak claw hand.

The radial nerve is most commonly injured in the mid-arm region where humeral shaft fractures damage the nerve trunk. A wrist drop develops due to paralysis of all the extensor muscles of the wrist.

Treatment

Any wound in which a nerve injury is suspected must be carefully explored. If the wound is clean and there are no other vital struc-

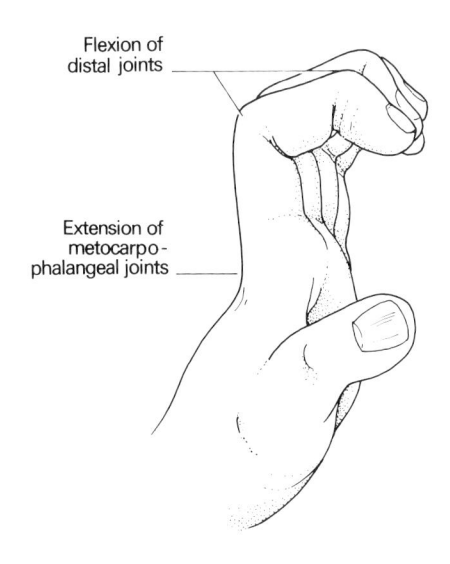

Fig. 22.38. Claw hand in ulnar nerve paralysis.

tures divided a primary repair of the nerve ends may be undertaken. Very fine suture material is necessary to approximate the nerve sheath and careful splintage of the wrist joint will be necessary to prevent undue tension of the repair site. The recovery of motor and sensory function will be slow for the regenerating nerve grows at a rate of approximately 1 mm per day. If the wound is dirty or tendons are divided then the nerve ends should be tagged with markers and a secondary repair undertaken at a later date.

REGIONAL ORTHOPAEDIC CONDITIONS

THE NECK

Torticollis

Torticollis is a lateral flexion deformity of the cervical spine. It is seen as a neonatal deformity due to a tear and then contracture of the sternomastoid muscle at the time of birth. In most cases simple stretching of the neck is effective, but in some babies the torticollis persists and operative release of the tight sternomastoid muscle is necessary. A torticollis may be acquired later in life and is then accompanied by pain and spasm in the neck. This condition is usually associated with osteoarthritic changes in the cervical spine.

Cervical spondylosis

Osteoarthritis of the cervical spine produces pain, stiffness, and sometimes a torticollis. The pain may radiate to the upper limbs for the nerve roots issuing from the lower cervical region become compressed by the degenerative osteophytes around the joints concerned. Physiotherapy, traction and mobilisation of the neck is helpful and a neck collar may be necessary if the symptoms are acute.

Brachial plexus injuries

Motor cyclists involved in high-speed injuries may damage the shoulder and the neck, avulsing or dividing the roots of the brachial plexus at the base of the neck. Partial division of the nerves will produce patchy paralysis and anaesthesia of the upper limb and recovery will recur to a variable extent. A completely paralysed and anaesthetic arm is a useless member and it may be an advantage to amputate the limb so that a prosthesis may be fitted.

THE SHOULDER

There are several inflammatory condition of the shoulder joint and its capsule which produce pain and stiffness:

1. *Acute bursitis.* A minor strain of the shoulder is followed by severe pain and swelling. On X-ray an area of calcification in the capsule develops (Fig. 22.39) and the shoulder becomes progressively stiff. An injection of hydrocortisone into the capsule may give complete relief but sometimes operative release of the tight, calcified plaque is required.

2. *Rupture of the supraspinatus tendon.* A strain of the shoulder may also produce this tendon tear. Abduction of the shoulder is impossible and there is considerable tenderness over the superior aspect of the joint. This condition always spontaneously recovers given time and and there is no indication for operative repair.

3. *Frozen shoulder.* The capsulitis which follows the acute bursitis or a minor tear of the capsule may progress despite treatment. Complete immobility of the shoulder joint may result. It frequently takes 2–3 years to resolve but a good prognosis can always be given to the patient, for full mobility will eventually return.

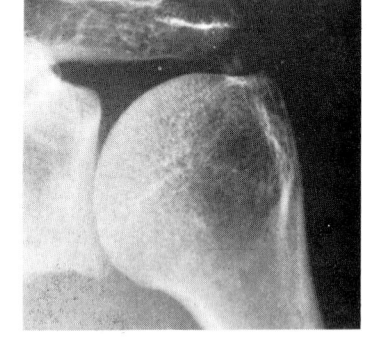

Fig. 22.39. Calcification in the capsule of the shoulder joint.

THE ELBOW

Tennis elbow

Pain and tenderness develops around the lateral epicondyle of the lower humerus at the elbow. Strain of the elbow joint region is usually described by the patient and eventually the pain may become so severe that it is difficult to even raise small objects with the extended wrist. The pain and tenderness is due to an inflammation of the forearm muscle attachment to the bony epicondyle and is treated by a local injection of local anaesthetic and hydrocortisone (xylocaine 4 ml of 1% + 25 mg of hydrocortisone).

Rarely operative release of this extensor tendon from the condyle is necessary in the chronic condition.

Loose bodies

Javelin throwers, fast bowlers and other sportsmen may avulse small portions of bone and articular cartilage from the capitellum and radial head (Fig. 22.40). Osteo-arthritic changes in the elbow may also produce loose bodies which result in an internal derangement of the joint with locking and recurrent painful episodes. Surgical removal of the loose bodies is necessary.

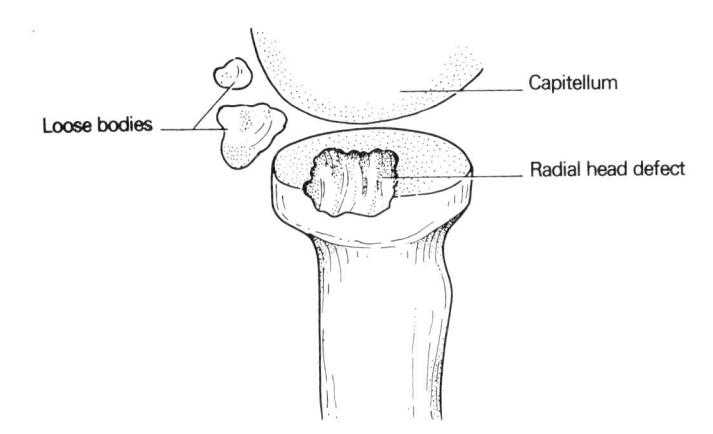

Fig. 22.40. Avulsion of loose bodies from the radial head.

THE WRIST AND HAND

De Quervain's stenosing tenosynovitis (Fig. 22.41)

The extensor tendons to the thumb run over the radial styloid within their own sheaths. At this point the sheath may become inflamed, producing extreme local pain and tenderness locally and there is increasing stiffness of the thumb due to entrapment of the tendon within this sheath. In the early stages an injection of 25 mg of hydrocortisone with xylocaine (1 or 2%) may be helpful, but surgical release is frequently required.

Dupuytren's contracture

This is a common condition in the elderly in which there is fibrosis of the palmar aponeurosis which produces a flexion deformity of the

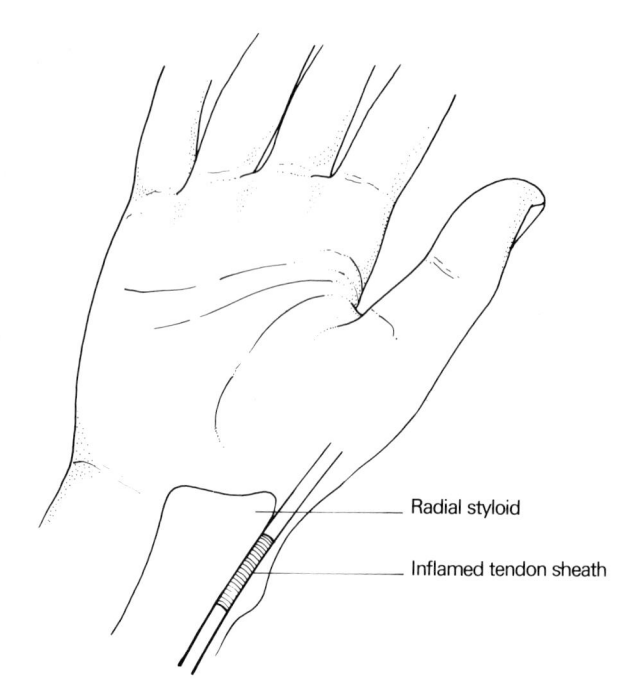

Fig. 22.41. De Quervain's stenosing tenosynovitis.

Fig. 22.42. Paronychia.

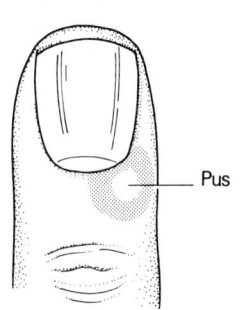

finger at the metacarpo-phalangeal and proximal interphalangeal joints, usually starting at the fourth digit and spreading to the fifth and sometimes the third finger. Since the aponeurosis only extends distally to the base of the middle phalanx, the distal interphalangeal joint escapes. The contracture is often bilateral.

Treatment Mild degrees of contracture are left alone, but if disability is caused the thickened fascia is excised.

Hand infections

1. *Paronychia*. This common infection involves the nail bed and frequently follows a 'hang-nail' (Fig. 22.42). At the early stage antibiotics may be given but after a few days pus develops and surgical evacuation will be required. An incision from the proximal corner of the nail through the infected area is made (Fig. 22.43) and in severe infections a portion of the nail will have to be removed. The whole nail must be removed if the infection has spread to the other side of the finger.

2. *Pulp space infections*. Needle points and other penetrating injuries readily infect the finger or thumb tips. The area becomes painful, swollen and red, and pus develops at an early stage. The

pulp space is divided by fibrous septa into multiple compartments and so surgical drainage must be extensive and complete. An incision on both sides of the pulp space is required and a through-and-through drain remains for twenty-four hours.

Tendon sheath infection. A needle may enter the tendon sheath, infecting the whole length of the tendon in the finger and the palm. The sheath quickly becomes distended with infected fluid or pus and must be drained as soon as possible. Any delay in releasing the infection may result in adhesion of the sheath to the tendon, producing a stiff finger or thumb.

Palmar infections. The palm is divided into three compartments—the thenar compartment on the thumb side, the hypothenar on the little finger side, and the mid palmar space between the two. Penetrating wounds may infect these compartments and drainage will again be necessary. When the mid palmar space is infected the whole hand becomes extremely swollen and the infection points into the web space where it may be drained by a surgical incision.

In all hand infections, surgical drainage is combined with immobilisation, elevation and antibiotic therapy.

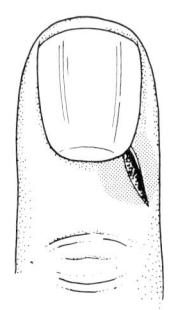

Fig. 22.43. Paronychia drained by an incision.

Tendon injuries

Lacerations affecting the dorsum of the hand and wrist in which the extensor tendons are divided present no real problem. The extensor tendons must be carefully sutured and the hand and wrist splinted in extension for three weeks. They always heal satisfactorily and function should return to normal.

The flexor tendons on the anterior aspect of the hand, however, constitute a much more difficult repair problem. Following their division, repair is very likely to produce adhesions to other tendons and surrounding tissues with a result that the hand or finger becomes stiff. In the proximal part of the hand and wrist direct repair of the divided tendon may be undertaken with an end-to-end suture (Fig. 22.44). If the wound is dirty or the wound exploration is extremely delayed then it is preferable to close the skin and to allow the wound to heal. Tendon suture is undertaken secondarily at a later date. If the wound is clean and it is within 6 hours of injury then primary repair of the tendon may be undertaken with antibiotic cover.

Fig. 22.44. Tendon repair by an end-to-end suture.

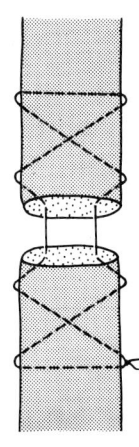

Laceration of the fingers affecting the flexor tendons within their tight flexor tendon sheath produce specific problems of adhesion and finger stiffness. In most cases it is better to cut out the lacerated tendons and insert a tendon graft which is taken from either palmaris longus in the forearm or one of the toe extensor tendons. This graft is attached distally to the distal phalanx of the finger and proximally to the flexor tendon in the palm or the wrist (Fig. 22.45). The hand should be completely immobilised for 3 weeks postoperatively with the fingers in flexion and then a prolonged course of physiotherapy is undertaken to mobilise the hand and the affected fingers.

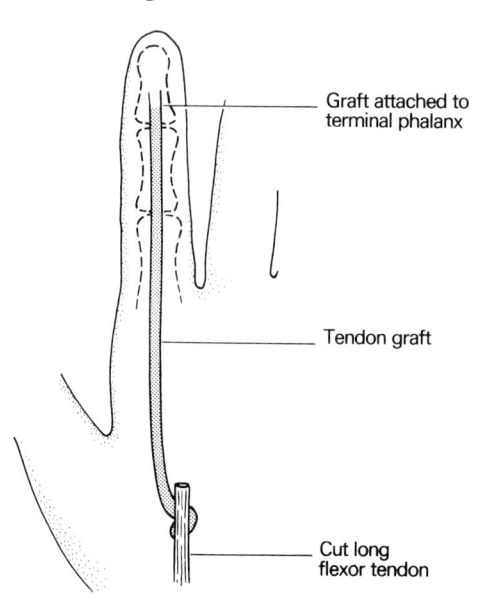

Fig. 22.45. Tendon graft.

THE SPINE

Backache

There are many causes of pain in the spine and these include infection, rheumatoid diseases, abnormalities of the retroperitoneum and posterior abdominal wall, and, most commonly, mechanical abnormalities. These mechanical derangements of the spine may be classified into (i) acute back strain, (ii) intervertebral disc syndromes, (iii) instability syndromes, (iv) chronic back strains.

1. *Acute back strain.* This condition is commonly seen in the nurses on the ward. When lifting a heavy patient pain may be experienced in the low lumbar region and there is tenderness where the paraspinal muscles insert onto the iliac crest. Acute pain and stiffness develops but resolve satisfactorily after adequate rest. An injection of local anaesthetic (xylocaine, 1%) into the tender area may be helpful.

2. *Intervertebral disc syndromes.* A prolapsed intervertebral disc produces low lumbar pain together with sciatica (pain radiating into

the leg). There is often a history of a heavy lift or injury and the pain may become very severe. The spine becomes curved with a scoliosis or a tilt (Fig. 22.46). Straight leg raising on the affected side is limited and neurological abnormalities may develop when the lumbar roots are compressed within the spinal canal. An x-ray may reveal a decreased disc space at the affected level.

The essential feature of the treatment of this condition is rest in bed. The mattress must be firm and the nurse should make sure that fracture boards are inserted beneath the mattress. Adequate sedation and analgesia is required and in most cases resolution of pain and the sciatic symptoms occurs over the next few weeks. If neurological signs such as weakness of the muscle group or complete anaesthesia persist, or if the bladder becomes affected by compression of the cauda equina in the spinal canal then there is an indication for operation. A myelogram is usually performed at this stage to confirm the site of the disc prolapse. Dye is injected into the subarachnoid space and its flow is altered by a disc prolapse. A laminectomy is performed to remove the posterior elements of the spinal canal and the disc is removed from around the nerve root.

3. *Instability syndromes.* A spondylolysis is a condition where a defect or fracture through the posterior elements of the vertebra occurs (Fig. 22.47). A spondylolisthesis—a slip of one vertebral body forwards on the next—may follow (Fig. 22.48). Chronic degenerative changes in one disc space may also produce a minor slip of one vertebra on the next. The symptoms of low lumbar spine pain and sciatica are controlled by a lumbar supportive corset and the strengthening effect of physiotherapy. If the slip continues or symptoms become severe in spite of this conservative treatment

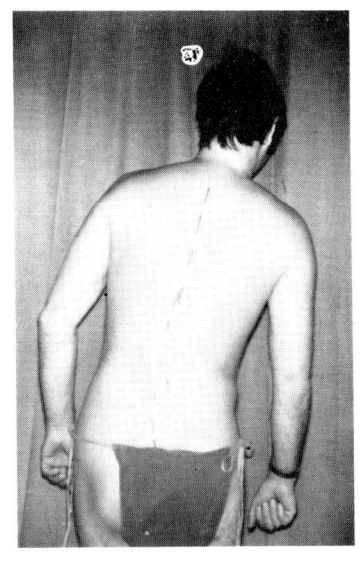

Fig. 22.46. Sciatic scoliosis.

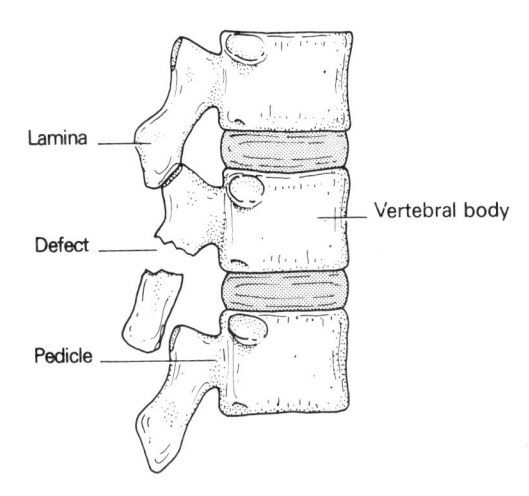

Fig. 22.47. Spondylolysis.

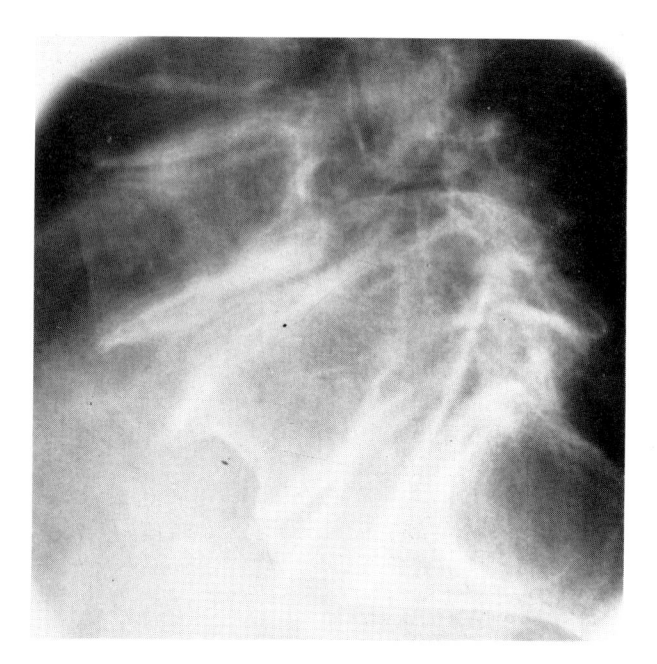

Fig. 22.48. Spondylolisthesis—a slip of one vertebral body forward on the next.

operation may be required to stabilise the segment. Fusion of the spinal vertebra will be required.

4. *Chronic back strain.* This is a common problem and frequently seen in the housewife who is required to undertake heavy housework and the frequent lifting of children. Pain is experienced in the low lumbar region and is aggravated by exercises. The pain sometimes radiates to the buttocks and thighs but true sciatica is not experienced. On X-ray there is usually no abnormality, but minor chronic degenerative changes may later develop. The physiotherapist will be very helpful to this patient, and a supportive corset is advisable when undertaking housework etc.

Osteomyelitis of the spine

Pyogenic organisms such as those seen in osteomyelitis (page 528) may travel via the blood stream to the vertebrae and produce infection within a disc space. Infection rapidly spreads to adjacent vertebral bone, which may collapse and produce a large paraspinal abscess. Pain is extremely severe. The spine develops extreme spasm and the patient becomes ill very rapidly with a high fever, raised white count, and a high E.S.R. The organisms may be identified on blood culture and appropriate antibiotics are given. The spine must be put at rest and to allow this to be as complete as possible the patient is confined to a plaster bed (Fig. 22.49), or alternatively

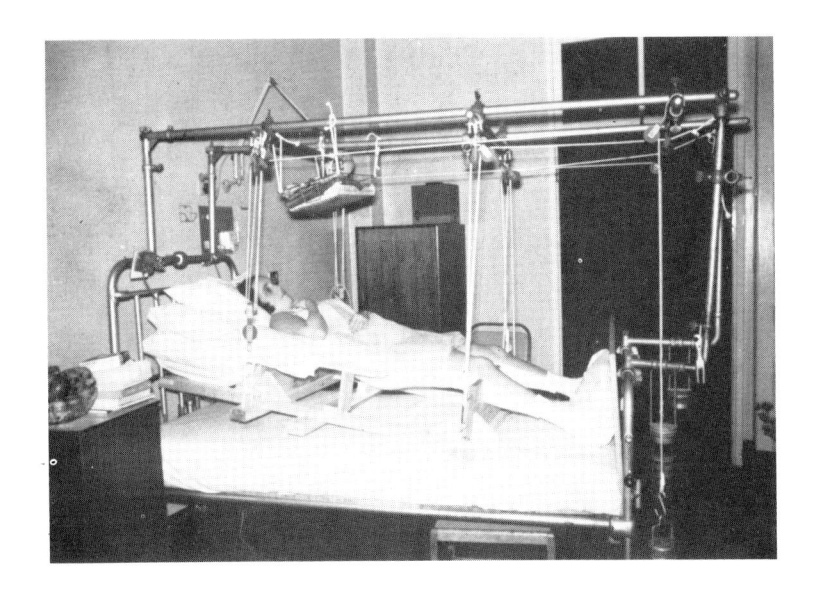

Fig. 22.49. Patient being nursed on a plaster bed.

nursed on a circle electric bed. This apparatus is very satisfactory from the nursing point of view and immobilises the spine to allow satisfactory resolution of the infection.

Tuberculous infection of the spine (Pott's disease) (Fig. 22.19)

The disc space and adjacent vertebral bodies are similarly affected. The abscess which develops may distend the psoas muscle sheath on either side of the vertebral column and sometimes may compress the spinal cord producing a paralysis of the lower limbs (Pott's paraplegia).

The infection is treated by appropriate rest and anti-tuberculous drugs. Exploration of the spine from the chest or abdomen may be necessary to eradicate the abscess cavity and to allow bone healing. Bone grafting may be required if a large cavity is present.

THE HIP

Perthes' disease (Fig. 22.50)

This an avascular necrosis of the femoral head and occurs in the child between the ages of 5 and 10 years. The cause of this avascularity is unknown but there is some evidence that the high pressure of synovial fluid within the hip joint may be responsible. There is obstruction of the vessels which supply the femoral head of the developing child with blood. The child limps and pain is experienced in the thigh and knee region (rarely in the hip and groin area). X-rays

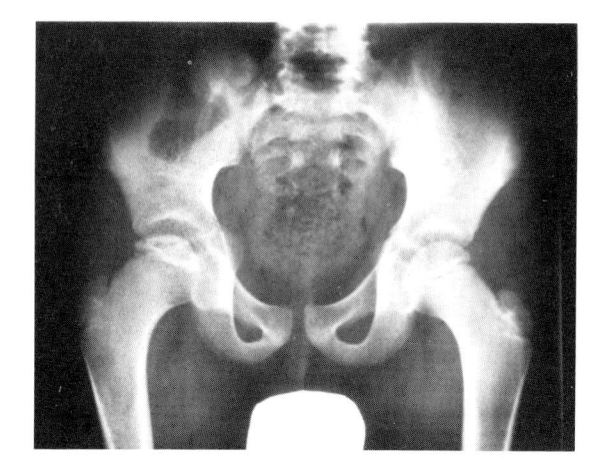

Fig. 22.50. Perthes' disease of the right hip.

reveal a sclerotic, fragmented and squashed femoral head and, if this poor shape persists, early osteoarthritis of the hip joint may result.

The *treatment* to be given depends on the extent of the avascularity. In many minor instances no treatment at all is required and the parents can be reassured that the hip will return to a normal functional state and a very good hip shape will be retained. Severe cases of Perthes' disease may require operation. An osteotomy of the upper femur is undertaken to contain the squashed mushroom-shaped head of the femur in a better position within the acetabulum.

Slipped femoral epiphysis

This occurs in children between the ages of 10 and 15 and produces symptoms and signs very similar to the sub-capital femoral neck fractures described on page 502. The children are frequently affected by endocrine abnormalities. They are frequently Fröhlich-like, grossly overweight and with poorly developed secondary sex characteristics. The slip of the epiphysis from the neck may occur suddenly and acutely (Fig. 22.51) or it may occur slowly in a chronic fashion. In the acute type the femoral head must be manipulated back on to the neck and internally fixed with fine pins (Fig. 22.52). In the chronic slip internal fixation with pins must be undertaken before the slip becomes too displaced.

THE KNEE

Internal derangements of the knee

Cartilage Tears. Rotational injuries of the knee most commonly occur on the football or athletic field but similar injuries to the joint may occur in men who have to crouch and work in confined spaces.

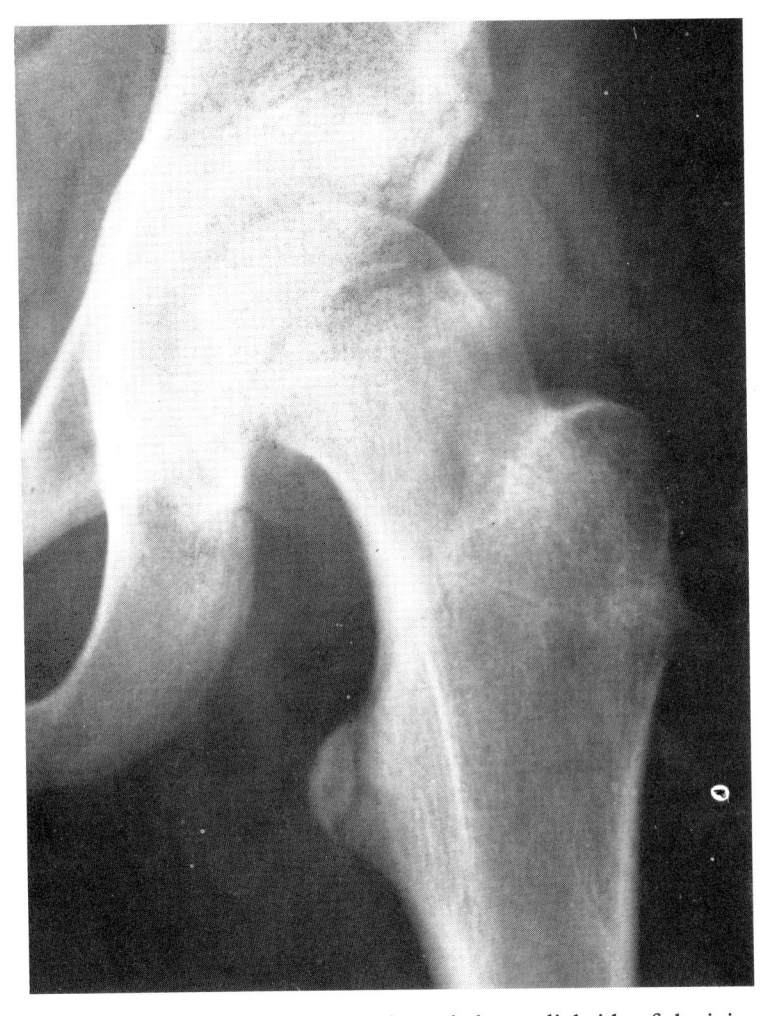

Fig. 22.51. Slipped femoral epiphysis.

Pain is experienced immediately and the medial side of the joint is most commonly affected. The footballer has to go off the field and swelling in the joint develops usually that evening or the next day. The joint may remain locked if a 'bucket-handle tear' of the cartilage is sustained with one segment of the meniscus being displaced into the centre of the joint (Fig. 22.53).

Alternatively the joint may spontaneously unlock and the symptoms gradually settle. Recurrent episodes of pain, swelling, locking and 'giving way' are characteristic of the torn meniscus. Repeated mechanical derangements will eventually produce joint surface damage and it is important to remove the torn meniscus.

When the diagnosis is definite, meniscectomy is advised. If the symptoms and signs are not so clear-cut a course of physiotherapy must be given to build up the knee musculature and to await events.

Fig. 22.52. The epiphysis has been repositioned and internally fixed with pins. ▶

Fig. 22.53. Bucket handle torn meniscus. ▼

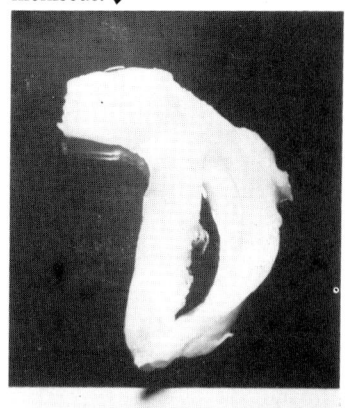

Some help may be given by the introduction of dye and air into the joint so that X-rays may be taken with the cartilage outlined: this technique being called arthrography (Fig. 22.54).

A small endoscope may be passed into the knee joint and with this instrument the internal structures can be visualised and tears of the cartilage actually seen. This instrument—the arthroscope—has improved the accuracy of diagnosis very greatly in the last few years.

Ligament Tears. The knee joint is stabilised by the medial and lateral collateral ligaments together with the anterior and posterior cruciate ligaments (Fig. 22.55). The medial collateral ligament is the most commonly torn, and strains of this structure are seen in soccer and skiing injuries.

A partial tear of this ligament will require treatment in a plaster cast with the knee immobilised for 6 weeks. Gross tears of the medial collateral ligament are often associated with anterior cruciate ligament tears and injuries of the meniscus. Conservative treatment of this injury with plaster will be unsatisfactory, for continued instability will result and will usually prevent a sportsman from returning to his games.

Operative treatment of the collateral ligament must be undertaken and the cartilage derangement must be treated. It is sometimes possible to repair the anterior cruciate ligament if it removes a small piece of bone from either end, but if the ligament is shredded, repair is ineffective. The stability of the joint then depends on the quality of the quadriceps muscle.

Loose Bodies. Osteochondritis dissecans is responsible for most of the loose bodies seen in the knee joint in a young person (Fig. 22.56). It is due to a fracture through the articular cartilage and underlying bone and the fragment may either remain in its crater causing symptoms of pain and instability or it may loosen and form a separate loose body which intermittently locks the joint.

Osteoarthritic changes may be the cause of a loose body in the elderly. Loose bodies which are repeatedly deranging the knee must be removed.

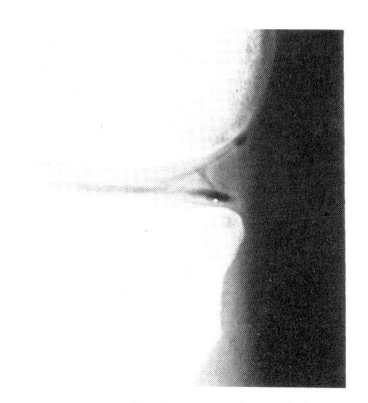

Fig. 22.54. Arthrography of the knee showing a cartilage tear.

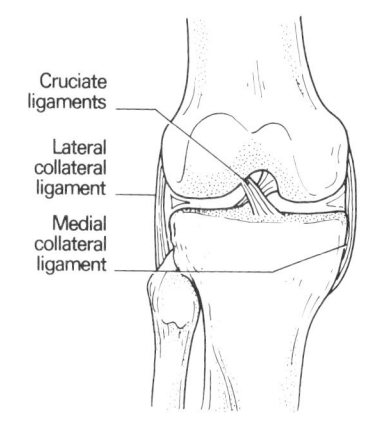

Fig. 22.55. The knee joint ligaments.

Fig. 22.56. Osteochondritis dissecans.

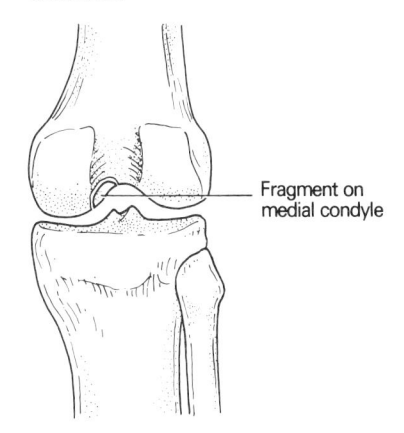

THE ANKLE

Sprains

Ankle sprains are due to a partial tear of the lateral collateral ligament. An inversion twisting injury of the ankle joint will rupture the front band of this ligament (Fig. 22.57) causing swelling, bruising, and local tenderness. If no fracture is detected on X-ray the essential treatment is rest and elevation of the ankle. After a day or two active exercises are started to return the muscle control of the ankle to normal as soon as possible. If the tear of the lateral collateral ligament is complete producing gross instability, a below-knee plaster is applied for 4 to 6 weeks.

Achilles tendon tears

The large Achilles tendon above the heel bone may rupture in sportsmen who are leaping to reach a ball. The unfit person who is performing strenuous, unaccustomed exercise may also be affected. There is a sharp, sudden episode of pain above the heel and the patient often describes the situation when he feels he has been 'shot in the heel'. Swelling and bruising rapidly develops and a gap in the Achilles tendon can be detected. The patient is unable to stand on tip-toes but simple plantar flexion of the foot is still possible for the other ankle flexors are intact.

If the tear is left untreated the patient's gait will be poor. It is advisable to operate and repair the tendon at this early stage. Fol-

554
Chapter 22

Fig. 22.57. Sprained ankle. Partial rupture of the lateral ligament.

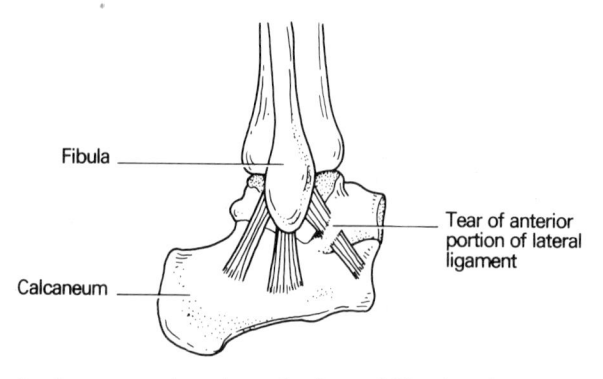

lowing operation 6 weeks immobilisation in a plaster cast will be necessary. If operation is contra-indicated a satisfactory result will be obtained if a below-knee plaster is applied with the foot in full plantar flexion.

THE FOOT

Hallux valgus

The great toe becomes displaced at the metatarso-phalangeal joint (Fig. 22.58). This condition is often inherited and is aggravated by

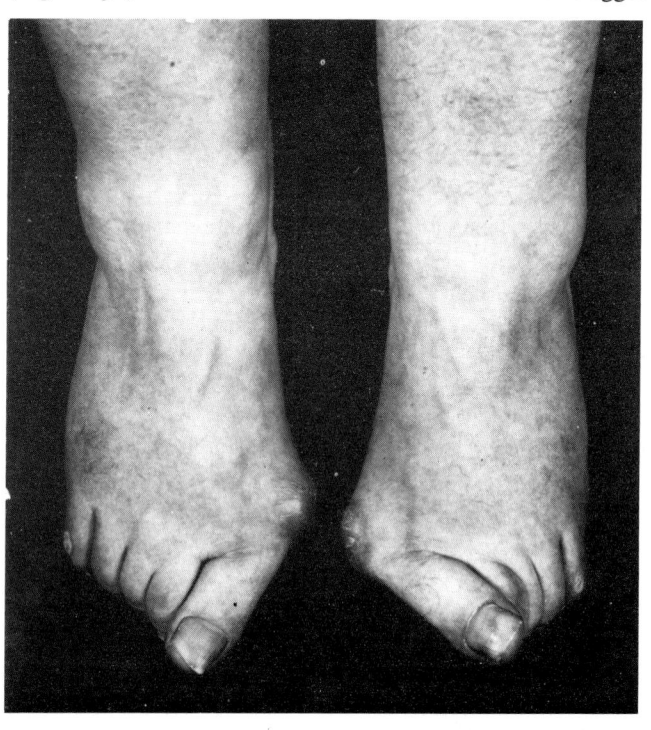

Fig. 22.58. Hallux valgus.

the use of inappropriate footwear. A bunion may develop due to the formation of an exostosis at the head of the metatarsal, and the second toe may become displaced at the metatarso-phalangeal joint. Pain and discomfort may be due to the bunion and if it persists the exostosis is removed.

A full correction of the deformity may be undertaken by arthrodesing the great toe metatarso-phalangeal joint. The proximal part of the great toe phalanx is removed in the Keller's operation and this will also straighten the deformity and remove the discomfort.

Metatarsalgia

Pain below the forefoot may be due to prominence of the metatarsal heads in the sole musculature. It may also be due to a pain from a neuroma between the metatarsal heads; this condition being called a Morton's metatarsalgia. A simple insole to redistribute the weight beneath the foot together with strengthening exercises of the intrinsic muscles will alleviate the symptoms in most cases. A neuroma must be removed surgically.

Hammer toes

The deformity shown in Fig. 22.59 may be corrected by fusion of the proximal joint.

Plantar fasciitis

Pain beneath the heel is a common condition and is due to inflammation of the plantar ligament where it is inserted into the calcaneum. A calcaneal spur may develop and treatment consists of injection of local anaesthetic and hydrocortisone. A moulded soft heel pad is helpful.

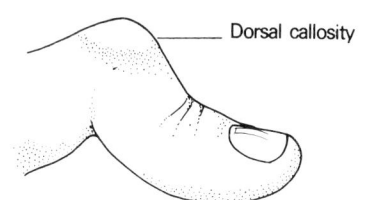

Fig. 22.59. Hammer toe.

Chapter 23. Transplantation

Introduction

Transplantation of human tissues has been a topic for popular discussion for a little over a decade now, mainly because of the use of organs such as kidneys, liver, heart or lungs taken from people who have recently died. But it should not be forgotten that transplantation has been undertaken for longer than this. Skin grafting has been a successful technique for many years as a means for obtaining cover for areas of skin surface denuded by burns.

Types of transplant

If a tissue is taken from one area of the body and is placed in another, this is known as an *autograft*. Examples of autografts are skin grafts, bone chips taken from the iliac crest to fill in bone spaces and the use of the long saphenous vein to bypass a block in the femoral artery. These types of graft will not be discussed further in this chapter.

A tissue taken from one individual in a species and placed in another of the same species is called an *allograft*. Examples of allografts are renal, liver, cardiac and lung transplants.

If an animal from one species donates an organ to an animal of another species this is known as a *xenograft*. This type of graft has been used in the past, for example baboon kidneys have been placed in humans but the problems posed, which will be discussed later, are too great and xenografting is not now used clinically.

Immunological rejection

In precisely the way that the body recognises and rejects an infecting organism, so it recognises and rejects an allograft and a xenograft.

The body contains protein and has the capacity to recognise 'self' in immunological terms. If a foreign protein (an *antigen*) enters the blood stream, *antibodies* against it are formed. The source of the antibodies are the small lymphocyte cells in the regional lymph nodes. When antibodies recirculate in the patient's blood stream and come into contact with the protein which stimulated their production, they react with this protein, altering its structure and function. This antigen-antibody reaction to foreign protein is the basic mechanism that underlies the immune response.

When skin is applied, as an autograft, from, say, the thigh to the arm in a patient with burns, no immune response occurs because the grafted skin contains precisely similar proteins to the skin which covered the grafted area. However, if skin is taken from one member of a species and is placed on a denuded and vascular area of another member of the same species, that is an allograft, antibodies against the graft form within 7 to 14 days and the graft is rejected. For the first few days the graft will be vascularised normally, but, as antibodies begin to form, the endothelium lining the blood vessels that supply the allograft is progressively destroyed because of the antigen–antibody reaction. This process of *rejection* is accompanied by some of the features of an inflammatory response. There is infiltration of the area with white cells and exudation of tissue fluid into the inter-cellular space. Thus, there are two arms of the rejection process, the first being the release into the circulation of foreign proteins with the formation of antibodies and the second being the recirculation of antibodies with an antigen-antibody reaction.

One interesting exception to the rejection seen in allografts is in the case of *identical twins*. It is possible to take tissue from one twin and to graft it on the other twin without there being any development of antibodies. Thus the grafted tissue is not rejected. This is because both twins arise from the division of one cell and both therefore have an identical genetic make-up.

In the case of a xenograft, the rejection process is more vigorous than in the case of an allograft. It is as if the proteins of a different species are more 'foreign' and produce a more rapid and profound antibody response.

Immunosuppression

It is possible to modify the production of antibodies by suppressing their manufacture. To do this it is necessary to interfere with the metabolism of the small, immunologically competent lymphocytes by means of drugs or it is possible to remove them physically. The drugs that are used to suppress the immune response are azathioprine, which interferes with the use by the lymphocytes of an amino-acid, purine, which is vital to their normal function, together with steroids to reduce inflammatory response. Occasionally other drugs such as actinomycin, which is related to the antibiotics, are used. Another form of drug therapy is the use of antilymphocyte serum. Lymphocytes are first removed from the patient and antibodies against them are raised in horses. These antibodies are concentrated and when injected into the patient the immune response so invoked will result in the destruction of the lymphocytes which were originally used to raise the antibodies. Actual removal of lymphocytes can be achieved by cannulating the thoracic duct and clearing the lymph so obtained of the cells before it is re-injected.

By these means it is impossible to suppress the immunological rejection process to the point where it is possible for an allograft to survive for a considerable length of time. There is, however, one other extremely important method whereby the rejection process is modified and this is by immunological donor-recipient matching.

Donor matching

It is possible to match the donor organ to the immunological type of the recipient with the result that the allograft protected by immunosuppressive therapy will survive for years—the longest survival time for an allograft kidney is now over 10 years. The first part of the matching process is to ensure that the blood groups of donor and recipient are the same. Following this, there are a number of antibodies that are recognised as being important to the rejection process. These antibodies, (of the HL-A system) are dependant for their existence on the genetic pattern and can be recognised by testing the lymphocytes of either the donor or the recipient against a number (50 to 60) of different types of serum obtained by the purification of serum from a panel of people whose antibody constitution has become known. It is thus possible to 'type' both a potential donor of organs and a potential recipient. If the donor and recipient have a similar immunological construction then the rejection of the transplanted organ has been clearly shown to be modified.

CLINICAL TRANSPLANTATION

Corneal transplantation

One of the forms of transplantation that has been successfully carried out for the longest time is that of the cornea. The reason for the success of this operation (where the cornea from the eye of a person recently dead is used to replace an opaque cornea) is that the grafted cornea is not revascularised. It is thus a privileged tissue nourished by means of tissue perfusion of nutrients and oxygen.

Renal transplantation
Ten years ago this was experimental but now this procedure is carried out in a number of centres throughout the world with good therapeutic results. Kidneys are particularly suitable for transplantation because of the development of the artificial kidney, because of their gross anatomical structure and because they are paired organs.

The artificial kidney means that it is possible to maintain life in the absence of any functioning renal tissue at all. The end-point of gradually deteriorating function is not therefore sudden death of the patient, so that it is possible to maintain a potential recipient in good health until a suitable donor kidney is available.

The gross anatomy of artery, vein and ureter makes it surgically simple to remove a kidney with preservation of the vital structures so that the artery can be re-anastomosed end-to-end to the up-turned internal iliac artery, the vein end-to-side to the common iliac vein and the ureter to the bladder of the recipient. It is usual to place the left donor kidney in the right iliac fossa and vice versa so that the renal pelvis of the donor kidney is always anterior.

The fact that the kidney is a paired organ has meant that it has been possible to remove one kidney from a healthy, live donor. This is probably not an important source of kidneys at the present time but in the development stage of transplantation it meant that kidneys were being transplanted between members of families with the result that a form of automatic tissue typing occurred.

The main problems associated with renal transplantation are, first, the obtaining of preservation of suitable donor organs, second the immunological problems already mentioned and finally cost.

There is no doubt now that kidneys for transplantation have to be obtained in most instances from cadavers. They must be removed from the body of the donor not more than 30 minutes after death. Obviously there are difficulties in obtaining permission for this to be done if this has to be sought from relatives. There are also difficulties in ensuring that there is someone who is competent at cadaveric kidney removal and storage present at the time of death. The ethical problems of permission will be debated in forthcoming years. One side points out the number of young or middle-aged adults who die per year from bilateral renal disease and who would be saved by renal transplantation and generally wish permission to be automatic, the onus being on a person, in life, to state clearly that he does not wish his organs to be used. The counter argument says that there is dignity in death as well as in life and are we, that is the doctors, so sure that we can define the precise point of death anyway? It is perhaps too simple merely to say that in death one would consent to the giving of one's organs because in near-death and death itself the suffering is borne by relatives. A more realistic approach is to consider giving permission for the removal of these vital organs from one's children should they be killed or die from some fatal disease.

Storage of kidneys is generally satisfactorily achieved by arterial perfusion, just after removal, with ice cold saline followed by packing of the organ in ice in a thermos flask. This method preserves the kidney for up to 12 hours.

One of the immunological problems which is very real is the question of donor-recipient matching and the logistical problems which arise. It is obviously unlikely that blood group and HL-A matching will occur by chance at one centre. Therefore a European Transplant Organisation has been established whereby potential donors are identified and are tissue typed. This typing is fed into a computer which contains details of the tissue types of all the recipients waiting for kidneys. The computer rapidly produces the most suitable recipients and it is then a logistical problem to transport the kidney from the point of its removal from the cadaver to the patient who is to receive it. Thus a fatal car crash in Switzerland can result in a kidney being flown to, say, Manchester and used there.

The cost of transplantation is high, as is the cost of maintaining a patient on intermittent renal dialysis. How far any country is prepared to support a transplant programme is a political decision but clearly there is a cost limit to the expansion of the service offered. In this country at the present time somewhere in the region of 250 renal transplants are being performed annually against a background of 3,000 deaths in young adults from bilateral renal disease a year.

Cardiac transplantation

The first human cardiac transplant was carried out in the United States by Dr. Hardy in Jackson, Mississipi in January 1964. The heart of a chimpanzee was used as the potential human donor did not die before the recipient reached the point of death and the operation was not successful. Four years later, in December 1967, Dr. Barnard in Cape Town carried out the first human to human cardiac transplant.

Since that time several hundred cardiac transplant operations have been carried out throughout the world with varying success. The consensus of opinion at the present time is that cardiac transplantation should only be carried out at one or two centres and that much more immunological knowledge of the rejection problem is required before satisfactory results justify the cost involved.

Liver transplantation

This has been performed in a number of centres. When it is realised that the liver has two blood supplies, one from the hepatic artery and one from the portal vein, that it is attached to the inferior vena cava and that it is tucked up underneath the diaphragm it will be appreciated that the technical difficulties are considerable. It remains a matter for continuing research in certain centres but at present it has no general clinical therapeutic application.

Lung transplantation

One or two cases, including an apparently successful one from Holland with reasonable, survival have been reported. But the immunological and infection problems with lungs seem to be more severe than with other tissues and are at present insurmountable.

Index

abdomen drains 30–1
abdominal hernia 268–78
abdomino-perineal excision 264–6, *265*
    pull-through anastomosis 250
abduction
    hips 505–6, 521
    splint 522, *522*
    traction 523, *523*
abscess 4–5, *5*, 9–10
    appendix 219, 221
    brain 452
    cerebral 137–8, *138*
    cold 128, *128*–9
    extradural *451*, 452
    lungs 77
    lymphadenitis 125
    paraspinal 548
    pelvic 224–5
    perianal 357–8, *358*
    pericolic 234
    peritonsillar 468–9
    pilonidal sinus 407
    psoas 528
    septum 460
    subdural 452
    subphrenic 224, 225
    treatment 9–10
    tuberculous 128, *129*
accidents
    care of patient 482–3

acetabulum
    fracture 500–1
    hip dislocation 522–3
achalasia of cardia 163, 167–8, *168*
Achilles tendon 524
    tears 553–4
acholuric jaundice 123, 294, 299
acid hypersecretion 187
acidosis 317
acoustic tumours 140
acromegaly 140, *141*
acromioclavicular separation 491, *491*
actinomyces israeli 17
actinomycin D 68, 558
actinomycosis 17, 288
Addison's disease 387
adenocarcinoma 172
adenoidectomy 467, *468*
adenoids 467
adenoma 52
    adrenal cortex *385*, 387
    parathyroid gland 381
adenomatous polyp
    colon 237
adenomyosarcoma 338–9
adrenal cortex 383–7
    adenoma *385*, 387
    physiology 383–4

adrenal glands 381–7
adrenal medulla 381–3
    ganglioneuroma 382
    neuroblastoma 382
    phaeochromocytoma 382
    tumours 382–3
adrenalectomy 385, 387
    breast cancer 399
adrenaline 39, 381–2, 440
adrenocorticotrophic hormone 384
adrenogenital syndrome 385–7
agranulocytosis 374, 469
air encephalography 141
airway maintenance 146–7, *148*
albumen synthesis 282
alcohol poisoning 303
alcoholism 196, 303
aldosterone 316, 384
    oversecretion 385, 387
aldosteronism 385, 387
alkaline phosphatase 282
alkalis 180
alkylating agents 68
allograft 556
alpha cells
    pancreas 301–2
alpha particles 65
aluminium hydroxide 171, 188, 197
amazia 389

amethocaine   439
amnesia   160
amoebiasis   18–9
amoebic colitis   1
amoebic dysentery   229
amoebic hepatitis   19, 289
ampicillin   221, 223
ampulla of Vater   301
amputation   110–1, 123
amylase   174, 302
   increase   304
anaemia
   acquired hæmolytic   299
   aplastic   299
   burns   46
   myelosclerotic   299
   sickle cell   299
anaesthetic recovery   26–7
anal canal   246–66, *247*
   anatomy   246–8, *247*
   atresia   *248*, 248–9
   condylomata   262
   dilator   255
   fissure   254–6, *255*
   fistula   258, *259*
   orifice   246
   sinus   258
   skin tags   262
   sphincter   260
   lax   263
   spasm   254
anal warts   260, 260–2
Anderson-Hynes pyeloplasty   *329*, 329
androgen production   385–7
androgen treatment
   breast cancer   399
aneurysm   94, 104–7, *105*
   grafting   *106*
   intracranial   143–4, *145*
angina pectoris   93, 98–9
angiocardiography   92, 96
angioma
   intracranial   144–5
ankle
   orthopaedic conditions   553–4
   Pott's fracture   511–3, *512–3*
   sprains   *553*, 554

ano-rectal atresia   *248*, 248–9
ano-rectal fistulae   259
ano-rectal gonorrhoea   262
anterior nasal packing   458, *459*
antibioticoma   222, 390
antibiotics   3, 68
   prophylaxis   8
antibodies   7–8, 124, 557
anti-catarrhal vaccine   461
anticoagulant drugs
   overdose   323
anticoagulant therapy   34–5, 196
anti-convulsant drugs   161
anti-diuretic hormone   316
antigens   124, 557
antilymphocyte serum   558
anti-metabolites   68
antithyroid drugs   373
antrostomy
   intranasal   462
   radical   463, *464*
anuria   316–9
   calculous   337
   reflex   336
   treatment   317–9
   urinary stone   336
anus
   imperforate   248
   pruritus   256–7
aorta
   coarctation   92–3, *93*
aortic aneurysm   94
   treatment   *106*
aortic stenosis   93
aortogram   325
aplastic anaemia   299
appendicectomy   221–2
appendicitis
   acute   218–222, 224
   left-sided   234
appendix   218–9, 219–25
   abscess   219, *221*
   differential diagnosis   220
   gangrene   218, *219*
   mass   221, 221–2
   perforation   218, *219*, 220–2
   peritonitis   220–1

aqueous humour   417
   blockage   428
Arnold-Chiari malformation   133
arterial embolism   111–3
arterial injury   102–3
arterial reconstructive surgery   108–9, *109*
arterial wall
   degeneration   105
arteries   100
arteriography   325, *326*
arteriosclerosis   102, 105, 107–11, 231
arteriosclerotic aneurysms   94
arterio-venous aneurysm   104, *105*
arthritis
   septic   528, *529*
arthrodesis   532
arthrography   552, *553*
arthroplasty   531–2
artificial kidney   318–9
artificial limbs   111
ascaris lumbricoides   283
ascites   54, *57*
   malignant   238
aspiration biopsy   143
aspiration pneumonia   163, 172
aspirin   181, 196
astigmatism   437
atherosclerosis   102, 105, 107–11, 231
atresia
   anal canal   *248*, 248–9
atrial septal defects   95, *95*
atropine methyl nitrate   178
audiogram   445, *445*–6
aural granulations   450
aural speculae   443
auricle   442
   congenital deformity   445
   epithelioma   447
   rodent ulcer   447
   trauma   447
Austin Moore prosthesis   504
autograft   556
auto-hæmorrhoidectomy   252

autoimmune diseases   379
avascular necrosis   498, 501–2, 503
azathioprine   557–8

BCG vaccination   16
baboon kidneys
  transplantation   556
bacillary dysentery   229
bacille Calmette-Guerin   16
back strain
  acute   546
  chronic   548
backache   546–8
bacteria   1
balanitis   367
Bárány noise apparatus   443, *443*
barium enema   229, *229*, 235, 239
  double contrast   239
barium meal   179, *179*, 184, 204–5, *204*
barium swallow   164
  and meal   169–70, *170*
barium treatment
  intussusception   218
Barlow's test   521, *521*
basal cell carcinoma   411–2, *412*
basal hour secretion   175
basal layer of skin   403
basophil adenoma   140
bat ears   445
bedsores   29–30, *30*, 148
Bennett's fracture   499–500, *500*
berry aneurysm   104, *105*, 143
beta cells
  pancreas   301–2, 307
beta particles   65
betamethasone cream   257
Bigelow evacuator   356, *356*
bile   292
bile canaliculi   281
bile ducts   279
bile ducts
  compression   283
  obstruction   283
  system   *281*

wall abnormality   283
bile salts   292
  non-absorption   205
bile secretion   282
biliary cirrhosis   283
biliary surgery   286, *286*
biliary tract   279–81
bilirubin   282–3, 293
Billroth I gastrectomy   181, *181*
biogastrone   180
birth trauma   538
bladder   342–6
  carcinoma   345, 345–6
  closed catheter drainage   355, 355–6
  congenital abnormalities   342
  golf ball   330
  inflammation   344–5
  irrigation   361
  pain   323
  papilloma   345, 345–6
  paralysis   525
  pelvic abscess   224
  rupture   342–4
  spinal injuries   519
  stones   334, *335*, 337–8
  tumours   320, 345–6
blade plate fixation   509, *509*
blepharitis   423, 423–4
blindness
  causes   429
blood count
  infections   6
blood glucose level   302
blood loss
  treatment   195–6
blood transfusion
  objections   24
blood urea   324
boils   89–9
bone
  diseases   538–9
  metastasis   534, *534*
  osteogenic sarcoma   86
  nibbling forceps   157, *158*
  tumours   534–7
bovine mycobacteria   201
bowel

gangrene   231
  tumour   61, *61*
Bowman's capsule   315, *315*
Boyle-Davis gag   469, *469*
brachial artery injury   494–5, *495*
brachial plexus injuries   542
brain
  abscess   452
  radiotherapy   66
  scan   141, *142*
  secondary deposits   138, 141
  space occupying lesions   135–7
  stem injury   160, *161*
  tumour   62
  ventricular system   132, *132*
branchial cyst   128
breast
  acute inflammation   389–90
  anatomy   388
  benign tumours   392–3
  Brodie's disease   392
  carcinoma   86, 127, 393–7, *394–5*
  cyst   391, *392*
  development   389
  duct papilloma   392
  fibroadenoma   392–3, *393*
  lymphatic drainage   388, *389*
  tumour   61
breast cancer
  clinical features   396
  clinical staging   396–7, *397*
  pathology   394–5
  screening   401
  special investigations   396
  spread   394–5
  treatment   397–9
Brodie's disease   392
bronchi   71, *71*
  mucus secretion   216
  neoplasms   83
bronchiectasis   80–1, *81*
bronchopleural fistula   74
bronchus
  adenoma   53
  carcinoma   77, 83–6

564

Buerger's disease   102
Burkitt's lymphoma   69
burns
   closed treatment   49–50, *50*
   exposure treatment   48, *49*
   full thickness   43–4, *44–5*
   general treatment   47–8
   local treatment   48–50
burns
   open treatment   48, *49*
   partial thickness   43–4, *44*
   pathology   43–7
   Rule of Nine   47, *48*
burr hole   157, 159
   exploration   151
bursitis   542
butazolidine   181, 196

cachexia   56–7, *57*
caecostomy   237
caecum   201, 218, 226
   volvulus   236–7
caesium 137   65
calcaneal spur   555
calcaneum   511
   fracture   513–4, *514*
calcium gluconate   305, 377
calcium oxalate calculi   334, *334*
calculous anuria   337
Caldwell-Luc procedure   463, *464*
calipers and braces   525, *525*
callus   485
calorie replacement
   anuria   318
calyces
   kidney   313
cancer   51
   telling patient   37
candida   1
   albicans   17
candidiasis   17
Cannon ring stripper   109, *110*
capitellum   543
carbachol   359
carbenoxalone sodium   180
carbimazole   374–5

carcinoid syndrome
   small intestine   207–8
carcinoid tumours   83
   colon   237
   rectum   263
carcinoma   52, 54
   basal cell   411–2, *412*
   bladder   345, 345–6
   breast   86, 127, 393–9, *394–5*
   colon   237–42
   gall bladder   294–5
   kidney   339–41
   large intestine   53
   lung   57–8, 83–6, *84–5*
   maxillary antrum   464, *465*
   nasopharynx   464–5
   oesophagus   171–3, *172*
   penis   368, *368*
   prostate   356–7, *357*
   rectum   238, 263–6, *264*
   squamous cell   410–1, *411*
   stomach   57, 182–5, *184*
   thyroid   373, 377–8
   tongue   65, *65*
   vocal cord   473
carcinomatous stricture
   colon   *240*
cardia
   achalasia   163, 167–8, *168*
   palliative intubation   59, 60
cardiac arrest
   temporary   90
cardiac catheterisation   95–6
cardiac defects
   congenital   94–7
cardiac surgery
   principles   88
cardiac transplantation   99, 560
cardiogenic shock   39–40
cardio-pulmonary bypass   90, 91, 94
carotid angiography   144, *145*, 157
carpal tunnel syndrome   540
cartilage tears   550–2
caruncle   416
castor oil   227

cataract   *429–31*, 429–31
   extraction   *430–1*, 430–1
   surgery   440
catarrh   466–7
catheters   360, 360–1
   central venous pressure   41
catheterisation   360–1
cauda equina injury   516
caval drip   41
cavitation   78–9
celbenin   390
Celestin tube   60, 173
cellulitis   10–1, *11*
   breast   389
cerebral abscess   137–8, *138*, 146
   angiography   137, 141, *142*
   arteriogram   151
   compression   149–51
   hernia   268
   palsy   538
   thrombosis   107
cerebrospinal fluid
   circulation   132–3
cerumen   447
cervical fusion   515, *516*
cervical oesophagostomy   165
cervical spine
   fracture dislocation   515
   injuries   514, *514–5*
   osteoarthritis   541
cervical spondylosis   541–2
cetrimide   361
Charnley total hip replacement   532, *532*
chest
   anatomy   70–1, *70*
   physiology   71–2
chlorambucil   68
chloramphenicol   440
chlorhexidine   404
chloride   174
   absorption   316
chloroquine   19
chlorpromazine   60, 160, 284
chlorpropramide   284
choana   465

565

choanal atresia   467
cholangiogram
   intravenous   296
   operative   297, *297*
cholangiography   288
cholangitis   283
cholecystectomy   296–7
cholecystitis
   acute   220, 222, 294, 296–7
   Murphy's sign   294
cholecystogram   295–6, *296*
cholecystography   285
cholecysto-jejunostomy   287, *287*, 307
cholecystokinin   186
cholecystostomy   297
cholera   200
cholestatic jaundice   284
cholesteatoma   450
cholesterol   282, 292–3
   stones   292–3
cholestyramine   205
chondroma   52, 535
chondrosarcoma   52, 537
chordae tendineae   88
chorioncarcinoma
   uterus   69
choroid   416
choroiditis   427
chromaffin cells   381
chromic acid   381
chromophobe adenoma   140
chylous ascites   125
chymotrypsin   302
ciliary body   416
cinchocaine   257
Circle of Willis   143
circlo-electric bed   515, *516*
circumcision   366–7
cirrhosis   289–92
   biliary   289
   cardiac   289
   portal   289
   treatment   290–2
claudication   107–8
clavicle
   fractures   490, 490–1
claw hand   540, *541*

closed treatment of burns   49–50, *50*
clostridium tetani   12
clostridium welchi   13
clot retention
   prostatectomy   355–6
club foot
   congenital   523–4, *524*
   treatment   524, *524–5*
coal-tar paste   121
coarctation of aorta   92–3, *93*
cobalt 60   65
cobalt beam therapy   63
Cock's peculiar tumour   405
codeine phosphate   205
colchicine   68
cold abscess   128, *128–9*
colectomy   59, 230
   partial   241, *241*
colitis
   ischaemic   231
   ulcerative   227–31
collar and cuff sling   493–4, *494*
Colledge tube   *474*
Colles' fracture   497–8, *497–8*
colon   226–46
   anatomy   226, *226–7*
   carcinoma   59, 229, 233–4, 238–42
   Crohn's disease   202
   diverticula   232–5, *232–3*
   diverticulitis   220
   drainpipe   229, *229*
   gangrene   224
   intussusception   217
   perforation   244
   preparation for surgery   240
   tumours   237
   ulcerative colitis   227–31
   volvulus   236–7, *237*, 244
colonic contraction   227
colonic interposition   165
colonic surgery
   preparation   26
colonoscopy   240
colostomy   242–6, *243*, 249, 265
   care   244–6

defunctioning   243, *243*
Devine   243
diet   245–6
double-barrelled   236, 243–4
loop   243, *243*
side   242–3, *243*
terminal   242, *243*, 265
transverse   234
coma
   causes   146
   progressive   149
comminuted depressed fracture   *153*
comminuted fracture   153
common cold   461
compound fracture   483
compound fracture of skull   153, *153–4*
compression plating technique   511, *512*
concomitant squint   435
conductive deafness   443–4, *444–5*
congenital megacolon   249
coning   152
conjugated bile salts   199
conjunctiva   422
   irrigation   438, *439*
conjunctival haemorrhage   154, *155*
conjunctivitis   422, 422–3
Conn's syndrome   385, 387
conscious level   150
consent form   20–1
constipation
   absolute   210
constrictive pericarditis   97
contact bleeding   228
cornea   416
corneal graft   426, *427*
   surgery   441
   microscope   429
   scar   426
   transplantation   558–9
   ulcer   423, 426, *426*
coronary thrombosis   35, 107
cortisone   181, 196, 383–4, 386–7

suppression test 381
therapy 190
Courvoisier's Law 284, *284*
cranial nerves
   injuries 155
   palsies 159
   tumours 140
craniotomy 144
cremaster muscle 363
cretinism 371
Crohn's colitis 205
Crohn's disease 202–6, *203–4*, 229
   acute 220
   surgery 206
   treatment 205–6
   x-ray changes 204–5
cross-eyes 435
Crutchfield tongs 515, *515*
Curling's ulcer 46
Cushing's syndrome 56, 140, *385*, 385–6
cyclophosphamide 68–9
cystadenocarcinoma 306
cystic duct 281
cystine stones 333
cystinuria 333
cystitis 344–5
   tuberculous 330
cystogram
   micturating 325
cystoscopy 24
   prostatectomy 354
   urinary tract *324–5*, 324–5
cysts 405–6
cytocrinia 412
cytotoxic therapy 59, 67–9

dacryocystectomy 425
dacryocystitis 423–5
dacryocystorrhinostomy 425, *425*
deafness 443–4
death
   telling patient 37
decerebrate rigidity 160, *161*
decortication 82
deep vein

   system 114–6
   thrombosis 33–5
deformity
   neurological conditions 537–8
defunctioning colostomy 243, *243*
degenerative joint disease 528
dendritic ulcer 426
depressed fracture of skull 153–4
dermis 403
Devine colostomy 243
diabetes 102, 108, 146, 256
   insipidus 323
   mellitus 302, 323
   retinal degeneration 432
diabetic neuritis 108
diabetic patients 22
dialysis
   anuria 318
Diamox 428, 431
diaphragm 70
diaphyseal aclasis 535
diarrhoea
   spurious 264
diathermy
   coagulation 261–2, *325*, 325
diazepam 164
dicoumarol 323
diphenoxylate 205
diphtheria 473
diphtheroids 403
dislocation 484, *484*
   elbow 495–6, *496*
   hip 500, 500–1
   shoulder 494
dissecting aneurysm 94, 104, *105*, 105
disseminated sclerosis 358, 429
diverticula of colon 232–5, *232–3*
diverticular disease 232–3, *233*, 235
diverticulitis
   acute 233–4, *234*
   colon 220

diverticulosis 232, *235*
Dohlman's operation 477
donor matching 558
Dormia basket *337*
drainage 30–1
drainpipe colon 229, *229*
dressings 32
duct of Santorini 301
duct of Wirsung 301
duct papilloma
   breast 392
Duke's classification
   rectal tumours 266
duodenal chyme 302
duodenal ulcer 176, 179, 186–90, *188*, 193, 196
   medical treatment 188
   perforated 190–3, *192–3*, 222
   surgical treatment 189–90, *190*
duodeno-gastric reflux 174
duodeno-jejunal junction 185
duodenoscope 188
duodenum 185–97
   anatomy 185–6, *186*
   erosions 196
   physiology 186
Dupuytren's contracture 543–4
Durabolin 399
Durham tube 480, *480*
dysentery 229
dysphagia 163, 172
dysuria 320, 323

ear 442–56
   anatomy 442–3
   clinical examination 443
   drum 442, *442*
   foreign body 447
   physiology 442–3
   suction clearance 456
   syringing *447*, 447–8
earache 454–6
Echinococcus granulosus 18, *18*
echo-encephalography 157
ectopia vesicae 342, 347

ectopic pregnancy
 ruptured   220
ectopic testis   363
ectopic thyroid   370, *370*
ectropion   423
elastic stockings   120
elbow
 dislocation   495–6, *496*
 orthopaedic conditions
   542–3
electro-encephalogram   137, 143
electro-magnetic radiation   65
embolectomy   35, 112, 206
embolism   102, 111
embolus   111
embryoma   338–9
emetine   19
empyema   78, 82, *83*
endarterectomy   98, *107*
endocrine pancreas   302
endocrine surgery   60
endoscopic prostatectomy
   353, 353–4, 358
endotracheal intubation   72–3,
   147, *148*
entamoeba
 histolytica   18
enteritis   177, 200
entropion   423, 425
 spastic   425, *425*
eosinophilic adenoma   140, *141*
epanutin   161
epidermis   403
epididymis
 cyst   365, *365*
 testis   361
epididymitis   364–5
epigastric hernia   268, 277–8
epiglottis   472
epilepsy   146
 persistent   161
epispadias   347
epistaxis   456–9
 arrest   457–8
 spontaneous   457
 surgical treatment   459
epithelial tumours   52
ergot poisoning   102

erythrocyte sedimentation rate
   6
erythromycin   390
Escherichia   1
eserine drops   428
ethmoidal artery
 ligation   459
European Transplant Organisation   560
eusol   258
Eustachian tube   442, 452
euthyroid state   370
Eve's tonsil snare   470, *470*
Ewing's sarcoma   537
exocrine pancreas   301–2
exomphalos   276
exophthalmos   371, *371*
exostosis   535
expiratory stridor   474
exposure keratitis   148
exposure treatment of burns
   48, *49*
extensor tendons
 repair   545
external angular dermoid   405
external auditory meatus   442
 congenital stenosis   447
 malignant disease   449
external ear
 malignant disease   455
extradural abscess   451, 452
extradural haematoma   156,
   158
extradural haemorrhage   155–8,
   158
extradural space   155
eye
 anatomy   416–9, *417–8*
 examination   420–2
 foreign body   439
 inflamed   422–9
 inflammation of inner eye
   426–9
 insertion of drops   438, *438*
 irrigation   438
 muscles   418, *418*
 surgery   440–1
 treatment   438

eyeball   416, *417*
eyelids   418–9, *419*
 eversion   420–1, *421*

facial paralysis   451, 452
faecolith   219
failing sight   429–35
falciform ligament   279
Fallot's tetralogy   96, 96–7
false aneurysm   104, *105*
familial polyposis coli   238
fat embolism
 fractures   486
feeding
 unconcious patient   147–8
 gastrostomy   172
femoral canal
 anatomy   274, *274*
femoral epiphysis   550, 551–2
femoral head
 avascular necrosis   549
 replacement   504–5
femoral hernia   268, 274–5, *275*
femoral neck
 fractures   501–6, *502–5*
 subcapital fracture   501,
   502, 503, 504–5
 subtrochanteric fracture   501,
   502, 502, 504
 transcervical fracture   501,
   502, 503
 treatment of fractures   503–6
 trochanteric fracture   501,
   502, 502, 504, 506
femoral osteotomy   523
femoral shaft
 fractures   506–9
 internal fixation   508–9, *509*
 supracondylar fracture   509,
   509
 treatment of fractures   507–8
femoral vein   274
fibrin   82
fibroadenoma
 breast   392–3, *393*
fibroadenosis   390
fibrocystic pancreatic disease
   215

568

fibro-liposarcoma 52
fibroma 535, *535*
fibula
    fracture 512
figure of eight bandage 491, *491*
filaria bancrofti 125
filariasis 125
filiform bougies 350, 350–1
fingers
    fracture 499–500, *500*
    laceration 545
fissure in ano 254–6, *255*
fissured fractures 153
fistula-in-ano 229, 258–60, *259–60*
    excision 260, *260*
fixation of fractures 488–9
flail chest 73, *73*
flexor tendons
    repair 545–6
fluid balance
    anuria 318
    prostatectomy 354–5
fluorescein 426
5-Fluorouacil 68–9, 242, 351
Fogarty balloon catheter 112
Foley balloon catheter 31, 348, *349*, 354–5, *355*, 360, 361
follicular tonsillitis 468
foot
    arthrodesis 538
    fractures 513–4
    orthopaedic conditions 554–5
foramen caecum 370
foreign bodies
    oesophagus 165–7
fossa ovalis 88
fractures
    care of patient 482–3
    closed 483, *483*
    complications 485–7
    compound 483, *483*
    delayed union 487
    fixation 488–9
    greenstick 483, *484*
    healing 484–5, *485*
    malunion 487

non-union 487
    principle of treatment 487–90
    reduction 487–8
    rehabilitation 489–90
    ribs 72–3
    simple 483, *483*
fragilitis osseum 539, *540*
freezing probe 434
Frog abduction plaster 522, *522*
frontal sinus
    obliteration 464
frontal sinusitis 463
    complications 464
fronto-ethmoidectomy 464
frozen shoulder 542
fundoplication 171
fungi 1
furunculosis 454
fusiform aneurysm 104, *105*

G cells 173, 175, 301
gall bladder 186
    anatomy 281, *281*
    carcinoma 294–5
    jaundice 284, *284*
gall stones 283, 292–7, 295–7
    clinical features 294–5
gall stones
    formation 292–3
    ileus 209, 294
    special investigations 295–6
    treatment 296–7
    types 292, *293*
Gallow's traction 507, *507*
galvano-cautery 457
gamma
    rays 65
    scan 137
ganglion 406, *406*
ganglioneuroma
    adrenal medulla 382
gangrene *101*, 101–2, 107–10, 113, 222
    hernia 269
    intestine 206, 210–1, 231
    piles 251

gas gangrene 13–4, 110
gastrectomy 197, 309
gastric acid hypersecretion 309
    aspiration 194, 223
    carcinoma 57, 182–5
    perforation 191
    chyme 302
    drainage 189, *190*
    erosions 181
    function tests 175–6, 188
    haemorrhage 182
    lavage 195
    peristalsis 194
    secretion 174–5
    transection 292
    tumours 196
    ulcer 176, 178–81, *178–80*, 196
    malignant 183, *183*
    medical treatment 180–1
    surgery 181
gastric volvulus 169
gastrin 173–5, 187
    Zollinger-Ellison syndrome 309
gastritis 181–2
gastro-colic fistula 183
gastro-colic reflex 227
gastroduodenoscope 305
gastroduodenoscopy 188
gastroenteritis 220
gastroenterostomy 185
gastro-intestinal haemorrhage 195–7
gastro-jejunostomy 189, *190*, 195
gastro-oesophageal continence 170
gastro-oesophageal reflux 168–71
gastroscopy 180, *180*, 185
gastrostomy 165, 197
gentamycin sulphate 49
germinal layer of skin 403
giant cell tumour 536
Gibbon's catheter 361
gigantism 140

glandular fever   127
glaucoma   423, *428*, 428–9,
   431–2, 431–2
   surgery   440–1
glioma   139, *139*
Glisson's capsule   279
glomerulus
   kidney   315
glomus tumour   410
glottic oedema   471
glucagon   301–2
glucocorticoids   383
   excess   385
glue ear   452–3
glycine   282
glycogen   282
glycosuria   316, 383
goitre
   non-toxic   *372*, 372–3
   physiological   *372*, 372
   toxic   372–5
gonorrhoea
   testis   365
   urethra   349
gout   332
Graves' disease   372
gravitational ulcer   121–3
Grawitz tumour   339–41
Great Ormond Street tube   480, *481*
great vessels
   surgical diseases   91–4
greater omentum   227
greater tuberosity
   fracture   492, *492*
greenstick fracture   483, *484*
griseofulvin   408
grommet   453, *453*
gum-elastic catheter   360, *361*
gumma   123, 136, 365

haemangioma   415
haemangiosarcoma   415
haematemesis   169, 195
haematoma
   auris   *446*, 447
   brain   135
   encapsulated   159

nail bed   409
peri-anal   253–4, *254*
spleen   299
haematuria   320, *322*, 323
   causes   321, *322*
haemochromatosis   289
haemodialysis   318–9, *319*
haemolytic anaemia   299
   -haemolytic streptococcus
   10–1, *11*
haemopericardium   97
haemophilia   196
haemorrhage
   fractures   485
   gastro-intestinal   195–7
   intracranial   155–9
   rectal   233
   tonsillectomy   470–1
haemorrhoidectomy   24, 251–3
haemorrhoids   250–3
haemothorax   76
hair
   follicles   403
   roots   403
hallux valgus   *554*, 554–5
halo-pelvic traction   526, *527*
hammer toes   555, *555*
hand
   infections   544–5
   orthopaedic conditions   543–4
hang-nail   544
Hanot's cirrhosis   289
Harrington distraction rod
   526, *527*
Hashimoto's disease   372, 379
haustra
   colon   226
   loss   228–9
head injuries   145–53
   complications   159–61
   indications for surgery   152
hearing tests   443–5
heart
   acquired diseases   97–9
   anatomy   87–8, *88*
   failure   39
   surgical disease   91
   valve replacement   98, *98*

heartburn   163, 168
heart-lung machine   90, *91*
heat exchanger   90
Heef test   15
heel fracture   513–4, *514*
Heller's operation   168, *169*, 235
hemicolectomy
   left   241, *241*
   right   241, *241*
   transverse   241, *241*
hemiplegia   538
heparin   34–5, 112
   overdose   323
hepatectomy   289
hepatic artery   279
   cell metabolism   281
   coma   146
   jaundice   282
   veins   279
hepatitis
   amoebic   289
   homologous   288
   infective   288
hepato-renal syndrome   286
hernia
   abdominal   268–78
   cerebral   268
   composition   267
   epigastric   268, 277–8
   femoral   268, 274–5, *275*
   gangrene   269
   hiatus   168–71, *169*, 196, 268
   incisional   268, 277, 278
   inguinal   268, 271–3, *272–3*
   irreducible   269, *270*
   para-umbilical   276
   reducible   269, *270*
   Richter's   275, *275*
   strangulated   211, 269–70, *270–1*
   umbilical   268, 275–6, *276*
   ventral   268, 277–8
herniotomy   272
herpes simplex   423
herpes zoster   220
hiatus hernia   168–71, *169–70*, 196, 268

570

Hibitane 361
Higginson's syringe 462
hilum
  kidney 312
hips
  abduction 505–6, 521
  central dislocation 501
  congenital dislocation 520–3, *522*
  fractures 501–6
  orthopaedic conditions 549–50
  osteoarthritis 502, *530–1, 530–2*
  posterior dislocation 500, *500*
  post-operative carde 505–6
  replacement 531–2
  rheumatoid arthritis 533
Hirschsprung's disease 249–50, *249–50*
Hodgkin's disease 52, 69, *130*, 130–1, 182
  pancreatitis 303
  spleen 300
homatropine 440
homograft valve 98
horse-shoe kidney 313, *314*
Horsley's wax 158
humerus
  fractures 492–5
  shaft 493–4, *494*
  humerus 492–3, *493*
  surgical neck 136
hydatid cyst 136
hydatid disease 18, 289
hydrocele 364–5, *365*
hydrocephalus 132–5, *134*
  acquired 133
  communicating 133
  congenital *133*
  obstructive 133
  spina bifida 524–5
hydrochloric acid 174
hydrocortisone 42, 383
  cream 257
hydronephrosis 320, *321*, 327–8, 328–9
  congenital 327

  obstructive 327
  pregnancy 327
  urinary stones 336
hydropneumothorax 76
hydrotherapy 530
5-hydroxyindole acetic acid 208
5-hydroxytryptamine 83, 207
hyperadrenocorticism 384–5
hyperbaric oxygen 14
hyperglycaemia 383
hyperglycaemic coma 146
hyperinsulinism 308
hypermetropia 437
hypernephroma *339*, 339–41
hyperostosis 140
hyperparathyroidism 303, 332–3, 380–1
hyperpyrexia 160
hypertension
  phaeochromocytoma 382
  retinal degeneration 432
hyperthyroidism 370–1, *371*
  clinical features 371
hypertrophic pyloric stenosis 176–8
hypoglycaemia 56, 308
hypoglycaemic coma 146
hypoparathyroidism 376–7, 381
hypopharyngeal diverticulum 477, *478*
hypopharynx 475–7
  foreign bodies 475–6, *476*
  malignant disease 476–7
hypophysectomy 386
  breast cancer 399
hypospadias 347, *347*
hypothermia 90
hypothyroidism 370–1, *371*
hypovolaemic shock 39, 506
hypoxia 486
hysterectomy
  anuria 317
hysteria 146

Icthopaste 121
identical twins 557

ileo-caecal region
  intussusception 217
ileo-caecal tuberculosis 201
ileo-caecal valve 218, 226
ileo-rectal anastomosis 230
ileostomy 230
  adhesive appliances 230–1, *231*
ileum 198, *198*
  stenosis 203
immunological rejection 556–7
immunosuppression 557–8
immunosuppressive therapy 206
imperforate anus 248
implantation dermoid 405, *405*
Imuran 206
incisional hernia 268, 277, 278
incontinence of urine 323
incubation period 7
incus 442
infarct 111
infection
  incubation 7
  mechanisms 4
  prophylaxis 7–8
  protecting mechanisms 6–7
  signs 4–7
  treatment 2, 7–8
  types 8–19
  wound 11–2
infective mononucleosis 127, 469
ingrowing toe nail 408
inguinal canal 271, *271*
inguinal hernia 268, 271–3, *272–3*
  acquired 272
  anatomy 271–2
  congenital 272
  direct 272
  indirect 271–2
  treatment 272–3
inhalation pneumonia 165
inspiratory stridor 474
instability syndromes
  spine 547–8
insulin 301–2
  test 176
insulinoma 307–9

intensive therapy units 38
interatrial septum 88
intermittent claudication 100, 123
internal ear
  malignant disease 455
interventricular septum 88–90
intervertebral disc syndromes 546–7
intestinal amoebiasis 18–9
intestinal obstruction
  acute 220
  congenital 177
  hernia 269
intestine
  rupture 222
  vascular disease 206–7
intra-abdominal pressure 170, 268
intracerebral haemorrhage 155
intracranial angiomas 144–5
  haemorrhage 155–9
  tumours 138–43
  vascular lesions 143–5
intradermal naevus 412, *413*
intralymphatic therapy 415
intramedullary nail fixation 508, *509*
intranasal antrostomy 462
intra-ocular pressure 431
intravenous infusions 29
intrinsic factor 199
intussusception 216–8, *217*
iodine
  thyroid 371
  treatment 373, 375
ionisation 65–6
iris 416
iritis 426–7, *428*
iron-deficient anaemia 167, 186
irradiation
  complications 66–7
  effects 65–6
  necrosis 67
irreducible hernia 269, *270*
ischaemic colitis 231
ischaemic ulcer 123

islet cell tumours 301, 307–10
islets of Langerhans 301
isonicotinic acid hydrazide 17

Jacksonian fits 157
Jaques' plastic catheter 361
jaundice 282–8
  acholuric 294, 299
  cholestatic 284
  hepatic 282
  obstructive 283–8
  patients' diet 22
  post-hepatic 283–8
  pre-hepatic 282
  surgery 285–8
jejunum 198, *198*
  sentinel loop 304
Jobson Horne wool carrier 448, *448*, 450
joints
  dislocation 484, *484*
  erosion 528, *529*
  stabilisation operation 538
  subluxation 484, *485*
junctional naevus 513, *513*

KCH speaking-valve 475
KCH tube 479, *479–80*
kala azar 299
Keen's aural dressing forceps 448, *449*
Keller's operation 555
ketosteroid excretion 385
kidney 312–41
  anatomy 312–3, *312*
  artificial 318–9
  carcinoma 86, 340–1
  congenital abscess 313
  congenital anomalies 313–4
  double 313
  embryology 313
  jaundice 286
  obstruction 320, *321*
  physiology 314–6
  polycystic disease 313–4, *314*
  rupture 326
  stones 334, *335*, 336

  storage 560
  transplant 559–60
  trauma 325–7
  tuberculosis 320, 329–32, 330
  tumours 338–41
knee
  arthrodesis 533
  fracture 510–1
  ligaments 552, *553*
  orthopaedic conditions 550–3
  rheumatoid arthritis 533
  septic arthritis 528
konakion 286

labelling patient 21
labyrinthitis 451, 452
lacrimal gland *418*, 419
lacrimal sac 419
  syringing 424, *425*
Ladd's band 214
lamblia 1
laminectomy 547
Langerhans
  islets 301
laparotomy 112, 200
  colon 234–7
  incisional hernia 277
  infection 222
  intussusception 218
  small intestine 213
  wounds 32, 36
large bowel
  carcinoma 229
  Crohn's disease 229
laryngeal diphtheria 473
laryngeal mirror 471
laryngectomy 473–4
laryngitis
  acute 472
  chronic 473
laryngoscopy 471, 472
laryngo-tracheo-bronchitis 473
larynx 471–5, *472*
  infections 472–3
  injuries 471–2
  removal 474
  tumours 473–4

lateral sinus thrombosis *451*,
    452
lazy eye 435–6
leather bottle stomach 183, *183*
leg
    anatomy of veins 113–6,
        114–5
    deep veins 114, *115*
    physiology of veins 116
    superficial veins 113–6,
        114–5
    thrombosis 33–5
    ulceration 121–2, *121–3*
leiomyoma
    oesophagus 172
    stomach 182
leiomyosarcoma
    oesophagus 172
    stomach 182
lens 417
lentigo 412
leptospirosis 288
leucotomy 455
leukaemia 52, 69, 469
    chronic lymphatic 130–1
Lichwitz trocar *461*, 461–2
ligament tears 552–3, *553*
ligation of veins 35
lignocaine 257
limb circulation
    impaired 102
linea alba 277–8
linear accelerator 64, *64*
lingual thyroid 370, *370*
linitis plastica 183, *183*
lipase 174, 302
lipoma 52, 415, *415*
lipoproteins 282
liposarcoma 52
Lister's metal bougies 350, *350*
lithotomy position 260
lithotrite 337–8, *338*
Little's area
    nose 457, *457*
liver
    anatomy 279–81, *280*
    carcinoma 289
    enlargements 288–9

microscopic anatomy 281
palm 290
physiology 282
transplantation 561
trauma 289
lobectomy 80–1
lobster-tail tube 480, *480*
lock-jaw 12
Lomotil 201, 205
long-sightedness 437
loop colostomy 243, *243*
loose bodies
    elbows 543, *543*
    knee 553
lotio plumbi 252
lower limb
    dislocations 500–11
    fractures 500–11
Lowenstein
        Jensen's medium 331
lumbar puncture 152
lumbar spine
    fracture dislocation 516–7
    fractures 20
    fusion 517, *517*
    injuries 516–7
lumbar sympathectomy 110
lungs
    abscess 77, 77–8
    anatomy 70–1, *70*
    carcinoma 57–8, 83–6
    hypoventilation 486
    neoplasms 83
    physiology 71–2
    secondary neoplasms 86
    transplantation 561
lymph nodes 124
    neoplastic 127
    ulceration 130
lymphadenitis 1, 10
    acute 125
lymphadenitis
    tuberculous 127–8
lymphadenopathies 126–31
lymphangioma 415
lymphangiosarcoma 415
lymphangitis 10
    acute 125

lymphatic leukaemia 130–1
lymphatics 124
    congenital abnormality 125
    malignant obstruction 126
lymphocytes 124
lymphoedema 125–6, *125–6*
lymphoid tissues
    tumours 130–1
lymphomas 52
lymphosarcoma 52, 69, 130–1
    colon 237
    rectum 263
    stomach 182

McKee Farrar total hip
        replacement 532, *532*
macular dystrophy 432, *433*
magnesium sulphate 9
magnesium trisilicate 171, 188
malabsorption 203–4
malaria 1, 299
maldescended testis 363
malignant disease
    clinical features 56
    diagnosis 57–8
    prognosis 60–3
malleoli 512–3
mallet finger deformity
    499–500, *500*
malleus 442
mammography 401
mannitol 152, 286
Mantoux test 15
maphenide acetate 49
Marfan's syndrome 94
Marjolin's ulcer 121, 411
masking
    hearing tests 443
mastectomy 58–9, 126, 398–9
    care of patient 399–401
mastitis 390–1, *391*
mastoid cells 442, *443*
mastoid infection 137
mastoidectomy
    cortical 450–1
    radical 451
mastoiditis *451*, 452, 454

573

maxillary antrum 461
   carcinoma 464, *465*
maxillary
   ligation 459
maxillary sinuses 462
maxillectomy 464
Mayo repair
   umbilical hernia 276, *277*
measles virus 1
Meckel's diverticulum 196,
   199, 199–200, 217
meconium 215, *217*
   ileus 215–6, *217*
median nerve 540
mediastinum 73–4
megacolon 249
megavoltage x-rays 65, 67
Meibomian cyst 424, *424*
Meibomian glands 419
melaena 195
melanin 290
melanocytes 412
melanoma 52, 412–5
   malignant 413–4, *414*
   subungual 410
melphalan 68
Meniere's disease 444
meningeal irritation 159
meningioma 139–40
meningism 143
meningitis 146, 160, *451*,
   452
menisectomy 551
6-Mercaptopurine 68
metabolic changes
   fractures 486–7
metacarpal fractures 499–500
metacarpal-phalangeal joint
   replacement 533
metacarpals
   chondromas 535
metanephric duct 313
metanephros 313
metastases 55, *55*
metatarsal fractures 514
metatarsal heads
   excision 534, *534*
metatarsalgia 555

metatarso-phalangeal
   joint 554–5
methicillin 390
methotrexate 68–9
methyl-testosterone 284
microlaryngoscopy 471
micturating cystogram 325
micturition
   disturbance 322–3
   frequency 320
middle ear
   conditions 449–51
   disease 444
   infection 137
   infection complications *451*,
   451–3
middle meningeal
   haemorrhage 155
mid-thigh perforator 115
miliary tuberculosis 15, 78,
   79
Milwaukee brace 526, *526*
mineral corticoids 384
mithramycin 68
mitral stenosis 97–8
mitral valve 88
mole 412
moniliasis 469
Morton's metatarsalgia 555
Moure-Lombard tube *474*
Mousseau-Barbin tube 60, 173
muco-perichondrium 460
mucoviscidosis 215
mucus secretion 215
multiple sclerosis 323
mumps
   orchitis 365
   pancreatitis 303
   virus 1
mycobacterium tuberculosis
   14, *16*, 78
myelogram 547
myelomeningocele 524–5, *525*
myelosclerotic anaemia 299
myopia 432, 437
myositis ossificans 496
myotomy 235
myringotome 450

myringotomy 449–450,
   449–450, 453
myxoedema 370–1, *371*

naevus 412
   intradermal 412, *413*
   junctional 413, *413*
nail bed haematoma 409
nail bed lesions 409–10
nail fixation
   hip 503, *505*
nails 407–10
   removal 408–9
nasal allergy 466
   catarrh 466–7
   packing 458, *459*
   polypi 465–6, *466*
   sepsis 450
   septum 457, *457*
   deflected 459–60, *460*, 466
   disorders 459–61, *460*
   snare 465, *466*
naso-gastric tube 148
naso-lacrimal duct 419
   obstruction 424–5
nasopharyngitis 424
nasopharynx 456–67
   carcinoma 464–5
neck
   orthopaedic conditions 541–2
Negus tube 480
neomercazole 374
neomycin 241
nephrectomy 327, 329, 336
   partial 327, 336
nephroblastoma 338–9
nephrolithotomy 336
nephron
   kidney 315, *315*
neruroglia 138
nerve damage
   fractures 486
nerve repair 541
Nettleship's dilator 439
neuroblastoma
   adrenal medulla 382
neurofibroma 415
neurofibrosarcoma 415

neurological conditions   537–8
neurosis
  post-traumatic   160
nipple
  Paget's disease   394, *394*
  retraction   396
Nitrogen mustard   68
nocturia   322–3
  prostatic enlargement   352
noradrenaline   39, 381–2
Normacol granules   255
normovolaemic shock   39–40
nose   456–67
  bleeding   456–9
  foreign body   456
  fracture   456–7
  infection   461–6
nylon darn repair
  hernia   272, *273*
nystatin   17

obstruction
  causes   209, *209*
obstructive jaundice   283–8
  features   283–5, *284*–5
  surgery   285–8
oesophageal atresia   163–5, *164*
oesophageal carcinoma   171–3, *172*
oesophageal disease
  investigations   164
  symptoms   163–4
  diverticulum   163
  pouch   167
  reconstruction   165
  resection   173
  transection   292
  varices   174, 196, 290–1
  web   167
oesophago-gastric junction   168
oesophagoscope   166
oesophagoscopy   164
osophagus   162–73
  anatomy   *162*, 162–3
  congenital abnormalities 164–5
  foreign bodies   165–7, *166*
  tumour   59, 60

oestrogenic hormones   282
olecranon
  fracture   496, *497*
oligaemic shock   46–7
oliguria   316–9
olivary-headed plastic bougies   350, *350*
onychogryphosis   408–9
oophorectomy
  breast cancer   399
oophoritis   1
open heart surgery   97
open treatment of burns   48, *49*
operating microscope   454, *454*
ophthalmoscope   420
opisthotonos   13
optic neuritis   429
orbicularis oculi   419
orbit   418
  exenteration   464
orbital haematoma   154
orchidectomy   357, 366
Ortolani's click test   521, *521*
osteitis fibrosa cystica   380
osteoarthritis   497, 528–32
  hip   502, 530–2, *530*–1
  wrist   498
osteoarthrosis   528
osteoblasts   485
osteochondritis dissecans   553, *553*
osteoclastoma   536
osteogenesis imperfecta   539, *540*
osteogenic sarcoma of bone   86
osteoma   535
osteomalacia   484, 538
osteomyelitis   490, 526–8, *528*
  acute   527
  chronic   527–8
  spine   548–9
osteophytes   529
osteoporosis   385, 484, 538
osteosarcoma   536, *537*
osteotomy   530–1, *531*
  femur   550
otalgia   454–6
  referred   455, 455–6

otitis externa   448
otitis media   449, 454
  chronic suppurative   450, *450*
  tonsillectomy   471
otorrhoea   449
  cerebrospinal fluid   154
otosclerosis   444, 453–4
otoscope
  electric   443
ovarian cyst
  ruptured   220
ovaries
  removal   399

Paget's disease
  bone   484
  nipple   394, *394*
palmar aponeurosis
  fibrosis   543–4
palmar infections   545
pampiniform plexus   362
pancreas   300–11
  anatomy   300–1, *300*
  carcinoma   284, *284*, 287, *287*, 306, 306–7
  cysts   310–1
  endocrine   302
  exocrine   301–2
  physiology   301–2
  removal   306
pancreatectomy   309
pancreatic cysts
  true   310
pancreatic ducts   301, *301*
  obstruction   303
pancreatic extract   216
pancreatic juice   301–2
pancreatic pseudocysts   310–1, *311*
  tumours   196
pancreaticoduodenectomy   307, *308*
pancreatitis   1, 295
  acute   303–5
  chronic   303, 305–6
  clinical features   303–4
  haemorrhage   304

pathology 303
  relapsing 303, 305
  special investigations 304
pancreatitis
  treatment 304–6
pancreatography
  operative 305
pancreozymin 186, 302
papaverine 103
papilloma 52
  bladder 345, 345–6
  colon 237
  skin 410
para-aminosalycilic acid 17
paracusis 453
paradoxical embolus 111
paraldehyde 147
paralysed patient
  rehabilitation 517
paralysis
  lower limbs 525, 525
paralytic ileus 28, 208–9,
  213, 304
paralytic squint 435
paranasal sinuses 456–67
paraphimosis 368
paraplegics
  kidney stones 333
paraspinal abscess 548
parathormone 379
  excess 380
parathyroid glands 369, 376
  adenoma 381
  anatomy 379, *379*
  physiology 379–80
parathyroid tumour 336,
  380–1
para-umbilical hernia 276
parietal pleura 71
paronychia 407–8, 544–5,
  544–5
  chronic 408
parotidectomy 24
parotitis
  postoperative 190
patellar fractures 510, *510–1*
patent ductus arteriosus *91*,
  91–2

Paterson-Kelly syndrome 167,
  476–7
Paul-Mikulicz operation 243–4
Paul's tubing 148
peak acid output 176
Pearson knee attachment 507,
  508
pelvic abscess 224–5
  cellulitis 11, 225
  fractures 518–9
  complications 519
  kidney 313, *314*
  osteotomy 523, *523*
  ring fractures *518*,
    518–9
  viscera
  damage 519
pelvis
  chronic inflammation 225
penicillin 174
penicillinoma 390
penicillium notatum 2
penis 366–8
  carcinoma 368, *368*
  paraphimosis 368
  phimosis 367
pentagastrin 175–6, 188
pepsin 174
peptic oesophagitis 166, 168,
  196
peptic ulcer 190, 193
  perforated 190–3, *192–3*,
    220
perceptive deafness 444, *444*,
  446
percutaneous transhepatic
  cholangiography 285, *285*
peri-anal abscess 257–8, *258*,
  259
peri-anal haematoma 253–4,
  254, 262
pericolic abscess 234
perimetry *421*, 421–2
peri-oesophageal abscess 166
peripheral arterial disease
  100–2
peripheral nerve injuries 540–1
peritoneal dialysis 318–9, 320

peritonitis 222–3
peritonsillar abscess 468–9
pernicious anaemia 181
persistent epilepsy 161
Perthes' disease 549–50, *550*
pethidine 304
petrositis 451, 452
phaeochromocytoma
  adrenal medulla 382
  excision 383, *384*
phagocytosis 6
phalangeal fractures 514
phalanges
  chondromas 535
pharyngeal pouch 167, 477,
  478
  sepsis 450
  ulceration 469
pharynx 468–71
phenobarbitone 147, 161
phenol 110
phenol in almond oil 252
phentolamine 383
phenylbutazone 530
phimosis 367, *367*
phosphatase
  carcinoma of prostate 357
  prostatic enlargement 353
phosphate excretion 380
phosphatic calculi 328, 333–4
phospho-lipids 292
photophobia 437
pigmented lesions
  treatment 414–5
piles 250–3
  clinical features 250–2
  injection treatment 252, *253*
  prolapse with strangulation
    251–2, *252*
  prolapsing 250–1, *251*
  sentinel 254, 255
  thrombosed external 253
  treatment 252–3
pilocarpine drops 428, 431, 440
pilonidal sinus 406–7, *406–7*
pin and plate fixation
  hip 504, *506*
pineal gland 141

pink-eye 422
pinna 442
   congenital deformity 445
   epithelioma 447
   rodent ulcer 447
   trauma 447
pituitary gland
   removal 399
pituitary tumours 140, *141*
   Cushing's syndrome 386
plantar fasciitis 555
plantar warts 410
plasma
   burns 46–7
   calcium level 379
   protein measurement 6
plasmodium 1
plaster
   backslab 498, *498*
   bed 548, *549*
   casts 488, *488*
pleura 70, 71
pleural effusion 54
pleurisy
   basal 220
plica semilunaris 416
Plummer-Vinson syndrome 167
pneumatic speculum 443
pneumaturia 233
pneumonia
   basal 220
pneumothorax 74–6, *74–5*
   treatment 75–6
podophyllin 261–2
poliomyelitis 524, 537
Polya gastrectomy 185, *185*, 189, 195
polyarteritis nodosa 303
polycystic disease 288
polycythaemia 289
polypoid carcinoma of stomach 183, *183–4*
polyposis coli
   familial 238
polyvinyl sponge wrap 263
pond fracture 153, 154
popliteal artery 109, *109*
portal hypertension 174, 196

cirrhosis 290
portal vein 279
portal venous system 298, *298*
Portex tube 480, *481*
porto-caval anastomosis 292, *292*
post-cricoid carcinoma 167, 173
post-hepatic jaundice 283–8
post-irradiation fibrosis 126
post-nasal plugging 458, *459*
post-operative adhesions 212
post-operative care 26–37
   chest 27–8
   drains 30–1
   drips 28
   fluids 28–9
   pain relief 26
   pressure areas 29–30
   rehabilitation 37
   skin 29–30
   smoking 27–8
   urethral caheters 31
   visiting 36–7
post-partum infection 223
post-traumatic neurosis 160
potassium 174
potassium iodide 373
Pott's disease of spine 527, 529, 549
Pott's fracture 511–3, *512–3*
Pott's paraplegia 528, 549
pouch of Douglas 225
prednisolone 257
prednisone 205–6
predsol 257
pregnancy
   hydronephrosis 327
   pancreatitis 303
pre-hepatic jaundice 282
pre-operative care 20–6
   bowels 26
   chest 24–5
   food 25–6
   nursing checks 22, 23
   nutrition 22
   premedication 25
   shaving 24
   smoking 24
   teeth 25

prepuce 367
   non-retractile 366–7
presbyopia 417, 436–7
pressure
   central venous 39, 41
   sores 29, 30
primary tuberculosis 15
probanthine 189
processus vaginalis 272, 362
proctitis 256
proctodaeum 248
proctofoam 257
proctoscope 251
proctoscopy 251
prostate 351, 351–8
   carcinoma 356–7, *357*
   surgical approaches *353*, 353–4
prostatectomy 354
   care 353–6
   clot retention 355–6
   complications 354–6
   prevention of infection 355
prostatic enlargement
   benign 351–6
   clinical features 352
   special investigations 352–3
   treatment 353–4
protamine sulphate 35
proteolytic enzymes 302
prothrombin 282
protozoa 1
pruritus ani 256–7
psoas abscess 528
pthallylsulphathiazole 241
pubic rami 518, *518*
puerperal infection 222
pulmonary embolus 35
pulmonary hypertension 91
pulmonary tuberculosis 15, 78–80
pulp space infections 544–5
pulse rate
   in infections 6
   sleeping 371
pupils 150, 151, 417
pure-tone audiometry *444*, 444–5

purine 558
pus 4, 6–7
   collection 82
pyelitis 344
pyelogram
   excretory 331
   intravenous *324, 324, 328, 328*
pyelography
   retrograde 325, 329
pyelolithotomy 336
pyelonephritis 220, 336
pyeloplasty 329, *329*
pyloric stenosis 193–5, *194*
pyloric tumour 176, 183
pyloric vein of Mayo 174
pyloroplasty 173, 181, 189, 190, 197
pylorus 174
pyoderma gangrenosa 229
pyonephrosis 328, 336
   tuberculous 330
pyrexia
   infections 5–6
de Quervain's stenosing tenosynovitis *543, 544*
quinsy 468–9

radial head 543
   fracture 496–7
radial nerve
   injury 493–4, 540
radial pulse
   absent 495
radiation sickness 66
radio-active fluorine 396
radio-active implants 63, 65
radio-active iodine 373, 375, 378
radio-active isotopes 63–5
radiotherapy 59
   principles 63–7
radium 64–5
   needles 65
raised intracranial pressure 136, 152
Ramstedt's operation 177, *177*, 235

Raynaud's disease 101–2, 113
von Recklinghausen's disease 380
rectal haemorrhage 233
rectal prolapse 262, 262–3
rectal tumour
   Duke's classification 266
   prognosis 266
recto-sigmoid region
   tumours 239
rectum 226, *247*, 246–66
   abdomino-perineal excision 264–5, 265
   aganglionic segment 249
   anatomy 246–8, *247*
   anterior resection 265
   carcinoma 238, 259, 263–6, *264*
   pelvic abscess 225
   polyvinyl sponge wrap 263
   prolapse 262, 262–3
   stenosis 264
   tumour 62
   ulcerative colitis 227–31
rectus sheath 276, *277*
recurrent laryngeal nerve injury 377, *377*
red cell destruction 299
reducible hernia 268–9, *270*
refractive errors 436–8
regurgitation 163
rehabilitation 37
rejection
   transplants 557
renal arteries
   aberrant 313, *314*
   artery 313
   colic 220
   ischaemia 92
   pelvis tumours 341
   physiology 314–6
   transplantation 559–60
   tuberculosis 329–32, *330*
   tubular necrosis 40, 286
   tumours 338–41
respiration 71–2
   nervous control 72
respiratory insufficiency 478–9

restlessness
   head injury 147
retention
   enemas 230
   urine 323, 336
reticuloses 127, 130–1, 289
reticulum cell sarcoma 130–1
retina 417
   haemorrhages 435
   thrombosis 434
retinal degeneration 429, 432
retinal detachment 432, 434, *434*
   surgery 440–1
retractile testis 363
retroperitoneal haemorrhage 208
retropubic prostatectomy *353*, 353–4
retrosternal thyroid 370, *370*
rheumatic heart disease 93
rheumatic pericarditis 97
rheumatism 427
rheumatoid arthritis 123, 127, 532–4
   treatment 532–4
rhinorrhoea
   cerebrospinal fluid 154
   excess 466
ribs 70
   stable fractures 72
   unstable fractures 73, *73*
Richter's hernia 275, *275*
rickets 539, *539*
rifampicin 17, 79
Rinnes test 444
Robert's pump *400*
rodent ulcer 411
   ear 447
Rose's cannula 462
rotating therapy 78
Roux-en-Y anastomosis 185, *185*

saccular aneurysm 104, *105*
salazopyrine 230
salmonella typhi 200
salpingitis 220, 222

Salt colostomy appliance 244, 246
salt metabolism 384
Salter's pelvic osteotomy 523, 523
Santorini
    duct 301
sapheno-femoral incompetence 117
saphenous veins 113
    graft 98, 110, *111*
sarcoidosis 127
sarcoma 52, 54
Savage decompresor 213
scalp
    laceration 152
scaphoid fracture 498–9, *499*
Schacht colostomy appliance 244, *245*
schistosomiasis 299
sciatic scoliosis 547, *547*
sciatica 525, 546–7
sclera
    eye 416
sclerectomy 431–2, *433*
sclerosant solution 118
sclerosis 529
scoliosis 525–6, *526*, 547
scopolamine 25
screening
    breast cancer 401
Scribner shunt 319, *319*
scrotum
    cysts 364–5
    hernia 271, *272*
sebaceous carcinoma 405
    cyst 404, 404–5
    glands 403
seborrhoeic keratosis 410
sebum 403
secondary carcinoma 128–30, *130*
secondary deposits 54, 55, 56–8
    effects 56–7
secondary invasion
    colon 237
secretin 186, 302

secretory otitis 452
segmental lobectomy 80
seminoma
    testis 365–6
Sengstaken tube 290, *291*
senile deafness 444
senile keratosis 410
Senokot 227
sentinel pile 254, 255
septal abscess 460
septal defects 94–5, *95*
septal haematoma 460
septal perforation 460
septic arthritis 528, *529*
septicaemia 40, 222
septicaemic shock 42
sequestrum 527–8, *528*
serotonin 207
sessile 54, *54*
sex hormone treatment 60
    breast cancer 398–9
sex hormones 383
shingles 220
shock
    aetiology 38–9
    clinical features 38
    septicaemic 42
    stages 40
    treatment 41–2
short-sightedness 437
shoulder
    calcification 542, *542*
    dislocation 494
    frozen 542
    injuries 492–4
    orthopaedic conditions 542
sialorrhoea 172
sickle cell anaemia 299
side colostomy 242–3, *243*
Siegle's speculum 443
sigmoid colon
    carcinoma 238
sigmoid volvulus 236, *237*
sigmoidoscope 227, 251, *251*
sigmoidoscopy 228, 251
silver nitrate 49, 457
silver sulphadiazine cream 50
simple fracture of skull 153, *153*

sinus
    pilonidal 406–7, 406–7
    tuberculous 128, 129
sinuses
    infection 461–6
sinusitis 461
    acute frontal 463–4
    acute maxillary 461
    chronic maxillary 461–3
skeletal traction 489, *489*
    apparatus 508
    cervical spine 515
    femoral shaft fracture 507
skin
    bacteriology 403–4
    function 403
    grafts 50, *50*, 556
    necrosis 67
    papilloma 410
    sensitivity tests 467
    squamous cell carcinoma 410–1, *411*
    structure 402, 402–3
    tags 262
    traction 488–9, *489*
    tumours 410–5
    unconcious patient 148
skip lesions
    Crohn's disease 202, 205
skull
    fractures 152, 153–5
    perforator 157, *157*
    space occupying lesions 135–7
    x-rays 151, *152*
sling
    collar and cuff 493–4, *494*
slipped femoral epiphysis 550, 551–2
slit-lamp 429
small bowel inflammation 201
small intestinal obstruction 208
    children 214
    clinical features 210–2
    pathology 210
    simple 210
    strangulation 210, *211*
small intestine 198–218

adynamic obstruction 208–9
  anatomy 196, *196*
  congenital atresia 214, *215*
  Crohn's disease 202, *203*
  dynamic obstruction 209
  intussusception 216–8
  necrotic 213
  physiology 198–9
  specific infections 200–2
  tumours 207–8
  volvulus 214–5, *216*
small vessel spasm 102
Smith-Petersen nail 503
Smith's fracture 498
smoking 84, 108, 180
Snellen's types 420
sodium 174
  absorption 316
sodium tetra-decyl-sulphate 119
Souttar's tube 60
spectacles 436–8
spermatic cord 271
  torsion 364
spherocytosis
  hereditary 294
sphincters
  unconcious patient 148
spina bifida 133, 524–5, *525*
spinal fusion 526, *527*
  injuries 514–7
  tumour 358
  vertebra fusion 548
spine
  orthopaedic conditions 546–9
  osteomyelitis 548–9
  tuberculosis 527, 529, 549
Spitz-Holter shunt 134, *135*, *525*
spleen 298–300
  anatomy 298, *298*
  ruptured 299
splenectomy
  conditions 299–300
splenic artery 298
splenic vein 298
spondylolisthesis 547, *548*
spondylolysis 547, *547*

sprains
  ankle 553, *554*
spurious diarrhoea 264
squint 418, 435–6, *435–6*
  concomitant 435
  operation 436, *436–7*
  paralytic 435
  treatment 436
staghorn calculus 329, 334, *334*
stapedectomy 454
stapes 442–3
  fixation 453
  prosthesis 454, *455*
staphylococcus albus 403
staphylococcus aureus 2, 2–3, 200, 389, 407
Starr-Edwards prosthesis 98, *98*
Steinmann pin 489, *489*, 507, 511
stelazine 202
sternomastoid muscle 541
steroid drops 423
steroid secretion 383
steroids
  Crohn's disease 206
  ulcerative colitis 230
stilboestrol 60, 357
  breast cancer 399
Still's disease 532
stomach
  anatomy 173–4, *173*, *175*
  carcinoma 182–5, *184*, 193
  erosions 196
  tumours 182
  ulcer 190, 193
stones
  urinary tract 332–8, *334–5*
strangulated hernia 269–70, 270–1
  treatment 272–3
strangury 323
stratum corneum of skin 403
streptococcus viridans 92
streptomycin 17
stress reaction
  burns 46
stricture formation 169

stridor 472, 474
string snig
  Crohn's disease 205
stroke 146
Stryker frame 515
stye 424, *424*
subacute bacterial endarteritis 92, 94, 104
subarachnoid haemorrhage 159
subarachnoid space 155
subconjunctival haemorrhage 154, *155*
subcutaneous tumours 415
subdural abscess 452
subdural haematoma 156, 158
  acute 158
  chronic 159
subdural space 155
subluxation 484, *485*
submucous resection 459–60, *460*, 463
subphrenic abscess 224, 225
subphrenic spaces
  pus 223
subtalar joint 514
subungual exostosis 409
subungual melanoma 410
succussion splash 193
sucking pneumothorax 75
suction clearance
  ear 450
suction drainage 400, *400*
sugar tolerance test 308
sulphadimidine 154
sulphamylon 49
sulphasalazine 230
sulphonamides 2
superficial vein system 114–6
supervoltage therapy 63, 67
supracondylar fracture
  femur 509, *509*
  humerus 486, *486*, 494–5, *495*
suprapubic catheter 348, *349*
suprapubic cystostomy 360
suprapubic region 323
suprarenal glands 381–7

supraspinatus tendon rupture 542
surgeons 21–2
sutures 32
swallowed foreign bodies 165–7, *166*
swinging pyrexia 5, *5*
sympathectomy 110, 113
sympathetic block 110
syphilis 104, 123, 127, 365, 469
systemic treatment of burns 2

T-tube cholangiogram 288
taenia coli 226–7
talipes equino-varus 523–4, *524*
talus 512
tarsal plate 419
taurine 282
tear-duct 419
   syringing 439–40
teflon tube 453, *453*
   graft 545–6, *546*
   injuries 545–6
   sheath infection 545
   suture 545, *545*
   transfers 538
tennis elbow 542–3
tension pneumothorax 74, *75*
teratoma 52
   testis 366
terminal colostomy 242, *243*
terminal ileum 226
   Crohn's disease 202–3
test meal 175
testicular descent
   abnormalities 363–4
testis 361–6, *362*
   cysts 364–5
   development 362
   gumma 365
   infection 365
   seminoma 365–6
   teratoma 366
   torsion 362, 364
   tumours 365–6
tetanus 12–3, 490
   toxoid 12–3

tetany 305, 378, 380
tetracyclines 19
tetralogy of Fallot 96, 96–7
thalassemia 299
thermography 401
thiotepa 68
thiouracil 284
Thomas' splint 507, *508*
Thompson prosthesis 504, *504*
thoracic spine
   injuries 515
   kyphosis 538, *538*
thoracotomy 165
thread worms 256
thrombocytopenic purpura 299
thromboendarterectomy 109–10, *110*
thrombophlebitis 120–1
thrombosed external piles 253
thrombosis
   deep vein 33–5
   lateral sinus 451, 452
   retina 434
thrombus 107, *107*
thrush 1, 17, 469
thumb
   fracture 499–500
thyroglobulin 370, 379
thyroglossal cyst 370, *370*
   fistula 370, *370*
thyroid 369–79
   anatomy 369, *369*
   carcinoma 373, 377–8
   congenital anomalies 370
   crisis 376
   cyst 373
   development 369–70, *370*
   function tests 371–2
   haemorrhage 376
   physiology 370
   types of enlargement 372
thyroidectomy 373, 381
   complications 375–7
   subtotal 375
thyrotoxicosis 370–1, *371*
   primary 372
   secondary 372
thyrotrophic hormone 378

thyroxine 370
   tests 372
   treatment 373, 375, 379
tibia
   fractures 510, *510–1*
tibial exostosis 535
Tiemann's catheter 360, *361*
Tilley's nasal dressing forceps 458, *458*
tinnitus 453
toes
   rheumatoid arthritis 534, *534*
Tom Smith's disease 528
tongue
   carcinoma 65, *65*
tonsil
   dissection 469–70, *469–70*
   position 147, *147*
tonsillectomy 469–71
   complications 470–1
   earache 456
   post-operative 470
tonsillitis 127, 468–9
tonsils 468–71
Torkildsen operation 135, *136*
torticollis 541
total hip replacement arthroplasty 531–2
toxaemia 146
   burns 46
toxoplasma 1
trabeculae carneae 87
trachea 71, *71*
   compression 376
tracheo-bronchial tree
   protection 478
tracheo-oesophageal fistula 165
tracheostomy 147, 471–3, 475, 478–81, *479*
   aftercare 480–1
   technique 479
   thyroidectomy 377
   tubes 479–80, *479–80*
trachoma 425
traction 488–9, *489*
transcoelomic spread 54–5
Translet colostomy appliance 246

581

transplantation
  cardiac 560–1
  corneal 558–9
  liver 561
  lung 561
  rejection 556–7
  renal 559–60
  types 556
transverse myelitis 358
transvesical prostatectomy 353, 353–4
trasylol 305
Trendelenberg operation 118
trichomonas vaginalis 4
tricuspid valve 88
trifluroperazine 202, 284
trigone 342
triiodothyronine 370
trimeprazine tartrate 25
trismus 468
trochanteric osteotomy 530–1, 531
Trousseau's sign 376, 380
true aneurysm 104, 105
truss 272
trypsin 216, 302
tryptic digestion 215
tuberculin 15
tuberculosis 14–7, 97, 201
  ileo-caecal 201
  pulmonary 78–80, 79–80, 82
  renal 329–32, 330
  spine 527, 529, 549
tuberculous abscess 128, 128–9
  cystitis 330, 344
  lymphadenitis 127–8
  peritonitis 16
  pyonephrosis 330
  sinus 128, 129
tubular necrosis 316–7
tubules
  kidney 315, 315
tumours
  anatomical situation 62
  classification 51–6
  clinical features 56

condition of patient 62–3
curative treatment 58–9
cytotoxic therapy 59, 67–9
diagnosis 57–8
differentiation 53–6, 53
endocrine surgery 60
epithelial 52
examination 57
extent of spread 61–2
history 57
intracranial 138–43
microscopic appearance 62
morale 60
pain relief 60
palliative treatment 58–60
pituitary 140, 141
prognosis 60–3
radiotherapy 59
sex hormone treatment 60
special investigations 57–8
supporting tissue 52
surgery 59
treatment 58–69
ulceration 54, 55
tunica albuginea 361
tunica vaginalis 361
tuning fork tests 443–4
turbinate hypertrophy 466
turbinectomy 463
tympanic cavity 442, 443
tympanic membrane 442, 442
tympanoplasty 451
typhoid 200

ulcerated tumour 123
ulcerative colitis 123, 205, 227–31, 228–9, 238
ulcers
  leg 121–3, 121–2
  self-inflicted 123
ulna
  fracture 496
ulnar neuritis 540, 541
ulnar styloid
  fracture 497
umbilical hernia 268, 275–6, 276
  acquired 276

  congenital 276
  Mayo repair 276, 277
unconcious patient
  blood pressure 151
  nursing care 146–8
  observations 149–50
  pulse 151
  pupils 150, 151
  respiration 151
  special investigations 151–2
underwater seal chest drain 76–6, 76
upper limb fractures and dislocations 490–9
upper respiratory obstruction
  tracheostomy 478
uraemia 146, 321
  diet 22
  prostatic enlargement 352
urate calculi 334, 334, 336
ureter 312–41
  anatomy 313
  congenital anomalies 313–4
  double 313, 314
  embryology 313
  stones 337
  tumours 341
ureteric colic 323
ureteric transplantation 342, 343
ureteroileostomy 342
ureterolithotomy 337
urethane 68
urethra
  bulbous 347–8
  congenital abnormalities 346–7
  dilatation 350–1
  male 346–51
  membranous 348
  obstruction 352, 358
  rupture 347–8, 348
  spinal injuries 519
  splintage 348, 349
  stones 334, 335
urethral bougies 348, 350–1
  catheters 31
  sphincter 342

stricture 349–51
valves 347
urethroscopy 324, 324–5
uric acid
  calculi 334
  excess 332, 336
urinary retention
  investigations 359
  management 358–60
  post-operative 359
  prostatic enlargement 352, 360
  treatment 359–60
  urethral stricture 360
urinary tract disease
  examination 323–5
  history 322–3
  investigations 319–25
urinary tract stone 332–8
  aetiology 332–3
  clinical features 334, 335
  complications 336
  special investigations 335–6, 336
  treatment 336–8
urine
  incontinence 323
  retention 323, 336
  tests 324
  tests for tuberculosis 331
uterus
  pelvic abscess 225
uvea 416
uveal tract 416
uveitis 426–8

vagina 225
  pelvic abscess 225
vaginal fistula 249
vagotomy 176, 181, 189, 190, 195, 197
  proximal gastric 191
  selective 189, 191
  truncal 189, 191
vagus nerves 174, 175
vallergan 25
valve replacement 94
vanillylmandelic acid 383

varicose eczema 117, 121
varicose ulcer 117, 121–2, 121–2
varicose veins 113–23, 117
  aetiology 116–7
  clinical features 117, 117–8
  complications 120–3
  external support 120
  haemorrhage 120
  treatment, injection 118–20, 119
  treatment, surgical 118
  ulceration 121, 121–3
vascular disease
  intestine 206–7
vasodilator drugs 113
vasomotor rhinitis 466
vasopressin 291
vasovagal syndrome 40
Vater
  ampulla 301
vein patch 110, 110
venous valves 116
ventilator 72–3
ventral hernia 268, 277–8
ventriculo-cisternotomy 135, 135
ventriculography 141
verruca vulgans 410
vesico-colic fistula 238
vesico-ureteric reflux 325
vibrio cholerae 200
vinblastine 68
Vincent's angina 469
vincristine 68–9
Vineberg's operation 98
virilism 385–7
virus
  hepatitis 196
  pericarditis 97
viruses 1
visceral pleura 71
viscopaste dressing 121
visiting
  post-operative 36–7
visual acuity
  testing 420, 420
visual field 421–2

loss 431
vitamin B$_{12}$ 282
  absorption 199
vitamin D deficiency 539
vitamin K 282
  injections 286
vitello-intestinal tract 199
vocal cords 471, 472
  benign tumours 473
  carcinoma 473
  paresis 475
Volkmann's contracture of hand 494, 495
volvulus
  caecum 236–7
  colon 236–7
  neonatorum 214–5, 216

Walford's silver cannulae 462, 463
Walsham's forceps 457, 457
warts
  anal 260, 260–2
water
  accumulation 317
  metabolism 384
  reabsorption 316
Waugh's tenaculum forceps 470, 471
wax 447
Weber's test 444
Westminster condylar
  replacement of knee 533, 533
Whipple's operation 307, 308
whooping cough
Wilm's tumour 338–9
Wilson's tonsil artery forceps 470, 470
Wirsung
  duct 301
wisdom teeth
  impacted 4
Woodman's operation 475
wound
  care 32–3
  dehiscence 36
  drains 30–1, 31

583

infection 8, 11–2, 33
wrist
  arthrodesis 538
  orthopaedic conditions 543–4
  osteoarthritis 498

x-rays 63–4
  therapy 65, 67
  tube 63
xenograft 556
xylocaine gel 253, 255

Zadek's operation 408–9, *409*
zinc sulphate 425
Zollinger-Ellison syndrome 187, 301, 309–10